Culture, Health and Illness

To my daughter Zoe

Culture, Health and Illness

FIFTH EDITION

Cecil G Helman MB ChB FRCGP Dip Soc Anthrop

Professor of Medical Anthropology, School of Social Sciences and Law, Brunel University, Middlesex, UK;

Senior Lecturer, Department of Primary Care and Population Sciences, Royal Free and University College Medical School, London;

Former Visiting Fellow in Social Medicine and Health Policy, Harvard Medical School, USA;

Former Visiting Professor, Multicultural Health Programme, University of New South Wales, Sydney, Australia.

HODDER
ARNOLD

PART OF HACHETTE LIVRE UK

First published in Great Britain in 1984 by John Wright and Sons Ltd
Second edition 1990
Third edition 1994, reprinted 1995, 1996, 1997 (twice) and 1998
Fourth edition published in 2000 by Butterworth Heinemann, reprinted by Hodder Arnold
This fifth edition published in 2007 by
Hodder Arnold, an imprint of Hodder Education, part of Hachette Livre UK
338 Euston Road, London NW1 3BH

http://www.hoddereducation.com

Whilst the advice and information in this book are believed to be true and accurate at the date of going to press,
neither the author nor the publisher can accept any legal responsibility or liability for any errors or omissions that
may be made. In particular (but without limiting the generality of the preceding disclaimer) every effort has been
made to check drug dosages; however it is still possible that errors have been missed. Furthermore, dosage schedules
are constantly being revised and new side-effects recognized. For these reasons the reader is strongly urged to consult
the drug companies' printed instructions before administering any of the drugs recommended in this book.

British Library Cataloguing in Publication Data
A catalogue record for this book is available from the British Library

Library of Congress Cataloging-in-Publication Data
A catalog record for this book is available from the Library of Congress

ISBN 978 0 340 914 502

3 4 5 6 7 8 9 10

Commissioning Editors:	Joanna Koster and Sara Purdy
Project Editor:	Clare Weber and Jane Tod
Production Controller:	Lindsay Smith
Cover Designer:	Laura DeGrasse
Indexer:	Laurence Errington

Typeset in 10/14 Sabon by Phoenix Photosetting, Chatham, Kent
Printed and bound in Spain

To visit the book's website, please go to www.culturehealthandillness.com

What do you think about this book? Or any other Hodder Arnold title?
Please visit our website at www.hoddereducation.com

Contents

Preface

Since the first edition of *Culture, Health and Illness* appeared in 1984, interest in cross-cultural issues in health, disease, and medical care has expanded out of all recognition. Hundreds of articles, books, and research projects on the subject have been published, in many different languages. New journals and websites have also appeared, and new courses on cross-cultural health issues have been developed at many universities, medical schools, and nursing colleges worldwide. *Culture, Health and Illness* itself has now been used as a textbook in over 40 countries (including in over 120 universities and colleges in North America) and translations have appeared in several different languages.

The enormous growth of the subject means that it has become increasingly difficult to describe all of the new developments within one book. Nevertheless, this fifth edition of *Culture, Health and Illness* does cover all the main developments of recent years. New material has been added to every chapter, and several entirely new chapters have been included, The book deals with increasingly important topics such as: globalization and migration, and their impact on global health and medical care; the growth of the internet, and of telemedicine; the importance of genetics in understanding patterns of human disease; the role of gender issues and sexuality; the worldwide increase in organ transplantations, and other new medical techniques, including biotechnology, genetic engineering and the new reproductive technologies; and the growing threat to human health of infectious diseases such as acquired immune deficiency syndrome (AIDS), malaria, severe acute respiratory syndrome (SARS), multidrug resistant tuberculosis, and many others. It deals particularly with the role of poverty and deprivation, including inequalities in access to medical care, in the causation of disease and human suffering. In many cases, these socio-economic factors are much more significant than cultural beliefs and practices.

The fifth edition is written in a very different world from 1984: more mobile, more inter-connected, more rapidly changing, and more diverse than any other period in human history. Currently, according to the United Nations, about 175 million people live outside their countries of birth or citizenship, and the rate of migration between, and within, countries is increasing rapidly. This has led, in many parts of the world, to a more diverse population, in terms of culture, social background, ethnicity and religion – and this, in turn, has increased the need for an understanding of these factors in medical and nursing care. To illustrate this, many different case studies, from over 90 countries, have been included in the text. In each case I have given the year when the study was published or carried out, to illustrate the historical depth of the subject, and its importance over many decades.

In writing this fifth edition, I would like to express my thanks to the following colleagues who have kindly sent me their papers, books or research findings, and which I have referred to in the text: Stephen Bach, Daniel Beck, Gillian Bentley, Maggie Burgess, J. Emilio Carillo, Susan M. Cox, Simon Dein, Maurice Eisenbruch, Carl Elliott, Gareth Enticott, Jiske Erlings, David Gellner, Robert A. Hahn, Suzette Heald, Elizabeth Hsu, Patricia Hudelson, David Ingram, Judith Justice, Sharon R. Kaufman, Robert C. Like, Gerald Mars, Alex Mauron, Jerry Menikoff, Susanna Hausmann Muela, Mervat Nasser, Lois Nixon, Melissa Parker, Mirilee Pearl, Joan Muela Ribiero, Hikaru Suzuki, Mark S. Tremblay, Elizabeth Panter-Brick, Irena Papadopoulos, Vikram Patel, Mary C.J. Rudolf, Andrew Russell, Clive Seale, Bob Simpson, Surinder Singh, Vieda Skultans, Stewart Skyte, Margaret Sleeboom, Johannes Sommerfeld, Mark Tremblay, Sandra Torres, Cassandra White and Sjaak van der Geest.

I also wish to acknowledge the help and support of Jane Tod, Sara Purdy and Joanna Koster of Hodder Arnold in the preparation of this book.

Cecil Helman

Companion website

The fifth edition of *Culture, Health and Illness* is accompanied by an exciting new website featuring book reviews, author biography, useful weblinks and further material:

- **Clinical Questionnaires** – covering each chapter topic these open-ended, qualitative questionnaires can be used in two ways. Faced with a clinical situation where socio-cultural factors might be relevant, health professionals can ask themselves these questions as a way of increasing awareness of these factors and acting accordingly. Each set of questions can also provide the basis for a small research project on a particular topic within the wider field of applied medical anthropology. In this latter case, it is suggested that the books and journals recommended at the end of each chapter be consulted for futher theoretical background before the project is attempted.
- **References** – cited at the end of each chapter in the book are the key references only; the full list of references cited is available on the website, divided by chapter.
- **Case studies** – each case study presented in the book is also available in electronic format.

To visit the book's website, please go to www.culturehealthandillness.com.

1

Introduction: the scope of medical anthropology

how, why, who

Medical anthropology is about how people in different cultures and social groups explain the causes of ill health, the types of treatment they believe in, and to whom they turn if they do get ill. It is also the study of how these beliefs and practices relate to biological, psychological and social changes in the human organism, in both health and disease. It is the study of human suffering, and the steps that people take to explain and relieve that suffering.

To put this subject in perspective, it is necessary to know something about the discipline of anthropology itself, of which medical anthropology is a relatively new offshoot. Anthropology – from the Greek, meaning 'the study of man' – has been called 'the most scientific of the humanities and the most humane of the sciences'.[1] Its aim is nothing less than the holistic study of humankind – its origins, development, social and political organizations, religions, languages, art and artefacts.

Anthropology, as a field of study, has several branches. *Physical anthropology* – also known as human biology – is the study of the evolution of the human species, and is concerned with explaining the causes for the present diversity of human populations. In its investigation of human pre-history it uses the techniques of archaeology, palaeontology, genetics and serology, as well as the study of primate behaviour and ecology. *Material culture* deals with the art and artefacts of humankind, both in the present and in the past. It includes studies of the arts, musical instruments, weapons, clothes, tools and agricultural implements of different populations, and all other aspects of the technology that human beings use to control, shape, exploit and enhance their social or natural environments. *Social* and *cultural anthropology* deal with the comparative study of present-day human societies and their cultural systems, respectively, though there is a difference in emphasis between these two approaches.

In the UK, *social anthropology* is the dominant approach, and emphasizes the social dimensions of human life. It sees people as social animals, organized into groups that regulate and perpetuate themselves, and it is a person's experience as a member of society that shapes his or her view of the world. In this perspective, culture is seen as one of the ways that Man organizes and legitimizes his society, and provides the basis for its social, political and economic organization. In the USA, *cultural anthropology* focuses more on the systems of symbols, ideas and meanings that comprise a culture, and of which social organization is just an expression. In practice, the differences in emphasis of social and cultural anthropology provide valuable and complementary perspectives on two central issues – the ways that human groups organize themselves, and the ways that they view the world they inhabit. In other words, when studying a group of human beings it is necessary to study the features of both their society and their culture.

Keesing and Strathern[2] define a *society* as comprising 'a total social system whose members share a common language and cultural tradition' – both of which usually mark it out from the surrounding populations. The boundaries between societies are sometimes vague but, in general, each has its own territorial and political identity. As mentioned below, most societies are becoming increasingly diverse, owing to immigration and other factors. In studying any society, anthropologists investigate the ways that members of that society organize themselves into various groups, hierarchies and roles. This organization is revealed in its dominant ideology and religion, in its political and economic systems, in the types of bonds that kinship or close residence creates between people, in its hierarchies of power and prestige, and in the division of labour between different people from different backgrounds and different genders. The rules that underpin the organization of a society and the ways that it is symbolized and transmitted are all part of that society's culture.

THE CONCEPT OF CULTURE

What then is *culture* (a word that will be used on many occasions throughout this book)? Anthropologists have provided many definitions of it, perhaps the most famous being Tylor's[3] definition, in 1871: 'That complex whole which includes knowledge, belief, art, morals, law, custom and any other capabilities and habits acquired by man as a member of society'. Keesing and Stathern,[4] in their definition, stress the *ideational* aspect of culture. That is, cultures comprise 'Systems of shared ideas, systems of concepts and rules and meanings that underlie and are expressed in the ways that human beings live'.

From these definitions one can see that culture is a set of guidelines (both *explicit and implicit*) that individuals inherit as members of a particular society, and that tell them how to view the world, how to experience it emotionally, and how to behave in it in relation to other people, to supernatural forces or gods, and to the natural environment. It also provides them with a way of transmitting these guidelines to the next generation – by the use of symbols, language, art and ritual. To some extent, culture can be seen as an inherited 'lens' through which the individual perceives and understands the world that he inhabits and learns how to live within it. Growing up within any society is a form of *enculturation*, whereby the individual slowly acquires the cultural 'lens' of that society. Without such a shared perception of the world, both the cohesion and continuity of any human group would be impossible.

The American anthropologist Edward T. Hall[5] has proposed that in each human group there are actually three different *levels* of culture. These range from the explicit manifest culture ('tertiary level culture') visible to the outsider, such as social rituals, traditional dress, national cuisine and festive occasions, to much deeper levels known only to members of the cultural group themselves. While the tertiary level is basically the public 'facade presented to the world at large', below it lies a series of implicit assumptions, beliefs and rules which constitute that group's 'cultural grammar'. These deeper levels include *secondary level culture*', where these underlying rules and assumptions are known to the members of the group but rarely shared with outsiders, and *primary level culture*'. The latter is the deepest level of culture 'in which the rules are known to all, obeyed by all, but seldom if ever stated. Its rules are implicit, taken for granted, almost impossible for the average person to state as a system, and generally out of awareness'.

In Hall's view, while the manifest, tertiary level of culture is easiest to observe, change and manipulate, it is the deeper levels (primary and secondary) that are the most hidden, stable and resistant to change. This in turn has major implications for applied social scientists, especially for those involved in aiding or educating populations from cultures different from their own.

One crucial aspect of any culture's 'lens' is the division of the world, and of the people within it, into different *categories*, each with their own name. For example, all cultures divide up their

Antivaxers...

members into different social categories – such as men or women, children or adults, young people or old people, kinsfolk or strangers, upper class or lower class, able-bodied or disabled, normal or abnormal, beautiful or ugly, mad or bad, healthy or ill. All cultures have elaborate ways of moving people from one social category into another (such as from 'ill person' to 'healthy person'), and of confining people – sometimes against their will – to the categories into which they have been put (such as 'mad', 'disabled' or 'elderly').

Anthropologists such as Leach[6] have pointed out that virtually all societies have more than one culture within their borders. For example, most societies have some form of social stratification into social classes, castes or ranks, and each stratum is marked by its own distinctive cultural attributes, including use of language, manners, styles of dress, dietary and housing patterns, and so on. Rich and poor, powerful and powerless – each will have their own inherited cultural perspective. To some extent, both men and women can have their own distinctive 'cultures' within the same society, and are expected to conform to different norms and different expectations. Children, adults and the elderly are all subject to different rules of behaviour, and have different views of the world. In addition to social strata, one can see that while most modern complex societies, such as those in North America and Western Europe have their own unique cultural traditions, they now include within their borders religious and ethnic minorities, tourists, foreign students, recent immigrants, political refugees and migrant workers, each of whom have their own distinctive culture. Many of these groups will undergo some degree of *acculturation* over time, whereby they incorporate some of the cultural attributes of the larger society, but others will not. In addition, an increasing number of the followers of different new religions, cults and lifestyles are beginning to appear in most Western societies, each with their own unique view of the world.

A further subdivision of culture within complex societies is seen in the various professional *subcultures* that exist, such as the medical, nursing, legal or military professions. In each case these people form a group apart, with their own concepts, rules and social organization. While each subculture is developed from the larger culture and shares many of its concepts and values, it also has unique, distinctive features of its own. Students in these professions – especially in medicine and nursing – also undergo a form of enculturation, as they slowly acquire the 'culture' of their chosen career over many years. In doing so, they also acquire a very different perspective on life from those who are outside the profession. In the case of the medical profession, its subculture also reflects many of the social divisions and prejudices of the wider society (see Chapters 4 and 6), and this might interfere with both health care and doctor–patient or nurse–patient communication, as illustrated later in this book.

All this means that most complex societies are never homogeneous, and are now a patchwork of different subcultures, with many different views of the world coexisting – sometimes uneasily – within the same territory. 'Culture' therefore is an increasingly fluid concept, which in most societies is undergoing a constant process of change and adaptation. Many individuals, families and even communities can now be said to occupy two, or even more, cultures at the same time. This *biculturalism* (and often bilingualism) is especially true of new migrants, where the traditional culture of the first generation often coexists with the very different cultures acquired by their children and grandchildren (see Chapter 12).

THE CONTEXT OF CULTURE

Overall, therefore, cultural background has an important influence on many aspects of people's lives, including their beliefs, behaviour, perceptions, emotions, language, religion, rituals, family structure, diet, dress, body image, concepts of space and of time, and attitudes to illness, pain and other forms of misfortune – all of which may have important implications for health and health care.

However, the culture into which you are born, or in which you live, is never the *only* such influence. It is only one of a number of influences on health-related beliefs and behaviours, which include:

- *individual* factors (such as age, gender, size, appearance, personality, intelligence, experience, physical state and emotional state)
- *educational* factors (both formal and informal and including education into a religious, ethnic or professional subculture)
- *socio-economic* factors (such as poverty, social class, economic status, occupation or unemployment, discrimination or racism, as well as the networks of social support from other people)
- *environmental* factors (such as the weather, population density or pollution of the habitat, but also including the types of infrastructure available, such as housing, roads, bridges, public transport and health facilities).

In any particular case, moreover, all of these factors will play some role, but in different proportions. Thus in some situations – depending on the context – people will act more 'culturally' than in others. At other times their behaviour may be determined more by their personality, economic status, what they have been educated to believe, or the characteristics of the environment in which they live.

Misuses of the concept of culture

The concept of culture itself has sometimes been misunderstood or even misused. For example, cultures are never homogeneous, and therefore one should always avoid using generalizations in explaining people's beliefs and behaviours. One cannot make broad generalizations about the members of any human group without taking into account the fact that differences among the group's members may be just as marked as those between the members of different cultural groups. Statements such as 'the members of group X do not do Y' (such as smoking, drinking or eating meat) may be true of some or even most members of the group, but not necessarily of all. One should therefore differentiate between the rules of a culture, which govern how one *should* think and behave, and how people actually behave in real life. Generalizations can also be dangerous, for they often lead to the development of stereotypes and then to cultural misunderstandings, prejudices and discrimination. Another reason not to generalize is that cultures are never static – they are usually influenced by other human groups around them, and in most parts of the world they are in a constant process of adaptation and change. Increasingly this is due to economic globalization and the growth of global communication systems such as radio, television and the Internet, as well as to jet travel, mass tourism and increased levels of migration (see Chapters 12 and 18). For some migrant communities this may mean that the previously close relationship between their culture and their geographical area of origin becomes looser over time, as they gradually assimilate into another cultural environment. For others, though, the choice may be to try maintain as much of their original identity as possible by, for example, always speaking their own language at home, eating their traditional foods and watching only satellite TV programmes from their home country. All this means that it is now difficult to generalize about cultural groups, especially in more complex societies. In this modern age of constant flux and population movements, what is true of a particular group's culture one year may not be true of it the next.

Therefore, the modern view of culture – as mentioned above – is to stress the importance of always seeing it within its particular *context*. This context is made up of historical, economic, social, political and geographical elements, and means that the culture of any group of people, at any particular point in time, is always influenced by many other factors. It may therefore be impossible to isolate 'pure' cultural beliefs and behaviour from the social and economic context in which they occur. For example, people may act in a particular way (such as eating certain foods, living in a crowded house or not going to a doctor when ill) not because it is their culture to do so, but because they are simply too poor to do otherwise. They may have high levels of anxiety in their daily lives, not because their culture makes them anxious, but because they are suffering discrimination or persecution from other people. Therefore, in understanding health and illness it is important to avoid 'victim blaming' – that is, seeing the poor health of a population as the sole result of its culture, instead of looking also at their particular economic or social situation.

In clinical care, a misuse of the concept of culture can occur when its influence is *over*emphasized in interpreting how some people present their symptoms to health professionals. Symptoms or behaviour changes may be ascribed to a particular person's 'culture' when they are really caused by an underlying physical or mental disorder.[7] For example, physical disorders of the brain (such as tumours or encephalitis) may be confused with mental illness in certain cultural and social contexts. Thus Weiss[8] has described how, in India and elsewhere, some cases of cerebral malaria have been mistakenly diagnosed as mental illness. Another serious misuse of the concept occurs when an individual's antisocial, dangerous or even homicidal behaviour is blamed on their 'culture', when it has nothing to do with it at all; an example of this is 'cultural camouflage' is described in Chapter 10.

SOCIO-ECONOMIC FACTORS: INEQUALITIES IN HEALTH

Economic factors and social inequality are some of the most important causes of ill health, since *poverty* may result in poor nutrition, overcrowded living conditions, inadequate clothing, low levels of education, housing (or work) sited in areas with greater environmental dangers (such as near factories producing toxic chemicals), as well as exposure to physical and psychological violence, psychological stress, and drug and alcohol abuse.

The unequal distribution of wealth and resources, and of access to health care facilities – both between countries and within each country itself – can also lead to this situation. An early study of these health disparities in the UK, the Black Report[9] of 1982, showed how health could clearly be correlated with income, and people in the poorer social classes had more illness and a much higher mortality than their fellow citizens in the more affluent classes. In recent years this situation in Britain has worsened, with a widening difference in life expectancy between the social classes. In England and Wales in 1972–76, the life-expectancy for those in professional occupations was 5.5 years longer for men, and 5.3 years longer for women, compared with those in unskilled manual occupations; by 1992–96, however, this class gap in life-expectancy had widened to 9.5 years for men, and 6.4 years for women.[10]

In many Western societies these disparities are particularly evident in ethnic or cultural minority groups, whether they are immigrants or native born. In the USA, several studies indicate that members of minority groups suffer disproportionately from conditions such as heart disease, diabetes, asthma, cancer, and other diseases.[11] The reasons for these health disparities are complex: they include the many effects of poverty, but also the biases and lack of flexibility of the health-care system itself. Also, as Betancourt and colleagues[11] report, ethnic minorities in the USA have much lower rates of coverage by health insurance: for example, while Latinos are only 13 per cent of the population, they represent 25 per cent of those without any health insurance. People with low incomes may not only be able to afford good health care, they may also be unable to take time off work to make use of whatever health care is available. A further factor in damaging the health of minority groups may be discrimination, racism or persecution by the 'host' population,[12] as well as a general unwillingness to take note of their health beliefs, practices and expectations.

In the developing world too, whatever the local culture, poor health is usually associated with a low income and poverty, since this influences the sort of food, water, clothing, sanitation, housing and medical care that people are able to afford.[13] Health disparities and the physical environment in which poorer communities live can directly impact on their health, resulting in, for example, an inability to afford a clean water supply, or adequate sewerage disposal. In 2005, the United Nations Development Programme estimated that 1.2 billion people still lacked access to safe drinking water, while 2.4 billion people had no access to proper sanitation, and that both situations could lead to increased rates of waterborne diseases, which already kill some 2 million children every year.[14]

An example of the relationship of inequality to health status was described in Unterhalter's[15] study of infant mortality rates among different ethnic communities in Johannesburg, South Africa, between 1910 and 1979. She found very much higher rates of infant mortality among blacks and other 'non-white' groups than among whites, and this clearly correlated with the economic and social inequalities imposed upon them by the *apartheid* system. Preston-Whyte[16] has described how the legacy of this political system of racism has made the control of acquired immunodeficiency syndrome (AIDS) in South Africa much more difficult today. This is because apartheid was a system that, in the rural areas, often separated men from their wives, sending them to work in the cities for many years. Here they lived in male-only hostels, and this helped institutionalize multiple-partner sex relationships for many of them. At the same time, in the rural areas poor women sometimes had to depend on selling sex in order to earn money for their own survival and that of their children.

The effects of social inequality on health and life expectancy can also apply to affluent societies; that is, deprivation can be *relative*, as well as absolute. Marmot[17] has described the 'status syndrome' in which, for people above a threshold of material well-being, *other* factors, such as the sense of autonomy and control over their lives, and opportunities for 'full social engagement and participation', are crucial for their health, well-being and longevity. Research indicates that the higher and more successful one is in the social hierarchy, or even within a particular organization, such as a business, corporation, or bureaucracy, the greater one's health and life expectancy. The lower the social ranking, the higher the health risks. For example, he quotes research showing that movie actors who win an Academy Award (an 'Oscar') live on average 4 years longer than their co-stars, and other actors who were nominated for the Award but never got it. This 'social gradient in health' seems to be found in all societies, rich and poor, where hierarchy or social inequality is a feature. An example of this from Britain was the famous 'Whitehall Study'[18] – a 25-year detailed study of the health of 18 000 government employees – which found a much higher morbidity and mortality, especially from heart disease, in the lower ranks of the bureaucracy. Top administrators and executive officers had much better health, and a greater life expectancy, than clerical or other lower staff. Factors such as income or level of education played a part in this, but so did the subjective sense of *control* that people had over their particular life circumstances – both at work, and at home. Marmot notes that a key factor here may be psychological, since 'the psychological experience of inequality has profound effects on body systems.' The subjective experience of stress, and of lack of control over it, may be a major factor in causing physiological changes, which in turn lead to the 'social gradient of health'. Furthermore, he notes that 'people at the same level in the occupational hierarchy with different amounts of control had markedly different rates of disease – low control consistently led to more disease.' Another factor is the degree of social cohesion that exists, and whether the individual is imbedded in supportive networks of family, friends, or workmates. On a national level, Marmot notes that societies that are characterized by high social cohesion, whether rich or poor,

Social hierarchy as a – Survival of the fittest
– Evolutionary tool
~ Survival tool

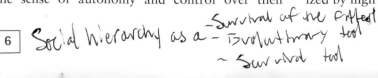

'have better health that others with the same wealth but lower social cohesion.'[19]

When poorer societies undergo rapid economic and social *development,* the health of many of their citizens may improve, but that of others may deteriorate. For example, a study in China in the mid-1990s[20] showed how for groups whose socioeconomic status improved, the odds of their having a healthier lifestyle actually decreased. New affluence meant a shift towards eating more processed food, rich in fats, salt and refined sugar, as well as a more sedentary lifestyle. Paradoxically, those groups who remained at a lower socioeconomic level seemed to maintain a healthier lifestyle, leading a more active life, and eating more natural foods such as fruits, vegetables and grains. This phenomenon of 'lifestyle transition' in poorer developing countries, may partly explain why 'nutrition-related noncommunicable diseases are more prevalent in the developing world among people with a higher socioeconomic status, whereas the opposite is found in developed societies'.[21] These 'new' diseases in the population include obesity, diabetes, and cardiovascular disorders (see Chapter 3).

Overall then, the conclusion of this section is that 'culture' cannot – and should never be – considered in a vacuum. 'Pure' culture hardly ever exits, for it is only as one component of a complex and diverse mix of influences on what people believe, how they live their daily lives, and whether they are healthy or ill.

MEDICAL ANTHROPOLOGY

Although *medical anthropology* is a branch of social and cultural anthropology, its roots also lie deep within medicine and other natural sciences, for it is concerned with a wide range of biological phenomena, especially in relation to health and disease. As a subject it therefore lies – sometimes uncomfortably – in the overlap between the social and natural sciences, and draws its insights from both sets of disciplines. In Foster and Anderson's[22]

useful definition it is: 'A biocultural discipline concerned with both the biological and sociocultural aspects of human behaviour, and particularly with the ways in which the two interacted throughout human history to influence health and disease'.

Anthropologists studying the socio-cultural end of this spectrum have pointed out that, in all human societies, beliefs and practices relating to ill health are a central feature of the culture. Often these are linked to beliefs about the origin of a much wider range of misfortunes (including accidents, interpersonal conflicts, natural disasters, crop failures, theft and loss), of which ill health is just one form. In some societies the whole range of these misfortunes is blamed on supernatural forces, or on divine retribution, or on the malevolence of a witch or sorcerer. The values and customs associated with ill health are part of the wider culture, and cannot really be studied in isolation from it. One cannot really understand how people react to illness, death or other misfortunes without an understanding of the type of culture they have grown up in or acquired – that is, of the 'lens' through which they perceive and interpret their world. In addition to the study of culture it is also necessary to examine the *social organization* of health and illness in that society (the health care system), which includes the ways in which people have become recognized as ill, the ways that they present this illness to other people, the attributes of those they present their illness to, and the ways that the illness is dealt with.

This group of 'healers' is found in different forms in every human society. Anthropologists are particularly interested in the characteristics of this special social group: their selection, training, concepts, values and internal organization. They also study the way these people fit into the social system as a whole: their rank in the social hierarchy, their economic or political power and the division of labour between them and other members of the society. In some human groups the healers play roles beyond their healing functions – they may act as 'integrators' of the society, who regularly reassert the society's values (see Chapter 9), or as agents of social control, helping to label and punish socially deviant behaviour (see Chapter 10). Their focus may not be only on the ill individual, but rather on his 'ill' family, community, village or tribe. It is therefore important when studying how individuals in a particular society perceive and react to ill health, and the types of health care that they turn to, to know something about both the *cultural* and the *social* attributes of the society in which they live. This is one of the main tasks of medical anthropology.

At the biological end of the spectrum, medical anthropology draws on the techniques and findings of medical science and its various subfields, including microbiology, biochemistry, genetics, parasitology, pathology, nutrition and epidemiology. In many cases it is possible to link biological changes found by using these techniques to social and cultural factors in a particular society. For example, a hereditary disease transmitted by a recessive gene may occur at a higher frequency in a particular population because of that group's cultural preference for endogamy (marrying only within one's own family or local kin group). To unravel this problem, one needs a number of perspectives:

- *clinical medicine,* to identify the clinical manifestation of the disease
- *pathology,* to confirm the disease on the cellular or biochemical level
- *genetics,* to identify and predict the hereditary basis of the disease and its linkage to a recessive gene
- *epidemiology,* to show its high incidence in a particular population in relation to 'pooling' of recessive genes and certain marriage customs
- social or cultural *anthropology,* to explain the marriage patterns of that society and to identify who may marry whom within it.

Medical anthropology tries to solve this type of clinical problem by utilizing not only anthropological findings but also those of the biological sciences – by being, in other words, a 'biocultural discipline'.

MEDICAL ANTHROPOLOGY AND THE HUMAN LIFE CYCLE

One important aspect of medical anthropology is the study of the human life cycle, and of all the stages from birth to death. The term *age-grade* is used in anthropology for the category of persons who happen to fall within a particular culturally defined age range (such as child, adult or elder).[23] Each of these age-grades is not just a universal biological stage of life; its beginning and end are also defined by the culture, as are the events expected within it. Furthermore, each age-grade also has profound social and psychological dimensions for those passing through it. In general, these define quite precisely how people within an age-grade should behave, and how other people should behave towards them. Just as every society has a profound split between the types of behaviour expected of males and of females, so are there major differences between what is expected of each of the age-grades.

Later in this book the two extremes of the human life cycle, birth and death, are discussed in more detail from the perspective of medical anthropology (Chapters 6 and 9). There is also further discussion of how, particularly in Western society, many of the normal milestones of the life cycle (such as puberty, menstruation, pregnancy, childbirth, menopause and even dying) seem gradually to have become 'medicalized' and turned into pathological, rather than natural states.

In recent years, medical anthropology has paid considerable attention to the cultural characteristics of two particular stages of human growth and development: childhood and old age. To some extent, both children[24] and the elderly[25] can be said to have their own cultures, or rather subcultures since they have their own unique view of the world and ways of behaving within it. Although each is always embedded within the wider culture, they also have certain distinct characteristics of their own.

8

CHILDHOOD

Like old age, the definition of childhood is not something fixed and finite and based only on biological criteria. Cross-cultural studies indicate there are wide variations in how childhood is defined, its beginning and end, and the behaviour considered appropriate for children and for those around them. James and colleagues[26] point out that definitions of childhood are always, to some extent, 'socially constructed', and this is why they tend to vary quite widely between different human groups. For example, different societies set different ages at which children can be educated, take part in certain religious rituals, work outside the home, have sexual relations, control their own finances, make independent decisions (about their health, education or place of residence), have their own identity documents or passports, take legal responsibility for their actions and so on. In some traditional cultures children were even expected to marry, and a betrothal ceremony would take place arranged by their parents and close kin. Although such arranged child marriages are now increasingly uncommon, especially in urban areas, in the past they existed in parts of India, China, Japan, Africa and southern Europe.[27] Among the Hausa of Nigeria, for example, childhood effectively ended for a girl when, at the age of 10 years, she was betrothed to her future husband and was expected to take on 'the social responsibilities of a wife'.[28] In other cultural settings, children have been expected to become full combatants in war – especially in civil wars and insurrections[29] – or to work full-time outside the home, often for very low wages.[29] The notion of childhood being a unique, protected time – a notionally carefree existence, with its own mores, leisure pursuits, dress codes, diets, treats, toys, books, computer programmes, movies, videos and magazines – seems to be a feature of economically more developed societies, where huge profits are being made from this conceptual 'separateness' of childhood. By contrast, in poorer societies children are in effect 'trainee adults', expected to perform almost all the usual adult tasks, such as child care, cooking, hunting, herding and earning money, as early as possible.

In the construction of childhood culture, both at home and at school, children are not just passive recipients of the process. They too develop their own lore and language,[24] and contribute to the development of their own identity. As James and colleagues[26] put it: 'children are not formed by natural and social forces, but rather … they inhabit a world of meaning created by themselves and through their interaction with adults'. Increasingly, medical anthropology is focusing on certain aspects of childhood culture that relate to health and illness – in particular, the needs and perceptions of the sick child, their beliefs about health and illness and their attitudes to medical treatment (see Chapter 5).

On the international level, the anthropological study of childhood is of growing importance because of the health implications of a number of contemporary social issues. These include the use of child labour,[29] the sexual and physical abuse of children,[30,31] the widespread prevalence of child prostitution,[29] the increased use of children in warfare[29] and the increasing numbers of 'street children' in many poorer countries.

Later in this book there will be discussion of some of those areas where medical anthropology has already contributed to a fuller understanding of infant and child health. They include the issues of disability (Chapter 2), male and female circumcision (Chapter 2), nutrition and infant feeding practices (Chapter 3), perceptions of illness (Chapter 5), pregnancy and childbirth (Chapter 6), self-medication and substance abuse (Chapter 8), family structure (Chapter 10) and immunizations, family planning and primary health care (Chapter 18).

OLD AGE

A relatively new branch of medical anthropology, *cross-cultural gerontology*, is the study of aging and social attitudes towards it across different cultures. It is of growing importance, since the number of aged people in the world is rapidly increasing. World-wide, the United Nations predict that the population aged 60 or over is expected to triple, from 606 million in 2000 to nearly 2 billion by the year 2050.[32] In more developed countries these people already constitute 20 per cent of the population (and have already surpassed the child population), and this will rise to 33 per cent by 2050. In developing countries, the percentage of aged will rise from 8 per cent to 20 per cent, with most of this growth expected to be in Africa, Asia and Latin America. Throughout the world, the 'oldest old' (aged 80 or older) are the most rapidly increasing age group among the older population, with a projected increase from 69 million in 2000 to 379 million in 2050.[32] This 'greying' of the population is likely to have major effects on society. Already, economic modernization, a falling birth rate, changing gender roles, and the mobility of populations have often led to the breakdown of the extended family structure, with more of the elderly than ever before being left to fend for themselves.

Anthropologists have pointed out that, in every culture, biological aging is not necessarily the same as social aging, or even as psychological aging. A particular chronological age defined as old in one culture may not be considered so in another. Similarly, behaviour defined by one group as inappropriate for the elderly, such as having sexual relations or wearing brightly-coloured clothes, may be considered quite normal in another. Also, self-perception and psychological aging are often independent of chronological age. Despite the body's physical decline, most older people retain within themselves a sense of what Kaufman[25] terms 'the ageless self'.

Cultures vary widely in the status that they give to the elderly. Unlike in Western industrial societies – where loss of productivity (and reproductivity) with age, usually means a steep drop in social status – the respect accorded to the elderly is usually much higher in traditional, more rural societies. In non-literate societies in particular, the elders are the living repositories of oral history and ancient traditions, and of cultural mores, beliefs, myths and ritual expertise. Under these circumstances, the unexpected death of a respected elder is almost equivalent to the effect of a library or university burning down in a more literate, developed society.

In general, modern Western industrial society, with its emphasis on youth, beauty, productivity, individualism, autonomy and self-control, is often quite intolerant of old people. They may even be seen by some as a burden, a drain on resources, an embarrassment, or even as unproductive parasites. As Loustaunau and Sobo[33] ironically put it 'Aging is unpopular in the United States' but this also is true of other countries. Increasingly, those societies that have entered the information age of computers, global telecommunications and artificial intelligence give an increased cultural importance to the brain (see Chapter 2). They especially value its cognitive functions: reasoning, memory, calculation, and the absorption and retention of large amounts of data. Such a cultural bias tends to devalue many of the elderly, especially if they suffer from some form of memory loss or cognitive impairment. This prejudice against the loss of cognitive skills is clearly seen in the presence of Alzheimer's or other forms of dementia (even if quite mild). In an age where the computer (with its advanced skills of memory, logic and calculation) has become the respected 'second self'[34] of much of the population, many of the normal signs of aging have become pathologized.

As Desjarlais and colleagues[29] point out, this attitude is in contrast to many other cultures, where dementia is not seen as such a major public health problem. Instead, it is regarded as an expected, or at least understandable, part of aging. In many non-Western societies, such as China, a certain amount of 'childishness' in the very old is seen as a condition to be tolerated and not as something abnormal and requiring medical treatment. Although Chinese families are generally very caring and supportive of the elderly, Desjarlais and colleagues point out that the increasing life expectancy (resulting in increased mental and physical disabilities) and the paucity of resources (such as homes for the elderly) is now creating considerable emotional and financial hardship for many families there. They quote another study from India that also suggests that senile dementia is less frequent or less severe there, either due to lower longevity or because there is greater tolerance for the demented aged there than in the West.

In his classic study of aging in India, Cohen[35] contrasts the Western view of dementia (especially Alzheimer's) as a discrete and serious 'brain disease' afflicting certain individuals with a view common among some Indians, that senility is not so much an individual pathology, but rather a result of the decline of the traditional supportive, extended family, owing to urbanization, modernity and Westernization. In their view 'modern India engenders senility' for 'in modern life old people are less respected and they become senile'. This difference of perspective is partly the result of different conceptions of the self; while Americans and Europeans 'act and experience themselves as autonomous and bounded entities, highly individuated selves within quite separate bodies', many Indians 'act and experience themselves primarily in terms of their relations with others, as linked and interdependent selves'. Thus a decline of close family ties is believed to have negative effects on the health and well-being of all its members, especially the aged.

In comparing aging cross-culturally it is important, however, not to over-romanticize the care of the elderly in non-industrialized societies. Although the elderly are generally well cared for by their relatives, they are sometimes abandoned or abused. In some societies, for example, demented old women can be in danger of being accused of being a witch and even put to death[36] (probably a similar situation to that which prevailed in the 'witch-craze' hysteria of sixteenth and seventeenth century England).

There are thus many different cultural definitions of 'successful ageing' found in different societies worldwide.[37] Some (especially in the Western world) may define it mainly as the ability to retain one's cognitive skills, economic self-sufficiency, and sense of optimism, while others may see it more as accumulating wisdom, serenity, tolerance, and a deeper understanding of the human condition. Psychiatrists, too, may experience difficulty in diagnosing dementia in a culturally diverse society because of language problems and the use of diagnostic instruments and questionnaires more suitable to Western populations.[38]

Overall, an aging population poses a growing challenge to the medical model, with its current emphasis on the dramatic 'quick-fix' types of treatment (see Chapter 4). In a world where an increasing number of the population will be suffering from chronic diseases (both physical and mental) this will require a major shift in the medical paradigm, with a move away from acute, more dramatic treatment towards longer-term, more holistic management: in other words, a shift from 'cure' to 'care'.

The 'medicalization' of old age

Human communities have always tried to find ways of extending the lifespan and staving off death, including the use of special diets, medications, prayers, rituals, and various forms of the 'elixir of youth'. In the industrialized world, however, old age has become increasingly 'medicalized' over the past century or so. That is, the physical and mental changes associated with ageing have come to be seen primarily as *medical* problems, which can best be dealt with by doctors, rather than by other groups in society. Within medicine, *gerontology* – the medical care of older people – is a relatively new profession, and dates particularly from 1881 when the French physician Jean Martin Charcot published his *Clinical Lectures on the Diseases of Old Age*.[39] Since then, ageing has increasingly been seen as a type of chronic disease; one that cannot be 'cured', only alleviated.

Parallel with this development has been the growth of a major commercial 'anti-aging' industry, offering the public a variety of products from glandular extract and vitamin supplements to special diets and exercise programmes. Medicine, too, has become part of this 'anti-aging movement. One type of medical science, *biogerontology*, has begun to explore various forms of 'life-extension' and has even raised the possibility that physical ageing itself can also be 'cured'.[40] As de Grey[41] puts it: 'Just as the purpose of oncology is to defeat cancer, the purpose of biogerontology is, and should be declared to be, to defeat ageing'. One aspect of this is the process known as 'compressed morbidity', which aims 'to forestall all chronic ailments of old age by intervening in the underlying molecular processes';[41] older people would therefore remain healthier for many more years of their life. Different types of research are being carried out in this area,[42] including research into the use of stem-cell therapy[43] and nanotechnology. However, because most of this research is taking place in richer, more developed countries, it raises the possibility of an even greater disparity between the life expectancies of rich and poor – between those who can afford to benefit from such research (the 'time rich') and those who cannot (the 'time poor').[44] Also, as Cetina[45] points out, all this emphasis on increasing longevity and enhancing the quality of life ('*life enhancement*') is largely stripped of any notion of moral improvement, and of the Enlightenment ideals of science leading to an expansion of human reason and to the perfectibility of human society. From the perspective of view of many religions, neither would it necessarily lead to the growth of greater spiritual wisdom or awareness.

A further aspect of 'life enhancement' – at least, in developed countries – is the growing use of medical interventions in older people, including transplants, and other surgery, and kidney dialysis. Kaufman and colleagues[46] describe this growing trend in American medicine, whereby 'the body seems open to unlimited manipulation, at any age, and the emphasis of the health professions is on the management and maximization of life itself'. Furthermore, 'medical practice in the past 15 years, especially, promotes the notion that aging is not inevitable (in the United States)'. They note how, since 1972 when Medicare benefits were extended to all person over 65 years with end-stage renal disease (ESRD), the numbers of elderly people on dialysis has risen greatly: from 16 000 in 1975 to 72 000 in 1995. By 2001, 20 per cent of all dialysis patients in the USA were over the age of 75 years, and 13 per cent were over 80 years. Similarly, the numbers of people over the age of 70 with ESRD who were receiving kidney transplants has also greatly increased. Such transplants are now routine in the seventh decade of life, and are sometimes performed on people in their early 80s. Many of these kidneys are donated by their adult children or other relatives.

For most people in the world, however, these advances in biogerontology will be largely irrelevant. In many poorer countries, 'old age' is a relative concept, and life expectancy is only 50 years or less. For these people, 'life extension' will mean at the very minimum overcoming such factors as poverty, poor nutrition, poor housing, polluted drinking water, and infectious diseases such as human immunodeficiency virus (HIV) infection, malaria or tuberculosis.

CLINICALLY APPLIED MEDICAL ANTHROPOLOGY

Within medical anthropology, some researchers have concentrated on its theoretical aspects while others (especially those involved in clinical practice, health education programmes or international medical aid) have focused more on its applied aspects in health care and preventive medicine. Interest in this field of *clinically applied medical anthropology* has grown steadily in the past few years. Medical anthropologists have become involved in a variety of projects, in many parts of the world, aimed at improving health and health care. They have worked both in the non-industrialized world and within the cities and suburbs of Europe and North America.

A number have become 'clinical anthropologists'[47] closely involved in patient care within a hospital or clinic setting, often as members of a multidisciplinary health care team. Here their role has been either that of teacher – raising their colleagues' awareness of the importance of cultural factors in health and illness – or of a health professional or therapist in their own right, with their own specific area of expertise.

Some have widened their focus beyond clinical care to include the more 'macro' influences on health. *Critical medical anthropology* focuses on the political and economic inequality between and within many of the societies in today's world, and especially on the close relationship between poverty and disease.[48,49] Other anthropologists have worked for international aid agencies, such as the WHO (World Health Organization) or (UNICEF) (United Nations International Children's Fund), on health problems in various parts of the non-industrialized world. Here they have helped in the planning and evaluation of different forms of health care and health education, or acted as advocates for particular patients or their communities. As well as monitoring the responses of various communities to health-care programmes, they have also studied the aid agencies themselves, observing how their organization and subculture can either help or hinder the success of the programmes.[50] In both the industrialized world and elsewhere, medical anthropologists have been especially involved in the areas of primary health care, family planning, maternal and child health, infant feeding, nutrition, mental illness, immunizations, the control of drug abuse and alcoholism, and the prevention of AIDS, malaria and tuberculosis.

The importance of cultural factors to many different aspects of international health was officially recognized in 1996 by the WHO and UNESCO, who declared it the Year of Culture and Health. In their joint declaration, the Directors General of both organizations proposed 'further avenues for cooperation so that health and culture can be developed in a mutually supportive manner which will benefit all peoples in all countries'.[51]

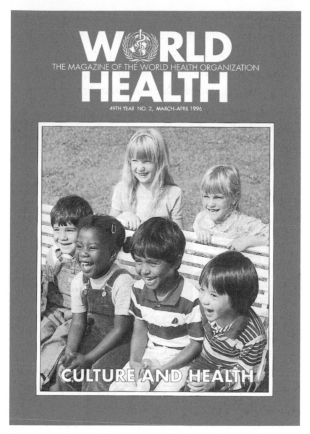

Figure 1.1 Cover of the journal *World Health*, in which the WHO and UNESCO declare 1996 to be the year of 'Culture and Health'. (Source: World Health Organization, front cover, *World Health*, No. 2, March–April 1996.)

To illustrate how medical anthropology may be useful in dealing with a particular health problem in a particular part of the world, take the example of diarrhoeal diseases. According to the WHO,[52] the high incidence of these diseases poses a major health problem world-wide, especially in the non-industrialized world. There they are usually associated with poverty and the resultant malnutrition, poor sanitation, contaminated drinking water and vulnerability to infection. They kill about 5–7 million people every year. A long-term solution to this problem is not in the hands of health professionals or social scientists, since it will involve major and comprehensive economic, social and political changes, both within those countries and in their relation to the rest of the world.

In terms of an immediate treatment, however, oral rehydration therapy (ORT) provides a safe, inexpensive and simple way to prevent and treat the life-threatening dehydration associated with the diarrhoea, in both infants and children. Despite this, mothers in many parts of the world are reluctant to use this relatively simple form of treatment, even when it is free and easily available to them. Anthropological research, as illustrated in the case study below has found that this is partly due to indigenous beliefs about the causes and dangers of diarrhoeal disease and how they should best be treated.[53]

of the infant's head or pushing up on the hard palate with a finger. Many mothers in the group saw diarrhoea as a 'hot' illness (see Chapter 3), which required a 'cold' form of treatment, such as a change in maternal diet or giving certain foods and herbs to the infant, in order to restore the sick infant to a normal temperature. They classified most Western medicines, such as antibiotics and even vitamins, as also 'hot', and therefore inappropriate for a diarrhoeal child. A few even rejected ORS (which contains salt) because they thought that salt 'was bad for diarrhoea'.

Case study: oral rehydration therapy in Pakistan

A study by the Mulls[54] in rural Pakistan in the 1980s showed widespread ignorance or rejection of oral rehydration therapy (ORT) by mothers. This was despite the fact that the use of ORT has been promoted on a national level by the Ministry of Health since 1983, and packets of oral rehydration solution (ORS) are available free of charge through government health outlets; also, more than 18 million packets of ORS are produced annually by Pakistan's own pharmaceutical industry. The researchers found that many of the mothers were ignorant of how the ORS should be used, and some of them saw the diarrhoea (which was very common in that area) as a natural and expected part of teething and growing up and not as an illness. Some believed it was dangerous to try to stop the diarrhoea, lest the trapped 'heat' within it spread to the brain and caused a fever. Others explained infant diarrhoea as caused by certain folk illnesses (see Chapter 5) such as *nazar* (evil eye), *jinns* (malevolent spirits) or *sutt* (a sunken or fallen fontanelle said to cause difficulty in infant sucking), which should be treated with traditional remedies or by traditional healers without recourse to ORT. Some of these mothers did not connect the fallen fontanelle with severe dehydration, and tried to raise it by applying sticky substances to the top

Although conducted some years ago, studies such as this remain as important reference points, for diarrhoeal diseases are still the major cause of child mortality in Pakistan, and a more recent (1991–92) nationwide survey in that country showed that local beliefs about diarrhoeal diseases were still important in dissuading women from using ORS for their children.[55] While 91 per cent of mothers in the survey had now heard about ORS, only 34 per cent had actually used it during their child's last episode of diarrhoea, and only 27.5 per cent kept some ORS at home.[55]

This and other case studies illustrate that health care programmes should be designed not only to address medical concerns, but also to involve community participation. They need to take into account the specific needs and circumstances of different communities, their social, cultural and economic backgrounds, and what the people living in them actually believe about their own ill health and how it should be treated. They also need to take into account that changes in knowledge do not necessarily result in changes in behaviour.

CULTURAL COMPETENCE

In recent years, the concept of *cultural competence* has become popular among health planners as well as doctors and nurses, especially in North

America.[56] This has largely resulted from the increasing cultural and ethnic diversity of the population, and the need to improve communication with minority and immigrant groups, and improve the quality of their medical care.[57] As Carillo and colleagues[58] note 'Despite the multitude of cultures in the United States, physicians are inadequately trained to face the challenges of providing quality care to socially and culturally diverse populations'.

According to the US government's Office of Minority Health (OMH) 'Cultural and linguistic competence implies an ability by health-care providers and organizations to understand and respond effectively to the cultural and linguistic needs brought by patients to the health care setting'.[59] 'Cultural competence' therefore has several different dimensions:

1 Improving the *sensitivity* of health professionals to the cultural beliefs, practices, expectations and backgrounds of their patients, and their communities[56–58,60] (such as beliefs about the origins of ill-health, the greater role of the family in making health-related decisions or the preference of some female patients to be examined only by a female health professional);

2 Improving access to health care by eliminating *structural barriers* to quality health care for minorities (such as providing interpreter services, hospital diets that accord with religious beliefs, shorter waiting times for appointments and culturally appropriate health education materials). Also included here are the difficulties that minority patients encounter in getting a regular doctor, or in being referred to a specialist;[11]

3 Reducing *organizational barriers,* such as the low numbers of health professionals, administrators and policy-makers drawn from minority communities, who might be helpful in designing more culturally appropriate health services. According to Betancourt and colleagues,[11] this lack of diversity at the policy-making level has led to 'structural policies, procedures and delivery systems inappropri-

ately designed or poorly suited to serve diverse populations'. They point out that in 1997 only 11 per cent of medical graduates in the USA were from minority ethnic groups.

Another aspect of cultural competence is the issue of *informed consent* for medical treatments, tests or research. Dein and Bhui[61] point out that the modern notion of presenting information to a patient, expecting them to fully understand that information, and then to decide freely whether or not to agree – may all be in conflict with the cultural values of some ethnic groups. They may refuse to sign an informed consent form because they are illiterate, or come from a society where verbal commitments are highly regarded, while written contracts are distrusted. They may also not share the Western notions of autonomy and individuality, whereby individuals make decisions by themselves, for themselves, instead of on behalf of a group.

A number of benefits are thus likely to arise from increasing the cultural competence of health professional. According to Genao and colleagues[62] it can improve not only physician–patient communication, but also patient satisfaction and compliance (such as fewer missed appointments). It can also have a positive impact on the diagnosis and treatment of ill-health, and the proper use of medical resources. It may also, in the long term, reduce disparities in health between minorities and the majority population.

Despite the obvious usefulness of the concept of cultural competence, it should be noted that it is not a substitute for *clinical competence*. Being culturally competent does not necessarily mean that one is a good doctor or a good nurse. Rather, it is an important supplementary skill that should be acquired by *all* health professionals, in whichever context they work. Aside from dealing with a diverse population, this skill is important because the relations between any health professionals and their patients – whatever their backgrounds – can often be described as 'culture-clash' in itself (see Chapter 5).

Furthermore, in an age of global mobility, cultural competence is often not just a one-way phenomenon. With the increasing numbers of health professions migrating from one country to another (see Chapter 12), the majority population themselves may have to learn new skills for communicating with professionals from abroad, and whose command of the local language and culture may not be the same as their own.

Overall, cultural competence is never enough to deal with health disparities within a society. Because health care never takes place in a vacuum, all the wider social, cultural and economic realities of the society – such as its relationships of power and inequality – always need to be taken into account when trying to improve the health care of all sectors of the society. Finally, as described in Chapter 5, cultural competence always requires *reflexivity* on the part of health professionals: the ability to honestly examine their *own* cultural 'baggage', such as prejudices or particular beliefs, that may interfere with the successful and humane delivery of health care.[60]

NURSING ANTHROPOLOGY

In many ways, anthropology has become better integrated into nursing than into medicine, especially in North America and Europe. Nurses have often been aware earlier than their medical colleagues of the need to adapt clinical practice to the realities of an increasingly diverse society. Since the 1980s, a focus on anthropology and cultural competence has become an essential part of the curriculum of many nursing colleges. The innovative work of Leininger,[63–65] Papadopoulos and colleagues,[66] Purnell,[67] Andrews and Boyle,[68] and others have all been important in this development.

Leininger[63] has defined *transcultural nursing* as: 'A formal area of study and practice focused on comparative holistic culture, care, health, and illness patterns of people, with respect to differences and similarities in their cultural values, beliefs and practices with the goal to provide culturally congruent, sensitive, and competent nursing care to people of diverse cultures'. While Papadopoulos and colleagues[66] define it as: 'The study and research of cultural diversities and similarities in health and illness as well as their underpinning societal and organizational structures, in order to understand current practice and contribute to its future development in a culturally responsive way'.

Thus, transcultural nursing focuses not only on the culturally sensitive care of clients from a variety of backgrounds, but also on the societal structures that construct and perpetuate inequality, and poor access to health care. It aims to empower its clients and enable them to take part in decisions regarding their own health care. In their model of transcultural nursing, Papadopoulos *et al.*[66] also emphasize the importance for nurses of developing reflexivity and self-awareness (including a knowledge of their own 'ethnohistory'), as well as knowledge of other cultures, as a prerequisite for delivering culturally sensitive care to their clients.

RESEARCH METHODS IN ANTHROPOLOGY

In studying societies and cultural groups around the world – including their health beliefs and practices – anthropologists have used two main approaches to research, both unique to anthropology. The *ethnographic* approach – also known as 'participant observation' – involves the study of small-scale societies or relatively small groups of people in order to understand how they view the world and organize their daily lives. The aim is to discover, in so far as this is possible, the 'actor's perspective'; that is, to see how the world looks from the perspective of a member of that society. To discover this, the anthropologists often carry out fieldwork, using the 'participant observation' technique. Here they live with and observe a group of people over a period of time (usually one or more years at least), and learn to see the world through their eyes while at the same time retaining the objective perspective of the social scientist. Although the work of anthropologists is 'concerned with meanings rather than measurements',[69] it often involves quantitative studies as well, such as counting the population, measuring their diet or income, or listing the inhabitants of various households. Ethnography then leads on to a second stage, the *comparative* approach, which seeks to distil the key features of each society and culture and compare these with other societies and cultures in order to draw conclusions about the universal nature of human beings and their social groupings.

In its earlier years, anthropology was mainly concerned with studies of small-scale tribal societies within or at the borders of the colonial empires. Modern anthropology, however, is just as concerned with performing ethnographies in complex Western societies. The 'tribe' of a modern anthropologist might easily be a sect in New York, a suburb in London, a group of surgeons in Los Angeles or patients attending a clinic in Melbourne. In all these cases, both the ethnographic and comparative approaches are used, as well as some of the interviewing and measurement techniques of sociology or psychology. Increasingly, modern anthropology now draws on other fields of study, such as history, literary criticism, semiotics, cultural studies, and genetics.

As detailed later in this book, the range of research techniques available to anthropology has steadily increased. As well as long-term 'participant observation', techniques now often include the use of open-ended questionnaires, videos or tape recordings, computer analyses, aerial photography, the compilation of family histories and analysis of genealogies, the collection of individual narratives and the examination of written or printed material such as diaries, letters, family photographs, newspaper articles, maps, census reports and local historical records.

More recently, to meet the increasing needs of international aid programmes, a number of 'rapid ethnographic assessment' techniques have been developed.[70] These usually involve a short, intensive period of research by a team of anthropologists and their assistants, and can last anything from several weeks to several months. They tend to focus on a particular problem (such as a high rate of diarrhoeal diseases) in a particular community or region. Used in conjunction with longer-term fieldwork, the data from these studies can be very useful in the planning and evaluation of international aid programmes.

Many of these new research methods now available to medical anthropology are described in more detail, in Chapter 19.

This book has been written by a medical anthropologist who is also a clinician. As such, its general approach arises mainly from the growing field of *clinically applied medical anthropology*, which has been briefly described above. Many examples of its application to real-life situations, especially in relation to contemporary health issues of global concern, are described in each of its chapters. Overall, the aim of the book is to demonstrate the clinical significance of cultural and social factors in illness and in health, in preventive medicine and health education, and in the actual delivery of health care.

KEY REFERENCES

5 Hall, E. T. (1984). *The Dance of Life*. Surbiton: Anchor Press, pp. 230–31.

10 Charlesworth, S.J., Gilfillan, P. and Wilkinson, R. (2004) Living inferiority. *Br. Med. Bull.* 69, 49–60.

11 Betancourt, J.R., Green, A.R., Carillo, J.E. and Ananeh-Firempong, O. (2003) Defining cultural competence: a practical framework for addressing racial/ethnic disparities in health and health care. *Publ. Health Rep.* 118, 293–302.

17 Marmot, M. (2004) *Status Syndrome*. London: Bloomsbury, pp. 1–36.

26 James, A., Jenks, C. and Prout, A. (1998). *Theorizing Childhood*. Cambridge: Polity Press, pp. 22–34.

35 Cohen, L. (1998) *No Aging in India*. Berkeley: University of California Press, pp. 15–20, 32–34.

Universal Nature

38 Livingston, G. and Sembhi, S. (2003) Mental health of the ageing immigrant population. *Adv. Psychiatr. Treat.* 9, 31–37.

46 Kaufman, S., Shim, J.K. and Russ, A.J. (2004) Revisiting the biomedicalization of aging: Clinical trends and ethical challenges. *Gerontologist* 44(6), 731–738.

47 Johnson, T. M. (1987). Practising medical anthropology: clinical strategies for work in hospital. In: *Applied Anthropology in America* (Eddy, E. and Partridge W., eds), 2nd edn. New York: Columbia University Press, pp. 316–39.

49 Baer, H. A., Singer, M. and Susser, I. (1997). *Medical Anthropology and the World System*, 2nd edn. Westport: Praeger.

53 Weiss, M. G. (1988). Cultural models of diarrhoeal illness: conceptual framework and review. *Soc. Sci. Med.* 27, 5–16.

56 Like, R. C., Steiner, R. P. and Rubel, A.J (1996). Recommended core curriculum guidelines on culturally sensitive and competent health care. *Fam. Med.* 28(4), 291–297.

 See http://www.culturehealthandillness.com for the full list of references for this chapter.

RECOMMENDED READING

Medical anthropology

Anderson, R. (1996) *Magic, Science and Health.* London: Harcourt Brace.

Foster, G. M. and Anderson, B. G. (1978). *Medical Anthropology.* Chichester: Wiley.

Hahn, R. A. (1995). *Sickness and Healing: an Anthropological Perspective.* New Haven: Yale University Press.

Sargent, C. F. and Johnson T.M. (eds) (1996). *Medical Anthropology.* Westport: Praeger.

Kleinman, A. (1981) *Patients and Healers in the Context of Culture.* Berkeley: University of California Press.

Landy, D. (ed.) (1977) *Culture, Disease and Healing.* Basingstoke: Macmillan.

Lupton, D. (1994) *Medicine as Culture.* London: Sage.

Nursing anthropology

Andrews, M. and Boyle, J. (2003) *Transcultural Concepts in Nursing Care*, 4th edn. Philadelphia: Lippincott.

Leininger, M. (2005) *Cultural Care Diversity and Universality: a Worldwide Nursing Theory.* Boston: Jones and Bartlett.

Papadopoulos, L. (ed) (2006) *Transcultural health and social care: developing culturally competent professionals.* London: Elsevier.

Social and cultural anthropology

Keesing, R.M. and Strathern, A.J. (1998). *Cultural Anthropology: A Contemporary Perspective*, 3rd edn. London: Harcourt Brace.

Peacock, J.L. (2001). *The Anthropological Lens*, 2nd edn. Cambridge: Cambridge University Press.

2 The body: cultural definitions of anatomy and physiology

To the members of all societies, the human body is more than just a physical organism fluctuating between health and illness. It is also the focus of a set of beliefs about its social and psychological significance, its structure and its function. The term body image has been used to describe all the ways that an individual conceptualizes and experiences his or her body, whether consciously or not. In Fisher's[1] definition, this includes 'his collective attitudes, feelings and fantasies about his body', as well as 'the manner in which a person has learnt to organize and integrate his body experiences'. The culture and background in which we grow up teaches us how to perceive and interpret the many changes that can occur over time in our own bodies and in the bodies of other people. We learn how to differentiate a young body from an aged one, a sick body from a healthy one, a fit body from a disabled one; how to define a fever or a pain, a feeling of clumsiness or of anxiety; how to perceive some parts of the body as public, and others as private; and how to view some bodily functions as socially acceptable and others as morally unclean.

The body image, then, is something acquired by every individual as part of growing up in a particular family, culture or society – although there are, of course, many individual variations in body image within any of these groups.

In general, concepts of body image can be divided into four main areas:

1 Beliefs about the optimal shape and size of the body, including the clothing and decoration of its surface.
2 Beliefs about the boundaries of the body.
3 Beliefs about the body's inner structure.
4 Beliefs about how the body functions.

All four are influenced by social and cultural background, as well as by individual factors, and can have important effects on the health of the individual.

THE SHAPE, SIZE, CLOTHING AND SURFACE OF THE BODY

In every society, the human body has a social as well as a physical reality. That is, the shape, size and adornments of the body are a way of communicating information about its owner's position in society, including information about age, gender, social status, occupation and membership of certain groups, both religious and secular. Included in this form of communication are bodily gestures and postures, which frequently differ between cultures, and between different groups within a culture. The body language of, for example, doctors, priests, policemen and salespeople is very different from one another and conveys different types of messages. Clothing is also of particular importance in signalling social rank and occupation; in the Western world mink coats, jewels and designer clothes are usually worn as displays of wealth, in contrast to the ragged, ill-fitting or mass-produced clothes of the poor. Similarly, the white coat of the Western doctor or the starched cap of the nurse not only have a practical aspect (cleanliness and the prevention of infection) but also have a *social* function, indicating their membership of a prestigious, powerful occupational group, with its own specific rights and privileges (see Chapter 9). A change in social position is often signalled by a change in clothing – the black dress and shawl adopted by widows in a Greek village is a public indicator of their transition from married woman to solitary mourner. Similarly, new graduates at a Western university wear, at least temporarily, a uniform of academic gown and mortarboard. Thus many aspects of the body's adornments, especially clothing, have both a social function (signalling information about an individual's current position in society) and the more obvious utilitarian function of protecting the body from the environment.

While the body is protected by its clothing, some areas of the body surface are sometimes considered to be more vulnerable to the environment than others. For example, in the author's study[2] of English lay beliefs about chills, colds and fevers, the body image included certain areas of skin (the top of the head, the back of the neck and the feet) considered more vulnerable than other parts to penetration by environmental cold, damp or draughts. You 'caught cold' if you went out into the rain without a hat on (or after a haircut), or stepped in a puddle or on a cold floor. At the same time, fevers were believed to result from the penetration of germs or bugs or viruses through other breaks in the body's surface, such as the anus, urethra, throat, nostrils or ears.

In addition to clothing, body posture and the control of bodily movements can also be an indicator of social position: high-status persons are usually associated with tight bodily control and low-status persons with its absence. At the same time, each profession controls its body in a subtly different way: the posture and movements of a sol-

dier, for example, are very different from those of a dancer or a doctor.

Artificial changes in the actual shape, size and surface of the body, which are widespread throughout the world, can also have a social function. This applies also to the more extreme forms of bodily mutilation, which will be mentioned below. Inherent in most of these are culturally defined notions of 'beauty' – usually of women – and of the optimal size and shape of the body. Polhemus[3] has listed some of the more extreme forms of body alteration practiced now and in the past, especially among non-industrialized peoples. These include:

- artificial deformation of infants' skulls in parts of Peru
- filing and carving of teeth in pre-Columbian Mexico and Ecuador
- scarification of the chest and limbs in New Guinea and parts of Central Africa
- binding of women's feet in Imperial China
- artificial fattening of girls in some parts of West Africa
- tattooing of the body in Tahiti and among some Native Americans
- insertion of large ornaments into the lips and earlobes in the Brazilian Amazon, East Africa and Melanesia
- the wearing of nose- and ear-rings among the people of Timbuktu, Mali.

The most widespread form of bodily mutilation is male circumcision. It has been common in some communities for almost 5000 years, and today is practised by about one-sixth of the world's population.[4] The most controversial is probably female circumcision in its various forms, now often called female genital mutilation (FGM).[5] It usually involves the removal of all or part of the external genitalia, and is carried out on girls ranging in age from 1 month to puberty. An estimated 80 million girls and women living today have undergone circumcision, especially in sub-Saharan Africa, the Arab world, Malaysia and Indonesia, and some immigrant groups in Western countries.[6] In many of these regions, and especially in rural areas, women who are not circumcised may be stigmatized and find it difficult to get married. In 1982 the World Health Organization (WHO) urged health professionals not to carry out female circumcision under any circumstances, but although it is now illegal in many different countries, FGM is still carried out on large numbers of women and girls.

The health risks of such bodily mutilations are obvious. Female circumcision, for example, carries with it the dangers of infection, haemorrhage, damage to adjacent organs, scar tissue formation and long-term difficulties with micturition, menstruation, sexual intercourse and childbirth[6]. However, some forms of bodily mutilation may bring health benefits to the population, even if indirectly. Early male circumcision was once believed to be one of the factors protecting women from developing cancer of the cervix, but this is now disputed.[7] However, it may protect against some infections in the penile area, as well as phimosis (tight foreskin), and possibly acquired immune deficiency syndrome (AIDS). In 2005, The Joint United Nations Programme on HIV (human immunodeficiency virus)/AIDS (UNAIDS) reported a study from Gauteng province, South Africa, on men aged 18–24 years, which suggested that adult male circumcision may be associated with a lower risk of HIV acquisition.[8] Interestingly, since 1991 some South African traditional healers have been advising their uncircumcised male clients to become circumcised as a way of preventing sexually transmitted diseases.[9] In addition, as has been found among the Mende of Sierra Leone, the use of ritual scarring by a community may make them accept the 'ritual scars' of vaccination more enthusiastically than other groups without these customs.[10] Both scarification and tattooing (which carry with them the dangers of local infection, hepatitis B and AIDS) are now less commonly seen in the West, except among sailors and servicemen, though recently the popularity of tattooing, and of various types of body piercing, has begun to increase again among adolescents.

As well as these cultural influences, medical or surgical treatments may also have a profound impact on body image. This applies particularly to operations such as amputations, mastectomies and plastic surgery, and to treatments such as radiotherapy and chemotherapy that may result in hair loss or other physical changes. Similarly, some women may, after a hysterectomy, experience a sense of the loss of their female identity, at least for a while.

MAKING THE BODY BEAUTIFUL

Various forms of body alteration and self-mutilation are used in Western societies, especially by women, to conform to culturally defined standards of beauty. These include the widespread use of orthodontics, plastic surgery, breast implants, liposuction, ear and body piercing, bodybuilding regimens and hair implants, and the use of false teeth, eyelashes and fingernails. It has been estimated that in 2003 surgeons in the USA carried out 1.8 million cosmetic operations – nearly double the figures for 1997.[11] Among these is the growing demand for cosmetic surgery of the female external genitalia, to make them conform to the culturally 'ideal' images that are commonly seen in adult magazines and films.[12] These operations include reduction of the labia minora, remodeling of the labia majora, vaginal reconstructions, 'pubis tuck', and – in some communities – hymenoplasty, or restoration of the hymen, in order to restore 'virginity' before marriage, as well as repair of previous female circumcision.

Also included as a form of body alteration are the various forms of dieting, used mainly by women, in order to reduce their weight to more 'attractive' dimensions and improve their health. About 1.5 million people attend approximately 46 000 meetings of Weight Watchers each week, in a total of 30 countries world-wide,[13] while another organization Slimming World has 5500 weekly groups in the UK, and report that in the past 30 years over 3 million slimmers have attended these groups, and in total have lost 60 million pounds in weight.[14] Both organizations seem to attract many more women than men.

It has been hypothesized that anorexia nervosa, often accompanied by loss of periods, is an extreme, pathological form of dissatisfaction with body image in a society which values and rewards female slimness.[15] Thus it can only be understood within the context of certain wider cultural values and influences, especially the 'ideal' body shape of the times.[16] This image is widely disseminated by the media, with magazines, adverts and books all carrying photographs of slim and beautiful models and actresses, and this may have a negative influence on the body image and self-esteem of some young women. However, there are many other sources of this imagery in modern society.[17] Rintala and Mutajoki[18], for example, have analysed the size, shape and proportions of the mannequins displaying women's clothing in the windows of fashion stores. They show how these have become progressively thinner over the past 80 years until they are now virtually anorexic in appearance. As women need at least 17 per cent of their weight as fat in order to begin menstruating and about 22 per cent in order to have regular cycles, they calculate that 'a woman with the shape of a modern mannequin would probably not menstruate', as she would be so underweight. Orbach[19] has suggested further that anorexia is not only a cultural phenomenon, but may even represent a symbolic 'hunger strike' by some women against their oppression in Western society.

A widening gap has developed between concepts of 'ideal' female size and the reality of an increasingly overweight female population. Ainsworth[20] reviewed studies that show that while the average weight of most women increased between 1950 and 1978, the average weight of the centerfold models in *Playboy* magazine decreased in the same period. She reports also that the popular 'Barbie' dolls are also now much thinner than the average woman, and that to become a 'life-sized Barbie' an ordinary woman would have to grow 50 cm taller, add 13 cm to her bust, and lose 15 cm from her waist.

This cultural emphasis on the 'ideal' body does not only apply to women. While the centrefold male models of *Playgirl* have also got leaner over the past few decades, they have also got more muscular, with more pronounced biceps and shoulder muscles – a trend towards a 'bodybuilder' physique that is also found increasingly among male movie actors, and some boys' toys such as 'GI Joe'.[20]

In contrast to this slimming down of body image in industrialized countries, in parts of West and Central Africa wealthy men frequently sent their daughters to 'fatting-houses', where they were fed on fatty foods, with minimal exercise, so as to be plump and pale – a culturally defined shape believed to indicate both wealth and fertility.[21] I have called this phenomenon of voluntary obesity, *cultural obesity*, and it is described further in Chapter 3. An example of this is the 'Fattening Room' of the Annang people of Nigeria.[22] In the Pacific, a similar process of fattening girls (*ha'a-pori*) was common in nineteenth and early twentieth centuries in both Tahiti and Nauru,[23] while among the Enga people of the New Guinea Highlands it has been reported that a 'sleek, fat body' was regarded as the most important physical asset of a young woman, and 'a thin girl is considered unlikely to make a good marriage'.[24] Men, too, often value a plump body shape, as a sign of health and affluence. Among the Massa people of Northern Cameroon, de Garine[25] has described how male 'fattening sessions' are common, and social attitudes to obesity are much more positive than in the Western world. Among this group, and in many of the surrounding peoples, neither fatness nor obesity are frowned upon, or considered 'conducive to psychological unrest and a passport to death'. Conversely, slim people are seen as weak and tired and their body shape as ugly and ridiculous. In some communities, a slim body may be seen as a sign of HIV/AIDS, and therefore stigmatized even further. In contrast, in the Western world, obesity is increasingly seen as a major health problem, and carries with it a significant social stigma. Ritenbaugh[26] points out that medical descriptions of the causes of obesity – overeating and under-exercising – are often just a modern, medicalized version of the traditional moral disapproval of gluttony and sloth (Chapter 5), as well as of a lack of self-control. The 'global obesity epidemic' is described in more detail in the next chapter.

Not only is body shape altered to fit in with culturally prescribed patterns of beauty, but special clothes are also worn that make this possible. These include women's corsets and other constrictive underwear, and high-heeled or platform shoes, all of which may have a negative effect on health. Cosmetics and deodorants, which may cause skin allergies or contact dermatitis, are also part of the Western mode of communication, where personal body odour is considered to be offensive – a belief not shared by many other cultures.

EATING DISORDERS AND 'WESTERNIZATION'

The Western emphasis on the 'ideal' slim female body can have a major impact on the incidence of eating disorders – especially anorexia nervosa and bulimia – in countries undergoing economic development, urbanization and 'Westernization'. Exposure to images of super-slim females on television, movies, and magazines – as well as encounters with foreign tourists – may all lead to some young women becoming dissatisfied with their body image. Thinness, as Nasser[27] points out, has come to symbolize 'beauty, health, achievement and control'. She notes how the global incidence of eating disorders has risen steadily over the past 50 years, and is now affecting many poorer countries as well, especially in Africa, the Middle East, Latin America and Eastern Europe, as well as ethnic minorities and immigrant groups within Western Europe and North America. This rise is also caused by changes in diet and lifestyle, as well changes in female gender roles. In South Africa, for example, a rising incidence of eating disorders and dissatisfaction with body image has been reported among young African girls. In a study in the province of Kwazulu-Natal, many Zulu schoolgirls

admitted to using laxatives and diet pills to control their weight, and wanting to look less 'like their mums anymore and more like western girls'.[28] Nasser and Di Nicola[29] points out, however, that these eating disorders are not just an imitation of Western body image; on a much deeper level, they are embodied metaphors for 'culture chaos' and 'social crisis' – a 'quest for self-redefinition' in relation to others in a rapidly changing world.

INDIVIDUAL AND SOCIAL BODIES

As the section above illustrates, each human being has, in a symbolic sense, two bodies; an individual body-self (both physical and psychological), which is acquired at birth, and a social body that is needed in order to live within a particular society and cultural group.[30]

The social body is an essential part of the body image, since it provides each person with a framework for perceiving and interpreting physical and psychological experiences.[30] It is also the means whereby the physical functioning of individuals is influenced and controlled by the society in which they live. This larger society, or 'body-politic', exerts a powerful control over all aspects of the individual body – its shape, size, clothing, diet and postures, its behaviour in sickness and in health, and its reproductive, work and leisure activities.[31]

Douglas[30] points out that there is a two-way relationship between bodily and social imagery, with each influencing the other. Not only does society shape and control the bodies within it, but the body also provides us with a collection of 'natural symbols' with which to understand society itself and how it is organized – from the 'head' of government and the 'heart' of a community', to the 'left' and 'right' sides of the political spectrum. Gordon[32] notes that this close relationship between bodily and social imagery means that different types of society produce very different images of the body. For example, Western society sees itself as made up of autonomous, individual citizens, and it assumes that the body, too, is made up of individual organs, which can be removed and replaced by spare-part surgery without threatening the survival of the whole. As described below, this Western body image is very different from that found elsewhere – for example, in Japan.

In practice, however, the body image derived from society is not really external to or separate from the individual body-self, or from its physical reality. As Csordas[33] points out, the body and culture (like body and mind) are not really separate from one another. To a large extent, individuals *embody* the culture that they live in. Their sensations, perceptions, feelings and other bodily experiences are all culturally patterned; as is the body's awareness of other bodies within that society, and the ways that it relates towards them. Bodily sensations and perceptions (the 'somatic modes of attention') are the means by which people are aware of other bodies, and are able to create and maintain the networks of relationships with them. Thus they are 'culturally elaborated ways of attending to and with one's body in surroundings that include the embodied presence of others'. In a general sense, therefore, the body *is* culture – an expression of its basic themes. A full understanding of any human body gives, at the same time, a fuller understanding of the culture embodied within it.

THE BOUNDARIES OF THE BODY

SYMBOLIC SKINS

In every human group the boundaries of individuals' sense of self are not necessarily the same as the boundaries of their body, and their sense of personal identity extends far beyond the borders of their skin. They are surrounded by a series of what I would term *symbolic skins* – some of them invisible, others not. Hall,[34] for example, has identified four invisible, concentric circles of space and distance that surround the bodies of middle-class Americans. They are:

1 *Intimate* distance (0–18 inches [0–45 cm]) – this can only be entered by those who have an intimate physical relationship with the individual.

2 *Personal* distance (18 inches to 4 feet [45–120 cm]) – this involves less intimate contact and relationships, but is still within the zone of personal space; it is 'a small protective sphere or bubble that an organism maintains between itself and others'.

3 *Social* distance (4–12 feet) [1.2–3.6 m]) – this is the distance at which impersonal business transactions and casual social interactions take place.

4 *Public* distance (12–25 feet or more [3.6–7.5 m or more]) – this is the distance at which no social or personal interaction is taking place.

Hall stresses that the size and shape of these invisible 'bubbles' varies widely between different social and cultural groups within the USA, as well as in different parts of the world – for example, between Americans, British, French, Germans and Arabs. In each case, penetration by a stranger (including a health professional) of one of these unseen skins, especially the inner two, may be experienced by the individual in that culture as rude, invasive or very threatening.

Other 'symbolic skins' that help define people's sense of self may include their cosmetics, clothing, jewelry, the walls of their rooms (or houses), their cars, the outer limits of their suburbs, cities or villages, their membership of an ethnic group or social class, or even the borders of their nation state (whose symbolic 'orifices' are airports, harbours and border posts). In those cultures where the group is considered to be more important than the individual, these skins usually include other people (members of the same family, clan, ethnic group, village or workplace), and sometimes even livestock, a dwelling or a piece of ancestral land. This collective sense of self, enclosed within a symbolic boundary far beyond the human body, is common in many parts of the world. For example, Tamura and Lau[35] note how, in Japan, the group is generally considered to be more central than the individual, and is thus intimately involved in the individual's sense of self – unlike the 'skin-encapsulated ego' common in the West. This in turn has implications when trying to define the moment of an individual's death, as discussed below. In many other societies, too, individuals do not necessarily 'own' their body in the way they would expect to in the West. Jadhav[36] describes how, in parts of northern India, the folk concept of *ārdha-angāni* ('half-body') can be found. Here, the left half of a married woman's body is believed to belong to her husband and his kinsfolk; in this cultural setting women may 'embody' any marital conflict by developing pain, paralysis or other symptoms of that side of their bodies.

The boundaries of an individual's body image are not static, however. They may alter with emotional state, disease or disability, surgery (amputations, mastectomies, breast augmentations, spare-part surgery) and medical treatments (radiotherapy, *in vitro* fertilization), as well as in physiological states such as pregnancy, obesity and weight loss. They also vary with age. In adolescence, an increasing body awareness is linked to the individual's need to develop the series of symbolic skins characteristic of their own culture or social group. These are acquired, one by one, as part of the transition from childhood to adult status. Often these new 'skins' are experienced as potentially fragile and easily disrupted by other people, especially adults. To most adolescents, an important boundary (or symbolic skin) of their sense of self is that of their peer group, and thus exclusion from it can be very traumatic for them.

In many traditional societies, the individual's status is physically 'written' onto the surface of their body. Tattooing, scarification, circumcision and piercing of ears, lips or other parts of the body are all permanent and visible forms of cultural skin. As well as status, they usually signal permanent membership of a particular community. Among groups such as the New Zealand Maori, for example, complex full-body tattoos were especially common. For

the Maori warriors they were even a type of spiritual armour that protected them, as well as an expression of deeper cultural and religious beliefs.[37] Thus to the anthropologist Claude Levi-Strauss,[38] the purpose of these tattoos was 'not only to imprint a drawing onto the flesh but also to stamp onto the mind all the traditions and philosophy of the group'. In Western society, however, tattoos are voluntary, but in recent years have become increasingly common. This phenomenon may represent – especially among younger people – a craving for a more permanent, fixed identity in an age of unpredictability and constant flux.

Changes in body image are common in certain severe, crippling diseases. For example, Kaufman[39] described the impact of a stroke on American patients as 'an assault on the taken-for-granted body – the "natural", "right" sense of self'. Faced with its crippling effects, and the fact that it cannot be cured, the neat equation between body and self often breaks down. The healthy self – determined to get better as soon as possible – finds itself in conflict with its permanently damaged body. Because contemporary US culture assumes that 'the individual can acquire the ability, through training and perseverance, to reverse disease outcomes and, in fact, to overcome nature',[39] the stroke victims' inability to master or cure their disability may be interpreted by them (and by others) as a sign of moral weakness, personal failure or loss of control.

THE INNER STRUCTURE OF THE BODY

To most people the inner structure of the body is a matter of mystery and speculation. Without the benefit of anatomical dissections, charts of the skeletal and organ structures or X-ray photographs, beliefs about how the body is constructed are usually based on inherited folklore, books and magazines, personal experience and theorizing. The importance of this 'inside-the-body' image is that it influences people's perception and presentation of bodily complaints. It also influences their responses to medical treatment. For example, a 20-year-old London woman was told, on the basis of her symptoms, that she was suffering from 'heart-burn', and an antacid mixture was prescribed. A week later, with the same symptoms, she saw another doctor and admitted she had not taken any antacid. Asked why she hadn't followed the first doctor's advice she replied, 'Of course I didn't take his mixture. How could he know I had heartburn if he didn't even listen to my heart?'

Several studies have been done on people's conceptions of what lies inside the body. In 1970 Boyle[40] studied 234 British patients, with the aid of multiple-choice questionnaires, to discover their knowledge of bodily structure and function, and then compared the answers with those of a sample of 35 doctors. He found a wide discrepancy between the two sets of answers, especially on the location of internal organs. For example, 14.9 per cent of the patients placed the heart as occupying most of the thoracic cavity, 58.8 per cent located the stomach as occupying the entire abdomen, from waist to groin, 48.7 per cent located the kidneys low down in the groin and 45.5 per cent saw the liver as lying in the lower abdomen, just above the pelvis. In another study in 1982, of 81 men and women in hospital awaiting major abdominal surgery Pearson and Dudley[41] found that, out of a total of 729 responses dealing with organ location, only 28 per cent were correct; 14 per cent were only vague answers, and 58 per cent were completely incorrect. Fifteen per cent equated the stomach with the abdominal cavity, 14 per cent marked in two livers on opposite sides of the body, and 18 per cent said the gallbladder was concerned with urine, or located it in the lower pelvic area, or both. Such bodily perceptions obviously influence how patients interpret, and present, certain bodily symptoms. For example, a vague discomfort anywhere in the chest may be interpreted as 'heart trouble', whether the doctor confirms this or not. A patient complaining of a pain in the stomach may be referring to virtually anywhere in the abdominal cavity.

Conceptions of what lies inside the body are also not static. They can vary with certain physical and psychological states, and seem to vary with age. A study by Tait and Ascher[42] in 1955 examined these conceptions in 107 hospitalized psychiatric patients, 105 candidates for admission to a US Naval Academy, 55 military men hospitalized in medical or surgical wards and 22 sixth-grade pupils in New York. Many of the drawings the psychotics produced 'exhibited disorderly arrangement, confusion, vagueness and pronounced and bizarre distortions of shape, relative size and position of [bodily] parts'. In the children's drawings the sexual organs were omitted, while the skeletomuscular system was prominently drawn. In

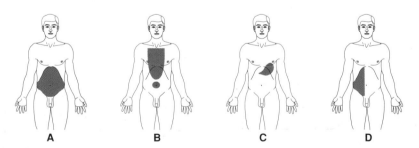

Distribution of positions of the stomach. **A**, 67 patients (58.8%), no doctors.
B, 22 patients (19.3%), no doctors. **C**, 23 patients (20.2%), 35 doctors (100%)
χ^2 43.21; D.F. 1; P < 0.0005 (doctors > patients).**D**, 2 patients (1.8%), no doctors

Figure 2.1 The position of the stomach: from a British study of doctors' versus patients' understanding of common anatomical terms.[40] (Source: Boyle, C.M., 1970. Difference between patients' and doctors' interpretation of some common medical terms. *Br. Med. J.*, ii, 286–9, Fig. 4. Reproduced with permission.)

medical and surgical patients there was a tendency to emphasize the organ or system involved in the illness for which they were hospitalized, such as the lung, the kidneys, or the skeletomuscular system. One patient with neurodermatitis drew the skin surface of the body, with only the faintest indication of ribs as the inside of the body.

Illness may also involve reifying a diseased organ or bodily part (thinking of it as though it were an 'it') – something partly alien to the body and only partly under its control.[43] In this way unpleasant or worrying bodily experiences can be denied, or separated from the type of body-image now idealized in the modern world; a body which is healthy, happy, independent and in full control of all its functions.[44] This is particularly the case in severe diseases, such as cancer, where both the disease and the affected body part are often seen as somehow separate or alien to the patient's body (see Chapter 5). In one study of psychosomatic disorders, for example, patients put the blame for their embarrassing symptoms (such as unexpected vomiting or diarrhoea) on a part of their body that was weak, unreliable and only partly under their control, such as an 'irritable colon', a 'nervous stomach' or a 'weak chest'.[44]

The effect of body image is also seen in the presentation of non-organic, i.e. psychogenic, signs and symptoms. In 1980, Waddell and colleagues[45] studied the distribution of physical signs for which no organic cause could be found in 350 British and American patients with low back pain. The distribution of these signs (such as numbness, weakness or tremor) did not match accepted neuroanatomical distribution. Instead, it corresponded to lay divisions of the body into regions such as knee, groin or waist. In another study by Walters,[46] hysterical pain or psychogenic regional pain was found to occur in distributions that matched patients' body images – especially their beliefs about parts of the body supplied by a particular nerve, rather than their actual anatomical innervation. Examples of this are the 'glove' or 'stocking' distribution of hysterical pain, numbness or paralysis.

Case study: internal body image in a patient in Boston, USA

Kleinman and colleagues[47] in 1978 described a case that illustrates the clinical significance of patients' beliefs about their bodies, and how these can affect their behaviour and the reactions of clinicians. A 60-year-old white woman was admitted to a medical ward in Massachusetts General Hospital, Boston, suffering from pulmonary oedema secondary to atherosclerotic cardiovascular disease and chronic congestive heart failure. As she began to recover, her behaviour became increasingly bizarre; she forced herself to vomit and urinated frequently in her bed. A psychiatrist was called in for an opinion. On close questioning he discovered that, from her point of view, at least, her behaviour made sense. She had been told by the doctors that she had 'water in the lungs'. She was the wife and daughter of plumbers, and her concept of the structure of the body had the chest connected by 'pipes' to the mouth and urethra. She was therefore trying to remove as much of the 'water in the lungs' as possible by vomiting and urinating frequently. She compared the latter to the effect of the 'water pills' that she had been prescribed, and which she had been told would get rid of the water in her chest by making her urinate. Once the actual 'plumbing' of the human body had been explained to her, using diagrams, her bizarre behaviour immediately ended.

THE FUNCTIONING OF THE BODY

While beliefs about the body's structure can have clinical importance, those about how it functions are probably more significant in how they affect people's behaviour. Beliefs about function usually deal with one or more of the following inter-related aspects of the body:

1 Its inner workings.
2 The effect on these of diet, environment and other outside influences.

3 The nature (and disposal) of the by-products of the body's functioning, such as faeces, urine and menstrual blood.

From the wide range of lay theories of physiology that have been studied, a few have been selected for closer examination.

BALANCE AND IMBALANCE

In all of these theories, the healthy working of the body is thought to depend on the harmonious *balance* between two or more elements or forces within the body. To a variable extent this balance is dependent on external forces such as diet, environment or supernatural agents, as well as on internal influences such as inherited weakness or state of mind. The most widespread of these theories is the *humoral* theory, which has its roots in ancient China and India but was elaborated into a system of medicine by Hippocrates, who was born in 460 BC. In the Hippocratic theory, the body contained four liquids or humours: blood, phlegm, yellow bile and black bile. Health resulted from these four humours being in optimal proportions to one another; ill health was caused by an excess or deficiency of one of them. Diet and environment could affect this balance, as could the season of the year. Treatment for imbalance/disease consisted of restoring the optimal proportion of the humours by removing excess (bleeding, purging, vomiting, starvation) or replacing the deficiency (by special diets, medicines, etc.). It also included a theory of personality types, based on the predominance of one of the humours, the four types being: sanguine (excess blood), phlegmatic (excess phlegm), choleric (excess yellow bile) and melancholic (excess black bile). Hippocratic medicine was restored and further elaborated by Galen (130–200 AD), a Greek physician living in Rome. In the centuries that followed, Galen's work gradually diffused throughout the Roman world and into the Islamic world. In the ninth century, under the Abbasid Dynasty of Baghdad, large portions of his work were translated into Arabic. Foster[48] has described how, during the Moorish occupation of the Iberian Peninsula, much of this humoral medicine was taken over by Spanish and Portuguese physicians and later carried by their descendants to South and Central America and the Philippines. However, some anthropologists believe that certain indigenous humoral and 'hot–cold' beliefs preceded the European conquest of Latin America,[49] although others dispute this claim.[50] In any case, humoral medicine remains the basis of lay beliefs about health and illness in much of Latin America, is also prominent in the Islamic world, and is a component of the Ayurvedic medical tradition in India.

In Latin American folk medicine, the humoral theory – often called the 'hot–cold theory' of disease' – postulates that health can only be maintained (or lost) by the effect of heat or cold on the body.[48] As Logan[50] points out, 'hot' and 'cold' here do not pertain to actual temperature but to a symbolic power contained in most substances, including food, herbs and medicines. In addition, all mental states, physiological states, illnesses, natural and supernatural forces are grouped in a binary fashion into 'hot' or 'cold' categories. To maintain health, the body's internal 'temperature' balance must be maintained between the opposing powers of 'hot' and 'cold', especially by avoiding prolonged exposure to either quality. In illness, health is restored by re-establishing the internal temperature balance by exposing oneself to, or ingesting, items of an opposite quality to that believed to be responsible for illness. Certain illnesses seen as 'hot' are believed to result from overexposure to sun or fire, or from ingesting hot foods or beverages. Both pregnancy and menstruation are considered to be hot states and, like other hot conditions, are treated by the ingestion of cold foods and medicines or by cold treatments such as sponging with cool water. Such beliefs can have dangerous effects on women's health. For example, postpartum or menstruating women from some parts of Latin America may avoid certain fruits and vegetables, which they classify as 'cold' and liable to clot their hot menstrual blood. The avoidance of such foods in women who already have a diet deficient in vitamins may eliminate even more of these vitamins from their diet. In one study from the USA,[51] a group of postpartum Puerto Rican women believed that if the lochia was 'clotted' by cold foods, it would be reabsorbed to cause nervousness or even insanity. As a preventive measure, they drank tonics containing 'hot' foods such as chocolate, garlic and cinnamon.

Humoral medicine is still one component of the pluralistic medical system in Morocco, as described by Greenwood,[52] but most of the emphasis is now placed on two of the humours: blood and phlegm. As in Latin America, this theory of health and illness relates the inner workings of the body to outside influences such as diet and environment. There are 'hot' and 'cold' foods and environmental factors, the imbalance of which in the body can cause hot or cold illnesses that are treated by foods of the opposite quality. Food is commonly used as a treatment, as most foods are considered hot and most illnesses cold. Excess blood is seen as a feature of 'hot' illnesses, and excess phlegm in the body as a feature of 'cold' ones. Most hot illnesses are caused by overexposure to sun, heat or hot winds, or by eating excess foods in summer. The heat then enters the blood, which rises to the head, causing flushing, fever and other symptoms. Treatment in this Moroccan humoral model is removal of the excess hot blood by cooling the body's surface, eating cold foods and using cupping and leeching at the neck to draw off some of the blood.

In the ancient Indian Ayurvedic system, there are similar highly complex concepts of the physiology of the body that equate health with balance. As described by Obeyesekere,[53] there are five bhūtas or basic elements in the universe; ether, wind, water, earth and fire. These are the basic constituents of all life, and also make up the three dōsas or humours (wind, bile and phlegm) and the seven dhātus or components of the body. Food which contains the five elements is 'cooked' by fires in the body and converted into bodily refuse and a refined portion, which is successively transformed into the seven basic components of the

body: food juice, blood, flesh, fat, bone, marrow and semen. The five elements also go to make up the three humours in the body; the wind element becomes wind or flatulence, fire appears as bile and water appears as phlegm. The harmonious working of the body results from an optimal balance of these three humours, and illness results from relative excess or deficiency of one or more of the humours. As in Latin America, there are 'cooling' and 'heat-producing foods' that are used to reduce excess of a humour; hot foods can cause excess bile, and thus illness must be treated by a diet of cold food and other medication. Ayurveda also includes a theory of temperament and its relationship to ill health. For example, a patient whose temperament results from an excess of bile is believed to be especially vulnerable to illness caused by an excess of this humour, and thus should avoid heat-producing food which may increase even further the amount of bile in the body.

Like Ayurveda, traditional Chinese medicine also saw health as a harmonious balance, in this case between two contrasting cosmic principles: yin, described as dark, moist, watery and female, and yang, which is hot, dry, fiery and male. The organs of the body were either predominantly yin (such as the heart, lungs, spleen, kidneys and liver) or yang (such as the intestines, stomach and gallbladder). Illness was believed to result from an imbalance, usually an excess of one principle within an organ, which might then have to be removed by acupuncture or moxibustion.[54]

The humoral concept has largely disappeared from the UK and other European societies, but concepts of restoring health by counteracting one element in the body with another still persist. In English folk beliefs about colds and chills, which are thought of as being caused by the penetration of environmental cold or damp into the body, a common treatment was to counteract cold by heat. Heat was administered in the form of warm drinks, warm foods (which help generate the body's own heat) and rest in a warm bed. The aphorism 'feed a cold, starve a fever' sums up this approach. To prevent colds and chills a variety of patent tonics were used, such as cod liver oil and malt extract, to generate heat inside the body. As one elderly patient put it me, if you went outdoors after taking a tonic 'you felt warm inside', for the tonic was an internal protection against excess cold.[10]

Humoral medicine has, of course, also disappeared from modern scientific medicine. Nevertheless, modern physiology does include numerous examples of diseases that are caused by a deficiency or excess of certain substances in the body, such as hormones, enzymes, electrolytes, vitamins, trace elements and blood cells, which can be corrected by replacing the deficient substance or counteracting the excess. The concept of the negative feedback loop in endocrinology, whereby an increase in one hormone in the bloodstream results in a decrease in another, might also be seen as a balance/imbalance view of ill health, though it also includes notions simultaneously of deficiency/excess. In everyday language, too, echoes of humoral thinking remain, in phrases such as 'he's a well balanced person', 'to eat a balanced diet', 'to be ill-humoured', 'everything in proportion', or 'he's too full of testosterone'.

SYMBOLIC ANATOMIES

In traditional systems of healing, such as traditional Chinese medicine, Tibetan medicine or Ayurveda, practitioners are working not only with concepts of balance but also with their own models of the body's structure and function. Usually, these are part of much wider cosmologies, linking the individual body to greater forces in the universe. Often they deal with the flow, blockage, concentration or imbalance of mystical forces (usually translated into our Western idiom as 'energy'). Being part of much larger cosmologies, these traditional 'maps' of the human body bear little relation to the illustrations in a Western anatomy textbook. In traditional Chinese acupuncture, for example, the body is crisscrossed by a series of meridians, or invisible channels,

along which flow *chi* – the vital energy or life force of the human body. Any interruptions or imbalances in its flow may be linked to disease, both physical and mental. Treatment is by needling some of the 309 acupuncture points along the meridians in order to restore the flow of *chi* and the harmonious balance between *yin* and *yang*.[54] In the Tantric tradition of both Hinduism and Buddhism, the *chakras* (or 'wheels') are concentrations and receptors of energy along the central axis of the body. Thus, in the Hindu version, the body is traversed by a number of channels (or *nadis*) along which flow a vital force, or *prāna*. The central one of these channels, rising from the anus up to the crown of the head, is the *sushumna*. Along it lie the seven *chakras*, each located at a key point for the body's functioning.[55] In Tibetan Buddhism, usually only five or six chakras are described.[56] In both traditions, healing – by means of certain rituals, yoga practices, herbs, acupuncture or moxibustion – aims to restore, strengthen or rebalance the flows of vital energy within and beyond the body, especially in relation to the *chakras*.

To the scientific medical mind, these 'maps' of the body are merely symbolic – mystical metaphors that bear no relation to physical reality. To the practitioners of these ancient forms of healing, however, they represent true models of how the body functions in both health and disease, and are rooted in religious traditions many thousands of years old.

THE 'PLUMBING' MODEL OF THE BODY

In the Western industrialized world, many contemporary concepts of the body's structure and function seem to be borrowed partly from the worlds of science and technology. Familiarity with drainage systems in the home, electricity, machines, computers and the internal combustion engine all provide the models in terms of which people conceptualize and explain the structure and workings of the body. A common version of this might be termed the 'plumbing' model, as illustrated in the case study above. Here the body is

Figure 2.2 Acupuncture charts on the walls of a clinic in Qinghai, China. The charts show the various acupuncture points on the body, and the meridians or channels along which flows its vital energy or chi (Source: © Catherine Platt/Panos Pictures. Reproduced with permission.).

conceived of as a series of hollow cavities or chambers, connected with one another and with the body's orifices by a series of pipes or tubes. The major cavities are usually the chest and the stomach, which almost completely fill the thoracic and abdominal spaces, respectively.

This type of subdivision of the body into large volumes with a single name was demonstrated in Boyle's[40] study in Britain, mentioned above, where 58.8 per cent of the sample saw the stomach as occupying the entire abdominal cavity. Lay vocabulary of ill health also reflects this conception; for example, 'I've got a cold on my chest' or 'my chest's full of phlegm'. The cavities are connected to each other and to the orifices by pipes such as the intestines, the bowel, the windpipe and the blood vessels. Central to this model is the belief that health is maintained by the uninterrupted *flow* of various substances, including blood, air, food, faeces, urine and menstrual blood, between cavities, or between a cavity and the body's exterior via one of the orifices. Disease, then, is seen as the result of blockage of an internal tube or pipe.

The implications of this model in clinical practice were well demonstrated in the example quoted from Kleinman *et al.*[47] A further example, in the

UK, is the widespread folk concept of the dangers of constipation – that is, of a 'blockage in the bowels'. In this model, more common in the older generation, the retained faeces were thought to diffuse into the bloodstream and somehow contaminate it with impurities and 'toxins' – and this then affected both the complexion and one's general health. Self-prescribed laxatives are still widely used in order to achieve a 'good clear out' and so preserve good health and a good complexion. The notion of a 'good clear out' is also applied to menstrual and postpartum blood, and will be described more fully below.

The plumbing model does not necessarily cover all aspects of the body's physiology and anatomy, but mostly deals with the respiratory, cardiovascular, gastrointestinal and genitourinary systems. It is not a coherent or internally consistent system, but rather a series of metaphors used to explain the body's functioning. Often, different physiological systems are lumped together if they occur in the same area (e.g. the chest). A man with nasal catarrh and cough, for example, described his self-treatment as 'I gargled with salt water to get the catarrh out – and I always swallow a bit of it to loosen the cough'.[17]

The model can also be used to express emotional states, especially lay notions of 'stress' or 'pressure' (see Chapter 11), in images borrowed from the Age of Steam: 'I blew my top', 'I need to let off steam', 'I almost burst a boiler'.

THE BODY AS A MACHINE

The conceptualization of the body as an internal combustion engine or as a battery-driven machine has become more common in Western society. These machine and engine metaphors are increasingly encountered by health professionals, who may in turn reinforce them, especially by the use of such explanatory phrases as 'your heart isn't pumping so well', 'you've had a nervous breakdown', 'the current isn't flowing so well along your nerves' or 'you need a rest – your batteries need recharging'. Central to the body as a machine concept is the idea of a renewable fuel or battery power needed to provide energy for the smooth working of the body. 'Fuel' here includes various foodstuffs or beverages, such as tea or coffee, and the large number of self-prescribed vitamins, tonics and other patent remedies. Some people may conceive of alcohol, tobacco or psychotropic drugs as forms of essential fuel without which they could not function in everyday life.

The machine model includes the idea that individual parts of the body, like the parts of a motor car, may fail or stop working, and may sometimes need to be replaced. Modern spare-part surgery (see below), with its widespread usage of organ transplants and artificial organs and body parts, as well as the use of electronic aids such as pacemakers and transistor hearing-aids, all help to reinforce the image of the body as a repairable machine, with treatment consisting of 'new parts for old'.[57] This, in turn, may result in unrealistic expectations of medical treatment. Certain diagnostic procedures such as electrocardiographs or electroencephalograms, which measure the body's 'electrical currents' or waves, as well as the use of foetal monitors in obstetrics (see Chapter 6), may all reinforce the machine

metaphor in the minds of both patients and health professionals.

Allied with this image of the body as a machine is that of the mind as a computer. The increasing use of computers has influenced the ways many people in the industrialized world think about themselves. We now live in a new psychological culture, in what Turkle[58] calls a 'computational culture', with new metaphors for the mind as mainly a processor and storehouse of information. In this model, thoughts, ideas, creativity, memory and personality are all seen as forms of 'software' or programs hidden inside the 'hardware' of the brain and the skull. Thus mental illness or deviant behaviour can now be conceived of as faulty wiring or programming of the individual brain, to be cured by merely reprogramming or rewiring – a new and simplified image of human thought and behaviour that has important social implications. At the same time, just as the mind is seen as a computer, so can the computer be seen as a sort of external mind – a second brain outside the skull, an advanced organ of memory, logic and calculation (what Turkle[58] terms a 'second self'). In the modern information age, loss of a computer or of its electronic memory can seem to some individuals almost as traumatic as a brain injury or a stroke.

THE BODY IN SPACE AND TIME

THE BODY IN SPACE

The concept of symbolic skins, outlined above, means that the body's existence is always shaped and altered by cultural notions of space. These usually extend the body's boundaries far beyond its natural, physical border of skin. In spatial terms, these symbolic skins – some of them invisible, others not – may enlarge the body (and the sense of self that it contains) by an enormous distance. Furthermore, some writers such as McLuhan[59] have argued that the media (radio, television) can now extend the body's special senses (listening, looking) to virtually every part of the world. With their help one can now 'hear' or 'see' events on the other side of the globe at the very moment that they occur. The phenomenal growth of the Internet, and of telemedicine, in recent years has also added to this process, and is described in Chapter 13.

Other cultural concepts of the body, described earlier, deal more with ideas of internal space. They include the arrangement of the bodily organs and systems or, in the case of *ārdha-angāni* the penetration of social categories to within the borders of skin. The recent growth of medical technology (see Chapter 4) has also altered the spatial reality of the human body. The use of X-rays, scans and magnetic resonance imaging (MRI) have now made the body 'transparent' both to medical science and to patients themselves. In a symbolic way, this may be slowly weakening or dissolving people's sense of their own skin as the first, most intimate and fixed border of the self.[60] Similarly, life-support systems and monitoring machines, as well as the development of the new reproductive technologies (see Chapter 6), all help to extend the body's boundaries even further. In the case of dialysis machines, for example, it is as if certain organs – in this case the kidneys – have now become external to the body itself.[60]

THE BODY IN TIME

The human body exists in *time*, as well as in space. This is partly due to cultural concepts of the development and changes of the body as it travels from birth towards death. Much of this Western medical model of *developmental time*[61] – of 'normal' physical and mental development – is based on a rigid, linear image of time, divided into a series of clearly defined milestones of development. Failure to achieve these milestones at exactly the right time (according to the textbook) is often regarded as a sign of abnormality; of being in some way undeveloped or even retarded. These ideas of developmental time determine many aspects of a child's life, such as when they immunized, or when they start school. Later it will define when young people are

considered 'developed' enough to vote, drive cars, inherit money or have sexual relations. It will also define at what age people are considered 'old', and are obliged to retire from work – whether this suits their life situation or not.[61]

Hall[62] has described the two concepts of time most common in Western countries. These are:

1 *Monochronic* time, which is linear, clock time. Here time is seen as a line or ribbon stretching from past to future, and divided into segments known as years, months or days. Every phenomenon is assumed to have a beginning and an end, and in between the two one can only do 'one thing at a time'. Monochronic time is a form of external social organization imposed on people, and is essential for the smooth functioning of industrial society. It is particularly strong in organizations and bureaucracies. In these settings, time is almost tangible; it can be spent, wasted, invested, bought or saved. Time can be converted into money, just as money can be converted into time. This type of time implies, however, a complete dominance over the body and its processes by clocks, calendars, diaries and schedules.

2 *Polychronic* time, in contrast, is much more human time, where personal relationships and interactions take precedence over the rigid schedules of the calendar and the clock. Time is not experienced as a line, but as a point at which relationships or events converge. Polychronic people are not so dominated by clock time; instead, they 'are oriented towards people, human relationships, and the family, which is the core of their existence'. In Hall's view, monochronic time in the USA is more public, 'male' time, while polychronic is more private, 'female' time – the time of the home, leisure and family life.[62] Polychronic time is more common in less-industrialized societies, where official meetings sometimes only take place 'when the time is right', rather than adhering to a rigid schedule – and clock-bound Westerners often find this very frustrating.

Both forms of time – but especially monochronic time – imply different types of cultural time pressure that impact upon the human body in modern society. An example of this is the damaging physiological effect of driving in heavy traffic during 'rush hours', to and from work, each day of the week. Some of the other effects of clock time, on heart disease for example, are discussed further in Chapter 11. In the case of the contraceptive pill, too, a rigid 28-day cycle of clock time is imposed onto the woman's physiology, and for some women this may possibly have emotional, or physical consequences. Throughout the Western industrialized world, moreover, monochronic time is a widespread feature of almost all medical institutions, including hospitals, clinics, doctors' offices and medical bureaucracies. In these health-care settings, this *bureaucratic time*,[61] the overuse of rigid schedules such as hospital visiting times or appointment systems, may be seen by some ill people as inhuman and impersonal. They, and their families, may see it as a way avoiding human contact, of not dealing immediately with their illness and the emotional reality of their situation.

Other forms of cultural time

Several *other* forms of cultural time also exist in most societies,[61] each of which can have major effects on human health and behaviour. These include:

1 *Calendrical time* – the division of the year, based on the natural world (usually the lunar or solar cycles) into days, weeks and months. This includes the annual spring, summer, harvest and winter festivals, the division of the year into 'work time' and 'vacation time', and into special festivals such as New Year's Day, or the summer equinox. Different points in the annual calendar may negatively affect the mental or physical health of different groups of individuals: students at examination time, accountants at the end of the tax year, businessmen struggling to meet a deadline, and academics under pressure to produce research papers or grant applications, within a limited time-frame each year.

2 *National time* – the time cycle specific to each individual nation state, and which includes its annual public holidays and special celebrations such as Thanksgiving Day in the USA, Bastille Day in France, or the Remembrance Day in the UK. For some people, celebration of these special days may involve over-eating and alcohol abuse, or other at-risk behaviours.

3 *Religious time* – the cycle of time linked to the weekly cycles of Sabbaths and workdays. However, it also includes the annual religious feasts, fasts and festivals of each religion, such as Saints' Days, Christmas, Easter, Yom Kippur, Passover, Ramadan, Diwali, etc. Religious time also includes the numinous or 'timeless' time of religious rituals, prayer, meditation and contemplation. It may involve intense emotional states, which can have major effects on psychological state, and in some cultures may also involve the use of powerful hallucinogenic drugs (see Chapter 8). Mass religious pilgrimages to holy sites may sometimes be linked to the spread of certain infectious diseases.

4 *Bureaucratic time* – the times of institutions, mentioned above, which prescribes the length and timing of the working day, the length of vacations, and the dates of annual reports, income tax returns, grant applications and office parties. Like developmental time, it also specifies when one can legally begin to work, and when one is obliged to retire – irrespective of the needs of the particular individual.

5 *Social relationship time* – the specific dates in an individual's personal social network, such as the dates of birthdays, anniversaries, weddings or memorial days when these social relationships need to be commemorated or reinforced by an exchange of gifts or cards. An example of the effects of this type of time are 'anniversary reactions' – often episodes of depression and anxiety – that some bereaved people experience on every anniversary of the death of their loved one.

Author is bias to the negative

6 *Symbolic-rebirth time* – the sense of changed time that can occur after major points of transition or crises in the life cycle – such as religious conversions (where individuals are 'born again'), major crises (such as accidents, assaults, or rapes), major illnesses (such as heart attacks, stroke or transplant surgery) or major life transitions (such as giving birth, or being bereaved). In each case individuals may have the sense of having a 'second life' (and identity) within their lifespan, and time may now be experienced as 'time before' and 'time after' that major event.

Together with monochronic clock time, each of these forms of cultural time are imposed upon the individual by the society in which they live, and can influence not only their behaviour and perceptions, but also their mental and physical health.

THE 'DISABLED' BODY

One of the key cultural categories, found in virtually all societies, is the division between the 'able' and the 'disabled' body. Despite this division, anthropologists have pointed out how these definitions vary widely between different social and cultural groups, as do the meanings they ascribe to these particular labels.

Some attempts have been made to standardize the classification of disabilities internationally, such as the WHO's *International Classification of Impairments, Disabilities, and Handicaps*[63] of 1980. From an anthropological perspective, however, it is the social dimensions of how people (whether disabled or not) interpret and respond to these cultural categories that is of the greatest interest. This phenomenon is of growing importance, since it was estimated in the 1980s that there were about 500 million severely disabled people in the world.[64] Since then this number has greatly increased, due partly to various wars and civil conflicts, and to the large numbers of landmine victims in Cambodia, Mozambique, Afghanistan and elsewhere.

'DISABILITY' VERSUS 'IMPAIRMENT'

The sociologist Michael Oliver[65], in a radical critique of the subject, makes a useful distinction between *impairment* and *disability*. The former describes a body lacking part or all of a limb, or having a defective limb or some other bodily mechanism, while the latter refers to the many social and other disadvantages imposed by society on people with physical impairments. He criticizes the medical model of disability, which focuses solely on the individual and their physical condition instead of on the society in which disability occurs. His model emphasizes how the very concept of disability is socially constructed, and how this category helps create a large number of people who are dependent, marginal and supposedly unproductive economically. Society's narrow definitions of physical normality lead it to ignore and marginalize those who do not fit within that definition. Thus it does not provide the facilities (such as ramps for wheel-chairs) for those who are physically different from the majority of the population. This radical model represents, therefore, a shift in focus from individual to social pathology. Disability is not seen as an individual problem, but as one of society. In some ways, therefore, this perspective resembles the 'socially labelling' model of psychiatric disorders described in Chapter 10. Furthermore, Oliver argues that, because disability is largely 'socially constructed', it follows that not all impaired people need necessarily be 'disabled': this state is not necessarily an inherent aspect of the individual, but is determined rather by the meanings that society ascribes to it and the state of dependency that it often imposes.

DISABILITY AND STIGMA

In many societies, anthropologists have described how people with different physical shapes, sizes and bodily functions are often subject to considerable *stigma*, as well as to prejudice and discrimination.[66,67] Even though the disabled body is not necessarily a sick body, these people often encounter a variety of social disadvantages – especially in finding a marriage partner. Misconceptions and prejudice about blindness are particularly common.[68] In Uganda, for example, Sentumbwe[69] describes how blind girls usually have much reduced marriage opportunities. It is widely assumed that, although they are able to have sexual ('lover') relationships, they will normally not be acceptable as a potential wife, since 'the management of a home requires sight and complete physical functioning'. Many men therefore see them merely as sexual objects, and try to exploit the situation. Despite this, Sentumbwe points out that many blind women in Uganda *do* get married, raise children, have employment and contribute towards the economic and social life of the community. He anticipates a time when, through public education, 'the sighted might come to see the blind as persons with a visual impairment rather than as people who are blind and therefore socially and physically handicapped'. Devlieger[70] also describes how, among women of the Songye people of the Democratic Republic of Congo (former Zaire), a major disability of the limbs which may inhibit daily domestic tasks can make getting married very difficult; however, this does not apply to men with similar disabilities. Similarly, anthropologists[70] have described the social difficulties of physically impaired young people in Dakar, Senegal, and how marrying off a disabled daughter means accepting a lower 'bridewealth' for her than would be paid for a 'normal' woman, but obtaining a wife for a disabled son requires the payment of a much larger than normal bridewealth – a sum that can take many years to accumulate.

The degree of stigma and the economic effect of physical impairment can depend on a number of factors. These include the type of impairment, the socio-economic position of the person and their family *vis-à-vis* the wider society, the types of rehabilitation or treatment available, and the level of technology and social organization of the society itself. In an age of computers, information technology, telecommunications and the Internet, for example, many types of physical impairment are no longer a barrier to a full working and social life. In other cultures, stigma can be avoided or lessened in different ways. In Botswana, Ingstad[71] has described how the parents of a physically impaired child are able to avoid the stigmatizing label of *mopakwane* – a disability believed to be caused by the parents having broken the taboo against having sexual relations while the baby is very young. They do this either by claiming that it is something that 'just happened' (that is, without any social cause), or that the child is *mpho ya modimo*, a 'gift from God'. Actually naming the child in this way can in some ways protect it from stigma in its future life.

POSITIVE ASPECTS OF DISABILITY

It should be emphasized, however, that the stigmatization of *all* physical impairment is not universal. In many cultures different forms of impairment are seen in a more positive light, and disabled people play a full role in community life. For example, Levinson and Gaccione[72] list several cultures where people with certain types of physical impairment are highly valued and believed to have special powers or abilities. In rural Korea, in a cultural tradition that goes back 1000 years, some blind men have been *pongsa* – a special group of diviners who act as fortune tellers, select sites for buildings and graves, pray for rain and place curses. They are believed to have a special type of sight, the 'eyesight of mind'. Among the Tiv people of Nigeria, too, blind people are often believed to develop this special type of sight, and are respected accordingly. Reynolds-Whyte and Ingstad[67] also note how, in many cultures, blind people are more likely to become learned religious men, storytellers or singers, such as the *Surdasi*, the blind singers of India. They also mention how, particularly in some very poor countries in Africa and Asia, physical disability can sometimes be turned to economic advantage. In these contexts, beggars often 'use their impairment as a tool to work for their families', and can sometimes earn more than the physically able.

THEORIES OF CAUSATION OF DISABILITY

As with other human problems, physical impairments are often blamed on a variety of causes – originating either in individual behaviour or in the natural, social or supernatural worlds (see Chapter 5). Supernatural theories are particularly common, even among the disabled themselves. In one study of 104 blind people in rural Ethiopia,[68] for example, 45 per cent of them blamed their blindness on a febrile illness and 15 per cent on accidents, but 33 per cent blamed supernatural forces such as 'curses' or divine punishment. In that same study, almost all the fully and partially sighted people in the community thought that blindness prevented education and that educational opportunities should not be given to the blind. In many other non-industrialized societies, too, considerable attention is paid to the *cause* of the impairment. Often a physical abnormality is seen as the result and expression of some abnormality in that person's relationships with their social or supernatural environment. Among the Songye people, for example, Devlieger[70] describes how physical impairment is often seen as 'a symptom of something more important'. It can be the result of sorcery (often resulting from social or familial conflict) or the breaking of taboos (such as those against sex during pregnancy), or from a lack of respect given to a dead ancestor. For example, a person with a club foot may be seen as having been born 'with the spirit of the ancestor', since this could mean that that the ancestor was not well buried and his coffin was too small so that his legs were compressed. If no other social cause can be found, the condition may simply be ascribed to the act of God (*Efile Mukulu*).

In general, but without over-romanticizing the picture, the ethnographic evidence suggests that in many small-scale societies the physically impaired are treated with more care – as a more normal, accepted part of everyday life – than in many Western, industrialized societies. But even within these Third World communities, attitudes towards disabled people are usually not uniform. Often those with different types of impairment are labelled differently and then treated in a different way. Devlieger,[70] for example, has described how, among the Songye, physically unusual or 'abnormal' children are divided into three categories: 'bad' (*malwa*) children include albino, dwarf and hydrocephalic children; 'faulty' (*bilema*) children include those with deformed upper or lower limbs (such as from polio or birth injuries) or congenital abnormalities (such as club foot); while 'ceremonial' (*mishinga*) children include twins, or children born with the hands or feet first or with the cord around their neck. Those in the last category are given special attention and a higher social status, and are believed to have special powers of healing. Conversely, the 'bad' children are treated as marginal, inferior beings that are not fully human. There is believed to be something supernatural about them, since their origin is believed to be associated with sorcery, and thus they were recently in contact 'with the anti-world of sorcerers'. Although given basic care, they are expected to die fairly soon, since 'they come into this world to stay for a short time and afterwards return to their own world'. The third, probably more common group, includes *mwana wa kilema* ('a child with a fault'). These children have distorted bodies and their condition is believed to arise from distorted relationships within their family or community. Little effort is made to improve their physical functioning, but they are not necessarily treated in a negative way. Instead, 'the person with a disability is seen not as an abnormal, a marginal or a deviant figure, but as a liminal one' (for discussion of such 'liminal' identity, see Chapter 9). Furthermore, they are often valued as confidants for their wisdom, and for their unique perspective on the world.

Finally, many of the supernatural explanations for the disabled body attach to congenital conditions rather than to those acquired later in life, where 'personhood has already been established'.[67] Despite this, an acquired physical impairment can have almost as dramatic psychological and social effects on the individual concerned. Two classic

Guilt to benefit the ...

monographs on this theme are those of the Dutch journalist Renate Rubinstein[73] and of Oliver Sacks,[74] the neurologist and writer. Rubinstein described her emotions of powerlessness when she developed multiple sclerosis, her new dependence on doctors and technology, and the feeling of being 'not quite human anymore' – at least in a social sense. Sacks, too, gave a poignant and graphic account of his experience of a severe leg injury, of the many shifts in body image and the sense of self that this involved, and how incomprehensible much of his experiences were to the doctors and nurses involved in his care.

Overall, then, the category of the disabled body is not fixed. It is a complex and variable one, and its definition depends on social, cultural, economic and historical context. In industrial societies, in particular, there is a concerted attempt to shift this definition from disability, with all the disadvantages this label implies, towards the more neutral definition of physical impairment.

'NEW BODIES' OF THE TWENTIETH CENTURY

Over several decades now a number of 'new bodies' – or new ways of conceptualizing the human body – have appeared in the Western, industrialized world. Each is the result of advances in both medical treatment and diagnostic technology. Their effect has been to alter radically the ways that the modern body, including its boundaries and interior, is conceived of, not only by doctors but also by much of the lay public. Six of these new conceptualizations are described below.

THE COMPOSITE BODY

As a result of the success of spare-part surgery, it has become possible to replace diseased or damaged organs or body parts either by implanting an artificial organ or by transplanting an organ from another person. Artificial body parts, made of metal, plastic, nylon or rubber, now include hips,

knees, arteries, larynx, limbs, teeth, heart valves, corneas and oesophagus. Transplanted organs include hearts, kidneys, corneas, cartilage, bone, hair, liver, lungs, pancreas and parathyroid. Many thousands of people, especially the aged, now have bodies that are partly artificial or are composites of parts of other bodies. Despite their obvious medical and psychological advantages, these spare parts may be subtly altering the contemporary body image and the sense of what is self and what is non-self.[57] They also create new links of 'kinship' between the donors and recipients of these organs, whether living or dead, and between the recipients of artificial organs and those who have manufactured or implanted them. In a sense the boundaries of the modern body have partly dissolved; as people get older, their bodies increasingly absorb the body parts of other people, or the prosthetic products of industry, in a way that was unknown to previous generations. Some of the implications of this new situation are discussed in more detail below.

THE 'CYBORG'

Cyborgs are advanced fusions of human beings and machines. Modern medical technology has enabled many people to be kept alive or to function better by attaching the body to a machine, large or small, for most of the time. These now include dialysis machines (for kidney failure), life-support systems (such as heart–lung machines and 'iron lungs'), incubators (for premature infants), artificial hearts, and smaller machines such as transistor hearing aids and heart pacemakers. By creating bodies that are partly machine – sometimes called 'bionic bodies',[75] medical technology has profoundly influenced the contemporary body image, a fact reflected in the imagery of popular culture.[60] For example, the *New Scientist* in 2004 reported the types of artificial parts for the 'bionic body' that are currently being developed, and claimed that 'some artificial body parts (will) work better than the originals.'[75] As well as the 'total artificial heart'

(TAH),[76] these new mechanical parts will include: penile implants, to help sexual dysfunction; cochlear implants, to restore hearing; electrodes implanted in the brain to treat Parkinson's disease, control behaviour, or improve memory; tiny muscle stimulators ('microstimulators') inserted in muscles, and controlled by an external electromagnetic coil, to help paralysed limbs regain movement; moveable bionic arms for amputees, which are connected directly to the person's nervous system, and will respond to nervous signals from the brain; artificial blood for transfusions, and to prevent the spread of infection; and prosthetic femurs for children, that will elongate as the child itself grows larger. All these developments concentrate on the repair or regeneration of injured or ageing bodies; however, further scientific developments, especially in bioengineering (genetic engineering), nanotechnology and information sciences (including robotics and artificial intelligence), are aiming to further 'enhance' healthy bodies so as to develop a new breed of 'posthumans'[77] – human beings with greatly improved physical, psychological and intellectual powers.[78] Furthermore, in some hospitals in the USA and elsewhere, both cardiac and urological surgery have been using a robotic extension of the surgeon's hands and instruments – the computerized 'da Vinci Surgical Robotic System'– which actually performs the operation, and which can be operated electronically by the surgeon, sitting at a console on the other side of the room. For many people, then, all of these innovations and research in both medicine and surgery are likely to further reinforce the concept of body-as-a-machine described above.

'Cyborgization' seems to involve not only turning humans into machines, or into part-machines, but also regarding machines as partly 'human'. Seeing the computer, for example, as a 'second self',[58] or a hearing aid, artificial limb or pacemaker as a new 'part' of the body, is only possible because of the blurring of boundaries between bodies and machines that is increasingly taking place.

THE VIRTUAL BODY

The development of communications media, and the Internet, have led to the possibility of a 'body' existing only in an abstract, immaterial form in 'cyberspace: as a 'virtual body'. An example of this is the Visible Human Project (VHP), begun in 1989 by the United States National Library of Medicine, and which consists of an online library of digital images of normal adult male and female anatomy, based on numerous MRI and computed tomography (EBCT) scans and anatomical images of two dead bodies.[79] They are what Csordas[80] has called *computerized cadavers*. These detailed images, many of them three-dimensional, are now available online to nearly 2000 licensees in 48 countries, and are used for educational, diagnostic and research purposes by many thousands of people worldwide.[79] Both the VHP and the Human Genome Project (HGP) are reconceptualizations of the body – not as flesh-and-blood but as *information* – potentially available to any user of the internet. In the words of Sandelowski[77] 'The body in these projects is data come to life on our computer screens'. This, to some extent, makes actual dissection of a real human body redundant, since 'the VHP and the HGP allow repeated excursions into virtual bodies without actually penetrating any body at all.' Both are examples of what she terms the new 'posthuman body': 'a disembodied informational structure with no clearly defined self.'[77]

The idea of a 'virtual body' can also refer to the new sense of the human body created by telephones, the media, computers and the Internet. It refers especially to the ways that the body's boundaries have now been extended into cyberspace. An early example of this, noted by McLuhan,[59] was the way that media such as television and radio now extend the range of an individual's central nervous system across the world, particularly their eyes and ears. The growing access to computers has also meant that for some people the computer itself has become a parallel brain outside the skull, to which they delegate many of the organic brain's functions of memory, logic and calculation. As

McLuhan put it, the modern human has become 'an organism that now wears its brain outside its skull and its nerves outside its hide'.[59] For some of these people, losing data from their computer's hard drive may seem almost as significant as losing their memory after a head injury or a stroke. To many others, the computer terminal linked up to the Internet may have become a new type of sensory organ – a means of interfacing, often at a great distance, with other people and other environments, and absorbing a whole new range of sensory data (auditory as well as visual). It provides a way of meeting and communicating with other people, as well as accessing new sources of information.

Increasingly, thanks to computers, more of our cerebral functions are taking place outside of our bodies: either within these computers or in cyberspace. Kurzweil[78] points out that the exponential growth of computers and information technologies means that 'non-biological intelligence is doubling in capacity each year, whereas our biological intelligence is essentially fixed'. Since more and more of our thinking is done by our computers, rather than by our brains, he calculates that by the 2030s the *non*-biological portion of our intelligence will predominate and by the 2040s it will be 'billions of times more capable than the biological portion'. However, it is unlikely that these new and expensive technologies will be equitably shared among the populations of the world or that they will equally available to the poor, as well as to the rich. Some of these developments, such as telemedicine, and their implications, are described in more detail in Chapter 13.

THE BRAIN

For several decades medical research and practice has focused increasingly on the study of the brain, and the monitoring of its functions. This has followed advances in neurophysiology and in diagnostic technologies such as the electroencephalogram (EEG). In symbolic terms, however, it seems to have resulted in a contemporary shift in body image – locating the true site of 'personhood' and the 'self' (as well as of the personality and the unconscious) within the brain itself, rather than in the body as a whole. This echoes cultural models, such as *phrenology*, from the nineteenth century, which emphasized the head and brain as the most important part of human anatomy, and the physical expression of its underlying moral character. This shift is illustrated by changing medical definitions of death. Since the late 1960s death has increasingly been defined as 'brain death': that is, the end of cerebral functions rather than the cessation of other bodily functions such as heartbeat or respiration.[81] In a sense, defining death primarily as the end of cognitive functions, and of the ability to think, echoes Descartes's remark three centuries ago: 'I think, therefore I am'. If you cannot think, you cannot exist.

In many Western countries it is now possible for comatose patients to be declared legally dead on the basis of an EEG, and their organs 'harvested' for transplantation to other people, even if their heart is still beating and they are still breathing with the aid of a life-support system.[82] Increasing focus on the brain is reflected in a huge increase in brain research, in the declaration by the US Congress of the 1990s as 'The Decade of the Brain',[83] and in the growth of the 'brain banks' (collections of brain and neural tissue for research) in the USA and elsewhere. For example, in 1993 the National Neurological Research Specimen Bank at Veterans Administration Wadsworth Hospital, University of California, Los Angeles, held more than 2000 brains and collected 150 more each year,[84] while in Russia in 1991 the Moscow Brain Institute still had 30 000 slices of Lenin's brain for study, as well as those of other prominent people.[85]

In Japan, however, Nudeshima[86] has pointed out that there is considerable cultural resistance to the Western approach to brain death, followed by organ harvesting. For this reason, many Japanese who needed a transplant have had to travel abroad to get one.[86] Despite the Organ Transplant Law of

1997,[87] which for the first time recognized brain death as the end of life, and the distribution of 23 million organ donor cards throughout Japan, a year later not a single transplant operation had been performed.[88] From 1999 onwards, however, a relatively small number of transplants have been carried out in Japan.[89] For Nudeshima,[86] this was because 'the traditional Japanese notion of person had a communal, not an individual, basis'; the death of an individual's brain was not necessarily equated with the actual death of that individual. Death was seen as a long process rather than as a single event, and was only recognized as being final after a series of rituals conducted by the family and community (see Chapter 9) and which sometimes lasted several years. Also, in a society where reciprocity and social relationships are very important, there may be some resistance to receiving organs from an anonymous donor; while Shinto and Buddhist beliefs, which locate the soul everywhere in the body, not just in the brain, also make it difficult to define an individual's moment of death merely by their death of their brain.[90]

THE MEDICAL BODY

The essential reductionism of modern medicine coupled with advances in diagnostic technology (see Chapter 5) has led to a focus on progressively smaller and smaller areas of the body. Medical diagnosis routinely deals with abnormalities at the biochemical, cellular and even molecular levels. This is reflected in the illustrations in medical textbooks over the past century or two. Gradually, they have shifted from gross anatomy to microanatomy; from depictions of the body itself to those of individual organs, and finally of cells or even of molecular structures within those cells, especially their genetic material. Arguably, the 'body' in which modern medicine is now most interested is that of the cell itself. Much of the medical discourse on AIDS, for example, focuses mainly on this cellular level, especially in relation to the immune system. Also, since 1895 the development of X-rays and, more recently, ultrasound,

CT and MRI scans has made the human body more 'transparent', with its structure and interior easily visible.[91] Many thousands of patients have been shown scans or X-rays of their own bodies, in hospitals, doctors' offices and antenatal clinics. Together with medicine's reductionist view of the body, which the public increasingly learns about via the media, magazines, the Internet, or during consultations with a doctor, this has undoubtedly influenced, in subtle ways. how people perceive their own bodies.

Recent advances in medical technology make possible a growing number of what Kaufman and Morgan[92] term 'liminal beings'. At the end of life, these ambiguous life forms include people who are 'not-dead-but-not-fully-alive', such as deeply comatose patients and 'brain-dead cadavers' – both of whom have their vital functions maintained, sometimes long-term, by life-support systems. Some of the implications of this are described in Chapter 14. Similarly, at the beginning of life medical technology now also makes possible another group of liminal beings, or 'new forms at the margins of life',[92] which include stem cells, DNA samples, fetal specimens, and frozen embryos, ova and sperm. In most cases, however, the benefits of these advanced medical technologies, such as stem cell research, are only available to those who live in richer nations and the wealthy elite of poorer countries.

THE EXTERNAL WOMB

Advances in the medical treatment of infertility (the new reproductive technologies), such as *in vitro* fertilization (IVF) or surrogate motherhood (see Chapter 6), have influenced the view many women have of their own bodies and reproductive functions.[93] For example, whereas ovulation, fertilization and pregnancy used to take place within the same woman's body, it is now possible for one or more of these to take place outside her body or even in the bodies of other women. A baby's gestation, birth and development may now involve three different women: the genetic mother, the

Figure 2.3(a,b) X-rays of the chest and hands: diagnostic technology now makes the body 'transparent' to both doctors and patients. (Figure 2.3a reproduced with kind permission from Jenkins P., *Making Sense of the Chest X-ray: a Hands-on Guide*, London: Hodder Education, 2005; Figure 2.3b courtesy of Dr P R Patel, reproduced with kind permission from Patel, K., *Complete Revision Notes for Medical Finals*, London: Hodder Arnold, 2006.)

carrying mother and the nurturing mother[94] – one supplying the ovum, another carrying the foetus during pregnancy and a third caring for the baby once it has been born. Although welcome to infertile women, these advances in reproductive technology, like spare-part surgery, have influenced both body image and assumptions about body boundaries. If one woman's child can be carried in the womb of another (an external womb, as it were), then traditional notions of what is body, self and non-self will all have been radically altered. For the ovum donor, moreover, the ova themselves can become an external body part – one that will soon blend into the body of another woman.[95]

TRANSPLANTS AND THE TRADE IN HUMAN BODY PARTS

Since the first successful kidney transplant in 1954, and the first heart transplant in 1967, there has been an enormous increase in the numbers of organ transplants done worldwide. About 65 000 now take place every year, around 45 000 of which are kidney transplants.[96] The remainder are of lung, liver, pancreas, and other organs. However, the number of available organs is still much less than the number of those who need a transplant, but cannot find a donor. Many of them will die before such an organ becomes available. Currently, organs for transplantation – whether from dead or living donors – are a rare commodity, and subject to the laws of the market place: the laws of supply and demand. They have been increasingly turned into objects for sale and barter: a process known as *commodification*.[90] However, human organs are never just neutral objects or 'things'. As parts of living people they carry with them a great deal of symbolism. Organs such as the heart or brain are also interwoven into everyday language, as powerful metaphors.[97] The heart, for example, is not just a muscular pump; it is also a universal symbol for love, emotion, personality, courage and will. For many people, it is the essence of 'personhood' –

someone can be described as 'good hearted', 'hard hearted' or 'broken hearted'. Thus, heart transplants, even today, can have a powerful symbolism for those who receive them, since it is a process where someone 'sick at heart' 'takes heart' from a donor, so that they can now be as 'hearty' as before.[97]

Transplants create new types of 'kinship' or connections between people. They can also create the sense of partial immortality, for even though the donor may have died, their organ continues to live on within another person. While this is welcome to some of their families, it may not be so to others: some may even see this process as lengthening their period of mourning, and delaying their emotional closure.

Like other medical procedures, organ transplants are always shaped, to some extent, by the context in which they occur. While the 'spare part' model of donated organs may be common the West, it is not the same elsewhere. In Sri Lanka, for example, Simpson[98] describes how among the Sinhalese population, Therevāda Buddhism has had an important influence in encouraging the donation of organs and tissues (including of eyes and blood). This arises from the Buddhist emphasis on charity or donation, given selflessly and without thought of gain, as one of the ways towards achieving *nibbāna*, the highest state of enlightenment. This dedicated act (known as *dāna upa paramitā*) of giving body parts to those in need has a long tradition behind it. For the donor, it reveals a healthy lack of attachment to the material world, including to their body. As one devout Buddhist man put it: 'I hope I die quickly and cleanly from a brain haemorrhage so that maximum use can be made of all my body parts.'

In a Western setting, Sharp's study in Indianapolis, USA,[99,100] revealed very different, and sometimes contradictory, views of transplantation among doctors, recipients and the families of organ donors. For the surgeons, the organs were seen as impersonal 'things', as 'mere muscles, pumps, filters, or bits of flesh'. They were like 'spare parts' necessary to make the body function

normally again. They tended to discourage any contact between the recipients and the donor's next-of-kin, and revealed as little information as possible about the donor. Increasingly, some also regarded these organs as commodities. Despite the fact that the US National Organ Transplantation Act of 1984 outlawed the commercialization of body parts, many surgeons still regarded these organs as rare and precious objects, to be bought and sold at the best possible price.

For the recipients, though, these organs were usually not seen as neutral 'things' – especially 'life saving' organs such as hearts, lungs or livers. Sharp[99] notes how receiving a transplant can have major psychological and social effects on the recipient. For some of them, having a part of someone else's body within their own 'can fragment their sense of self'. Many try to 'restructure' their identities after the operation, by developing a private, idealized, fantasy image of the donor, and the type of person that they were, and then try to integrate this into their new self-image. Some (especially children) may even fear that the organ will carry with it the attributes (especially the negative ones) of its former owner, hidden within its 'cell memories'. Receiving an organ also means that a new biography is grafted on to the old one. Not only is the person 'reborn' after the operation (the *symbolic rebirth* mentioned above), but in a sense the organ carries with it its own biography, its own history.[99] The recipient may ask Where does it come from? What is its history? Who is the donor? What sort of person were they? How did they die? – though in most cases the never learn the answers. In Sharp's study,[99,100] many of the recipients felt they were the fortunate recipients of a 'gift of life', and would have liked to reciprocate in some way to the donor's family, but this was frustrated by the donor's anonymity and the attitudes of the medical staff. As a way of indirectly 'paying back', many of them, after their operation, became involved in voluntary work, among people less fortunate than themselves.

The family of organ donors often have a very different attitude to transplantation. Many of them may want to make personal contact with the recipient, as they feel a sense of ownership, or kinship with the person in whom their loved one's heart is now beating, or lungs expanding. According to Sharp they 'feel they have the right to control how recipients use *their* parts or *their* organs'.[100] But like the recipients they, too, are usually discouraged by the hospitals from making this social connection.

Organ transplantation raises many new ethical questions about what exactly constitutes the end of 'life', and the moment of 'death', especially in different cultures. Is it the death of the entire body, its heart, lungs, senses, pain sensations, movements – or just the death of its brain? As noted above in the case of Japan, the notion of 'brain death' is not necessarily accepted universally. Currently, as Lock[101] points out, still only about 1 per cent of deaths in the developed world are recognized as 'brain death', rather than – as in previous years – the death of the cardiac or respiratory systems. Furthermore, the diagnosis of brain death always depends on very advanced technology, which is not always available. Even when it is available, the potential donor is in an ambiguous state. For their family, the notion that their loved one is a 'brain-dead cadaver', a 'living cadaver' or a 'neomort' in an 'irreversible coma' may be very difficult to accept while they still look 'alive', have good skin colouring and a regular pulse, their nails and hair are still growing, and they are still breathing (albeit with the aid of a life-support system). Furthermore, the question arises: who now 'owns' this 'neomort' and their body parts, and who can now give informed consent for them to be 'harvested'?

In Lock's view,[101] Western medicine and its diagnostic technology have invented a 'new death' – or rather an entirely new way of defining the moment of death. This gives doctors a tremendous power over the exact timing of the comatose body's 'second death' – the moment at which they decide to 'switch off' the life-support system. It also gives them the power of deciding what should be done with the neomort's organs. Nevertheless,

even some doctors are uneasy about this situation. Among the intensive care doctors she interviewed, 'not one believes that a diagnosis of brain death signifies the end of biological life, despite the presence of irreversible damage and knowledge that this condition will lead, usually sooner rather than later, to complete biological death'.

COMMODIFICATION OF BODY PARTS

One major contemporary issue in transplantation is the *commodification* of human organs, and the international trade in them, both legal and illegal. They have increasingly been turned into 'products' or objects that can be bought and sold around the world.[90,101] The supply of human organs for transplantation has become a major multi-million dollar industry, with many international ramifications. Many thousands of people are now involved in the selection, removal, transport, storage, procurement and sale of organs from thousands of 'brain-dead cadavers' in many different parts of the world.

Reviewing the current status of this international trade, Scheper-Hughes[102] states that: 'The organs trade is extensive, lucrative, explicitly illegal in most countries, and unethical according to every governing body of medical professional life. In some sites, the organs trade links the upper strata of biomedical practice to the lowest reaches of the criminal world. The transactions can involve police, mortuary workers, pathologists, civil servants, ambulance drivers, emergency room workers, eye bank and blood bank mangers, and transplant coordinators.' She gives examples of how organs, such as kidneys, now flow in increasingly large numbers from poorer countries to richer ones, and how this 'bio-piracy' is just another example of global inequality, and of the exploitation of the poor by the rich. Often donors in the developing world are forced to part with a kidney or other organ because of their poverty, since it is the only 'collateral' that they possess. In parts of India, it has become common in some communities to trade a kidney in order to pay for the dowry of a daughter, or for some other necessary expense. In Brazil, too, she found poor people willing to sell either a kidney or an eye as they needed the money, and 'because I have two of them'. In many poorer countries, a large black market now exists to sell organs to rich foreigners, especially those from the Middle East, Europe, and North America. In some cases, these organs have been removed without the consent of the donor or their family. She cites allegations that in China organs from executed prisoners have been 'harvested' and then sold to foreigners, and that in South Africa under *apartheid*, and Brazil under military dictatorship, organs were taken from dead donors without permission. As a result of this, rumours of 'organ-stealing' by the authorities, or by foreigners, have become rife in many countries.

In some cases, the state may seek to control the supply of body parts by 'nationalizing' it. This was the case in Brazil in 1997 when, in order to deal with the under-supply of organs, and reduce the commercial trade in them, a Federal law was passed of 'presumed consent' that 'makes all Brazilian adults into universal organ donors at death unless they officially declared themselves to be "nondonors of organs and tissues"'. According to Scheper-Hughes, this caused panic in some poor Brazilians, who feared that the 'the new law is just another bureaucratic assault on their bodies', and that if they were ill doctors seeking organs for transplantation might not be so active in keeping them alive.[102]

Whatever the source of organs for transplantation, their recipients can perceive these new organs in many different ways, as described in this case study from Sweden.

Case study: perceptions of organ transplantation in Sweden

Sanner[103] examined peoples' attitudes to organ donation in Sweden in 2001. She found two main conceptions of the body, each of which influenced people's willingness or unwillingness to either receive or donate organs. First, the view that the body was merely an objective 'machine-like' entity, and did not really represent 'the self'. This made it easier for them to see donated organs merely as 'spare parts'. Second, the view that body and 'self' are closely inter-related, so that a new organ could 'transfer' the donor's qualities, such as their personality and behaviour, into the recipient. Within these two conceptions, she identified seven discrete attitudes towards organ donation itself:

1 *Willingness both to receive, and to give* – this was associated with the machine-model of the body, and with a willingness to both donate and receive organs (or blood). This group did not associate their sense of self with their organs ('What is me is not depending on whose kidney I have received').

2 *Willingness to receive, but not to give* – these also had a machine model, but had a strong anxiety about death, and their ambition was to survive at any price. Thus they were willing to receive an organ, but not to risk their lives by donating one to someone else.

3 *Willingness neither to receive nor to give* – these were people who felt that exchanging organs was somehow 'unnatural', 'against nature', and 'would breach the borders that nature has determined'. Many were also opposed to transplanting animal organs into humans ('My body would let me know that an animal organ didn't fit. It's contrary to nature').

4 *Willingness neither to receive nor to give: the 'influencing organ'* – these believed that the organ might change one's personality, and personal identity, since the 'qualities' of a person resided in their body and organs. They firmly refused either to accept an organ, or to donate one, as 'they did not want to become part of an unknown individual' or vice versa ('Everything is in the heart; I neither want to give it nor take it'). They also rejected organ donation from an animal ('I would perhaps look more piggish with a pig's kidney').

5   *Willing neither to receive nor to give: the 'reincarnated body'* – this group held a very concrete view of reincarnation, believing that resurrection would not be possible if the body was incomplete, and lacking some vital organ.

6   *Mixed feelings about receiving, willingness to give to family members* – like (4) this approach expressed initial anxiety about the 'influence' of an organ received from a stranger ('What if it comes from a sinful man?'), but eventually they would agree to accept one, especially from a relative. They were also willing to donate their own organs, but only to close family members.

7   *Mixed feelings about receiving, but willingness to give* – this last group were willing to donate organs to strangers, but were anxious about how receiving an organ would change their own body image: would they recognize themselves afterwards? Would artificial parts turn them into a 'cyborg'?

THE BODY DURING PREGNANCY

All cultures share beliefs about the *vulnerability* of the mother and fetus during pregnancy; to a variable extent, this extends after birth, usually throughout the early postpartum or lactation period. Cultural concepts of the physiology of pregnancy are often evoked after the child is born, in order to explain *post hoc* any unwanted outcomes of pregnancy such as a deformed, ailing or retarded child. In most cultures it is believed that the mother's behaviour – her diet, physical activity, state of mind, moral behaviour, use of drink, drugs or tobacco – can directly affect the physiology of reproduction and cause damage to the unborn child. Anthropologists have argued that not all the taboos and restrictions surrounding pregnant women can be explained as protecting the mother and foetus from physical damage; the pregnant woman is also in a state of *social* vulnerability and ambiguity. She is in a state of transition between two social roles; those of wife and mother.[104] In this marginal state, as in other states of social transition (see Chapter 9), the person involved is seen as somehow in an ambiguous and 'abnormal' state, dangerous both to herself and to others. The rituals and taboos surrounding pregnancy therefore serve both to mark this transition and to protect mother and foetus during this dangerous period.

FOLKLORE OF PREGNANCY

Several studies were carried out in the 1970s by Snow and colleagues[51,105,106] at public antenatal clinics in Michigan, USA, into lay beliefs about the physiology and dangers of pregnancy. In many cases these beliefs were markedly different from those of the clinicians involved in their care. In one study of 31 pregnant women,[105] 77 per cent of them believed that the foetus could be 'marked' – that is, permanently disfigured or even killed – by strong emotional states on the part of the mother, as divine punishment for behavioural lapses, by the 'power of nature' or by the evil intentions of others. The Mexican-American women in the sample believed that too much sleep or rest during pregnancy would harm the baby by causing it to 'stick to the uterus', making delivery difficult or impossible. They also feared the effect on the child if they saw a lunar eclipse, believing that if a pregnant woman goes out unprotected at this time her child may be born dead, or with a cleft palate or part of the body missing. Wearing a key suspended around the waist was thought to be adequate protection at this time. Many in the study also believed that excessive emotion in the mother – fear, hate, jealousy, anger, sorrow, pity – could all be dangerous to the unborn child. If the pregnant woman saw something that frightened her, like a cat or a fish, the child might be born resembling that object. One woman frightened by a fish during her pregnancy gave birth to a child that 'has two holes in the roof of her mouth and can swim like a fish'. Foetal damage could also result from behavioural lapses on the part of the mother; making fun of a cripple or retarded person during pregnancy could result in God afflicting the infant with a similar disability. Finally, the malevolence of another person could cause foetal damage and even death. Similar lay beliefs are found throughout the world, with local variations.

Beliefs about the effects on the foetus of maternal diet were also investigated in one of the Michigan studies.[51] Ninety per cent of a sample of 40 women thought that pregnant women should change their diets in some way, while 38 per cent believed that food cravings could 'mark' the child permanently if these cravings were not satisfied. In most cases the baby was believed to be marked by unsatisfied food cravings. One woman thought that if a pregnant woman craved chicken but did not get it, the baby could be born 'looking like a chicken'. Other beliefs related to the effect of particular types of food on the foetus; for example, a baby might be born with red spots if the mother ate too many cherries or strawberries during pregnancy, or have a 'chocolate mark' if she ate (or even sat upon) any chocolate. Snow points out that some of these dietary beliefs may be dangerous in pregnancy, as they may provide the rationale for undesirable eating habits by the women. Another factor among some Latin American women is the use of 'hot' or 'cold' foods in pregnancy, irrespective of their nutritional properties, in order to maintain their internal 'balance'. Similar beliefs are found among women from the Indian subcontinent. Homans[104] quotes a British-born Asian woman as saying, 'my mother said not to have "hot" things, not to sit in front of the heater and not to have Coca Cola … The body acquires too much heat and this can lead to miscarriage'.

Beliefs about the state of the uterus during pregnancy can also affect a pregnant woman's health. In one of the Michigan studies,[105] a widely held belief was that the uterus was a hollow organ that was 'tightly closed' during pregnancy to prevent the loss of the foetus. One woman believed that pregnant women could not contract venereal disease (and therefore did not need to take precautions against it) during pregnancy as 'the uterus is closed and germs cannot enter'.

Beliefs about the physiology and dangers of pregnancy have social, psychological and physical aspects. They set pregnant women apart as a special category of person surrounded by what their culture tells them are protective taboos and customs, and these help to explain retrospectively any physical damage or deformity in newborn children. Both aspects, as illustrated above, may have damaging effects on the pregnant woman and her unborn child.

BELIEFS ABOUT BLOOD

To illustrate further some of the clinical implications of cultural conceptions of physiology, a number of beliefs about the nature and function of human *blood* are described below. The human experience of blood – as a vital liquid circulating within the body, and which appears at the surface at times of injury, illness, menstruation or childbirth – provides the basis for lay theories about a variety of illnesses. In general, these illnesses are ascribed to changes in its *volume* ('high blood', caused by too much blood), *consistency* ('thin blood' causing anaemia), *temperature* ('hot illnesses' caused by 'heat in the blood' in Morocco), *quality* ('impurities' in the blood, from constipation) or *polluting power* (menstrual blood causing 'weakness' in males). It should also be remembered that lay concepts of blood deal with much more than its perceived physiological actions; blood is a potent image for a number of things, social, physical and psychological. It is what Turner[107] calls 'a multi-vocal symbol', that is, it signifies a number of elements at the same time. Among the cluster of meanings associated with blood cross-culturally are: an *index* of emotional state (blushing or pallor); personality type (hot-blooded, cold-blooded); illness (flushed, or feverish); kinship ('blood is thicker than water'); social relationships ('bad blood between us'); physical injury (bleeding, bruises); gender (menstruation); danger (menstrual[108] and postpartum blood); and diet ('thin blood' from a bad diet).

For many reasons, then, the clinician should be aware of the possible hidden symbolism in any lay conceptualizations of blood. These beliefs may even influence whether people are willing to have blood tests in hospital, or donate blood for transfusions. They are especially important now because of the growth of the AIDS pandemic, as well as spread of other infectious diseases such as hepatitis B and C.

Case study: beliefs about blood in South Wales, UK

Skultans[109] in 1970 studied the beliefs about menstruation among women in a mining village in South Wales. She found two types of belief about menstrual blood. The first was that menstrual blood is 'bad blood', and menstruation the process by which the system is purged of badness or excess. The emphasis was on losing as much blood as possible, as this was the method whereby 'the system rights itself'. The women said they felt huge, bloated, slow and sluggish 'if they do not have a period or if they do not lose much'. One woman felt 'really great' after a heavy period, and most insisted on the value of having a monthly 'good clearance'. Skultans found that this group had relatively undisturbed and stable married lives, and regarded the menstrual process as 'essential to producing and maintaining a healthy equilibrium' by regular purging of badness. These women also saw menstruation as a state of increased vulnerability, and particularly feared anything that might stop the flow; this would obviously give them a pessimistic attitude towards the menopause, while at the same time they might not worry about menorrhagia or an exceptionally heavy bleed, regarding it instead as 'a good clearance'. The second group of women believed that menstruation was damaging to their overall health, and were fearful of 'losing their life's blood'. They wished to cease menstruating as early as possible and, unlike the first group, were much more positive about the menopause and its attendant symptoms. Skultans found that this group, who viewed periods as 'a nuisance', seemed to be associated with irregular or disturbed conjugal relationships.

Case study: beliefs about menstruation among the Zulu of South Africa

Ngubane[110] in 1977 described beliefs about menstrual blood among the Zulu people of South Africa. Menstruating women are believed to have a contagious pollution, which is dangerous both to other humans and to the natural world. Men's virility may be weakened by this blood, especially if they have intercourse with a menstruating woman. A menstruating woman should also avoid sick people or their medicines during her period, and crops may be ruined or cattle fall ill if she walks among them. In other African societies, women may be confined each month to an isolated 'menstrual hut' to protect the community from their dangerous pollution. Similar beliefs about the 'uncleanness' and polluting powers of menstrual blood are found, especially among men, in cultures and religious groups in many parts of the world.

Case study: beliefs about menstruation in Michigan, USA

Snow and Johnson,[51,106] in the 1970s, examined beliefs about menstruation of a group of low-income women, in a public clinic in Michigan. Many of them saw menstruation as a method of ridding the body of 'impurities' that might otherwise cause illness or poison the system. They believed that the uterus was a hollow organ that was tightly closed between periods while it slowly filled with 'tainted blood', and then opened up to allow the blood to escape during the period. As a result, they reasoned that one could only get pregnant just before, during or just after the period, 'while the uterus is still open'. During this time, the women believed themselves to be particularly vulnerable to illness caused by the entry of external forces such as cold air or water, germs or witchcraft. One woman in the group speculated that one should not attend a funeral during menstruation lest the germs that caused the deceased's death enter the open uterus and cause disease. A recurrent fear among the group was of stopped or impeded menstrual flow, or of the flow of blood in the postpartum or postabortion period. Latin American women in particular feared that certain 'cold' foods (or cold water or air) might clot the 'hot' blood, and interrupt the flow. The stopped flow might then 'back up' in the body and cause a stroke, cancer, sterility or 'quick TB'. 'Cold' foodstuffs included fresh fruits, especially citrus, tomatoes and green vegetables. As one Mexican-American woman put it '*Le da mucha friadad a la matriz*' ('Such things make the womb very cold').[51] The researchers point out that avoidance of such foods during vaginal bleeding associated with menstruation, postabortion or postpartum states can eliminate much-needed vitamins from a diet which, for many low-income women, is already deficient in vitamins. The fear of impeded menstruation may also lead some women to avoid some methods of contraception (oral contraceptives, intrauterine contraceptive devices) that may cause changes in menstruation.

Case study: 'high blood' in the Southern United States

Snow,[111] in 1976, described a common lay belief among low-income patients in the Southern USA, both black and white, called 'high blood'. The central belief was that the blood went up or down in volume depending on what one ate or drank, and this could cause either 'high blood' or 'low blood'. 'Low blood' was believed to result from eating too many acid or astringent foods, such as lemon juice, vinegar, pickles, olives, sauerkraut and Epsom salts, and caused lassitude, fatigue and weakness. It was thought to occur particularly in pregnant women and should be treated by ingesting certain red foods or drink, such as beets, liver, red meat, grape juice and red wine. In contrast 'high blood' resulted from eating too much rich food, especially red meat. Home remedies included taking lemon juice, vinegar, sour oranges, Epsom salts and the brine from pickles or olives. The clinical implications of this belief were not only the effects on health of

this type of diet (for example, one with a very high salt content), but also the effect on compliance with a doctor's instructions by one who confused 'high blood' with high blood pressure. Patients who interpreted a diagnosis of high blood pressure as 'high blood' might increase the amount of salt in their diet and reduce the intake of red meat in a diet that may already be deficient in protein.

Case study: 'sleeping blood' in the Cape Verde Islands

Like and Ellison[112] in 1981 described the case of a 48-year-old woman from the Cape Verde Islands who was admitted to a neurology ward in a hospital in the USA. She was suffering from paralysis, numbness, pain and tremor of her right arm. It was discovered that 2 years previously she had suffered bilateral Colles' fractures of her wrists, and after that her neurological symptoms gradually appeared. No physical cause for her illness could be found, until it was realized that she believed herself to be suffering from a Cape Verdean folk illness, 'sleeping blood' (*sangue dormido*). In this lay model, traumatic injuries (in this case, her wrist fractures) may cause a person's normal 'living blood' (*sangue vivo*) to leak out into the skin, turn black (i.e. form a haematoma) and become 'sleeping blood'. It is feared that deeper deposits of blood develop between the muscles and the bones and, if not removed, their volume may expand over time and obstruct the circulation distal to the traumatized area. In addition, the internal 'living blood' may dam up and cause various disorders such as pain, tremor, paralysis, convulsions, stroke, blindness, heart attack, infection, miscarriage and mental illness. The patient explained her neurological disabilities as due to the blockage resulting from the 'sleeping blood'. She was eventually treated by withdrawing 12 ml of blood from her right wrist (the *sangue dormido*) on two occasions, and by the application of cold packs, after which her tremor, paralysis and pain completely disappeared.

Case study: blood as a non-regenerative liquid

Foster and Anderson[113] pointed out that the belief that blood is a non-regenerative liquid which, when lost through injury or disease, cannot be replaced, leaving the victim permanently weakened, is common in many parts of the world. In parts of Latin America people are most reluctant to part with their precious blood, and this may be one of the reasons why blood banks are less successful in getting donations of blood than in the USA and in Europe.

Case study: 'dirty' or 'lost' blood among the Mende of Sierra Leone

Bledsoe and Goubaud[114] in 1988 described how, among the Mende people of Sierra Leone, blood was seen as a vital liquid that was almost impossible to replace if lost. Debilitating sicknesses, injuries and infestation with small organisms and worms (*fulu-haisia*) were all said to make blood 'dirty', or to drain it. Blood could also be 'lost' by having blood samples taken at hospital, or by donating blood; thus 'the Mende view with great fear the attempts of hospital workers to induce them to give blood'. Attempts were made to replace, build or purify the blood by the use of certain foods (especially palm oil and greens such as spinach or potato leaves) and certain medicines (especially those that are red in colour). *All* red medicines were considered desirable, whatever they contained, provided that they were red, brown or even orange in colour – for example, Fanta, Guinness stout or Vimto are also taken during illness. Because palm oil was the favourite remedy for dirty or inadequate blood, young children might be fed only soft rice (which develops the body) and palm oil (which makes it produce blood) until well into their second year.

KEY REFERENCES

3 Polhemus, T. (1978). Body alteration and adornment: a pictorial essay. In: *Social Aspects of the Human Body* (Polhemus T., ed.). London: Penguin, pp. 154–73.

20 Ainsworth,C. (2004) Vital statistics. *New Scientist* 184(2471), 40–31.

27 Nasser, M. (2003) Eating disorders across cultures. *Psychiatry* 11(11),12–14.

30 Douglas, M. (1973). *Natural Symbols*. London: Penguin, pp. 93–112.

48 Foster, G.M. (1994). *Hippocrates' Latin American Legacy: Humoral Medicine in the New World*. Reading: Gordon and Breach.

53 Obeyesekere, G. (1977). The theory and practice of Ayurvedic medicine. *Cult. Med. Psychiatry* 1, 155–81.

58 Turkle, S. (1984). *The Second Self: Computers and the Human Spirit*. St Albans: Granada, pp. 281–318.

65 Oliver, M. (1990). *The Politics of Disablement*. London: Macmillan, pp. 78–94.

77 Sandelowski, M. (2002) Visible human, vanishing bodies, and virtual nursing: Complications of life, presence, place, and identity. *Adv. Nurs. Sci.* 24 (3), 58–70

88 Hadfield, P. (1998). No spare parts: cultural qualms are undermining Japan's transplant efforts. *New Scientist*, 31 October, p. 13.

92 Kaufman, S.R. and Morgan, L.M. (2005) The anthropology of the beginnings and ends of life. *Annu. Rev. Anthropol.* 34, 317–314.

103 Sanner, M.A. (2001) Exchanging body parts or becoming a new person? People's attitudes toward receiving and donating organs. *Soc. Sci. Med.* 52, 1491–1499.

See http://www.culturehealthandillness.com for the full list of references for this chapter.

RECOMMENDED READING

de Garine, I. and Pollock, N.J. (eds). (1995) *Social Aspects of Obesity*. Reading: Gordon and Breach.

Helman, C. (1992) *The Body of Frankenstein's Monster: Essays in Myth and Medicine*. New York: W. W. Norton.

Ingstad, B. and Reynolds-Whyte, S. (eds) (1995) *Disability and Culture*. Berkeley: University of California Press.

Nasser, M., Katzman, M.A. and Gordon, R.A. (eds) (2001) *Eating Disorders and Cultures in Transition*. Hove: Brunner-Routledge.

Sacks, O. (1991). *A Leg to Stand On*. Picador.

RECOMMENDED WEBSITES

TransWeb.Org (website dealing with organ transplantation): http://www.transweb.org

3

Paper Topic

• Hunger in America

!

Essay

Food is more than just a source of nutrition. In all human societies it plays many roles and is deeply embedded in the social, religious and economic aspects of everyday life. For people in these societies it also carries with it a range of symbolic meanings, both expressing and creating the relationships between man and man, between man and his deities, and man and the natural environment. Food is an essential part of the way that any society organizes itself, and of the way it views the world that it inhabits. To some extent you are what you eat – or what you refuse to eat.

The anthropologist Claude Levi-Strauss[1] argued that, just as there is no human society that does not have a spoken language, so also is there no human group that does not in some way process some of its food supply through cooking. In fact, the constant transformation of raw into cooked food is one of the defining features of all human societies, a key criterion of *culture* as opposed to *nature*.

Anthropologists have further pointed out how cultural groups differ markedly from one another in many of their beliefs and practices related to food. For example, there are wide variations throughout the world as to what substances are regarded as food and what are not. Foodstuffs that are eaten in one society or group may be rigorously forbidden in another. There are also variations between cultures as to how food is cultivated, harvested, prepared, served and eaten. Each culture usually has a set of implicit rules that determine

who prepares and serves the food and to whom, which individuals or groups eat together, where and on what occasions the consumption of food takes place, the order of dishes within a meal, and the actual manner of eating the food. All of these stages in food consumption are closely patterned by culture, and are part of the accepted way of life of that community.

In most parts of the world the actual preparation of food is usually the task of women,[2] but in many societies they are also closely involved in its production: milking animals, caring for poultry and livestock, and planting, tending and harvesting a wide variety of crops. In many rural parts of the Third World women also play a leading role in the retail marketing of food, such as the famous 'market women' of West Africa, the Caribbean and parts of Latin America.

CULTURAL CLASSIFICATIONS OF FOOD

Because of the central role of food in daily life, especially in social relationships, dietary beliefs and practices are notoriously difficult to change, even if they interfere with adequate nutrition. Many well-meaning nutritionists, nurses and doctors have discovered this fact in dealing with cultures other than their own. Before these beliefs and practices can be modified or improved, it is important to understand the way that each culture views its food and the way that it *classifies* it into different categories. In general, six types of food classification systems can be identified, though in practice they overlap, and several of them usually coexist within the same society. They are:

1 Food *versus* non-food.
2 Sacred *versus* profane foods.
3 Parallel food classifications.
4 Food used as medicine, and medicine as food.
5 Food as poison.
6 Social foods (which signal relationships, status, occupation, gender or group identity).

Their clinical significance is that they may severely restrict the types of foodstuffs available to people, and that diet may be based on cultural rather than nutritional criteria.

FOOD VERSUS NON-FOOD ①

Each culture defines which substances are edible and which are not, although this definition often leaves out substances that *do* have a nutritional value. In the UK, for example, snakes, squirrels, otters, dogs, cats and mice are all edible, but are rarely classified as food. In France snails and frogs' legs are food, but usually not so in the UK. In parts of the Far East dogs and cats are commonly eaten, but this does not occur in the Western world. Irrespective of cultural background, however, virtually no human groups in the world define human flesh as food.

In some cases, the definition of substances as non-food may result from their historical associations; for example, Jelliffe[3] suggested that the spleen is rarely eaten in Britain because, in the ancient Galenic humoral system, it was the prime seat of the melancholic humour. Definitions of what is considered edible and what is not tend to be flexible, however, especially under conditions of famine, economic deprivation and foreign travel. In addition, there is a spectrum among the substances defined as food ranging between those that are regarded as nutritious, and are eaten during meals, and those eaten between meals as snacks. In some cases the manufacturers of certain of these snacks, such as sweets, candies, chocolates and cakes, have sought to promote their products as a nutritious food – something that 'fills the energy gap' between proper mealtimes.

Whatever the origins of these definitions, classifying a substance as non-food on cultural grounds may leave out useful nutriments from the diet, and this seems to be a universal phenomenon. 'No group', as Foster and Anderson[4] put it, 'even under conditions of extreme starvation, utilizes all available nutritional substances as food'.

SACRED VERSUS PROFANE FOODS ②

The term 'sacred' foods is used here to refer to those foodstuffs the use of which is validated by *religious* beliefs, while foodstuffs expressly forbidden by the religion can be termed 'profane'. This latter group is usually the subject of strict taboos that not only prohibit ingestion of the food but also forbid physical contact with it. In most cases, this profane food is also seen as unclean and dangerous to health. The sacred/profane dichotomy applies to much more than food, since it is usually part of a wider moral framework including dress, behaviour, speech and certain ritual actions, such as regular prayers, or ritual bathing and other rites of purification. The priestly castes and officiators within these groups are more likely to be subject to these strict rules, which maintain their purity and holiness, than the average worshipper. On certain occasions or fasts, all, or certain foodstuffs are considered profane, and must be avoided. Examples of this are the annual 25-hour fast of the Jewish *Yom Kippur* or Day of Atonement, observed on the tenth day of the Hebrew month of Tishri, and the Muslim fast of *Ramadhan* where, for the ninth month of the lunar year, food and drink are avoided between dawn and sunset by all Muslims above the 'age of responsibility' (15 years for boys, 12 years for girls) unless they are ill, menstruating, pregnant or lactating. Ramadhan ends with the festival of *Eid ul-Fitr*. Regular food abstentions are also a feature of Hinduism and, according to Hunt[5], many observant Hindus spend 2 or 3 days a week 'fasting' – that is, eating only 'pure' foods such as milk, fruit, nuts and starchy root vegetables like cassava and potatoes.

Strict taboos against certain types of food are characteristic of a number of religious faiths:

Hinduism – orthodox Hindus are forbidden to kill or eat any animal, particularly the cow. Milk and its products may be eaten, since they do not involve taking the animal's life. Fish and eggs are infrequently eaten.

Islam – neither pork nor any pig products may be eaten. The only meat permitted is that from cloven-hooved animals that chew the cud, and it must be *halal* (ritually slaughtered). Only fish that have fins and scales may be eaten, and shellfish, shark and eels are therefore forbidden.

Judaism – as with Islam, all pig products are forbidden, and also fish without fins or scales, birds of prey and carrion. Only animals that chew the cud, have cloven hooves, and have been ritually slaughtered are *kosher* and may be eaten. Meat and milk dishes are never mixed within the same meal.

Sikhism – Beef is strictly forbidden, but pork is allowed though it is rarely eaten. The meat must also be slaughtered in a special ritual way known as *jhatka*.

Rastafarianism – many Rastafarians are vegetarian, although some follow dietary restrictions similar to Judaism.[6] As with many other religious groups, alcohol is strictly prohibited.

A more secular example of food taboos is found in the contemporary *whole food* movement in the UK and USA. Here the sacred/profane dichotomy is between 'whole foods' on the one hand and 'junk foods' on the other, but also between natural and artificial, between the purity of the past and the pollution of the present. Junk foods are associated with ideas of uncleanliness and danger, especially from their additives, dyes, preservatives and other pollutants. In the ideology of the movement these additives are often associated with the supposed evils of modernity, and of the urban, industrial way of life. Similarly, the modern movement of *vegetarianism*, which Twigg[7] sees as offering 'a this-worldly form of salvation in terms of the body', sees meat and its various products as dangerous and profane. This movement associates a vegetarian diet with purity, lightness, wholeness and spirituality while, in contrast, meat and blood are associated with aggressiveness, base sexual instincts, an 'animal nature' and a disharmonious world.

As will be illustrated below, all these forms of food taboos may exclude much-needed nutriments from the diet by classifying some foodstuffs as profane and therefore forbidden. They may also result in some forms of medication being rejected on religious grounds – for example, insulin made from beef or pork is unacceptable to many Hindus and Muslims.

PARALLEL FOOD CLASSIFICATIONS

The division of all foodstuffs into two main groups, usually called 'hot' and 'cold', is a feature of many cultural groups in the Islamic world, the Indian subcontinent, Latin America and China. In all these cultures, this binary system of classification includes much more than food; medicines, illnesses, mental and physical states, natural and supernatural forces, are all grouped into either hot or cold categories. The theory of physiology on which this is based, and which equates health with *balance* between these two categories, has been fully described in Chapter 2.

In many cases this view of health and illness represents a survival of the humoral theory of physiology, especially in Latin America and North Africa. In China and India, while hot/cold dichotomies are also found, they have a different genealogy – from the yin–yang and Ayurvedic systems respectively. The notions of hot and cold do not refer to actual temperature, but rather to certain symbolic values associated with each category of foodstuffs. Because health is defined as a balance between these categories, ill-health is treated by adding hot or cold foods or medicines to the diet in order to restore the balance. For example, among some Latin American groups living in the USA, a 'cold' disease such as arthritis may be treated by hot foods or medications, while in Morocco, 'hot' illnesses such as sunstroke are treated by cold substances. In most cases these parallel food classifications are not based on a logically consistent principle, nor are foodstuffs that are classified as hot in one culture or region necessarily seen as hot in another.

Local historical and cultural factors, as well as personal idiosyncrasies, may play a part in assigning foods to these two categories. For example, in his study in Morocco, Greenwood[8] found significant disagreements among his informants as to which foods were 'hot' and which were 'cold', though they all agreed on the tastes, physiological effects and therapeutic value expected of the two categories. In some cases the choice of category was based mainly on personal experience. For example, one man noted that goat's meat tasted sour and caused indigestion and joint stiffness (cold conditions) and that goats could not tolerate being outside in the winter; however, cattle could, and therefore goat's meat was cold while beef was hot.

Parallel food classifications sometimes include intermediate categories such as cool, warm or neutral, so that there is a spectrum between hot and cold rather than a clear division. In the 1970s Harwood[9] described an example of this form of classification among a small group of immigrants from Puerto Rica in New York City. While diseases were grouped into hot and cold categories, foodstuffs and medications were divided into hot (*caliente*), cool (*fresco*) or cold (*frio*). Arthritis, colds, menstrual periods and joint pains were all cold diseases, while constipation, diarrhoea, rashes, tenesmus and ulcers were all hot. The hot medicines included aspirin, castor oil, penicillin, cod liver oil, iron and vitamins, while cold medicines were bicarbonate of soda, mannitol, nightshade and milk of magnesia.

The three categories of foods are shown in Table 3.1, though this division is not necessarily typical of all Puerto Ricans today, whether in New York or elsewhere. Harwood noted how the classification he described was not based on relative temperatures – iced beer, for example, was still considered hot because it is an alcoholic beverage.

Cold illnesses were sometimes blamed on eating too many cold foods, which cause a stomach chill or *frialdad del estomago*. Similarly, a person with a cold may refuse to drink fruit juices recommended by a physician as they are also classified as cold.

During pregnancy a woman in this group would avoid hot foods or medications (including iron and vitamin supplements) lest her child be born with a hot illness, such as a rash. After delivery and during menstruation cold foods would be avoided lest they clot the blood and impede the flow, causing it to go backwards into the body and cause nervousness or insanity.

In Tann and Wheeler's[10] study of a group of London Chinese in 1980, mothers believed that their diet should be modified according to the general health of the infant receiving their breast milk. If the baby had a cold illness, they avoided cold foods that might turn the breast milk cold and thus aggravate the illness. In some cases this led to a considerable restriction in the sources of nutrition available to the mother.

Table 3.1 Hot–cold classification of foods among some New York Puerto Ricans, USA

Hot (caliente)	Cool (fresco)	Cold (frio)
Alcoholic beverages	Barley water	Avocado
Chili peppers	Bottled milk	Bananas
Chocolate	Chicken	Coconut
Coffee	Fruits	Lima beans
Cornmeal	Honey	Sugar cane
Evaporated milk	Raisins	White beans
Garlic	Salt-cod	
Kidney beans	Watercress	
Onions		
Peas		
Tobacco		

Source: Harwood (1971).[9]

In the 1970s Hunt[5] described the hot–cold classification system among some Asian immigrants (from India, Pakistan and Bangladesh) living in the UK, including both Hindus and Muslims. Their classification of foodstuffs into hot and cold is shown in Table 3.2. As with the Puerto Rican example, illnesses were treated by restoring the balance of hot and cold forces within the body; a febrile illness, for example, is treated with cold foods such as rice, greengram and buttermilk. A more recent study by Chowdhury and colleagues[11] of British Bangladeshis, revealed that *two* different parallel food classification could be held at the same time: in this case 'weak' versus 'strong' foods, and 'digestible' (*loghu pak*) versus 'indigestible' (*guru pak*) foods. This classificatory system is described in more detail later in the chapter.

The importance of these types of parallel classificatory system, especially those used as a form of self-medication, is that in some circumstances they may prove damaging to health and well-being.

Table 3.2 Hot–cold classification of foods among some Asians in the UK

Hot	Cold
Wheat	Rice
Potato	Plantains
Buffalo milk	Cow's milk
Fish	Buttermilk
Chicken	Greengram
Horse gram	Peas
Groundnut	Beans
Drumstick	Onions
Bitter gourd	Green tomatoes
Carrots	Pumpkin
Radish	Spinach
Fenugreek	Ripe mango
Garlic	Bananas
Green mango	Guava
Paw-paw	Lemons
Dates	

Source: Hunt, 1976[5].

FOOD AS MEDICINE, MEDICINE AS FOOD

This category system usually overlaps with parallel food classifications when the two coexist in the same society, as in the cases of Morocco, India and Puerto Rico quoted above. However, in other societies special diets may also be seen as a form of 'medicine' for certain illnesses or psychological states. Some examples of this have been quoted in the previous chapter, such as 'feed a cold, starve a fever' in the case of common viral or bacterial infections, or the use of certain foods or vitamins (a form of concentrated food) to prevent colds and chills. In the case of special physiological states (such as pregnancy, lactation and menstruation) certain foods are sometimes avoided, or else prescribed to aid in the physiological process. The effect of hot and cold foods on these states has already been described in the case of women from Latin America. In a 1978 study[12] of 40 women attending a public clinic in Michigan, 11 believed the foetus could be 'marked' if the mother's food cravings were not satisfied, 12 thought that the diet should be altered in the postpartum period and four believed it should be changed during lactation. Twelve women in the sample admitted to having eaten starch, clay or dirt during pregnancy – as one pregnant woman put it, it was a good idea to eat earth since it acts as 'a scrub brush through the organs'. One woman believed that, during lactation, the supply of breast milk could be increased by drinking red raspberry tea and avoiding acid foods and cabbage. In many of these cases, cultural prescriptions about the appropriate food and drink to 'treat' or advance a physiological process may have negative effects on the patients' health.

The American folk illness 'high blood' (and its opposite, 'low blood'), described in Chapter 2, is a further example of food as medicine. 'High blood' is treated by taking lemon juice, vinegar, sour oranges, pickles, olives or sauerkraut, while the treatment of 'low blood' involves an increased consumption of beets, grape juice, red wine, liver and red meat. Where a patient confuses the diagnosis of high blood pressure with 'high blood', much needed sources of protein may be cut from the diet and replaced with foods with a high salt content – which may be dangerous in a case of hypertension.

Etkin and Ross[13] studied the use of plants, both as medicine and as food, among the Hausa people of Northern Nigeria. They found that many of the plants were used as folk medicines and as food. For example, cashew nuts were chewed for treatment of intestinal worms, diarrhoea and dyspepsia, but were also added to soups and used as a condiment in vegetable foods. By analysing both the nutritional and pharmacological properties of many of these substances, they concluded that many plants taken as medicine may in fact also have nutritional value, while some of the plants used mainly as food also have a medicinal effect. Therefore, only by examining all the many uses of plants can an estimation of their overall nutritional value be made. They also suggest that agricultural development programmes that attempt to reduce crop diversity in order to maximize calorie and protein availability may reduce the range of nutrients available to food-producing populations, as well as the plants available both as medicines and as dietary constituents.

More recently, and especially in the USA, there has been increasing interest in 'nutriceuticals' – foods or nutritional supplements that are believed to prevent or treat a variety of physical and mental disorders. When included in the diet, these 'functional foods' or are said to give a variety of health benefits beyond basic nutrition. These include olive oil or oily fish eaten to reduce cholesterol levels, green teas drunk for their antioxidant properties, and high-roughage foods eaten to prevent bowel cancer, diverticulitis, haemorrhoids or constipation. Included here, too, is the wide variety of 'health foods', 'whole foods' or 'organic foods' (see above) now on sale in most industrialized societies.

Medicines, whether medically or self-prescribed, may also come to be regarded as a form of food or nutriment without which the patient might weaken or die. Examples of this are certain cardiac or hypotensive drugs, insulin therapy, and thyroid and other hormone replacement therapy. When these drugs are regularly taken at mealtimes, they may become incorporated into the meal as a symbolic form of food. Other substances such as vitamins and tonics, alcohol, tobacco and psychotropic drugs, if taken regularly, might also come to play this role (see Chapter 8).

In some cases, the consumption of certain foods can be perceived not as a medicine but as a form of 'immunization' against disease. Enticott[14,15] describes how in some rural English communities, there has been opposition to the introduction of pasteurized milk, which is seen as 'artificial' and 'unhealthy'. Conversely, local unpasteurized milk, with all its bacteria and impurities, is seen as 'immunizing' the body against disease by exposing it regularly to the pure, beneficial, protective, 'vital force' of 'Nature' – the environment in which these communities work and live. It is thus also an assertion of the values of their rural lifestyle vis-à-vis those of the townspeople.

FOOD AS POISON

This refers to a relatively new phenomenon in affluent countries, with abundant food supplies, namely, a growing concern about food safety, with regular 'food scares' that sweep through the population every few years. In these situations, a certain type of foodstuff is classified – often temporarily – as a 'poison': a substance dangerous to health, or causing disease, and which should be avoided. In the UK in recent years, several 'food scares' have focused on chemical additives – such as colourings, dyes (such as Sudan 1), antibiotics, dioxins, mercury in fish, organophosphates and their metabolites in fruit and vegetables, phthalates in infant formula feeds, bisphenol A in various canned products, acrylamide (a potential carcinogen) in a range of fried and baked foods, and hormone residues with oestrogenic activity in different foodstuffs (which can affect sperm counts). Other 'scares' have focused on microbial contamination – such as bovine spongiform encephalopathy (BSE) ('mad cow disease'), food poisoning from *Escherichia coli* or *Salmonella*, or contamination of chickens by *Campylobacter*, or on the perceived risks of genetically modified (GM) foods and crops.[14] The notion of 'junk food' or 'fast food' as being dangerous to health because of their relatively high levels of salt, sugar and fat should also be included here. Although these 'scares' are usually based on proven scientific information, public responses to them often have a strongly symbolic aspect. Enticott,[15] for example, notes how in some rural areas of England some people now choose food which they see as 'natural', 'traditional', 'organic' or 'local' in preference to prepacked, processed and mass-produced 'artificial' foods, because they symbolize for them a more 'natural' state of moral purity, pre-industrial innocence and local *communitas* – even though these 'natural' foods can sometimes have health dangers of their own.

SOCIAL FOODS

Social foods are those that are consumed in the presence of other people, and which have a *symbolic* as well as nutritional value for all those concerned. A snack eaten in private is not a social food, but the constituents of a family meal or religious feast usually are. In every human society, food is a way of creating and expressing the *relationships* between people. These relationships may be between individuals, between the members of social, religious or ethnic groups, or between any of these and the supernatural world. Food used in this way has many of the properties of the ritual symbols described later in this book (Chapter 9). In particular, when food is consumed in the formalized atmosphere of a communal meal it carries with it many associations, telling the participants much about their relationship with one another and with the outside world. Most meals have a ritual aspect in addition to their purely practical role in providing nutrition for a number of people at the same time. Like all ritual occasions, they are tightly controlled by the norms of a particular culture or group. These norms, or rules, determine who prepares and serves the food, who eats

together, and who clears up afterwards. They also determine the times and setting of meals, the order of dishes within a meal, the cutlery or crockery used, and the precise way in which the food may be consumed (table manners). The food itself is subject to cultural patterning, which determines its appropriate size, shape, consistency, colour, smell and taste. Both the formal occasion of a meal and the types of food served within it can therefore be viewed as a complicated *language*, which can be decoded to reveal much about the relationships and values of those sharing in the food. Each meal is a restatement and recreation of these values and relationships.

Different types of meal convey different messages to those taking part in them. Farb and Armelagos[13] point out that, in North America, cocktails without a meal are for acquaintances or people of lower social status, meals preceded by alcoholic drinks are for close friends and honoured guests, and a cold lunch is 'at the threshold of intimacy' but not quite there. Social intimacy is symbolized by invitation to a complete meal, with a sequence of courses contrasted by hot and cold; the buffet, the 'cookout' and the barbecue extend friendship to a greater extent than an invitation to morning coffee, but less so than an invitation to a complete sit-down meal.

Social status

Meals can also be used to symbolize social *status*, often by serving rare and expensive dishes – what Jelliffe[3] calls 'prestige foods'. According to him, these are usually protein (and often animal), are difficult to obtain or prepare (as they are rare, expensive or imported) and are often linked historically with a dominant social group (such as venison, which was the preserve of the upper classes in Europe during the Middle Ages). Among the prestige foods that can be identified are venison and game birds in Northern Europe, the T-bone steak in America, caviar in much of the Western world, the camel hump among Bedouin Arabs, and the pig in New Guinea. Status can also be acquired by giving enormous feasts, where large amounts of food are conspicuously eaten or wasted. A well-known example of this, from the anthropological literature, is the *potlach* feast of the Indians of north-western USA and Canada. Here, different families competed with one another to throw huge, lavish feasts, each one greater than the next, and where large amounts of food were wasted. The aim was to humiliate rival families by throwing a feast that could not be matched by them.

In other societies, the display and sharing of food is also used to obtain prestige, but without the wastage characteristic of the *potlach*. In the Trobriand Islands off Papua New Guinea, for example, a farmer who has produced much food during a season is regarded as having shown great skill and prowess in farming, and to have been especially favoured by supernatural powers. He is then able to demonstrate his success and increase in status by displaying large piles of food he has grown at any of the tribal group ceremonies (such as harvest or mourning rituals), and to distribute this food to relatives and friends that he wishes to honour. Belshaw[17] pointed out that this does not result in a gluttonous feast, since the food, when distributed, is cooked and eaten in the home of the recipient.

In other social systems, such as the Hindu caste system in India, social rank is usually marked by the types of food prepared and eaten by each caste. The highest prestige is given to raw foods, which are considered suitable for the priestly Brahmins and other upper castes. Cooked food is less valued unless it contains *ghee*, a form of butter from which the water has been removed. Inferior cooked foods include pickles, cheap curries and barley cakes, all of which lack *ghee*. Food may not be accepted from, or prepared by, the members of lower castes, although food can travel downwards in the caste system as payment for goods or services. In this society, food functions both as a form of currency and as an indicator of social position.

In many parts of the world, light-coloured foods such as white bread or white rice have a higher status than dark-coloured foods. In Europe, it was the peasants who ate rough, brown bread while the aristocracy ate white bread or cakes, and the same pattern existed elsewhere. In the Third World, as Trowell and Burkitt[18] note, westernization has led to the increased status of white bread and rice and other refined foods. Cereals are increasingly refined to produce low-fibre white wheat flour and polished white rice, resulting in a decreased intake of dietary fibre. Some of the Western diseases that possibly result from this change will be mentioned below.

Group identity

As well as signalling status, food can be used as a badge of *group identity*, whether the group is based on regional, familial, ethnic or religious criteria. Each country has its national dish, and often regions within those countries are known by their local cuisine. Many of these well-known 'ethnic cuisines' have actually been imported from other countries: for example, according to Goody,[19] pasta probably originated in China, before entering Europe via Germany and then becoming a 'typical' Italian dish only from the fourteenth century onwards. Today, however, food produced and eaten locally is closely identified with the sense of continuity and cohesion of the community, and its dietary practices are often carried to other countries when members of the community emigrate. In their new countries, the immigrants may continue to eat their traditional diet – with its familiar taste, smells and mode of preparation – or merely revert to it only on special occasions. For example, Jerome[20] studied the changes in diet and the pattern of meals in African-Americans who had migrated from rural areas in the South to large cities in the North. The traditional Southern pattern consisted of two meals: breakfast, which comprised fried meats of various kinds, rice, grits, biscuits, gravy, fried sweet Irish potatoes, coffee and milk; and the 'heavy boiled dinner', which took place in the mid-afternoon and comprised boiled vegetables or dry legumes seasoned with a variety of meat items. The main dish was accompanied by cornbread, potatoes, a sweet beverage or milk, and an occasional dessert or fruit. In the Northern, urban environment, under the influence of occupational schedules, the pattern changed. The heavy boiled dinner was now served at 4–6 p.m. and renamed 'supper' while the large breakfast usually persisted for about 18 months after migration, with lunch consisting of leftovers from it. Eventually a new pattern was established with three meals: breakfast, comprising eggs, or bacon or sausage with eggs, hot biscuits, 'light' bread and coffee; lunch of sandwiches, soup, crackers, raw fruits and a fruit drink; and dinner, either 'heavy boiled' or fried food. The traditional large breakfasts were reserved for weekends, 'off-days' and holidays.

In some cases, the persistence of traditional diets and patterns of food consumption habits among migrants may conflict with the advice of their doctors and nutritionists, especially in the case of diabetes. This is described below in the case of British Bangladeshis (see case study),[21] but it has also been described in many other groups, including Vietnamese immigrants to the USA,[22] and Tongan immigrants to New Zealand.[23]

As Jerome's study[20] illustrated, the internal structure and content of meals can be remarkably uniform within a social or cultural group. A similar study, of working-class British meals, was carried out by Douglas and Nicod[24] in 1974. They found that meals, unlike snacks, were highly structured events, with certain combinations of foods served in the appropriate sequence. Breakfast, where the dishes were served in any order, was not usually regarded as a meal. At meals, careful combinations were made between salty and sweet, moist and dry, and hot and cold foods. When food was very hot it had to be accompanied by a cold drink, while a dessert taken with a hot beverage had to be cold, dry and solid (cake or biscuits). Douglas and Nicod were able to decipher the underlying recurrent grammar of these meals, and point out that improvement in their nutritional qualities had to take this structure into account rather than trying to impose the opinions of the middle-class dietician.

Feasts and festivals

Because of their central role in defining and recreating group identity and cohesion, communal meal, feasts or festivals mark many of the important occasions in the life of the group. Examples of this are feasts associated with weddings, christenings, circumcisions, wakes, *barmitzvahs* and religious festivals and services.

Foods consumed during religious occasions are more likely to have a symbolic rather than a nutritional significance – for example, the Communion wafer or Host, or the Passover unleavened bread or *matzoh*. Consuming these foods confirms and re-establishes the relationship between man and his deity, as well as between man and man. More sec-

Figure 3.1 The wedding cake as symbolic food: bridal couple with their wedding cake in Gorizia, northern Italy. (Source: © J Tod. Reproduced with permission.)

ular group festivals, where the group's history and experiences are celebrated, also utilize special foods – for example, the turkey eaten at the American Thanksgiving. Farb and Armelagos[25] note how the pumpkin, originally a commonly used vegetable, has gradually assumed more symbolic and less nutritional significance as a decoration at Halloween or Thanksgiving. They estimate that every autumn nearly three million pumpkins are sold in Massachusetts, and that 90 per cent of them will never be eaten, instead being carved into 'jack-o-lanterns', or used to decorate front porches, window-sills and dining tables. Similarly, every August in the town of Buñol, eastern Spain, over 125 000 kg of tomatoes are thrown by revelers at one another, in the annual festival of *La Tomatina* – a popular tradition that began in 1945.[26]

A further example of a social food with ritual, rather than nutritional significance is the British wedding cake. Charsley[27] suggests that the wedding cake, comprising three tiers, each covered with smooth white icing and surrounded by elaborate ornaments and decorations (silver or gold horseshoes, slippers or flowers), is symbolic of the bride herself, in her long white dress and veil. Furthermore, the joint cutting of the 'virginal white' cake by the new bride and groom has a sexual significance, symbolic of the couple now 'becoming one flesh'.

These many examples of social foods illustrate the multiple roles that food plays in human society: creating and sustaining social relationships; signalling social status, occupation and gender roles; marking important life changes, anniversaries and festivals; and reasserting religious, ethnic or regional identities. Because of their many social roles, dietary beliefs and practices are sometimes difficult to discard, even when they are dangerous to health.

CULTURE AND MALNUTRITION

The six systems of food classification described above illustrate how food may be eaten for cultural as well as nutritional reasons. From a clinical perspective, these cultural influences may affect nutrition in two ways:

1 They may exclude much-needed nutriments from the diet by defining them as non-food, profane, 'poison', alien or lower-class food, or food on the wrong side of a hot/cold dichotomy
2 They may encourage the consumption of certain foods or drink, by defining them as food, sacred, 'medicine', 'whole food', or as a sign of social, religious or ethnic identity, which are actually injurious to health.

When both of these influences co-exist there is likely to be an increased risk of *malnutrition* – manifesting either as *under*nutrition (a deficiency of vitamins, proteins, energy sources or trace elements) or as *over*nutrition (especially obesity and its consequences). Other cultural factors can also have an indirect effect on nutrition, such as beliefs about the structure and functioning of the body, its optimal size and shape, and the role of diet in health and disease. Also, the rules of food use and distribution within a family may contribute towards malnutrition – for example, by giving larger portions of food to male members of the family than to females.

THE ROLE OF DEPRIVATION

It should always be remembered that cultural influences alone *do not* account for the vast majority of malnutrition world-wide, although they may be one of the factors contributing towards it. To be fully understood, malnutrition should always be placed in its wider social, political, economic and environmental context. For example, various forms of *deprivation* – that is, the lack of available food or of the means to obtain what food there is – accounts for most cases of undernutrition, especially in the developing world. Such deprivation may result from a number of factors, especially:

- poverty, caused by the unequal distribution of resources within a society or between societies
- natural disasters, such as floods, tidal waves, tornadoes and drought
- wars (especially civil wars) and other forms of violent social upheaval
- crop failures, caused by locusts and other insects or parasites.

Another factor, fully described by Keesing and Strathern,[28] is the international *political economy* of food production and consumption. They note how in many parts of the Third World, both under colonialism and afterwards, people were encouraged and sometimes forced to grow commodities for export (such as tobacco, sugar cane, coffee or cotton) rather than staple foods for internal consumption. In large areas of the developing world, more and more land was devoted to producing these 'cash crops' for export. In the 1970s, for example, cash crops occupied an estimated 55 per cent of the cropland in the Philippines, 80 per cent in Mauritius and 50 per cent of all cultivated land in Senegal. Many developing countries are therefore at the mercy of fluctuations in the world market for their cash crops, and are also increasingly reliant on imported food for subsistence. Furthermore, advertising from firms in the industrialized countries has promoted the use of less nutritious and more expensive artificial foods, such as soft drinks, canned foods and infant formula feeds (see below). In many countries an overemphasis on the production of raw materials, such as coal, copper, tin, gold or oil, or even on the tourist industry, may play a similar role to cash crops: increasing dependence on international markets, and reducing the land and population available for food production.

Recently, more attention has been paid to the phenomenon of *globalization* (see Chapter 12) and its effect on global diet.[29,30] This process involves the diffusion of Western modes of food production, marketing and consumption to many parts of the world, especially to poorer countries. One effect of this is to concentrate power over these processes into fewer and fewer hands, especially in the Western corporate sector. This in turn implies a shift in power from the producer of food – the farmer, peasant, or agricultural worker – to the distributor of that food (often a multinational corporation or 'agribusiness').[29] Overall, the effects of this process on nutrition include the rapid change of centuries-old traditional diets, the introduction of a variety of nutritionally inadequate fast foods ('burgerization'[29]), and a shift towards high-fat, high-salt, and high-calorie diets as part of this 'nutrition transition'[30] (see below).

In many cases of malnutrition, therefore, the causes lie outside the control of individuals, their families and their communities. Thus cultural factors, as well as personal factors such as ignorance or idiosyncrasy, are only one part (though they may be an important part) of the complex mix of influences on the individual that determine whether his or her diet is nutritionally adequate or not.

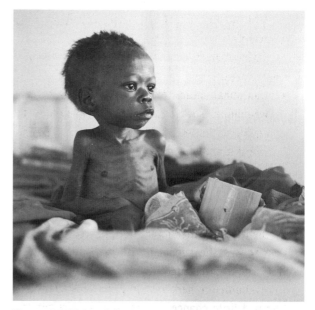

Figure 3.2 Malnutrition is a major cause of death among children in developing countries. (Source: © Jann Banning/Panos Pictures. Reproduced with permission.)

Case study: malnutrition among children in Farimabougou, Mali

Dettwyler[31] in 1992 described some of the 'intricate web of interacting factors' that contribute to child malnutrition in Farimabougou, near Bamako, Mali. Based on a sample of 136 children, her study indicates that relative poverty alone cannot completely explain variations in diet and nutritional status within the community. Other studies in Mali also indicate that 'rising income is not correlated with an increase in quantity or an improvement in the nutritional quality of the diet'. In each case of severe malnutrition, therefore, 'a variety of biological, social, and cultural factors' – *in addition* to low incomes – has contributed to the child's poor growth, a situation that she terms 'socio-cultural malnutrition'. These factors include:

- differences in maternal age, experience, competence and attitudes to child-rearing
- the support networks available to mothers and the breakdown of the extended family unit under the influence of the wage economy
- maternal illness, such as malaria or measles
- marital problems, family conflicts and the difficult position of women in a polygamous society
- decisions on how household resources are to be allocated
- traditional infant feeding practices, such as weaning as soon as the mother gets pregnant again, or letting children themselves decide whether and how much they want to eat.

In one case, a 16-year-old unmarried mother with twins, living as a low-status foster child in another family's compound, was given little help by them with either infant feeding or childcare; neither was she supported by the father of her children. She resented the twins because 'they were a burden to her', and with two small children 'she had little chance of marrying'. As a result of these and other factors, the children were neglected and failed to thrive. In another case, a father spent most of his income on his moped and on clothes for himself and his wife, leaving little over to pay for the children's food.

Dettwyler thus pointed out that, although in some circumstances one factor – such as drought, famine or war – may be responsible for malnutrition, 'the vast majority of malnutrition in Third World populations does not have one primary cause'. Since 'all poor people are not the same', she warns against simplistic solutions of the problem. Poverty, however, does play a crucial role in the 'web of causation' of childhood malnutrition in Mali. Apart from having less money to spend on food for the children, a contaminated environment (due to the complete lack of sewage and garbage disposal) and inadequate primary health care both contribute to frequent childhood diarrhoea and other causes of poor health. Furthermore, in a situation of deprivation, ill, malnourished or stressed parents are less able to deal with the demands of childcare and to ensure adequate nutrition of their children.

To illustrate further the contributory role of culture in malnutrition, three topics are discussed below, with examples.

IMMIGRANTS AND ETHNIC MINORITIES IN THE UK: SOME NUTRITIONAL PROBLEMS

Most immigrant groups bring with them their own dietary culture, with their traditional beliefs and practices relating to food. Not only does this ensure a sense of cultural continuity with their countries of origin, but it also plays many symbolic, religious and social roles in their daily lives. Food habits are one of the important indicators of acculturation, together with dress, behaviour and family structure, and are often among the last cultural traits to go if immigrants seek to discard their original cultures. In addition to dietary habits, other factors beyond the control of the immigrants themselves may affect their health and nutrition.

These include: discrimination or rejection by the host community; unemployment; physical violence or racial harassment;[32] substandard or overcrowded living conditions; low incomes; little leisure time; long working hours; social isolation; and the stressful effects of culture change itself (see Chapter 12).

Stroud[33] in the early 1970s reviewed the commonest nutritional problems of southern Asian (India, Pakistan and Bangladesh) and West Indian immigrants in the UK. These included osteomalacia and rickets among Asians, various forms of anaemia among both Asians and West Indians, and overnutrition (obesity) in some communities, including from the Caribbean. Today some, though not all, of these nutritional problems persist, especially rickets in some parts of the Asian community.[34]

It should be noted that many of the studies on immigrant nutritional health applied mainly to the first generation of immigrants, rather than to their descendants who were born and raised in the UK. Among both immigrant groups and the majority populations, cuisines are in a constant state of flux as increasing numbers of people adapt to new types of food, and to new forms of food preparation. It is important, therefore, not to stereotype – or stigmatize – the diets of immigrant communities.

RICKETS

Considerable research has been done on Asian rickets in the UK, which has occurred at a much higher rate than among the white population. The problem was first described in the 1960s, but is still believed to be widespread today.[34] It is especially common among those aged 9 months to 3 years, 8–14 years, and among pregnant and lactating Asian women.[35,36] Several factors have been blamed for this high incidence, including:

- a deficiency of vitamin D and calcium in the Asian vegetarian diet[34,37]
- the phytate content of Asian diets (in chapattis and cereals),[37] which binds with calcium and prevents its absorption

- skin pigmentation (skin pigments absorb ultraviolet light, with consequent reduction in vitamin D production)
- genetic factors
- a lack of exposure to ultraviolet light due to poor inner-city housing, confinement of women indoors, and types of female dress which cover large areas of skin surface.[34,38]

While the lack of dietary vitamin D is not the sole cause of rickets (one should include, for example, the fear of racial attacks which may keep some Asian women indoors),[32] it is still an important cause of the condition. Hunt[5] points out that the Asian diet supplies about 1.5 μg of vitamin D daily, compared with 2.9 μg daily in the rest of the UK population (Iqbal and colleagues[34] give this figure as 3.0 μg daily), who derive most of their vitamin D from margarine and fish – both of which are hardly used by Asians. Hindus reject fish for religious reasons, while some Muslims believe that margarine contains pig fat. The lack of dietary vitamin D is especially important in girls during their growth spurt at puberty and in pregnant women; in both cases, social seclusion and dress also play a part. Rickets in infancy has also been blamed on the Asian practice of weaning babies directly onto cow's milk, without using vitamin drops or vitamin D-enriched baby foods. Stroud[33] points out that cow's milk and human milk contain 20–40 IU/L of vitamin D, while the recommended allowance for infants of this vitamin is 400 IU/day (10 μg); therefore, a baby fed entirely on human or non-proprietary cow's milk will have much less than the recommended daily allowance.

Vitamin D supplements have therefore been suggested for both infants and pregnant Asian women. According to an editorial in the *Lancet*[39] in 1981, doctors in the UK should 'regard all pregnant Asian women as potentially osteomalacic and ensure that they receive adequate supplementary vitamin D (400 IU daily) throughout pregnancy and lactation', though some obstetricians were not convinced of the value of these supplements.[40] More recently, Pettifor[37] suggests that the best way of preventing Asian rickets in the UK would be by increasing vitamin D intake, or by reducing the phytate content, or both. Where cases of vitamin D deficiency with rickets or osteomalacia are found, Iqbal and colleagues[34] suggest that other members of their families be screened as well because they too may be suffering from vitamin D deficiency.

From a different perspective, Mares and her colleagues[41] have argued against the overemphasis on the role of the 'Asian diet' in causing rickets among south Asian communities in the UK. They suggest that in fact only about one-quarter of British Asians – mainly Hindus, but usually not Muslims or Sikhs – are, to a lesser or greater extent, actually vegetarian, that many Asians do in fact eat large amounts of dairy products, and that the positive role of vegetarian diets in protecting against heart disease and many other disorders should also be emphasized.

Nutritional rickets has also been described among some West Indian infants whose parents belong to the Rastafarian religion. In 1982, Ward and colleagues[42] described four cases of children aged between 11 and 20 months who were found to have clinical rickets. Their parents were strict Rastafarians, and ate a vegetarian diet that also excluded fish. They were breast-fed until the second half of the first year of life, when they were weaned on an essentially vegetarian diet known as *I-tal*. None had received vitamin supplements during infancy; neither had they completed a full course of immunizations. Like many Asians, they had low incomes and lived in depressed inner-city areas where opportunities for outdoor play were few and exposure to sunlight was likely to be limited.

The global perspective

From a global perspective, more recent research suggests that in many developing countries in Asia and Africa, where the population relies heavily on cereal-based staples (often unrefined cereals, which are high in phytates) with few or no dairy products in the diet, the major cause of nutritional rickets in children beyond infancy is a deficiency of *dietary*
calcium, rather than only a deficiency of vitamin D. According to Pettifor:[37] 'nutritional rickets, a disease once thought to be attributable solely to vitamin D deficiency, should be viewed as having as having a spectrum of mechanisms, with classic vitamin D deficiency, as observed among breast-fed infants, at one end and dietary calcium deficiency… at the other'.

Between these two extremes, it is likely that a combination of vitamin D insufficiency with a low dietary calcium or high phytate intake, is 'the most frequent cause of rickets globally.'

ANAEMIA

Stroud[33] also reported higher rates of iron-deficiency anaemia among both Asian and West Indian infants and children. In part this may have resulted from prolonged breast-feeding or weaning directly on to cow's milk, since both types of milk are deficient in iron, containing only 0.3 mg/L and 1.0 mg/L respectively. According to Hunt[5] in 1975, the diet of adult Asians is devoid of easily assimilated iron from animal sources; although iron is added to chapatti flour, only about 3 per cent of it is absorbed when eaten as part of an Asian diet. In some cases the anaemia may result from hookworm (ankylostoma) infestations, because of the demands such infestations may make on body proteins; however, according to Stroud this is rare in the UK in all communities. Hunt also pointed out that megaloblastic anaemias – caused by folic acid or vitamin B_{12} deficiency – was more common among Asians in the UK, especially Hindus. Asian cooking habits may destroy much of the folic acid, for example by boiling pulses for about an hour, or by the prolonged gentle heating of finely cut-up foods. In addition, the habit of boiling the milk, tea leaves and water together for 5 minutes when making tea is thought to destroy much of the vitamin B_{12}, which is especially important in Hindus, whose vegetarian diet lacks other sources of vitamin B_{12}. However, it should be noted that traditional cuisines of some immigrant groups often change gradually over time, to adapt to their new environment, and this may well include a change in their cooking habits.

OVERNUTRITION

Based on this I am overweight

A final problem among some immigrants in the UK is that of overnutrition, a condition that is *not*, by any means, confined to immigrant or ethnic minority communities. For example, in 1971 Taitz[43] studied 261 normal full-term British infants born in Sheffield at birth and again at 6 weeks. The study found that only 21 were breast-fed, and that at 6 weeks the majority of the artificially fed infants (40.4 per cent of the males, 37.3 percent of the females) were substantially overweight, and above the 90th percentile for their age on the Tanner centile charts. Taitz ascribed this overnutrition to encouragement by doctors, welfare clinics, health visitors and grandmothers, and to 'the popular notion of the "bonny" baby with bloated cheeks and limbs, protuberant belly, and the various signs of the "Michelin Tyre Man" syndrome'. In addition, 'the apparently low resistance of present-day mothers to the crying infant and the tendency to provide instant gratification in a caloric form may also play its part'. Taitz pointed out the danger of overnutrition in infancy, since it may result in obesity in later childhood and adulthood – a prediction that seems to have come true in the present day.

Some of the wider issues relating to today's world-wide increase in obesity, especially in childhood, are discussed below.

THE GLOBAL OBESITY EPIDEMIC

In recent decades, *obesity* has become one of the major causes of death and disease in many parts of the world. According to the World Health Organization (WHO)[44] there is now a 'global obesity epidemic' with about 1 billion overweight adults worldwide, at least 300 million of whom are clinically obese. The WHO definitions of 'overweight' or 'obese' here depend on the individual's *body mass index* (BMI), which is defined as that person's weight in kilograms divided by the square of their height in metres (kg/m^2). A BMI of 25 kg/m^2 is defined as overweight, and one of over 30 kg/m^2 as obese.[44]

A key characteristic of obesity is that it is associated with an increased risk of developing many other medical conditions. These include Type 2 diabetes (also known as non-insulin dependent diabetes mellitus, NIDDM, or T2DM), cancer (especially of the breast, colon, prostate, or endometrium), heart disease, gall bladder disease, stroke, respiratory disorders, infertility, obstructive sleep apnea and osteoarthritis.[44] Sometimes it is also associated with psychological problems, such as depression or low self-esteem.[45] Overall, the WHO estimated in 2002 that approximately 58 per cent of diabetes, 21 per cent of ischaemic heart disease, and 8–42 per cent of certain cancers globally were attributable to a BMI above 21 kg/m^2.[44] The obesity epidemic, and its associated diseases, is affecting not only the richer, industrialized world, but also many poorer countries as well (see Table 3.3). For these countries, the public health and economic implications of this epidemic are enormous. The WHO have estimated that 115 million people in these developing countries suffer from obesity-related problems, and that they account for 2–6 per cent of their total health costs.[44] Perhaps most importantly, obesity accounts for 58 per cent of the global burden of *diabetes*, especially of Type 2, and this in turn can cause many other health problems. The WHO estimate that the number of people with diabetes will more than double over the next 25 years, to reach a total of 366 million by 2030, and most of this increase will occur as a result of a 150 per cent rise in developing countries.[46]

A major aspect of this problem is the huge rise in *childhood obesity*,[44–46] with an estimated 22 million children under 5 years old now classified as being overweight.[44] One British cohort study, for example, carried out on school children in Leeds between 1996 and 1998, found that as many as 30 per cent of 11-year olds were overweight (> 85th percentile) and 17 per cent were obese (> 95th percentile), with a significant rise over the 3-year period.[47] Similarly, a study in the USA showed that approximately 14–15 per cent of all 15-year-olds were obese, and that the prevalence of childhood obesity was particularly high among African-Americans, and some Hispanic and Native American groups.[48] The danger of this situation is that this in turn can result in a variety of disorders, psychological as well as physical,[45,49] and that many of these obese children will grow into obese adults, with all the associated health risks. To reduce the possibility of this happening, the WHO recommend promoting an active lifestyle for children, restricting their television viewing, reducing their intake of packaged snacks and sweetened soft drinks, and increasing their intake of fruit and vegetables.[44,46]

What has caused this rise in obesity worldwide? As explained below, it is blamed mainly on major changes in dietary patterns (the 'nutrition transition') that have occurred in recent decades, coupled with the increasingly sedentary nature of modern life, especially in communities newly undergoing westernisation, urbanization, and economic development.[44,45] It is also linked to patterns of infant feeding, and the use of artificial formula feeds (see below). Obesity is also often correlated with low socio-economic status, and with low levels of education. However, genetic factors may also play a role. A large study by Tremblay and colleagues[50] examined reasons for

Table 3.3 Percentage of obese adults (> 15 years old) in selected countries

Country	Men	Women
India	0.3	0.5
China	2.4	3.4
Switzerland	7.9	7.5
Brazil	8.9	13.1
Vanuatu	12.2	19.6
United States	25.8	19.6
Marshall Islands	38.5	52.7
Samoa	48.4	67.9

World Health Organization (2005).[44]

the wide differences in rates of obesity and being overweight in different Canadian ethnic groups, compared with whites. They found significantly higher rates among Native Canadians (Indians and Inuit) compared with whites, but lower rates among East Asians, South-east Asians, Arabs, and blacks (though the rates for black and white women did not differ significantly). These differences in weight between (non-immigrant) ethnic groups remained significant, even when the effects of age, household income, educational level, physical activity, and birthplace were taken into account. They suggest that this is due to a combination of genetic predisposition, different social pressures on different groups, and different cultural norms related to ideal body size, diet, and level of physical activity. Among immigrants to Canada, the study also revealed differences in the prevalence of obesity and being overweight, which related to the time since immigration, with a higher prevalence in long-term immigrants (11 years or more), than in more recent immigrants (10 years or less). Among all ethnic groups this 'healthy immigrant' effect thus seems to fade within a decade of arrival, as they are exposed to a new diet and lifestyle, though the differences between these groups still remain. Significantly though, a low BMI, for example, among Asian ethnic groups, may be misleading, as it does not in itself indicate the level and distribution of body fat or predict the subsequent consequences for health. The authors suggest that, after adjusting for BMI, Asians generally have a higher percentage of body fat than their white counterparts, and therefore a BMI threshold of $25\,kg/m^2$ may be too high to identify people in those communities at increased risk of disease, and therefore this threshold may have to be reduced.

Ironically, this worldwide rise in obesity, whether among native or migrant populations, is taking place at the same time as a greater cultural emphasis than ever before on the social value of a slimmer body (especially among women). This contradiction between facts and expectations has led, among other things, to a global epidemic of diets and dietary fads.

'CULTURAL OBESITY'

Although the health risks of obesity have been clearly demonstrated by epidemiological studies, one should always be cautious in applying large-scale population studies to any particular individual case, given the normal variations in body size and shape found in any community, and the stigma attached to a label of 'obesity'. Furthermore, not all forms of obesity are the result of poor diet, inadequate lifestyle, or genetic factors. Neither is obesity seen everywhere as the same stigmatized, unfortunate condition: a sign of low self-control and low moral status (a modern version of the deadly sins of Gluttony and Sloth). As described in Chapter 2, there are many areas of the world where people actually *welcome* a large body size, especially among women, as a sign of sexual attractiveness, healthiness and material wealth, and will do everything they can to achieve it. The result of this is what I would term *cultural obesity*. This may explain, in part, the wide difference in the obesity prevalence, in different parts of the world (Table 3.3). Pollock[51] has described several examples of voluntary obesity from West Africa, Central Africa and the Pacific, including the nineteenth century fattening rituals (*ha'apori*) for young people in Tahiti and Nauru, and the huge body size of contemporary groups such as the Sumo wrestlers of Japan. This long history of cultural obesity – well before Western intervention – indicates that obesity cannot be blamed only on modernity.[51] It also suggests why 'ideal' body shapes and sizes from the northern hemisphere are not necessarily welcomed in the southern hemisphere, and why there may be considerable cultural resistance to health messages that promote dieting, exercise and the losing of weight, as indicated by the case study from The Gambia.

Case study: urban obesity in The Gambia

Prentice[52] in 2000 described the effects of demographic transitions, such as urbanization, on average body weight in The Gambia. In the rural areas obesity is almost unknown, and childhood under-nutrition is a major problem. In contrast, in the new urban townships obesity and its associated diseases – especially Type-2 diabetes – have become increasingly common, with middle-aged urban women now showing over 30 per cent prevalence of clinical obesity. These two very different types of health problem – undernutrition and overnutrition – together impose a major economic burden on the country, as they do elsewhere in Africa. Explanations for this rise of obesity in The Gambia range from genetic to socio-economic theories. In particular, Prentice mentions how migrants to the city, as they enter the wage economy and become more affluent, tend to make major changes to their diet (what he calls 'coca-colonisation'), and to their levels of physical activity. They begin to eat a higher proportion of fatty foods, 'fast foods' and cheap vegetable oils. Also, unlike in the rural areas, they no longer walk up to 10 km to their fields or draw water by hand from the wells and carry it on their heads, or work for 8 hours at a stretch before returning home. Instead, they now have the leisure time to watch television. Escaping from hard physical labor is seen as a badge of success, and exercise as 'an unwelcome reminder of a poorer past'. Furthermore, as elsewhere in West Africa 'fat is beautiful', a sign of wealth as well as of health (and especially of not having human immunodeficiency virus [HIV]/acquired immune deficiency syndrome [AIDS]). For all these reasons, he suggests that convincing people to lose weight in this situation will be difficult to do.

In cases such as obesity in The Gambia, a change in diet, lifestyle and body image may be difficult to achieve if nutritionists and dieticians focus only on a 'numerical' approach: the 'calorie count' of foods, the weight of different foodstuffs, the percentages of fat or sugar in the diet, the exact timing of meals, the weight of the person and the circumference of their waist. All these numerical measurements – characteristic of the 'disease' approach to ill-health (see Chapter 5) – ignore the *meanings* and social significance of food, meal-times, and the body itself for the people concerned, as illustrated in the case study of British Bangladeshis.

Case study: beliefs about food and diabetes among British Bangladeshis, London, England

In two studies, in 1998 and 2000, Greenhalgh and colleagues,[11,21] studied beliefs about diet and diabetes mellitus among a group of 40 Bangladeshi immigrants in London. While some of these beliefs overlapped with the medical model, others were very different. The whole group recognized the importance of diet in diabetes control, and believed that one of the main causes of diabetes was too much sugar. They also blamed heredity, 'germs' and stress. In terms of foodstuffs, however, they divided them into two symbolic categories in terms of their perceived 'strength' (nourishing power), and 'digestibility'. Strong foods were perceived as energy-giving, and included white sugar, lamb, beef, *ghee* (derived from butter), solid fat and spices. Such foods were considered crucial to maintain or restore health, and essential for certain festive occasions. They were considered dangerous, however, for the old or the debilitated (including diabetics), for whom weak foods (such as boiled rice or cereals) were more appropriate. Raw foods, and those baked or grilled, were considered indigestible, as were all vegetables that grow under the ground. They were considered unsuitable for the elderly, the very young or those who were very ill. Thus, the recommendation that diabetics should bake or grill their foods rather than fry them would not accord with their food beliefs. In contrast, molasses – a dark form of raw sugar, liquid at room temperature – was considered safe for diabetics to eat, and very different from lighter coloured white sugar, butter, *ghee* and solid fat, which was forbidden. The whole sample believed that the onset and control of diabetes depended on the *balance* between food entering the body and emissions from the body, such as semen, sweat, urine and menstrual blood. An excess of any of these emissions was believed to cause illness and weakness, as in diabetes. In the Bangladeshi community, because communal feasts, festivals and social occasions are common (and usually involve the consumption of sweets and rich foods), a calculated compromise between social obligations and dietary compliance had to be made by both diabetics and their families. Finally, the value of physical exercise and weight-reduction had little cultural meaning for the sample. In general, larger body size (but not obesity) was viewed as an indicator of more health, while thinness was a sign of less health.

INFANT FEEDING PRACTICES: CROSS-CULTURAL COMPARISONS

The care and feeding of infants is a central concern in every human group. There are widespread differences, however, in the techniques of infant feeding, whether breast, bottle or artificial feeds are used, and in the age and technique of weaning. Despite medical advice that, for a variety of physiological and emotional reasons, 'breast is best', breast-feeding has declined in most countries in the world this century. This is particularly the case in urban, industrialized societies or in non-Western societies undergoing modernization and urbanization. In most cases, moving from the countryside into the city results in a decline in breast-feeding. For example, the 1984 *World Fertility Survey*,[53] based on data from 42 developing countries, found that rural women in those countries breast-fed an average of 2–6 months longer than their urban counterparts. As Farb and Armelagos[54] put it, 'mothers in many parts of the world often consider breast-feeding to be a vulgar peasant custom, to be abandoned as soon as the bottle can be afforded'.

This decline in human lactation has been described as the greatest nutritional crisis in the world today.[28] Several reasons have been advanced for the shift from breast to bottle, including urbanization, the breakdown of the extended family and the increased employment of women outside the home.[55] A further factor in some non-industrialized countries, especially those in Africa, are the huge advertising campaigns in favour of bottle-feeding, promoted by the Western manufacturers of artificial infant foods. These campaigns have been heavily criticized for depriving babies of the nutritional and immunological advantages of breast milk, and for increasing the dangers of malnutrition and the risk of diarrhoeal diseases. In many areas mothers may not have the facilities to prepare infant feeds with properly boiled water and sterilized bottles, thus increasing their babies' risk of infection.

A reverse trend is appearing in many industrialized countries, as the past few years have seen a gradual return to breast-feeding among many mothers in the upper socio-economic classes. For example, according to the United Nations International Children's Fund (UNICEF),[56] from 1995 to 2000 the proportion of babies breastfed in the UK rose by 3 per cent, with the largest increases in Northern Ireland (9 per cent) and Scotland (8 per cent), while in England and Wales the increase was only 2 per cent. In 2000 the lowest rate of breast-feeding in the UK was in Northern Ireland, where only 54 per cent of babies were breast-fed at least once, compared with 63 per cent in Scotland and 71 per cent in England and Wales.[57] Overall by 2000, 69 per cent of all British babies were breast-fed at birth, though this had dropped to 22 per cent by the age of 6 months. As well as these regional differences within the UK, there were also class differences: breast-feeding was much more common among mothers who were more middle class, educated and aged 30 years or older. At 6 months, only 13 per cent of babies from poorer social classes were still being breast-fed, compared with 31 per cent in the more affluent social classes.[58]

Figure 3.3 Despite medical advice that for a variety of emotional and physical reasons 'breast is best', many women are unable or unwilling to breast-feed their infants. (Source: © iStockphoto.com/Tim Osborne. Reproduced with permission.)

A different picture emerges from the poorer, developing world – especially in Sub-Saharan Africa – where many women who are HIV positive are now being advised *not* to breast-feed. This is because an estimated half of all mother-to-child HIV transmissions in developing countries occurs during breast-feeding.[57] In many cases this new advice has created confusion in the minds of many mothers as to whether they should breast feed or not. Thus the overall picture is of breast-feeding declining in some communities, but rising in others – sometimes within the same country. In 2005 UNICEF[59] provided an overview of the situation worldwide. They estimated that during the 1990s there was a slight increase in exclusive breastfeeding in the first 4 months of life, with rates in the developing world rising from 48 to 52 per cent, though the proportion of children still breastfeeding at 1 and 2 years increased only slightly. The highest rates of exclusive breastfeeding were in East Asia and the Pacific (57 per cent), and the lowest in the CIS (Commonwealth of Independent States) region (17 per cent). Although the rates of breastfeeding in Latin America and the Caribbean remained low, there were substantial improvements in both those regions.

In any particular country or community, there is always a range of factors – social, cultural, personal and economic – that influence whether and for how long women breast-feed their infants, how they explain a failure to breast-feed to themselves and to others, and when and how they wean their infants. Like other human activities, breastfeeding does not take place in a vacuum; it is always shaped by the cultural, social, religious and economic environment in which it takes place. This is illustrated by the case study example from Egypt.

Case study: beliefs about breast-feeding and weaning in a poor urban neighbourhood in Cairo, Egypt

Harrison and colleagues[60], in a study in 1993 of 20 mothers in Boulaq El Dakrour, Cairo, found a range of beliefs about whether a woman could breast-feed or not. All the women aimed to breast-feed their babies well into the second year of life, but did not assume that ability to breast-feed was automatic. Successful breast-feeding was believed to require patience, time, a sense of responsibility, good luck, a healthy mental state and specific changes in diet and behaviour. They cited many reasons why some women could breast-feed and others not. Some believed that adequate breast milk is a 'gift from God', and that only 'a lucky mother can breast-feed'. Others saw maternal emotional state as very important, since they believed that unhappiness turns the maternal body and its breast milk 'hot', and that this 'sadness milk' or 'grief milk' could cause diarrhoea in the infant. Thus, some mothers going through a stressful time would express much of their milk manually and discard it. In contrast, several would increase their breast-feeding if the baby was ill. The child itself was believed to influence the amount of milk that was available; certain children were seen as more 'blessed', a characteristic that ensures a plentiful supply of breast milk. Nursing another woman's baby of the same age as one's own was also common in this community, as elsewhere in Egypt. This act had considerable symbolic significance, creating a quasi-kinship relationship between the women and babies involved and resulting in a lifetime prohibition against marriage between children breast-fed by the same woman. There was also a range of beliefs about when to wean the infant. Many based their decision on the infant's developmental milestones, such as when it had all its teeth, or was able to walk or eat adult food. Others cited maternal illness, pregnancy, employment outside the home, medical advice and the use of oral contraceptives as reasons to stop breast-feeding. Seasonal and religious factors also had an influence on when to wean; some mothers preferred summer to winter, some stopped breast-feeding because they had decided to fast during *Ramadhan*, while others avoided *Muharam* (the first month of the Islamic calendar), which was thought to be an unsuitable time for weaning.

'Milk Kinship' in Islamic societies

One aspect of the Egyptian case study is the 'milk kinship' created by a woman wet-nursing another woman's baby. Although this has been reported from other societies, both Islamic and non-Islamic, Khatib-Chahidi[61] describes how Islamic law in particular defines three types of kinship: relationships by blood, by marriage, or by milk (*al-rida'a* in Arabic, *shiri* or *reza'i* in Farsi). The fact of a woman (the 'milk mother') breast-feeding another woman's child, rather than just rearing it, is what creates this form of symbolic kinship. She describes the complex rules in Shi'ite Iran whereby the child who was wet-nursed is subject to a range of prohibitions regarding whom they can marry when they grow to adulthood. These include the 'milk mother' herself, as well as her husband, siblings, children, and parents. However, if she herself was wet-nursed as a baby, the marriage prohibitions also extend to include all *her* 'milk relatives' (such as her own 'milk mother' and 'milk father', their siblings, and their children). A number of rules also govern the choice of a wet-nurse (*dayeh*), who should be intelligent, of good character (*ba e'fat*), attractive and devout. Khatib-Chahidi points out, however, that the introduction of formula infant feeds to Iran many decades ago has gradually undermined the traditional institution of milk kinship, especially among those social classes who were affluent enough to afford these artificial feeds.

Breast-feeding among different communities in the UK

The five case studies that follow, from the period 1977–2003, indicate the range of infant feeding practices among different communities in the country, and the effects this may have on the babies' health. The reasons for choosing one type or amount of infant feeding over another are many, and include the influence of cultural factors on maternal diet (and therefore on the infant's health).[60] Some of these socio-cultural factors have been described above, but they include cultural conceptions of what a healthy, bonny baby should look like, the type of lifestyle the mother should follow after delivery, and whether public breast-feeding is acceptable or not. It should also be remembered that in some parts of the world lactation is seen as an effective contraceptive, and this may influence the choice of type of infant feeding. In some of these societies this is backed up by taboos that prohibit sexual intercourse until the infant is weaned (see Chapter 6). Where breast-feeding is optional, and other forms of contraceptive are available, cultural beliefs and fashions, as well as economic factors, will determine whether most mothers choose this form of infant feeding or not.

A further factor, described by Ball,[62] is mothers' expectations of whether not their babies should sleep throughout the night, without feeding. This expectation can come from other people, or even from their physicians. She notes that, for physiological reasons, bottle-fed infants are more likely to begin to sleep through the night without waking, and from an earlier age, than breast-fed babies. Mothers who see this as both desirable and 'normal' often cite it as a reason for giving up breastfeeding, and then using artificial feeds. Ball suggests that both frequent breastfeeding and closer mother–baby physical contact (such as sleeping in the same bed), is more physiologically appropriate as we are a 'frequent suckling species', and are 'physiologically adapted for close mother–infant contact day and night,' To promote breastfeeding, she suggests that mother and infant share a bed, provided that this is done safely, as this eliminates the need for either of them to wake fully for a feed. It also halves the average intervals between feeds, enhances the overall production of breast-milk, and makes giving up feeding on the grounds of insufficient milk much less likely.

Case study: breast-feeding versus bottle-feeding in London, UK

Jones and Belsey[63] in 1977 surveyed 265 mothers of 12-week-old infants in the London Borough of Lambeth. Sixty-two per cent of the mothers had attempted to breast-feed (compared with 16 per cent in Dublin, 39 per cent in Newcastle and 52 per cent in Gloucestershire). The different communities showed different rates of breast-feeding; British 58 per cent, African 86 per cent, West Indian 84 per cent, Asian 77 per cent, European 59 per cent, and Irish 64 per cent. The ethnic background of the mothers was an important influence here, since in many communities breast-feeding was the accepted norm. Several reasons were given for not breast-feeding, especially because they 'disliked the thought of breast-feeding'; 54 per cent of bottle-feeders said this, while 44 per cent thought bottle-feeding was more convenient since it required less privacy than breast-feeding. Only 13 per cent of the bottle-feeders thought that the method they had chosen was the healthiest for the baby, compared with 85 per cent of the breast-feeders. Social, as well as ethnic factors were important in the choice of feeding technique, though the two were related; mothers were more likely to continue breast-feeding after 6 weeks if they had friends that had breast-fed. African and West Indian mothers more often had friends that breast-fed successfully than mothers in other ethnic groups, as did women in the upper socio-economic classes. Little evidence was found that either antenatal or postnatal medical advice affected the type of feeding chosen by mothers.

Case study: infant feeding practices in Glasgow, UK

Goel and colleagues[64] in 1978 studied the infant feeding practices of 172 families from various communities in Glasgow. These included 206 Asian, 99 African, 99 Chinese and 102 Scottish children. It was found that, after arrival in the UK, most immigrant mothers did not want to breast-feed their babies. Those immigrant children born outside the UK were more likely to have been breast-fed than those born within the UK; 83.7 per cent of Asian, 79.2 per cent of African and 80.9 per cent of Chinese children born abroad had been breast-fed. Ninety-nine per cent of the Scots children had been exclusively bottle-fed. The commonest reasons given by the immigrant mothers for not breast-feeding were embarrassment, inconvenience and insufficient breast milk. Two-thirds of the breast-fed Asian children were fed for at least 6 months and only 5 per cent of the African babies were breast-fed for more than 1 year, but Chinese mothers often breast-fed for 1–3 years, and many of their children were not given solid foods till they were 1 year or older. Asian children born in the UK usually had solids by 6 months

(but were given these at 1 year if they had been born abroad). Both African and Scottish children were given solids at 6 months. The authors suggest that all Asian children be given vitamin D supplements, since 12.5 per cent of the Asian children in the sample were found to have rickets.

Case study: feeding patterns in Chinese children, London, UK

Tann and Wheeler[65] in 1988 assessed feeding patterns and growth rates of 20 London Chinese children, aged between 1 and 24 months, over a period of 6 months in 1988. All the families had originated from the New Territories, a rural area of Hong Kong. With one exception, all the children were bottle-fed, and soft canned food and rusks of the British type were introduced at between 1 and 6 months. Subsequent to this, at 6–10 months, most mothers introduced congee, a traditional Chinese weaning food prepared by boiling rice in large quantities of watery meat broth. Soft, boiled rice was introduced at about 10 months, and then gradually the full range of Chinese foods was introduced. The mothers had chosen not to breast-feed mainly because of the 'inconvenience', although in Hong Kong nearly 60 per cent of mothers wholly or partially breast-feed their children. Most of the sample believed that milk quality was affected by the quality of the food eaten by the mother after delivery; in Hong Kong, Chinese mothers were usually confined at home for 30 days after delivery, during which nutritious (i.e. meaty) food was served to them by female relatives – a process known as 'doing the month' (see Chapter 6). In London they could not afford such a luxurious post-confinement period, as they had to get on with work or household chores. As a result, they believed they were not sufficiently well nourished to produce good milk for the babies. Meat served in hospital after delivery was not considered nourishing enough, since it should have been cooked in a traditional way with special spices, herbs and wines. The authors found that despite this, all the Chinese children in the sample were well nourished. The role of 'hot–cold' foods in the mother's diet has been mentioned previously.

Case-study: infant feeding practices of Pakistani mothers in England and Pakistan

Sarwar[66] in 2002 compared the infant feeding practices of two groups of Pakistani mothers –one living in Nottingham, England, the other in Mian Channu, Pakistan. Despite having very similar socio-cultural backgrounds, there were marked differences between the two groups. In Pakistan, 73 per cent of the mothers chose breast-feeding as the initial method of feeding, compared with only 24 per cent in England. Overall, breast-feeding was much more commonly practiced in Pakistan, and for a much longer period, compared with England, where bottle-feeding predominated. The reasons for this shift included the easy availability of artificial feeds in England, peer pressure, and the fact that the mothers felt that exclusive breast-feeding restricted their lives, and was too demanding. While both groups of mothers commenced weaning their babies between 3 and 4 months with rice, cereals and eggs, in Pakistan this progressed to fruit, vegetables and family foods, but in England it moved on to fruit, vegetables, meat, and convenience foods (some of them very sweetened). The study indicated, therefore, how migration – as well as changes in social and economic context – are influencing mothers' decision whether to breast-feed or not. If they do decide to breast-feed, it also influences for how long they will continue this feeding.

Case-study: perceptions of breast-feeding in Northern Ireland, UK

Stewart-Knox and colleagues[57] in 2003 studied a sample of mothers in Northern, Ireland, and their reasons for not breast-feeding. The study had important implications, since Northern Ireland has the lowest rate of breast-feeding in the UK, as well as being low compared with many other regions in Europe. The mothers described a series of barriers to breast-feeding, which included: (1) it tied them to the home, and restricted their freedom of movement; (2) they felt embarrassed to breast-feed, even in the presence of family and friends; (3) they found that going back to work made breast-feeding almost impossible; (4) they felt that breast-feeding required prolonged unpaid maternity leave, and this also made them feel more dependant on others; (5) they often lacked practical and emotional support from family members and partners; (6) they perceived breast-feeding as tiring, and associated with difficulty in establishing a routine; (7) they complained about a lack of provision in public buildings for nursing mothers; (8) they felt that promotion materials for breast-feeding were unrealistic, and often made them feel guilty or pressurized; and (9) they felt that all these barriers meant social isolation for a woman who chose to breast-feed. The authors place all these beliefs and attitudes in the context of the changing role of women in society. This major cultural shift has meant many more women in the workplace, and a higher value being placed now on their freedom and independence.

THE 'NUTRITION TRANSITION': GLOBALIZATION, DIETARY CHANGES AND DISEASE

THE 'NUTRITION TRANSITION'

An area of growing importance to nutritionists is the *globalization* of the human diet. In particular, they have studied the impact of social and economic change on nutrition and health, especially in those communities throughout the world that are undergoing urbanization, industrialization and westernization. As incomes rise in these societies, and their populations become more urbanized, they enter the different stages of what has been called the *nutrition transition*.[29,30] Both economic growth and the enormously rapid increase in urbanization world-wide (see Chapter 18) have had major effects on global dietary habits. Compared with rural diets, urban diets – especially in developing countries – are usually characterized by the consumption of more polished grains (rice and wheat, instead of corn or millet), more fats and animal products, more refined sugar, more processed foods, and more food consumed away from home.[30] Analysing data from 1962–1994, Drewnowski and Popkin[30] have shown how the global availability of cheap vegetable oils and fats has led to a greatly increased consumption of fat, and to a lesser extent sugar, among low income countries. One of the first stages of the nutrition transition is usually a major increase in the domestic production and imports of oilseeds and vegetable oils (including soyabean, sunflower, rapeseed, palm and peanut oils), rather than increased imports of meat and milk. Between 1991 and 1997, for example, global production of vegetable fats and oils rose from 60 million to 71 million metric tonnes. As a result, vegetable oils now contribute more energy to the human food supply than do meat or animal fats. Previously, high-fat diets were a privilege of the richer countries, but this is no longer the case. Throughout Asia, for example, despite the fact that there is now a greater diversity of foodstuffs available, the diets of both rich and poor countries show a decline in the proportion of energy derived from complex carbohydrates and a corresponding increase in the energy derived from fats. In Japan, for example, in the years 1946–1987, the fat content of the diet almost tripled from 9 per cent to 25 per cent of the total energy. The overall impact of this nutrition transition is seen especially in child health, with a significant rise in obesity world-wide.[44] In many parts of the world now, such as Latin America, the Caribbean and even the USA, 'the poor are more likely to be obese than the rich'. Drewnowski and Popkin predict that a diet that contains about 30

per cent of energy from fat may well become the global norm, and this will have major health implications in the future.[30]

Lang[29] has criticized the economic basis of globalization and its impact on global nutrition, especially in poorer countries. He points out that while there is nothing new in the exchange of foods, diets, recipes and products between different parts of the world – a process that began with the birth of agriculture – modern globalization is significantly different. What is new is the pace and scale of change, and the systematic way in which control over global food production and distribution can now be exercised. For the first time, also, such control is concentrated in relatively few (and mainly Western) hands. The growth of a global food market has shifted power away from the local producers of food and towards the multinational corporations who closely control its processing, distribution and sale. Farmers who produce food are encouraged to increase the size of their lands or herds, and to compete not only with other farmers locally but also globally. The implications of this, and the growth of cash crops in many poorer countries, have been discussed above. Globalization also makes possible the world-wide diffusion of new types of foods from the West, such as genetically modified products or branded processed foods. American-style fast food chains are now found all over the world; McDonalds, for example, now has more than 30 000 local restaurants or franchises in 119 countries on five continents.[67] Lang calls the spread of fast-food outlets 'burgerization'.[29] It is a process that is likely to contribute to the disappearance of local cuisines and dietary traditions, and may also have important impacts on health.

GLOBALIZATION OF CUISINES

The influence of 'Westernization' on the global diet is by no means one-way. In recent decades, most northern industrialized countries have imported food habits from the poorer south – such as Mexican food in the USA, south Asian curries in

Britain, and North African couscous in France. This globalization of 'ethnic' cuisines has had a major, and mostly welcome, impact on eating habits in the West, as well as providing employment opportunities for many members of ethnic minority communities. The new diversity of available foodstuffs can be seen not only in stores and supermarkets, but also in the range of restaurants. In the USA, the *Chinese Restaurant News* estimated that in 2005 there were 40 889 Chinese restaurants in the country, employing about 1 million people, and with total annual sales of $15.5 billion.[68] In the UK, there are approximately 7600 Chinese food outlets, 5932 Italian restaurants (the pasta market alone is worth £571 million), 600 Thai restaurants, and 550 Greek or Cypriot restaurants.[69] Probably the most popular ethnic restaurants in the UK are the 'curry houses' – mainly from India, Pakistan and Bangladesh. Curry first appeared in England in 1773, and the first Indian restaurant, the 'Hindostanee Coffee House', was established in London as early as 1809.[69] By 2000 there were about 8500 curry houses in Britain, employing some 70 000 people, turning over more than £2 billion annually, and serving 175 million meals each year.[70] In 2000 the London *Times* estimated that that there were more Indian restaurants (most of them run by Bangladeshis) in London than in Delhi and Bombay combined, and that more people are employed in the UK curry industry than in coal-mining, shipbuilding and the steel industry put together.[70]

The globalization of cuisine requires a complex system of trade and information flow to move cuisines, recipes and foodstuffs all around the world. Bestor,[71] for example, describes how Japanese food such as sushi has now become international, and how dishes such as wasabi mashed potatoes, sashimi grade tuna steaks, and sushi ginger relish are now common in many expensive restaurants in the USA. At the same time, frozen bluefin tuna fish from all over the world, including from the USA, are imported into Japan – where tuna is considered a great delicacy – and traded in Tokyo's vast Tsukiji fish market, often for huge sums of money. In some cases, Spanish tuna has to be imported into the USA to replace the tuna exported to Japan, or else some of the best quality American tuna is actually reimported back into the USA from Japan, via the Tsukiji market.

It should be remembered that the international trade of foodstuffs is not new, and that it has been going on for many centuries. However, what *has* changed enormously is the speed, complexity, and volume of this trade. This in turn has depended on a series of technological innovations, which have enabled food to be preserved, purified, packaged, and then safely transported around the globe. This process began on an industrial scale in the late eighteenth and early nineteenth centuries with the development of bottling and canning of food,[19] followed later by methods of transporting frozen foods packed in ice, and later in refrigerated containers. Goody[19] points out that innovations in transport in the nineteenth and twentieth centuries, especially in roads, railways, shipping, and air cargo, all aided the mass distribution of these packaged foods, from the point of production to the point of sale and consumption.

Overall, therefore, the effect of all these complex trends means that we now live in an age of rapid nutrition transition; global diet is in a constant state of flux, and the health implications of this are only now beginning to emerge.

THE 'DISEASES OF WESTERN CIVILIZATION': DIETARY CHANGES AND DISEASE

Burkitt[72] in 1973 examined many of the diseases that had become common in the Western industrialized world, particularly in Europe and the USA, over the previous century. These same diseases are rare or unknown in traditional, non-Western societies, but they increase in frequency under the influence of culture change – that is, where Western customs and lifestyles are adopted. These 'new' diseases include: appendicitis, diverticular disease, benign colonic tumours, cancer of the large bowel, ulcerative colitis, varicose veins, deep vein thrombosis, pulmonary embolism, haemorrhoids, coronary heart disease, gallstones, hiatus hernia, obesity and diabetes.

Burkitt saw obesity as the 'commonest form of malnutrition in the West', and it is also associated with some of the other 'Western diseases'. He estimated that over 40 per cent of people in the UK were overweight, and the problem was just as serious in the USA. He related the dramatic increase in frequency of the various diseases to dietary changes in the previous century. Between the years 1860 and 1960, fat consumption increased by less than 50 per cent while sugar consumption doubled. Over the past 100 years, the quantity of fibre consumed in the diet has markedly dropped. In 1860 the fibre content of white flour was 0.2–0.5 per cent and the amount of fibre supplied daily in bread was between 1.1 and 2.8 g. With bread consumption halved and the fibre content of white flour reduced to 0.1–0.01 per cent, the daily fibre intake from bread is about 10 per cent of the pre-1860 level. In addition, porridge oats, with a high fibre content, had gone out of fashion and been replaced by low-fibre packaged cereals. In non-Western societies that become Westernized, traditional diets are usually changed by the addition of sugar, the substitution of white bread for high-fibre cereals and, often, an increase in meat consumption. Burkitt pointed out, however, that in none of the 'Western diseases' is fibre deficiency a *sole* causative factor, but that it might be one important aetiological factor, although its precise link to these diseases, and the actual types of fibre (such as fruit and vegetables) that protect against them remain unclear.

Burkitt's 1973 study suggested therefore how changes in technology and dietary culture might possibly be related to the increased incidence of certain diseases. However, a more recent study[73] in the USA has cast doubt on whether a high-fibre diet could actually reduce the risk of colorectal cancer and adenomas in women, and therefore much further research into the precise role of fibre in certain diseases still needs to be carried out.

DIET AND CANCER

The study of a culture's dietary patterns and preferences is not only important in the search for malnutrition, or for any one of the 'Western diseases' listed by Burkitt and others. A number of studies suggest that, in some cases, different types of diet may be linked to certain forms of cancer. It has been suggested that one-third or more of all cancers may be related to dietary and nutritional factors.[74] In 1976 Lowenfels and Anderson[75] reviewed the evidence for this hypothesis, and found that differences in food intake patterns could be positively correlated with differences in the incidence of various cancers in world populations. This was especially the case in colonic and gastric cancer. In addition to the food consumed, variables such as total caloric intake, nutritional excess or deficit, the exposure to carcinogens and the consumption of alcohol also increase the risk of cancer. Many of these dietary factors, as noted earlier, may be affected by cultural beliefs and practices. In another review of the subject, Newberne[76] also cited evidence linking dietary patterns to a number of cancers, including cancers of the stomach, colon, oesophagus and breast (which has been linked to an increased intake of fat in the diet). He pointed out that, in the USA, food habits had gradually changed in the previous 40 years, a period in which cancer has increased in some populations. A further study by Kolonel and colleagues[77] examined the incidence rate of stomach cancer in four populations: Japanese in Japan; Japanese in Hawaii; Caucasians in Hawaii; and the general population of American whites. The highest rates were in Japanese in Japan, followed by the Hawaii Japanese, with the white groups at a much lower level. There was a positive association of high rates of the cancer with consumption, early in life, of the traditional Japanese foods of rice, pickled vegetables and dried/salted fish. It was postulated that stomach cancer might be caused by endogenous nitrosamines formed from dietary precursors – the nitrates, nitrites and secondary amines that are at high levels in the Japanese diet.[78]

Other studies indicate that in India and other parts of Asia, the high incidence of cancers of the oral cavity (lips, tongue, pharynx, floor of mouth and the salivary glands) may be related to chewing mixtures of tobacco, betel nuts and other substance.[79] In India a chewing mixture called *pan* (containing betel leaf, betel nut, tobacco, lime and aromatic substances), and in parts of Afghanistan and the former Soviet Central Asia a mixture known as *nass* (containing betel, tobacco leaf and lime treated with certain oils) have both been implicated in causing these cancers.[79] A diet rich in fats (especially saturated fats) and in calories has been blamed for increasing the risk of colon, breast and other cancers.[77] Certain food contaminants, especially the *aflatoxins* (found in mouldy peanuts or grains), have been linked to high rates of liver cancer in parts of Asia and Africa.[74] In contrast, certain types of diet may actually *protect* against some forms of cancer. A high intake of fresh fruits and vegetables (see below) has been found to reduce the incidence of cancers of the oral cavity, oesophagus, stomach and lung, while a low-fat, high-fibre diet may protect against cancers of the breast and colon.[74] A more recent study in Shanghai, China, found that a diet rich in certain vegetables, garlic and fruits (especially oranges and tangerines) was protective against laryngeal cancer, but the risk of laryngeal cancer was increased by eating salt-preserved meat and fish, as well as by other factors.[80] Relating specific dietary components to the causation of specific cancers still remains problematic, however. A recent survey of the subject by oncologists[81] agreed that 'although diet is likely to be a very important factor in carcinogenesis, there are not yet sufficient data to allow classification of specific nutritional factors among the established carcinogens'. Nevertheless, there was evidence that some nutrients and food groups may be involved in either increasing or decreasing cancer risk. Overall, they concluded that:

It is important that although no causal relation has been definitely established between any nutritional factor and any of the indicated cancers, a clear pattern of protection appears to characterize a high intake of fruits and vegetables, whereas a less clear pattern of increased risk appears to characterize positive energy balance and excessive intake.[82]

A more recent, comprehensive review of the subject by the World Cancer Research Fund and the American Institute for Cancer Research[81] concluded that 30–40 per cent of cancer cases throughout the world, or 3–4 million cases a year, could be prevented by dietary means. This particularly applies to cancers of the mouth, pharynx, stomach, colon, rectum, liver and breast. As with several other studies, their recommendations included:

1 The basic diet should be adequate and varied, and based mainly on foods of plant origin, including vegetables, fruits, and pulses (legumes), as well as minimally processed starchy staple foods.
2 The diet should always include a high intake of fruits and vegetables, which should provide 7 per cent or more of total energy
3 Total fats and oils in the diet should provide not more than 15–20 per cent of total energy; thus fatty foods (especially of animal origin) should be avoided.
4 If eaten at all, red meat should provide less than 10 per cent of the total energy.
5 Dietary salt from all sources should amount to less than 6 g/day (0.25 oz) for adults, so herbs and spices rather than salt should be used to season food.
6 A variety of starchy or protein-rich foods of plant origin should provide 45–60 per cent of energy, and these include cereals (grains), pulses, roots, tubers, and plantains.
7 Intake of refined sugar should be limited, and should provide less than 10 per cent of total energy.
8 Perishable food, if not consumed promptly, should be frozen or chilled, and stored in ways that minimize fungal contamination.
9 Meat and fish should be cooked at relatively low temperatures and not charred or grilled,

and cured and smoked meats should be avoided.

10 In the presence of an adequate, balanced diet, dietary supplements (such as vitamins) are 'probably unnecessary, and possibly unhelpful' for reducing cancer risk.

In addition to these dietary changes, they also recommended adequate physical exercise, avoiding being overweight, and drastically reducing alcohol intake and tobacco smoking.

SUMMARY

As the examples in this chapter indicate, a large number of diseases can be linked to dietary beliefs and practices, though these cultural factors are mainly relevant where enough food is available for nutrition in the first place. Attempts to modify or improve diets should therefore take into account the important cultural roles that food plays in all societies and cultural groups.

KEY REFERENCES

1 Levi-Strauss, C. (1970). *The Raw and the Cooked*. London: Jonathan Cape, pp. 142, 164.

8 Greenwood, B. (1981). Cold or spirits? Choice and ambiguity in Morocco's pluralistic medical system. *Soc. Sci. Med.* 15B, 219–35.

11 Chowdhury, A.M., Helman, C. and Greenhalgh, T. (2000) Food beliefs and practices among British Bangladeshis with diabetes: implications for health education. *Anthropol. Med.* 7(2), 209–226.

15 Enticott, G. (2003) Lay immunology, local foods and rural identity: defending unpasteurised milk in England. *Sociologia Ruralis* 43(3), 257–270.

21 Greenhalgh, T., Helman, C. and Chowdhury, A. M. (1998). Health beliefs and folk models of diabetes in British Bangladeshis: a qualitative study. *Br. Med. J.* 316, 978–83.

28 Keesing, R. M. and Strathern, A.J. (1998) *Cultural Anthropology*, 3rd edn. London: Harcourt Brace College Publishers, pp. 440–4.

29 Lang, T. (1999). Diet, health and globalization: five key questions. *Proc. Nutr. Soc.* 58, 335–43.

30 Drewnowski, A. and Popkin, B. M. (1997). The nutrition transition: new trends in the global diet. *Nutr. Rev.* 55, 31–43.

44 World Health Organization (2005) Obesity and overweight. *WHO Global Strategy on Diet, Physical Activity* and Health: http://www.who.int/dietphysicalactivity/publications/facts/obesity/en (Accessed on 14 July 2005)

49 Speiser, P.W., Rudolf, M.C.J, Anhalt, H. *et al.* (2005) Consensus statement: Childhood obesity. *J.Clin. Endocrinol. Metab.* 90, 1871–87.

51 Pollock, N.J. (1995) Cultural elaborations of obesity – fattening practices in Pacific societies. *Asian Pacific J. Clin. Nutr.* 4, 357–60.

60 Harrison, G. G., Zaghoul, S. S., Galal, O. M. and Gabr, A. (1993). Breastfeeding and weaning in a poor urban neighbourhood in Cairo, Egypt: maternal beliefs and perceptions. *Soc. Sci. Med.* 36, 1–10.

See http://www.culturehealthandillness.com for the full list of references for this chapter.

RECOMMENDED READING

Counihan, C. and van Esterik, P. (eds) (1997) *Food and Culture: a Reader*. London: Routledge.

Dettwyler, K. A. (1992). The biocultural approach in nutritional anthropology: case studies of malnutrition in Mali. *Med. Anthropol.* 15, 17–39.

Farb, P. and Armelagos, G. (1980). *Consuming Passions: the Anthropology of Eating*. Boston: Houghton Muffin.

Lang, T. (1999). Diet, health and globalization: five key questions. *Proc. Nutr. Soc.* 58, 335–43.

Maher, V. (ed.) (1992) *The Anthropology of Breast-Feeding*. Oxford: Berg.

World Cancer Research Fund/American Institute for Cancer Research (1997) *Food, Nutrition and the Prevention of Cancer: A Global Perspective*. London: WCRF/AICR.

World Health Organization (2003) *Diet, Nutrition and the Prevention of Chronic Disease*. (Technical Report Series 916). World Health Organization.

RECOMMENDED WEBSITES

Food and Culture: http://lilt.ilstu.edu/rtdirks/GEN-ERAL.html

Food Standards Agency (UK): http://www.food.gov.uk

Nutritional anthropology: http://lilt.ilstu.edu/rtdirks/NUTRANTH.html

UNICEF Statistics: Breastfeeding and Complementary Feeding: http://www.childinfo.org/eddb/brfeed

4

Caring and curing:
the sectors of health care

In most societies people suffering from physical discomfort or emotional distress have a number of ways of helping themselves, or of seeking help from other people. They may, for example, decide to rest or take a home remedy, ask advice from a friend, relative or neighbour, consult a local priest, folk healer or 'wise person', or consult a doctor, provided that one is available. They may follow all of these steps, or perhaps only one or two of them, and may follow them in any order. The larger and more complex the society in which the person is living, the more of these therapeutic options are likely to be available, provided that the individual can afford to pay for them. Modern urbanized societies, whether Western or non-Western, are more likely, therefore, to exhibit *health-care pluralism*. Within these societies there are many people or individuals, each offering the patient their own particular way of explaining, diagnosing and treating ill health. Though these therapeutic modes coexist, they are often based on entirely different premises and may even originate in different cultures, such as Western medicine in China, or Chinese acupuncture in the modern Western world. To the ill person, however, the origin of these treatments is less important than their efficacy in relieving suffering.

HEALTH CARE PLURALISM: SOCIAL AND CULTURAL ASPECTS

Anthropologists have pointed out that any society's health-care system cannot be studied in isolation from other aspects of that society, especially its social, religious, political and economic organization. It is interwoven with these, and is based on the same assumptions, values and view of the world. Landy[1] points out that a system of health care has two interrelated aspects: a *cultural* aspect, which includes certain basic concepts, theories, normative practices and shared modes of perception; and a *social* aspect, including its organization into certain specified roles (such as patient and doctor) and rules governing relationships between these roles in specialized settings (such as a hospital or a doctor's office). In most societies one form of health care, such as scientific medicine in the West, is elevated above the other forms, and both its cultural and social aspects are upheld by law. In addition, this official health-care system, which includes the medical and nursing professions, there are usually smaller, alternative systems such as homeopathy, herbalism and spiritual healing in many Western countries, which might be termed *health-care subcultures*. Each has its own way of explaining and treating ill health, and the healers in each group are organized into professional associations, with rules of entry, codes of conduct and ways of relating to patients. Health-care subcultures may be indigenous to the society or they may be imported from elsewhere; in many cases immigrants to a society often bring their traditional folk healers along with them, to deal with their ill health in a culturally familiar way. In the

UK, examples of these healers are the Muslim *hakims* or Hindu *vaids*, sometimes consulted by immigrants from the Indian subcontinent. In looking at health-care pluralism, wherever it occurs, it is important to examine both the cultural and social aspects of the types of health care available to the individual patient.

In this chapter the pluralistic health-care systems of complex, industrialized societies will be examined, in order to illustrate:

1 The range of therapeutic options available in these societies
2 How and why choices are made between the various options.

Health-care pluralism in the UK will also be discussed, and the implications of this for the delivery of health care.

THE THREE SECTORS OF HEALTH CARE

Kleinman[2] has suggested that, in looking at any complex society, one can identify three overlapping and interconnected sectors of health care; the *popular* sector, the *folk* sector and the *professional* sector. Each sector has its own ways of explaining and treating ill health, defining who is the healer and who is the patient, and specifying how healer and patient should interact in their therapeutic encounter.

THE POPULAR SECTOR

This is the lay, non-professional, non-specialist domain of society, where ill health is first recognized and defined and health-care activities are initiated. It includes all the therapeutic options that people use, without any payment and without consulting either folk healers or medical practitioners. Among these options are:

- self-treatment or self-medication
- advice or treatment given by a relative, friend, neighbour or workmate

- healing and mutual care activities in a church, cult or self-help group
- consultation with another lay person who has special experience of a particular disorder, or of treatment of a physical state.

In this sector the main arena of health care is the *family*; it is here that most ill health is recognized and then treated. It is the real site of primary health care in any society. In the family, as Chrisman[3] points out, the main providers of health care are women, usually mothers or grandmothers, who diagnose most common illnesses and treat them with the materials at hand. It has been estimated that about 70–90 per cent of health care takes place within this sector, in both Western and non-Western societies.[4] In most societies, the women are the guardians of a wide range of traditional remedies and ways of treating ill-health, passed down over many generations, from mother to daughter. In the Brazilian Amazon, for example, it is only the women who have the specialized knowledge of all the local plants and herbs, and who know how to use them to treat their families, and themselves.[5]

People who become ill typically follow a 'hierarchy of resort', ranging from self-medication to consultation with others. Self-treatment is based on lay beliefs about the structure and function of the body, and the origin and nature of ill health. It includes a variety of substances such as patent medicines, traditional folk remedies or 'old wives' tales', as well as changes in diet or behaviour. Food can be used as a form of medicine (see Chapter 3) in folk illnesses: for example, in 'high blood' in the southern USA, where certain foods are used to reduce the excess volume of blood, which is believed to cause the condition, or in parts of Latin America and Asia, where certain foods are used to counteract 'hot' or 'cold' illnesses and to restore the body to equilibrium. In both the UK and USA, self-prescribed vitamins are commonly used to restore health when one is 'feeling low'. The changes in behaviour that accompany different forms of ill health can range from special prayers, rituals, confession, fasting, or the use of talismans and charms to resting in a warm bed for a chill or cold.

The popular sector usually includes a set of beliefs about *health maintenance*. These are usually a series of guidelines, specific to each cultural group, about the 'correct' behaviour for preventing ill health in oneself and in others. They include beliefs about the healthy way to eat, drink, sleep, dress, work, pray and generally conduct one's life. They also include beliefs about the 'healthy' functioning of the body: how often one should defecate, for example, and at what times of the day.[6] In some societies health is also maintained by the use of charms, amulets and religious medallions to ward off bad luck, including unexpected illness, and to attract good luck and good health.

Most health care in this sector takes place between people already linked to one another by ties of kinship, friendship or neighbourhood, or membership of work or religious organizations. This means that both patient and healer share similar assumptions about health and illness, and misunderstandings between the two are comparatively rare.[3] The sector is made up of a series of *informal* and unpaid healing relationships of variable duration, which occur within the sufferer's own social network, particularly the family. These therapeutic encounters occur without fixed rules governing behaviour or setting; at a later date the roles may be reversed, with today's patient becoming tomorrow's healer. There are certain individuals, though, who tend to act as a source of health advice more often than others. These include:

1 Those with long experience of a particular illness or type of treatment.
2 Those with extensive experience of certain life events (such as women who have raised several children, or breastfed).
3 The paramedical professions (such as nurses, pharmacists, physiotherapists or doctor's receptionists) who are consulted informally about health problems.
4 Doctors' wives or husbands, who share some of their spouses' experience, if not training.
5 Individuals such as hairdressers, salespeople or even bank managers who interact frequently with the public, and sometimes act as lay confessors or psychotherapists.
6 The organizers of self-help groups.
7 The members or officiants of certain healing cults or churches.

All of these people may be considered as resources of advice and assistance concerning health matters by their friends or families. Their credentials are mainly their own *experience* rather than education, social status or special occult powers. A woman who has had several pregnancies, for example, can give informal advice to a newly pregnant younger woman, telling her what symptoms to expect and how to deal with them. Similarly, a person with long experience of a particular medication may 'lend' some to a friend with similar symptoms.

Individuals' experiences of ill health are sometimes shared within a *self-help group*, which may act as a repository of knowledge about a particular ailment or experience to be used both for the benefit of other members and for the rest of society. Self-help groups can bring many other benefits to members, such as sharing advice on lifestyle or coping strategies, or acting as a refuge for isolated individuals, especially those suffering from stigmatized conditions such as obesity or alcoholism. In industrialized countries, self-help groups have become an increasingly important part of the popular sector. Their roots lie originally in the USA, with the founding there of Alcoholics Anonymous (AA) in 1936.[7] There are currently an estimated 500 000 self-groups in the USA, and about 18 per cent of the American population have participated in one of them.[7] In Germany between 2 and 8 per cent of the population belong to a self-help group, while in Scandinavia that figure is lower at between 0.2 and 0.7 per cent.[7] One of the largest and oldest international self-help groups is AA, which has more than 100 000 groups in 150 countries, and over 2 million members.[8]

Experiences of ill health and suffering may also be shared within a healing cult, church or other religious group. For example, McGuire[9] has described some of the healing groups that are now found in middle-class suburban USA. These include movements such as Christian Science, the Unity School of Christianity, various other Christian groups (such as charismatic Catholic and Protestant Pentecostal groups), Human Potential groups (such as Scientology, EST, Progoff Process and Cornucopia), Eastern meditation and yoga groups (based on Zen or Tibetan Buddhism, Jainism or Hinduism), and the many types of spiritualist church and 'healing circles' that practise occult or psychic healing for their members. Many of these are based on the 'New Age' movement,[10] which emphasizes personal development, self-care and a holistic approach to health care, encompassing mind, body and soul. In non-Western societies too, self-help groups often have a religious basis. 'Spirit possession' cults, for example, are common in parts of Africa, especially among women. In these cults, women who have been 'possessed' and made ill by a particular spirit form what Turner[11] calls 'a community of suffering', the members of which ritually diagnose and treat those in the rest of society suffering from possession by the same malign spirit. Lewis[12] sees some of these spirit possession cults, like the Hausa *bori* cult in Northern Nigeria, as essentially women's protest movements against their social disadvantages. Membership of the cult brings prestige, healing power and special attention from their menfolk, who lavish gifts on them to appease the possessing spirits.

All aspects of the popular sector (and of the other two sectors) may sometimes have negative effects on people's mental and physical health. The family, for example, may either facilitate or impede health care. In Taiwan, according to Kleinman[13], the family's usual response to a sick member is to attempt to contain him, his sickness and the social problems that it generates within the circle of the family instead of sharing it with an outsider such as a medical practitioner.

In general, ill people move freely between the popular and the other two sectors and back again, often using all three sectors at once, especially when treatment in one sector fails to relieve physical discomfort or emotional distress.

THE FOLK SECTOR

In this sector, which is especially large in non-industrialized societies, certain individuals specialize in forms of healing that are either *sacred* or *secular*, or a mixture of the two. These healers are not part of the official medical system, and occupy an intermediate position between the popular and professional sectors. There is a wide variation in the types of folk healer found in any society, from purely secular and technical experts such as bone-setters, midwives, tooth extractors or herbalists, to spiritual healers, clairvoyants and shamans. Folk healers form a heterogeneous group, with much individual variation in style and outlook, but sometimes they are organized into associations of healers, with rules of entry, codes of conduct and the sharing of information.

Most communities include a mixture of sacred and secular folk healers. For example, in her study in the late 1970s of African-American folk healers in low-income urban neighbourhoods in the USA, Snow[14] described 'herb doctors', 'root doctors', spiritualists, 'conjure' men or women, Voodoo *houngans* or *mambos*, healing ministers and faith healers, neighbourhood prophets, 'granny women' and vendors of magical herbs, roots and patent medicines (Figure 4.1). Spiritual healers, who operate out of temples, churches or 'candle shops' are particularly common, and deal with illnesses believed to be caused by sorcery (hexing) or divine punishment. More secular illnesses are dealt with by self-medication, or by neighbourhood granny women or herb doctors. In practice, though, there is some overlap between their approaches and techniques. In another community, the Zulu of South Africa, there is also an overlap between sacred and secular healers. While sacred divination is carried out by female *isangomas*, treatment by

African herbal medicines is by male *inyangas*; both, though, will gather information about the social background of the victim as well as details of his or her illness before making a diagnosis.[15]

An example of a purely secular healer is the *sahi*, or health worker, as described by the Underwoods[16] in Raymah, Yemen Arab Republic. These healers have only appeared in Yemen in recent years, and their practice consists mainly of giving injections of various Western drugs. They have little training (usually a brief association with a health professional; in one case a month's work as a hospital cleaner), limited diagnostic skill, and they utilize few counselling or psychological skills. To the inhabitants of Raymah, however, the *sahi* practises what is considered to be the quintessence of Western medicine: 'the treatment of illness by injections'. The growing popularity of injections has been described in many Third World countries,[17,18] as has the proliferation of untrained *injectionists* (also known as injection doctors, needle men or shot givers) like the *sahi*. Other examples of this trend have been described by Kimani[19] in Kenya. There, untrained bush doctors administer medicines and injections, and 'street and bus-depot doctor boys' hustle antibiotic capsules acquired through the black market.

Most folk healers share the basic cultural values and world view of the communities in which they live, including beliefs about the origin, significance and treatment of ill health. In societies where ill health and other forms of misfortune are blamed on social causes (witchcraft, sorcery or 'evil eye') or on supernatural causes (gods, spirits, ancestral ghosts or fate), sacred folk healers are particularly common. Their approach is usually a holistic one, dealing with *all* aspects of the patient's life, including relationships with other people, with the natural environment and with supernatural forces, as well as any physical or emotional symptoms. In many non-Western societies all these aspects of life are part of the definition of health, which is seen as a *balance* between people and their social, natural and supernatural environments. A disturbance of any of these (such as immoral behaviour, conflicts within the family or failure to observe religious practices) may result in physical symptoms or emotional distress, and require the services of a sacred folk healer. Healers of this type, when faced with ill health, often enquire about the patient's behaviour before the illness and about any conflicts with other people. In a small-scale society the healer may also have firsthand knowledge of a family's difficulties through local gossip, and this may be useful in reaching a diagnosis. As well as gathering information about the patient's recent history and social background, the healer may employ a ritual of *divination*. There are many forms of this worldwide,[20] including the use of cards, bones, straws, shells, sticks, special stones and tea leaves, the arrangement of which is closely examined by the

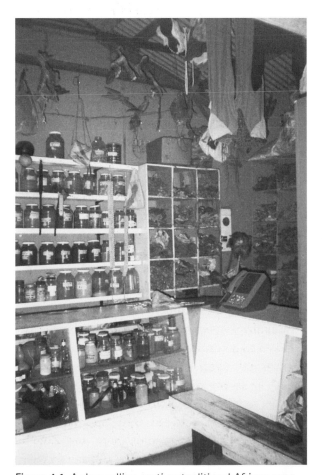

Figure 4.1 A shop selling *muti*, or traditional African remedies and folk medicines, in Johannesburg, South Africa.

healer for evidence of any underlying pattern. There is also examination of the entrails or liver of certain animals or birds, interpretation of dreams or visions, or direct consultation with spirits or supernatural beings by going into a trance. In each case, the divination aims to uncover the supernatural cause of the illness (such as witchcraft or divine retribution) by the use of supernatural techniques. The Zulu *isangoma*, for example, is consulted by the relatives of a sick person, who remains at home. Her diagnosis is made by going into a trance and communicating with spirits, who tell her the cause and treatment of the illness.[15]

The shaman

Another form of diviner is the *shaman*, who is found in different forms, in many different cultures. The shaman is a healer who mediates between the material and the spiritual worlds. Lewis[21] defines them as 'a person of either sex who has mastered spirits and can at will introduce them into his own body'; divination takes place at a séance, where the healer allows the spirits to enter him and through him diagnose the illness and prescribe the treatment. Because the shaman has 'mastered' these spirits that have entered him, he or she can then use them to help diagnose people possessed by these same, or similar malevolent spirits. In some cases the shaman may only enter their trance with the aid of powerful hallucinogenic drugs (see Chapter 8). This, and other forms of divination, sometimes take place in the presence of the patient's family, friends and other social contacts. In this public setting, the diviner aims to bring conflicts within a community – which may have led to witchcraft or sorcery between people – to the surface, and to resolve these conflicts in a ritual way. Sacred healers also provide explanations and treatment for subjective feelings of guilt, shame or anger by prescribing, for example, prayer, repentance or the resolution of interpersonal problems. They may also prescribe physical treatments or remedies at the same time.

Trance divination is common in non-industrialized societies, but is becoming increasingly common in the West, among mediums, clairvoyants, 'channellers', 'neo-shamans' and the members of certain healing charismatic churches. Even in less developed regions, shamanic healers who practice trance divination and healing are increasingly found in urban, as well as rural areas, as described in the case study from Siberia.

Case study: urban shamans in Ulan-Ude, Siberia, Russian Federation

Humphrey[22] studied the emergence of urban shamans in the city of Ulan-Ude, in the Buryat Republic of Siberia, since the fall of Communism. She describes the post-Soviet city, with its impersonal atmosphere, its shabby concrete buildings, and large anonymous apartment blocks, where most people find themselves living among strangers, instead of among kin. Most Buryats moved into the city from the countryside in the 1960s. This migration, plus the State's promotion of atheism, and the suppression of Buddhism and traditional spirit beliefs, meant that many lost touch with their rural roots and traditional culture. Once in the city, most had little choice as to where they lived or worked, and this also helped fragment their sense of identity and community. The Buryat shamans that have emerged are mostly city born, and cater mostly for educated clients. They tend to explain illness and misfortune as being due to the client's ancestral spirits, from the wilderness and steppes beyond the city. They often ask them about their genealogy, in order to identify the offending spirit so that it can then be exorcised or placated. To do this they often encourage them to find out more about their ancestors, and the areas from which they came. In some cases they encourage them to go back to these areas, to a particular mountain or tree where the spirit now resides, in order to perform a special ritual (*alban*) to placate it. Thus 'by insisting on these country links, the shamans reconceptualize and segment the city, so that it is now composed of individuals belonging to familial or decent groups, whose origins lie far away'. In this way, by 're-linking individual city people through half-forgotten familial ties with sacred–scary places in the countryside', they are helping them adapt to their post-Soviet urban reality. At the same time, they help them adapt to the new, bigger context in which they find themselves. In their sessions the shamans evoke not only clients' ancestral spirits, but also a less parochial and more eclectic range of 'deities' such as Archangel Gabriel, Japanese Samurai and even 'Autopilots of the Cosmos'. Buryat urban shamans act therefore not only as lay psychotherapists and counsellors but by linking clients to their roots, and to a wider context, they also make them more comfortable in the new, anonymous urban spaces that they now inhabit. As Humphrey notes, the shamans' 'perception of evil and misfortune in the city implies an awareness of relational flows of spirit power from the outside'.

Advantages and disadvantages of folk healing

For those who use it, folk healing offers several advantages over modern scientific medicine. One of these is the frequent involvement of the family in diagnosis and treatment. For example, as Martin[23] has pointed out, in Native American healing the patient's sickness places a responsibility on both patient and family to participate in healing rites. The focus of attention is not only the patient (as in Western medicine), but also the reaction of the family and others to the illness. The healer himself is usually surrounded by helpers, who take part in the ceremony, give explanations to the patient and his family, and answer any of their queries. From a modern perspective, this type of Native American healer with helpers, together with the patient's family, provides an effective primary health-care team, especially in dealing with psychosocial problems. Fabrega and Silver[24] have examined the advantages to the patient of another type of folk healer, the h'ilol in Zinacantan, Mexico, over Western doctors. In particular, there

is a shared world view, closeness, warmth, informality and the use of everyday language in consultations, and the family and other community members are involved in treatment. Also, the h'ilol is a crucial figure in the community and is believed to act for the benefit of the patient and the community as well as the gods; he can influence society at large, particularly the patient's social relationships, and he can influence the patient's future behaviour by pointing out the influence of past actions on his present illness. Finally, his healing takes place in a familiar setting, such as the home or a religious shrine. Because folk healers such as the h'ilol articulate and reinforce the cultural values of the communities in which they live, they have advantages over Western doctors, who are often separated from their patients by social class, economic position, gender, specialized education and, sometimes, cultural background. In particular, these healers are better able to define and treat illness – that is, the social, psychological, moral and spiritual dimensions associated with ill health, as with other forms of misfortune (see Chapter 5). Unlike in the Western world, where different types of misfortune are dealt with by different types of healer – physical problems by physicians, psychological problems by psychiatrists or therapists, social problems by social workers, and spiritual problems by ministers of religion – this type of healer deals with all these dimensions simultaneously. Furthermore, they often link them all together, into a single causal explanation. They also provide culturally familiar ways of explaining the cause and timing of the misfortune and its relation to the social and supernatural worlds.

In many countries today such folk healers are often used in parallel with medical treatment, even though both are based on very different premises. In Mexico, for example, Finkler[25] has described the differences, as well as the similarities, between doctors and spiritual healers (who heal with the aid of spirits that possess them). She shows how people use both systems, but for different purposes. As in many other cultures, the doctors tend to tell their patients what has happened, while the healers tell them why. Healers explain ill health in wider, more familiar cultural terms, involving the social, psychological and spiritual aspects of their patients' lives, while doctors concentrate mainly on physical diseases and the pathogens or behaviours said to cause them. This is despite the fact that the doctors spend twice as long (about 20 minutes) with first-time patients compared with the healers. However, there are some similarities between the two approaches. Both have a dualistic view of the patient, the doctors using a mind and body approach and the healers a spirit and body approach. Both attempt to peer inside the patient's body in order to diagnose ill health, the doctors with the aid of technology and the healers by means of the spirits that possess and aid them. Their therapeutic settings, however, are very different. The healing of *Espiritualismo* takes place in a temple in the presence of family and other members of the community, while doctor–patient interactions take place in the sterile isolation of a small cubicle, occasionally in the presence of strangers such as nurses or medical students. Finkler notes also that, unlike the doctors, spiritual healers rarely give their patients a specific diagnosis but rather an assurance that the spirits know everything about their affliction. To many patients this explanation is satisfying, since on some level it matches their own expectations and subjective emotional experience of ill health. While doctors tend to place the patient's ill health in a limited temporal frame, and to localize it in a particular part of the body, the omniscient spirits that aid the healer 'transcend time and space in the same way that the patient's sickness transcends temporal and spatial dimensions'.

Like other forms of health care, folk medicine has its disadvantages and its dangers. For example, folk healers may ignore, misdiagnose or mistreat the signs of serious physical disease or mental disorder, such as confusing psychosis, epilepsy or a brain tumour with 'spirit possession'. They may use forms of treatment, such as exorcisms, strong herbal concoctions, special diets, or extreme forms of prayer or fasting, which can cause physical or psychological damage to their clients. Some may use unsterilized needles or instruments in circumcisions, ritual scarifications, acupuncture or other treatments, leading to the spread of infections such as human immunodeficiency virus (HIV) or hepatitis B. Both male and female circumcisions, carried out by folk practitioners, may sometimes lead to a major haemorrhage, especially in those with a bleeding tendency, as well as to local infections or even septicaemia. Some traditional birth attendants may use unsterilized instruments in childbirth, or advise new mothers to discard their colostrum, or place pieces of dung on the baby's umbilical stump after birth – leading to neonatal tetanus (see Chapter 6). Some folk healers may also use the credulity and vulnerability of their clients to exploit them financially, emotionally, or even sexually. All of these examples mean that folk healers should be seen realistically, and not over-romanticized. For the people who consult them they undoubtedly have many advantages over biomedical doctors, but they can also have both disadvantages and dangers.

Training of folk healers

In general, folk healers have little formal training equivalent to the Western medical school. Skills are usually acquired by apprenticeship to an older healer, by experience of certain techniques or conditions, or by the possession of inborn or acquired healing power. People can become folk healers in a number of ways, such as:

1 Inheritance – being born into a 'healing family', sometimes of many generations of healers.
2 Position within a family, such as the 'seventh son of a seventh son' in Ireland.
3 Signs and portents at birth, like a birthmark, or 'crying in the womb' or being born with the amniotic membrane across the face (the 'caul' in Scotland).
4 Revelation – discovering one 'has the gift', which may occur as an intense emotional experience during an illness, dream or trance. In extreme cases, as Lewis[21] points out, the voca-

tion may be announced by 'an initially uncontrolled state of possession: a traumatic experience associated with hysteroid, ecstatic behaviour'.

5 Apprenticeship to another healer – a common pattern in all parts of the world, though the apprenticeship may last for many years.

6 Acquiring a particular skill on one's own, like the Yemeni *sahi*, the Kenyan bush doctors and other forms of injectionists. Modern would-be folk healers may now be able to acquire their healing knowledge from books, correspondence courses, or even the Internet.

In practice, these pathways into folk healing tend to overlap; for example, someone born of a 'healing family' and with certain signs and portents at birth may still need to refine their 'gift' by a lengthy apprenticeship to an older healer. In a few cases, healers may also be qualified as nurses or other health professionals. One study[26] has estimated, for example, that in South Africa almost 1 per cent of African nurses also work part-time as traditional healers.

While most folk healers work individually, informal networks or associations of healers do exist, and these provide for the exchange of techniques and information and the monitoring of each other's behaviour. Such a network among Zulu diviners or *isangomas* is described by Ngubane.[15] Meetings take place regularly between diviners to share ideas, experiences and techniques; each diviner has the opportunity to meet the ex-students, teacher and neophyte of each of her neighbouring diviners, as well as more distant ones. It is estimated that, over a period of 3–5 years, a diviner might make contact with over 400 fellow diviners all over southern Africa (though, recently, as mentioned below, they have begun forming their own professional organizations, and become subject to government moves to licence and regulate them). In other settings, such as low-income black neighbourhoods in the USA, several healers might be ministers of a spiritualist church, which also acts as an association of healers. In the suburban

healing circles described by McGuire,[9] almost all the participants have the chance to be both healer and patient at various times; therefore these groups overlap the boundary between folk and popular healing, and provide a venue for the exchange of information and experiences among a group of healers.

However, despite their many advantages it is important not to over-romanticize folk healers in general. Like all other health-care providers, including doctors and nurses, their ranks may include those that are incompetent, ignorant, arrogant or greedy, or have a very reductionist view of ill health and how it should be treated. Furthermore, not all folk healers come from the community in which they work or are familiar with its inner social workings. Some of the techniques they use may also be very dangerous to their patients. The use of unsterilized needles by injectionists, for example, may lead to severe skin abscesses, as well as to the spread of hepatitis B or acquired immune deficiency syndrome (AIDS). Some of their herbal remedies have been reported to cause severe illness, or even death.[27] It is important therefore to see folk healers in a balanced way, and to avoid both over-idealization and over-criticism of them. On one hand, one should avoid what Lucas and Barrett[28] term the Arcadian view – seeing them and the communities they work among as somehow 'natural' and holistic, living in peaceful harmony with nature and with one another. But on the other hand, the 'barbaric' view – seeing them and their communities as somehow primitive, degenerate, incompetent and underdeveloped – is also inaccurate. In most cases of folk healing, the truth lies somewhere between the two.

'Professionalization' of folk healers

The relationship between folk and professional sectors has usually been marked by mutual distrust and suspicion. Most doctors have tended to view folk healers as quacks, charlatans, witch doctors or medicine men, who pose a danger to their patients' health.

Increasingly (and often reluctantly), however, the medical authorities have recognized that, despite their shortcomings, folk healers *do* have some obvious advantages to the patient and their family, especially when dealing with psychological problems. In many developing countries, traditional folk healers are becoming incorporated into the margins of the medical system – sometimes against their will. The initiative for this has usually come from the World health Organization (WHO), or from national governments, or sometimes from the healers themselves. In 1978, the WHO issued its famous Alma-Ata declaration of 'Health for All by the Year 2000'. Its main proposal was for the worldwide provision of comprehensive primary health care (PHC), which would provide preventive, curative and rehabilitative services at an affordable cost.[29] However, with scarce resources, growing populations and limited medical manpower the task was almost impossible, and has recently become even more difficult because of new diseases such as AIDS. One result of this was a fresh look at traditional medicine, redefining it as a potential ally of the medical system rather than as an enemy. In 1978 the WHO recommended that traditional medicine be promoted, developed and integrated wherever possible with modern, scientific medicine,[30] but stressed the necessity to ensure respect, recognition and collaboration among the practitioners of the various systems concerned. The manpower resources that WHO hoped to enlist included herbalists, Ayurvedic, *Unāni* or Yoga practitioners, Chinese traditional healers such as acupuncturists, and various others. Special attention has been paid to the selection and training of traditional birth attendants (TBAs),[31,32] who already deliver about two-thirds of the world's babies (see Chapter 6).

Last[33] points out that now, as a result of these two declarations, 'the potential professionalization of indigenous practitioners is firmly on the agenda'. He notes that there has been a rapid growth in the number of practitioners' organizations, especially in Africa. Some (like the Zulu *isangomas*) operate mainly as informal networks, others as pressure groups or healing churches or cults. Several, such as the Zimbabwe National Traditional Healers' Association, have become recognized by government as professional bodies in their own right, with exclusive powers to educate, evaluate, license and discipline their members. In South Africa, the government's Traditional Health Practitioners Bill of 2004 has created a Council to oversee the licensing and regulation of the country's estimated 200 000 African traditional healers – who are consulted by about 70 per cent of the population – with the aim of ensuring 'the efficacy, safety and quality of traditional health care services.'[34]

For many folk healers, the process of forming a 'profession' (see below) has also often been a response to unequal competition from the medical system. By creating a professional association, they hope to advance their interests and those of their clients, improve standards, raise their prestige and earning power, gain official support and define an area of health care that only they can provide.

However, this is often problematic. For one thing, there is evidence that in many developing countries the actual number of traditional healers is declining, owing partly to education, urbanization and the breakdown of communities. Also, as Last[33] notes, traditional healers (especially of the sacred kind) are too diffuse a group, and their knowledge and practice too rooted in local contexts, to be effectively standardized. They also have specific notions of legitimacy, which derive mainly from the traditions of their community and their own charisma and not from some distant government bureaucracy. For many of their clients, 'the legality of a practice is less important than the practitioner's moral standing or trustworthiness'.

To some extent, this professionalization of traditional healers parallels a similar process that is ocurring among alternative and complementary healers in Western societies (see below). In Eastern Europe, since the eighteenth century, the Russian *feldshers* have also progressed along a lengthy road from local folk practitioners (often ex-army medics) to their more recent status as physician's assistants who often work in primary care, or obstetrics, especially in rural area.[35] By contrast, their equivalents in other Eastern European countries, such as the *cyruliks* of Poland, have largely disappeared.[35]

Velimirovic[36] sees the WHO initiative on traditional medicine as well-intentioned but misguided. He argues that its integration into the formal (professional) sector of health care since 1978 'has contributed virtually nothing to solving the monumental health problems of the developing world', or to the attainment of 'Health for All by the Year 2000'. This is partly because, in the WHO proposal, the definition of traditional medicine was never clear or consistent. Neither was its uncritical assumption of the efficacy of traditional medicine justified, since it ignored its many failures and shortcomings, such as its inability to cure malaria, cholera, yellow fever and other diseases. In many cases, the views of traditional healers on disease, and their treatments, were so detrimental to health that they themselves were part of the problem. Furthermore, in many developing countries traditional medicine 'is often not as popular with the people themselves as health planners believe'. Given the choice, many people prefer to consult Western-style doctors rather than traditional healers or untrained community health workers – even if this involves much expense and travelling a great distance to see them.

Despite this view, it should be emphasized that there *are* examples of the successful collaboration between traditional healers and the official medical system, especially in relation to AIDS prevention,[37] TBAs,[32] family planning,[38] the promotion of oral rehydration therapy,[39] the treatment of mental illness[40] and the treatment and rehabilitation of drug addicts.[41]

Traditional medicine in China and India

In countries such as India and China, strong indigenous systems of healing enjoy almost the same legitimacy and popularity as Western medicine and now, with government support, offer the population parallel systems of health care. They are already to some extent 'professionalized'. In China, despite several shifts of government policy, traditional Chinese medicine – including acupuncture, moxibustion and herbal remedies – still provides a complementary system of health care for much of the population, especially in rural areas, and exists alongside biomedical clinics and other facilities. In India there are 91 recognized Ayurvedic (Hindu) and 10 Unāni (Muslim) medical schools, and Ayurvedic medicine serves a large proportion of the population. The Indian Medicine Central Council Act of 1970 set up a Central Council for Ayurveda, which established a register of qualified practitioners and oversees the training of new ones. They grant a 3-year Bachelor of Ayurvedic Medicine and Surgery degree, followed by 3 years' postgraduate study.[42] However, by the late 1980s only 12 per cent of Ayurvedic practitioners had obtained the degree of a recognized teaching institution, 54 per cent had degrees from unrecognized schools, and 33 per cent had no qualifications at all.[42] A similar process has taken place with homoeopathy (which reached India in the 1830s)[43] and which since 1973 is overseen by a Central Council for Homoeopathy. This has recognized 200 000 homoeopathic practitioners, and supervises 104 colleges which run undergraduate courses in the subject. Postgraduate degrees are issued by the National Institute of Homeopathy in Calcutta, and there are 130–150 homoeopathic hospitals and 1500 homoeopathic dispensaries in India, all supported by the government. Homoeopaths outnumber Ayurvedic practitioners in several states, and homoeopathy is particularly widespread in the state of West Bengal, but also in Uttar Pradesh, Bihar, Tamil Nadu and Kerala, and tends to be more prevalent in urban than in rural areas.[43]

Srinavasan[44] noted in 1995 that Ayurveda was losing popularity to Western (allopathic) medicine in many parts of the country. One all-India survey showed that while 80 per cent of households in urban areas used allopathic medicine only 4 per cent used Ayurvedic, while in rural households 75 per cent used allopathy and 8 per cent Ayurvedic. This applied to most social classes. In contrast, in

Sri Lanka, Srinavasan has noted that government policy has strongly encouraged traditional Ayurvedic medicine, and that there are now 13 000 Ayurvedic physicians (1 per 1400 population) there, compared with 380 000 (1 per 2200 population) in India.[44]

Alternative and complementary medicine

In most Western countries a special form of health care – alternative or complementary medicine (sometimes known as CAM) – overlaps both folk and professional sectors. Its many types of healers usually include acupuncturists, homoeopaths, chiropractors, osteopaths, herbalists, naturopaths, spiritual healers, hypnotists, massage therapists and meditation experts. One of the most popular forms of CAM is acupuncture (which is now used in at least 78 countries worldwide).[45]

Unconventional medicine in Europe and Asia

In Europe, the CAM sector of health care is rapidly growing in popularity. In 1981, for example, an estimated 6.4 per cent of the population of Holland had visited a therapist or doctor practicing complementary medicine, and this had risen to 15.7 per cent by 1990, and 47 per cent of Dutch general practitioners now use a complimentary therapy.[46] In Germany, many thousands of *Heilpraktikers* (naturopaths who practise 'nature cure' and hydrotherapy) often also practise acupuncture, herbalism or chiropractic.[47] These naturopaths have been given official recognition since 1939, and according to Wirsing[48] there were about 7000 of them practising in Germany in 1996. He also estimated that there were about 2000 physicians who practiced homoeopathy, and another 1000 who practiced 'anthroposophic' medicine, based on the teachings of Rudolf Steiner.[48] In addition, 77 per cent of pain clinics in Germany now use acupuncture.[46] According to the WHO, 90 per cent of German's population have used a 'natural remedy' at some stage of their lives, and between 1995 and 2000 the number of doctors that had undergone special training in natural remedy medicine had almost doubled to 10 800.[45]

There are wide variations among the European countries as to which branch of alternative medicine they prefer. According to Fisher and Ward,[46] while anthroposophy is popular in all the German-speaking countries, about 50 per cent of the population in Belgium consult homoeopaths (apparently the highest rate in Europe), reflexology is particularly popular in Denmark (31 per cent of CAM users), massage is popular in Finland, spiritual healing is popular in Holland, and in France the most popular form of complimentary therapy is homeopathy, the use of which rose from 16 per cent of the population in 1982 to 36 per cent in 1992.

Outside of Europe, the WHO[45] estimates that 60–70 per cent of medical doctors in Japan also prescribe *kampo* medicine (traditional herbal remedies), 46 per cent of the Australian population have used some form of CAM, and that in Malaysia the use of traditional forms of Malay, Chinese and Indian medicines is common. Overall, these figures indicate that, even in developed and industrialized countries, a large proportion of the population prefer to use *other* forms of health care – either instead of, or in addition to biomedicine.

Unconventional medicine in the USA

In the USA, Eisenberg and colleagues[49] estimated that in 1990 almost one in three people used some form of unconventional medicine, most frequently for back problems (36 per cent), headaches (27 per cent), chronic pain (26 per cent) and cancer or tumours (24 per cent). The most common treatments they used were relaxation techniques, chiropractic and massage. In most cases (89 per cent) they saw these practitioners without the recommendation of their doctors, and 72 per cent never told them. Overall, they estimated that Americans made about 425 million visits to the unconventional practitioners in 1990, a figure exceeding the total number of visits to all US primary-care physicians (388 million). Furthermore, they paid about $10.3 billion 'out-of-pocket' for these therapies, compared with the $12.8 billion paid for all the hospital care in the USA. Most users of unconventional therapies were found to be between 25 and 49 years old, but they came from all socio-demographic groups. According to the WHO,[50] in the year 2000 158 million of the adult population in the USA used some sort of complementary medicines, and US $17 billion was spent on them. Acupuncture was particularly popular, and there were 12 000 licensed acupuncturists, while the practice of acupuncture was legal in 38 states.[45] The WHO also estimated that about 75 per cent of people living with HIV/AIDS in San Francisco used some form of traditional or alternative therapy (a similar proportion to London, England, and to South Africa).[50] Some of the more unorthodox forms of therapy used for HIV/AIDS in the USA are described in Chapter 16.

Kaptchuk and Eisenberg[51,52] have reviewed the steady rise of alternative medicine in the USA from 1800 to the present day. They quote one national study that shows that from 1990 to 1997 the number of respondents who used at least one of 15 representative alternative therapies during a 12-month period, rose from 34 per cent to 42 per cent. They point out that medical pluralism in the USA is now a fact and can no longer be suppressed or ignored by the medical profession. There is now an emerging dialogue between conventional and alternative medicine, and a growing recognition of the new cultural, religious and ethnic diversity in the country, as well as the growing power of consumer choice. In 1991 the National Institutes of Health set up an Office of Alternative Medicine (OAM), and an estimated 75 US medical schools now offer courses on alternative medicine.[53] Kaptchuk and Eisenberg[50,51] also provide a useful taxonomy of alternative ('unconventional') healing practices in the USA:

- *Professionalized or distinct medical systems* with their own distinct theories, practices, institutions, and methods of training. These include practitioners of chiropractic, acupuncture, homeopathy, naturopathy, massage, as well as conventional medical doctors who also practice these healing systems

- *Alternative dietary and lifestyle practices* (also known as '*Popular Health Reform*' systems) which include the 'health food' movement; the use of mega-vitamins, botanicals and nutritional supplements; and those who follow a macrobiotic, organic food, or vegan diet.

- *New Age Healing* is a disparate range of beliefs and practices – many drawn from Eastern religions or from paganism – and which often focus on esoteric 'energies', and on achieving a balance between them. It includes consultations with spirits or mediums and Oriental forms of healing such as Reiki or Qi-Dong, as well as the use of healing crystals or magnets.

- *Psychological interventions: Mind Cure and 'Mind–Body'* medicine range from more conventional forms of psychotherapy to the use of guided visualizations, meditations, affirmations and hypnotherapy; these focus on the notion that 'the mind is the most dominant energy for restoring well-being and maintaining health', and therefore that negative emotions can cause, or exacerbate, serious physical diseases.

- *Non-normative scientific enterprises* are forms of medical treatments or medications, or forms of diagnosis, that are not validated by the scientific establishment, and which are often resorted to by those with severe diseases such as terminal cancer. They include iridology, treatment with 'anti-neoplastons', 'hair analysis' to detect diseases and nutrient imbalance , and 'chelation therapy' to reverse arteriosclerotic disease.

- *Parochial unconventional medicine* are specific folk practices with deep cultural roots in certain groups in the USA. It includes spiritism among Puerto-Ricans, *curanderismo* among Mexican-Americans, *vodun* among Haitian-Americans, and various Native American forms of healing. Also included here are indigenous American folk medicine (sometimes from specific regions, such as southern Appalachia), and many different forms of spiritual and religious healing, such as Christian Science, and a variety of Pentecostal and charismatic churches.

THE PROFESSIONAL SECTOR

This comprises the organized, legally sanctioned healing professions, such as modern Western scientific medicine, also known as *allopathy* or *biomedicine*. It includes not only physicians of various types and specialties, but also the recognized paramedical professions such as nurses, midwives and physiotherapists. Every society has its own *ethnomedicine* – that part of its cultural system that deals specifically with sickness and healing[54] – and biomedicine can be regarded as the ethnomedicine of the Western, industrialized world. As such, it not only arises from this society, it also expresses (and constantly helps recreate) some of its basic cultural premises, including its ways of looking at the world, its social hierarchies and organization, gender roles, and attitudes towards illness and suffering.

Over the past century or so, this Western biomedicine has spread to cover much of the globe, so that it is now the dominant form of healing found worldwide, and in most countries forms the basis of the professional sector. However, in certain countries traditional medical systems may also become professionalized to some extent, and so be able to compete with biomedicine; examples of this are the Ayurvedic and Unāni medical colleges in India, which receive governmental support, and whose graduates are regularly consulted by many millions of people.

It is important to realize that for all its power and prestige, Western biomedicine provides only a small proportion of health care in most parts of the world. Medical manpower is often a scarce resource, with most health care taking place in the popular and folk sectors. In 2005 the WHO *World Health Statistics* report[55] illustrated the huge variations in the availability of doctors – as well as of nurses and midwives – throughout the world (Table 4.1). Based on data from 1997–2003, they showed considerable variation between countries in the supply of medical manpower, ranging from countries such as Uganda with 0.1 physicians per 10 000 population, to India with 5.9, China with 16.4, the UK with 21.3, the USA with 27.9, and the Russian Federation with 42.5. A comparison of the six main regions of the world (Table 4.2) graphically shows how varied, and unequal, is the distribution of the numbers of doctors, nurses and hospital beds available to the populations of these different regions.[56]

These figures, however, probably overestimate the numbers of doctors actually involved in direct patient care, as many of them work in research and administration rather than in clinical practice. In addition, the distribution of doctors is not uniform; in many non-industrialized societies they tend to cluster in cities, where facilities are better and practice is more lucrative, leaving many in the countryside to rely on the popular and folk sectors of care. In Mozambique in 1994, for example, 52 per cent of the country's doctors were concentrated in the capital city Maputo, while most of the rest practiced in the next largest cities.[57] In many of these countries, the proportion of doctors that work in the private sector has steadily increased, thus reducing even further the number available to provide low-cost health care by the state. In Zimbabwe in 1993, for example, 66 per cent of doctors worked in the private sector, while 59 per cent did so in South Africa and 25 per cent in Papua New Guinea.[58] Private medical practice has greatly increased in Malawi and Tanzania, following changes in government policy, while in Uganda, Bennett[58] has argued that the increase in private practitioners has 'created a culture in which good care has come to be associated with the availability of injections and other drugs, regardless of medical appropriateness'.

In most countries, especially in the Western world, the practitioners of scientific medicine form the only group of healers whose positions are upheld by law. They enjoy higher social status, greater income and more clearly defined rights, and obligations than other types of healers. They have the power to question and examine their patients, prescribe powerful and sometimes dangerous treatments or medication, and deprive certain people of their freedom and confine them to

Table 4.1 Relation of physicians, nurses and midwives to population in selected countries

Country	Physicians per 10 000 population	Nurses and midwives per 10 000 population
Malawi	0.1	2.6
Niger	0.3	2.7
Uganda	0.5	0.9
Afghanistan	1.9	2.2
India	5.9	7.9
Jamaica	8.5	16.5
Philippines	11.6	61.4
China	16.4	9.6
Mexico	17.1	10.8
Japan	20.1	86.3
United Kingdom	21.3	54.0
Egypt	22.2	26.5
United States	27.9	97.2
Ukraine	30.1	82.8
Greece	33.5	73.0
Russian Federation	42.5	85.1

World Health Organization (2005).[55]

Table 4.2 Relation of physicians, nurses and midwives, and hospital beds to population in different regions of the world

Region	Physicians per 10 000 population	Nurses and midwives per 10 000 population	Hospital beds per 10 000 population
Africa	1.8	8.8	?*
South-East Asia	5.0	7.4	17.0
Eastern Mediterranean	10.1	13.7	13.0
Western Pacific	15.8	19.7	34.0
The Americas	21.8	40.8	26.0
Europe	33.1	72.0	67.0

World Health Organization (2005).[56]

*Figures for hospital beds in Africa are not included in the report.

hospitals if they are diagnosed as psychotic or infectious. In hospital, they can tightly control their patients' diet, behaviour, sleeping patterns and medication, and can initiate a variety of tests, such as biopsies, X-rays or venesection. They can also label their patients (sometimes permanently) as ill, incurable, malingering, hypochondriacal, or as fully recovered – a label that may conflict with the patient's perspective. These labels can have important effects, both social (confirming the patient in the sick role) and economic (influencing health insurance or pension payments).

The medical system

As stated earlier, the dominant system of health care of any society cannot be studied in isolation from other aspects of that society, for the *medical system* (or professional sector of health care) does not exist in a social or cultural vacuum. Rather, it is an expression of, and to some extent a miniature model of, the values and social structure of the society from which it arises. Different types of society therefore produce different types of medical systems and different attitudes to health and illness, depending on their dominant ideology – whether this is capitalist, welfare state, socialist or communist. One society may see free (or relatively inexpensive) health care as a basic right of citizenship, or the basic right only of the poor or the very old, while another may see medical care as a commodity to be bought only by those who can afford it. In this latter case, the pursuit of profits in health care will exclude many of those poorer members of society who do not have the resources to pay for it. Whatever the type of society, the medical system not only reflects these basic values and ideologies, but in turn helps also to shape and maintain them.[59]

As an example of this, critics of the medical systems in the Western world have pointed out how the internal organization of the professional sector reflects some of the basic inequalities in those societies, especially in relation to gender, social class and ethnic background. Within the medical system most doctors are male (and usually white) and, as in the wider society, occupy many more of the prestigious, powerful and well-paid jobs than female doctors and nurses. Also, the personnel within this sector are arranged in hierarchies similar to the social strata of the wider society. In its dealings with the population the medical system may reproduce many of the underlying prejudices of society, as well as cultural assumptions as to what constitutes good and bad behaviour. For example, it has been suggested that racial prejudice plays an important role in how some Afro-Caribbean patients in the UK are classified by psychiatrists as 'mad', even when there is evidence to the contrary[60] (see Chapter 10). A similar process operated in the former USSR, in state psychiatry's attitude to political dissent.[61]

Other critiques of the Western medical system include that by Illich,[62] who has claimed that high-tech modern medicine has become increasingly dangerous to the population's health by reducing their autonomy, making them dependent on the medical profession and damaging their health by the side-effects of drugs and surgical interventions. In addition, the medical system is in a symbiotic relationship with the manufacturers of pharmaceuticals and medical equipment, and this relationship is not necessarily in the patient's interest.

Like Illich, other critics of the medical system have maintained that modern medicine, as well as controlling microorganisms, also seeks to control the behaviour of the population, especially by 'medicalizing' deviant behaviour, as well as many of the normal stages of the human life-cycle. Stacey[63] and others have suggested that this phenomenon is particularly evident in the case of women, especially during pregnancy and childbirth (see Chapter 6). Furthermore, much of the ill health in Western society that may be caused by other factors such as poverty, unemployment, economic crises, pollution or persecution is often ignored by the medical system, because its main focus is increasingly on the *individual* patient (or even on the individual organ) and the risk factors in his or her own lifestyle.[64]

Thus, in understanding any medical system, one must always see it in the *context* of the basic values, ideology, political organization and economic system of the society from which it arises. In that sense, the professional sector of health care, like the other two sectors, is always to some extent 'culture-bound'.

Comparison of medical systems

One can illustrate this culture-bound aspect, in the case of Western medicine, by comparing the medical systems of different Western countries with similar levels of economic development.

Obviously, these countries vary in whether health care lies mainly in the private or the public sectors, in the distribution of medical resources, their arrangements for health insurance and so on, but their professional sectors are all rooted in the same tradition of Western scientific medicine, and there is considerable exchange of medical data and techniques between them.

Despite Western medicine's claim of universality, however, various studies have illustrated significant differences in the types of diagnosis given and the treatment prescribed between different Western medical systems. For example, in 1984 a comparison of the patterns of prescribing of five different European countries (the UK, Germany, Italy, France and Spain)[65] found marked variations between them – and which could *not* be explained solely by disparities in the health of their populations. The study examined the 20 leading diagnostic categories and 20 leading types of drug prescribed in each of these countries. In the UK, for example, the major group of drugs prescribed was tranquillizers, hypnotics and sedatives (8.6 per cent of the total number of prescriptions), compared with 6.8 per cent in France, 6.0 per cent in Germany, 3.1 per cent in Italy and 2.0 per cent in Spain. In the UK, neuroses were among the commonest of diagnoses (5.1 per cent of the total number of diagnoses given), compared to 4.1 per cent in France, 3.2 per cent in Italy and 1.7 per cent in Spain. These differences may represent not only differences in morbidity between the five countries, but also major differences in nomenclature, in the criteria of diagnosis, and in *cultural* attitudes to certain types of behaviour and how they should be dealt with. Other studies, some of which are described later in this book, have shown differences between UK and US psychiatrists and between UK and French psychiatrists in the criteria they use to diagnose and treat schizophrenia (see Chapter 10); differences between UK, Canadian and US rates of various surgical operations, including Caesarean sections (see Chapter 15); and differences in the medical use of spas and hydrotherapy (*la thermalisme*) in France and in Germany (the *kur*),[66] but not in countries such as the UK or the USA.

A closer look at these national differences in the perception, diagnosis, naming and treatment of disease may suggest some of the cultural values that underlie those differences. For example, Payer[67] has examined the medical systems of the USA, France, Germany and the UK. She has described some of the diagnostic categories that have no clear equivalents in other countries, such as *crise de foie* and *spasmophilia* in France, *Herzinsuffizienz* and *Kreislaufkollaps* in Germany, or chilblains or 'bowel problems' in the UK. Furthermore, in understanding these variations she has related certain medical beliefs and practices to core cultural values in each of those societies. In the USA, for example, she sees a relation between the high rate of coronary bypass operations and other types of surgery and the American view of the body as a repairable 'machine', and one that needs to be repaired and overhauled at regular intervals. She describes the dominant attitude of US doctors to sickness as an aggressive and 'can-do' approach, part of the legacy of the frontier spirit: 'Americans not only want to *do* something, they want to do it *fast*, and if they cannot they often become frustrated'. As a result, US doctors do more diagnostic tests on their patients and perform surgery more often than do doctors from the other three countries. According to Payer, they often eschew drug treatment in favour of more aggressive surgery, and if they do use drugs, they tend to use higher doses than their European colleagues. In psychiatry, for example, the doses of some drugs used in the USA are up to 10 times higher than those used elsewhere. The reasons for these approaches to medical care are various, including the types of payment US doctors get for their services and the threat of malpractice suits against them. However, like doctors from the three European countries, it is the underlying *cultural* values of their society that play a part in determining how ill health is diagnosed and then treated.

The medical profession

Within the medical system those who practise medicine form a group apart, with their own values, concepts, theories of disease and rules of behaviour, as well as organization into a hierarchy of healing roles; this group therefore has both cultural and social aspects. It can be regarded – like lawyers, architects and engineers – as a *profession*. Foster and Anderson[68] define a profession as being 'based on, or organized around, a body of specialized knowledge [the content] not easily acquired and that, in the hands of qualified practitioners, meets the needs of, or serves, *clients*'. It also has a *collegial organization* of conceptual equals, which exists to maintain *control* over their field of expertise, promote their common interests, maintain their monopoly of knowledge, set qualifications for admission (such as the licensing of new physicians), protect themselves from incursions or competition by outsiders, and monitor the competence and ethics of their members. Although conceptually equal, the profession is arranged in hierarchies of knowledge and power, such as the ranks of professors, consultants, senior and junior registrars, (residents) and house officers (interns) in the UK. Below them are the paramedical professionals: nurses, midwives, physiotherapists, occupational therapists, medical social workers, etc. Each paramedical group has its own body of knowledge, clients, collegial organization and control over an area of competence but, overall, has less autonomy and power than the physicians.

The doctors themselves are divided into specialized subprofessions, which duplicate on a smaller scale the structure of the medical profession as a whole. Examples of this are the surgeons, paediatricians, gynaecologists and psychiatrists. Each have their own unique perspective on ill health, their own area of knowledge and their own internal hierarchy, from experts to novices. Medical specialities vary in status depending on whether they deal primarily with acute or chronic diseases, and the part of the body that they specialize in. In general, those who treat acute conditions, such as surgeons or internists, have a higher status than those who treat more chronic conditions, such as oncologists, geriatricians, psychiatrists and rheumatologists. That is, doctors who can 'cure' have a higher status than those who can only 'care'. Among surgeons, there is a status hierarchy that depends on the part of the body that they operate on. Because of the higher symbolic value our society gives to the brain and the heart, neurosurgeons and cardiac surgeons have a much higher status than, say, proctologists or gynecologists.

Pfifferling[69] has examined some of the assumptions and premises underlying the medical profession in the USA. In his view, it is:

1 *Physician-centred* – the doctor, and not the patient, defines the nature and boundary of the patient's problem; diagnostic and intellectual skills are valued above communication skills; settings for health care, such as doctors' offices, are often located for the benefit of doctors, far from their patients' homes.
2 *Specialist-orientated* – specialists, rather than generalists, get the highest prestige and rewards.
3 *Credentials-orientated* – those with higher credentials can rise in the medical hierarchy, and are considered to possess greater clinical skills and knowledge.
4 *Memory-based* – feats of memory (of medical facts, cases, drugs, discoveries, etc.) are rewarded by promotion and the respect of one's peers.
5 *Single-case-centred* – decisions are made on a single case of a disease, based on cumulative descriptions of previous clinical cases.
6 *Process-orientated* – evaluations of the doctor's clinical skill are made by measuring their impact on quantifiable biological processes in the patient over time (such as a fall in blood pressure).

One could add to this list the increasing emphasis on diagnostic technology rather than on clinical evaluations, and the growing influence of the corporate take-over of many hospitals throughout the country and its implications for health care. Many of these points are now beginning to apply equally to physicians in European countries, such as the UK.

In many industrialized countries the professional sector is also composed of local general practitioners or family physicians who, unlike many hospital doctors, are often deeply rooted within a community. There is some resemblance between these doctors (and nurses) and healers in the folk sector, particularly in their familiarity with local conditions and with the social, familial and psychological aspects of ill health, even though their healing is based on entirely different premises.

The hospital

In most countries, the main institutional structure of scientific medicine is the *hospital*. Unlike in the popular and folk sectors, the ill person is removed from family, friends and community at a time of personal crisis. In hospital they undergo a standardized ritual of depersonalization (see Chapter 9), being converted into a numbered 'case' in a ward full of strangers. The emphasis is on their physical disease, with little reference to their home environment, religion, social relationships or moral status, or the meaning they give to their ill health. Hospital specialization ensures that they are classified and allocated to different wards on the basis of *age* (adults, paediatrics, geriatrics), *gender* (male, female), *condition* (medical, surgical or other), *organ* or *system* involved (e.g. ear, nose and throat, ophthalmology, dermatology) or *severity* (intensive care units, casualty departments, emergency rooms). Patients of the same sex, similar age range and similar illnesses often share a ward. All these patients have been stripped of many of the props of social identity and individuality, and clothed in a uniform of pyjamas, nightdress or bathrobe. There is a loss of control over one's body, and over personal space, privacy, behaviour, diet and use of time. Patients are removed from the continuous emotional support of family and community and cared for by staff they may never have seen before. In hospitals, the relationship of health professionals – doctors, nurses and technicians – with their

patients is largely characterized by distance, formality, brief conversations and, often, use of professional jargon.

Hospitals have been seen by anthropologists such as Goffman[70] as 'small societies', each with their own unique culture; their own implicit and explicit rules of behaviour, tradition, rituals, hierarchies and even language. Patients in a ward form a temporary 'community of suffering', linked together by commiseration, ward gossip and discussion of one another's conditions. However, this community does not resemble or replace the communities in which they live and, unlike the members of self-help groups, their afflictions do not entitle them to heal others, at least not within the hospital setting.

The hospital, like the rest of the medical system itself, does not exist in a vacuum. It too is heavily influenced by cultural, social, and economic factors, at both the local and the national levels. Although the elements of the hospital may appear to be universal – doctors, nurses, wards, clinics, white coats, laboratories, high-tech equipment – they are actually very different in different countries, and a wide variety of 'hospital cultures' can be found throughout the world.[71] For example, hospitals in North America and northern Europe tend to be more socially separated from the communities they serve than elsewhere in the world. With the exception of some paediatric and obstetric wards, members of the patient's family or community are rarely allowed to stay overnight in the ward with a sick person, provide them with food, wash and dress them, or contribute to their nursing care. In most cases they are only allowed to visit the patient at often rigidly scheduled visiting hours, under the watchful eye of nurses and doctors. In contrast, in many parts of southern Europe, Asia and Africa, the boundary between hospital and community is much more porous; family members often spend many hours around the sick bed, washing, feeding and tending to the patient's intimate needs. In hospitals in the USA and northern Europe, these roles are usually carried out exclusively by nurses as part of the temporary quasi-family (nurse = mother, doctor = father, patient = child) of health professionals[72] described in Chapter 6.

There are many different ways of viewing the hospital and the many roles it plays in different countries, cultures and communities. For example, as well as a place where disease is cured and suffering alleviated, it can also be seen as:

1 A *refuge* – offering asylum (as it did in the Middle Ages) to those unable to cope in the outside world due to mental or physical ill health or old age.
2 A *factory* – an industrial institution that produces 'cured' people out of the raw material of 'sick people'.
3 A *business* – orientated (especially in the private, corporate sector) to making maximum profit out of the provision of health care.
4 A *temple* – dedicated to a particular religious cosmology (such as Ayurveda) or healing tradition, or to the transcendent power of science over the forces of disease and death.
5 A *university* – dedicated not only to the training of doctors and nurses, but also to the moral instruction of patients, teaching them *post hoc* how their ill health was the logical result of a previous lifestyle, and what they can do to prevent it happening again
6 A *prison* – protecting society by confining those regarded as mad, dissident or very unconventional, against their will.
7 A *city* – a miniature metropolis with each ward a 'suburb', and with its own administration, bureaucracy, workers, security personnel, chapels and stores, together with a constantly changing and involuntary citizenry of patients.

Whatever its local variations, and however it is viewed, the hospital remains the pre-eminent institution of biomedicine(Figure 4.2). It is, as Konner[73] terms it, a 'temple of science'. However, with their large staff and bureaucracy, and advanced diagnostic and treatment technologies, most modern hospitals are extremely expensive to run and are becoming more so. In the USA, for example, hospitals are the biggest spenders of health-care money,

spending about $1000 per American in 1990; nearly a quarter of hospitals' money is spent on administrative costs.[74] In 1960, in the USA, there was one administrator for every 3.17 patients, but by 1990 this had risen to one patient for every 1.43 administrators.[74] In the developing world particularly, these rising costs – and the fact that most of the huge, high-tech hospitals are sited in cities, far from the rural areas where most people live[75] – have led to a reevaluation of the hospital's role. A modern trend has been the development of smaller district hospitals, serving a local community, often in partnership with a network of local primary health-care providers (see Chapter 18), while fewer, large hospitals, with specialized skills and high technology, are reserved for more serious conditions. Despite this shift, in many countries most of the medical resources are still concentrated in large metropolitan hospitals, which are also the main sites for medical technology.

There is a wide variation, however, in the numbers of hospital beds available in different regions of the world, as illustrated by the 2005 *World Health Statistics*[55], even though these do not include numbers of hospital beds in Africa. Overall, these statistics of hospital beds available are probably misleading in the case of some poorer countries, where hospital capacity is often forced to expand beyond the available numbers of beds, and to accommodate extra patients in the corridors, on mattresses or chairs, or even on the bare floor.

The rise of medical technology

Technology can be seen as an extension of the human senses, and of their motor and sensory functions. Just as McCluhan[76] described the media (radio, television) as 'extensions' of the central nervous system and its functions (listening, looking), so does much of medical technology also provide more efficient ways of looking and listening to the human body and to its inner processes.

In every age, and in every society, healers have always made use of some form of equipment – knives, splints, scalpels, probes, spatulas or more

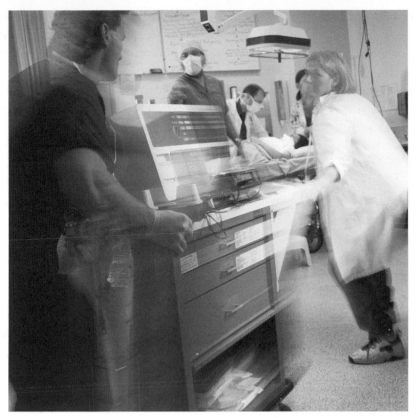

Figure 4.2 With its emphasis on technology and its treatment of severe diseases, the hospital is the main institution of modern, scientific medicine. (Source: EyeWire® by Getty Images™.)

magical items used in rituals. However, modern Western medicine is unique in the increasingly important role, both practical and symbolic, played by technology in both its diagnosis and treatment. Despite the growing cost and complexity of these machines, this 'technological imperative' is increasing every year.

Medical technologies, as complex systems of design and function, are not just physical objects used for a particular purpose. They are also cultural products, telling us something about the social, economic and historical values that produced them at a particular time and in a particular place. They have a range of meanings for those who use them professionally, and for patients who come to depend upon them. In a Western context, this technology expresses modern medicine's desire to master and control the body, its natural processes and its various diseases. However, in other parts of the world the same technology or

equipment may have very different meanings for the people who use it, depending on the social and cultural context. In many non-industrialized societies, for example, even the simple syringe is seen by the 'injectionist' and his clients (see above) as being, in some way, the very embodiment of modern Western medical science.

Foucault[77] has described how in European medicine, the 'medical gaze' of the late eighteenth century began increasingly to focus more on events and changes *within* the patient's body. The doctor concentrated less on the patient's subjective symptoms and visible signs, and instead 'began to perceive what was immediately behind the visible surface... and to map the disease in the secret depths of the body'. Undoubtedly, this shift was aided a few decades later by the invention of new diagnostic equipment. Tenner[78] has described how this process – from Laennec's humble stethoscope in 1816, to Roentgen's discovery of X-rays in 1895 and Herrick's invention of the electrocardiogram in 1918 – led to a greater ability to *localize* disease processes within the body. Sites of pathology could now be pinpointed with greater accuracy than ever before. Although of great benefit to both patients and clinicians, this process has also contributed to a narrowing of medical vision – to the reductionism, mind–body dualism and objectification of body so characteristic today of the disease perspective.

In other ways, too, medical technology has radically altered our sense of the human body. It has had major effects on our perceptions of the body in space, as well as in time. For example, one result of both diagnostic and life support technology is to blur the boundaries of the body; to dissolve the skin as the true border of the individual self.[79] X-rays, magnetic resonance imaging (MRI) scans, ultrasound scans, computed axial tomography (CAT) scans and advanced fibre-optics have all made the body more 'transparent'. Its interior has become more visible, and in some sense exterior. One can now examine its inner structure without any need to cut through the barrier of skin. Furthermore, the increasing use of life-support systems, dialysis machines, monitoring equipment and incubators – as well as the new reproductive technologies (see Chapter 6) – can also contribute towards a blurring of the boundary between self and non-self. Joined to the body, these machines can help create temporary or permanent *cyborgs*, becoming, in effect, external organs (lungs, heart, kidneys, etc.) of the body, and extending it beyond the borders of skin. Commonly this process is linked to the modern metaphor of the body as a machine, kept healthy by spare-part surgery.[79] The effects of this machine dependency, and particularly its violation of the normal body boundaries, has been movingly described by Kirmayer[80] in the case of a haemodialysis patient. Here the patient has to witness his own blood leaving his body, then travelling through plastic tubes into the depths of the machine. Somehow in this electronic being it is mysteriously 'transformed', before once again being returned into the privacy of the body. In a sense the body is turned inside-out; that which is normally inside is now put outside it. A private, hidden physiological process – the circulation of the blood – is now on full public view. The boundaries between self and non-self are no longer as clear as they once were.

In obstetrics, Davis-Floyd[81] also noted the negative effects of this process. She argues that obstetric hospitals in the USA have become like high-tech factories, dedicated to the mass production of perfect babies. In this environment, the overuse of technology conveys a message to the pregnant woman that her own body is merely a defective machine – one that needs to be controlled and directed by (medical) technicians, but not by herself. This in turn can have major emotional consequences for her. Despite this process, Browner[82] notes that many American women still remain ambivalent about the value of technology in their own pregnancies and childbirth (see Chapter 6).

In terms of time, some technologies can widen the gap between social and biological birth and death (see Chapter 9). For example, the development of ultrasound scans for prenatal diagnosis can help create a social identity for the foetus, in the eyes of its parents and doctors, many months before its actual delivery. Social birth can thus precede biological birth, reversing the normal order of events, and this in turn has had an effect on the abortion debate. In contrast, in the care of the dying, life-support systems can extend the gap between biological death (increasingly defined as brain death) and social death (the final death of personhood). In this comatose state, and until the life support system is switched off, the body can be maintained for months or even years. Konner[83] argues that in the case of the very elderly this can create an ethical dilemma, by extending the *quantity* of life, but often only at the expense of the quality.

Modern medical technology has thus had major social and economic costs for those who use it. Furthermore, it is increasingly expensive to buy, operate, maintain and repair. It is labour intensive, and requires specially trained technicians, maintenance workers, repairers and supervisors, as well as a constant supply of electricity and a reliable source of spare parts. As these machines become more complex and advanced, the possibility of their malfunction also increases proportionately.[78] In hospital settings, these complex technologies make health professionals increasingly dependent on outsiders, namely, the highly paid community of experts and engineers who service, maintain and repair them. When introduced into any clinical environment, the machines often require major adjustments in people's behaviour and how they relate to one another. For example, Barley[84] has described the introduction of computed tomography (EBCT) scanners into two hospitals in Massachusetts, USA, and the problems this caused for radiologists, technicians, and patients. Technical breakdowns and malfunctions required numerous social, behavioural and psychological changes, including new rituals, superstitions, and explanatory models for breakdowns, in order to integrate them into daily hospital life.

In poorer, developing countries, the purchase of these expensive technologies can have major impacts on public health policy. They may force a shift of scarce resources away from longer-term preventive medicine and health promotion towards high-tech solutions to social and health problems; from a community-based approach and district hospital system (see Chapter 18) utilizing more 'appropriate' and smaller-scale technologies, towards a focus on acute care in an expensive metropolitan hospital. In countries that cannot afford to maintain or repair them, these technologies may thus be completely inappropriate, often creating dependence on the large overseas companies that produce and maintain them, and supply their spare parts.

Diagnostic technology has also led to the creation of a new tier of 'patients'. These are the products of technology, such as strips of electrocardiogram (ECG or EKG) paper, X-ray plates or printouts of blood tests. Sometimes they are the focus of more medical attention than the patients themselves. For some health professionals these 'paper patients' are as interesting – or even *more* interesting – than the patients themselves. They are easier to interpret, control, quantify and monitor over time, and there is no danger of their being uncooperative. They are also free of such ambiguous, unpredictable aspects of illness as cultural or religious health beliefs. In many cases, though, the increasing overuse of medical technology has been forced on doctors, especially by the fear of being accused of medical malpractice.

Today, in many teaching hospitals, the presentation and discussion of these 'paper patients' – or their electronic equivalents – has become the most common way of teaching medical (and nursing) students about disease. Increasingly, grand rounds, case presentations and teaching sessions, focus more on slides, videos, photographs or computer graphics of the patients' condition – rather than on examining, or questioning, the actual patients themselves.[85]

A final and paradoxical effect of diagnostic technology is that, in some cases, it may make diagnosis, treatment and communication with patients, *more* difficult to achieve.[86] This has resulted from the shift, noted by Feinstein,[87] in how doctors make a medical diagnosis. In the past, doctors diagnosed disease based on what the patient told them about their symptoms (the history) and what they found on physical examination (the examination), as well as on the results of certain tests they performed. To make a complete diagnosis, they often also added in information they had gathered about the patient's lifestyle, family and social background. In contemporary medicine, however, the process of diagnosis has increasingly shifted from this collection of subjective or clinical information (gathered by listening, looking, touching and feeling) towards the use of notionally objective or 'paraclinical' information (gathered by the machines of diagnostic technology). Abnormalities can now be detected by these machines at the cellular, biochemical or even molecular level, even when patients have no abnormal symptoms at all and no subjective sense of anything being wrong with them. This has led to a widening gap (and increased possibilities for conflict) between medical definitions of *disease* and patients' subjective definitions of *illness* – a process described further in Chapter 5. Furthermore, doctors trained mainly to detect paraclinical disease may be less competent to interpret the complex, changing, clinical presentations found in real patients, in real life.[86] This complexity is partly due to the fact that the *same* paraclinical disease as revealed by technology (such as AIDS, cancer, or hypertension) may manifest itself in a variety of *different* clinical forms (such as weakness, pain, swelling, headaches or loss of appetite). Also, different paraclinical diseases (such as hiatus hernia and coronary artery disease) may present with almost identical clinical pictures (such as retrosternal chest pain). For all these reasons, therefore, knowledge of how to interpret both clinical *and* paraclinical data is essential for successful diagnosis, though the over-emphasis on the latter may mitigate against this.

Thus medicine's many new technologies have had major impacts, both positive and negative, on how it is practised. They have influenced how doctors diagnose and treat ill health, and how they relate to their patients. They may also have contributed, in some ways, towards alienation between patients and health professionals. In 1983, an Editorial[88] in the *Journal of the American Medical Association* posed the question: 'Has the machine become the physician?' It was suggested – as many others have since agreed – that this was, in fact, slowly happening (especially in the USA), and that it was having a major emotional effect on patients. The message the patient was now receiving was that of an 'impersonal, technology-dominated (medical) system'. Furthermore: 'The fact that the health care provided in the system may be improved as a result of the technology does not have as much impact as the subtle and hidden message that the machine has become the physician: the definitive adviser. The specialist-physician is metamorphosing into a technocrat and a businessman. The physician retreats behind the machine and becomes an extension of the machine'.[88]

In modern biomedicine, therefore, the machine is now an intrinsic part of almost every doctor–patient interaction. The professional relationship between doctor and patient can now be described as:

Doctor
Patient —— Machine

Whether the machine is be used for diagnosis (CAT scans, X-rays), treatment (dialysis or anesthetic machines), or communication (computers, telephones), it has become the key professional symbol of Western medicine. However, this process may have two negative effects on the doctor–patient relationship: the blurring of boundaries between doctor and machine (as *JAMA* suggests), and those between patient and machine. In the latter case, the patient's body may come to be seen increasingly in mechanical terms, as merely a type of 'soft machine' (see Chapter 2), and the machine itself as a sort of 'patient'. In some hospital wards now, patients have to compete for attention with the monitor machines at their bedside, and their doctors may give closer attention to those machines, and what they are 'saying', than to the patient lying on the bed besides them. Of all the machines used in medicine, though, the most pervasive is undoubtedly the computer – a situation described in more detail in Chapter 13.

Despite the disadvantages of this new situation, however, what Koenig[89] terms the 'technological imperative' of modern medicine still remains, especially in Western societies. In some ways it may also have contributed to the crisis of contemporary medicine.

The 'crisis' in Western medicine

Although it is the dominant ideology of healing world-wide, many believe that biomedicine is in crisis – at least in the Western world[73,75,90]. This is despite its many successes in preventing and treating disease, alleviating suffering, and increasing life expectancy. In recent years a growing public dissatisfaction has been reflected in increasing complaints against doctors, and litigation, media campaigns against the medical profession, and the increased popularity of non-medical and alternative healers.

There are several reasons for this. Paradoxically, some result from the very success of medicine itself. Over the last century, medicine has largely eradicated the major killer infectious diseases in most Western countries, such as smallpox, diphtheria, polio, tetanus, measles and many bacterial infections. Infant and maternal mortality has dropped, and life expectancy increased. As a result, more people are now living long enough to suffer from the *chronic* diseases – a situation that Tenner[78] terms 'revenge of the chronic'. These diseases include diabetes, hypertension, arthritis and Parkinson's disease, as well as other conditions that, like cancer, are diseases of later life. In most cases, a 'quick-fix' cure for these conditions is simply not possible. Instead, one needs a longer-term *care* model. This in turn requires a more cooperative approach to health care; one very different from the current rather authoritarian 'disease' perspective. In chronic diseases such as diabetes, patients have to become *co-healers*, monitoring their own condition and treating themselves on a daily basis, in collaboration with health professionals.[91] This increases the need for increased patient education,[92] and for a deeper understanding of the patient's needs, health beliefs and the realities of their daily lives.

At the same time, the costs of medical care are growing because of the escalating costs of hospitals, technology, drugs, medical bureaucracies, staff salaries, training, litigation and malpractice insurance. It has been estimated that in 2002 spending on health in the USA increased by 9.3 percent to reach the enormous figure of $1.6 trillion.[93] In most societies these rising costs exaggerate the effect of the already unequal distribution of health resources in the population, dividing them even further into those that can afford full medical care and those that cannot.[90] Also, the emphasis on more expensive, high-profile curative procedures – such as heart transplants – rather than on cheaper, more long-term health promotion campaigns to prevent heart disease in the first place, adds to the overall cost of the medical system.

Biomedicine's *iatrogenic* effects are now widely known to the public via the media. In addition to the thalidomide tragedy, many other drug side-effects have recently been reported, as well as a growing dependence on prescribed psychotropic and other medications. In hospital settings, more complex operations and diagnostic procedures all now increase the risk of complications and unwanted side-effects.[78] These include infections from antibiotic-resistant bacteria (which infect about 6 per cent of all hospitalized patients in the USA),[78] and many other adverse events. One detailed study[94,95] of over 30 000 hospital records in New York in the 1980s showed that adverse events occurred in 3.7 per cent of them. They were mainly caused by drug complications (19 per cent), wound infections (14 per cent) and technical complications (13 per cent). Of these adverse events, 70.5 per cent gave rise to disability lasting less than 6 months, 2.6 per cent to permanent disability and 13.6 per cent to death. The study estimated that, among the 2 671 863 patients discharged from New York hospitals in 1984 during the study period, there were 98 609 adverse effects, 27 179 of them involving negligence.

Chronic and resistant diseases

In terms of treatment, a growing range of infectious diseases cannot be cured by medicine and its 'magic bullets'. These include: *viral* diseases, such as HIV/AIDS, hepatitis B and C, Creutzfeld–Jacob disease (CJD) and some forms of influenza; *parasitic* diseases such as new strains of drug-resistant malaria; and *bacterial* diseases such as multidrug-resistant tuberculosis, resulting from the overuse of antibiotics in the past, and other drug-resistant bacteria. The rapid diffusion of infective agents or their vectors through jet travel and mass tourism has also made this situation much worst.

At the present time, control of diseases such as HIV/AIDS and malaria can only be successfully achieved by altering patterns of human behaviour (see Chapters 16 and 17), rather than by vaccines or antimicrobial drugs. This is especially relevant, since in most industrialized societies there is now an increasingly diverse patient population, especially in urban areas. This includes tourists, immigrants, foreign students, expatriate workers, immigrants and refugees, as well as the followers of different cults, religions and lifestyles. Each of these groups often has its own specific view of health and illness, and of how it should be treated. In socially and culturally mixed societies, therefore, a single inflexible model of health education and biomedicine may no longer be acceptable. For these reasons, medicine has to become more of an applied social science as well as an applied medical science.

Changes in the medical role

Doctors in Western medical systems are undergoing major changes in their traditional roles and in what is expected of them. Like other health professionals, they are now expected to be competent in a wide variety of roles. These include those of manager, educator, computer specialist, bureaucrat, government (or medical insurance company) employee, technologist, writer, financial expert, businessman, judge, ethical expert, advocate for patients, family friend and confidant, as well as that of healer. Many feel that their clinical autonomy has been reduced by the growing pressures of government bureaucracies, insurance companies, hospitals, medical schools and health maintenance organizations.[96] The historical successes of medical science, together with the decline in organized religion, has also led to exaggerated expectations of doctors. Often they are expected to behave as secular 'priests', in their own 'temples of science',[73] even when they have no pastoral training to do so. A further issue for the medical profession is that of *information overload*. According to Haines[97], there are currently over 20 000 medical journals world-wide, and these publish a total of two million articles each year. (If stacked on top of another, the pile would be 500 m high.) He estimates that a general physician would have to digest 19 original articles *every day* in order to keep up to date in his subject.

All these factors add up to major changes in the contemporary medical system, how it is perceived, and the role that it plays in any situation of health care pluralism. If the critics of biomedicine are correct, and the system *is* in crisis, then a very different paradigm for the practice of medicine will be required in the future.

THERAPEUTIC NETWORKS

In any society, people who become ill and who are not helped by self-treatment make choices about who to consult in the popular, folk or professional sectors for further help. These choices are influenced by the context in which they are made, including the types of helper actually available, whether payment for their services has to be made, whether the patient can afford to pay for these services, and the 'Explanatory Model' that the sick person uses to explain the origin of the ill health. This Model, described fully in Chapter 5, provides explanations for the aetiology, symptoms, physiological changes, natural history and treatment of the illness. On this basis, patients and their families choose what seems to be the appropriate source of advice and treatment for the condition. Illnesses such as colds are treated by relatives, supernatural illnesses (such as 'spirit possession') by sacred folk healers and natural illnesses by physicians, especially if the illnesses are very severe. If, for example, the ill health is ascribed to divine punishment for a moral transgression, then, as Snow[14] points out, 'Prayer and repentance, not penicillin, cure sin', though both may be used simultaneously: a doctor for treating physical symptoms and a priest or faith healer for treating the cause.

In this way, ill people frequently use several *different* types of healer and healing at the same time, or in sequence. This may be done on the pragmatic basis that 'two (or more) heads are better than one'. For example, Scott[98] describes the case of an African-American woman from South Carolina, living in Miami, Florida. Believing that she had been 'fixed' (bewitched), she treated herself with olive oil and drops of turpentine on sugar cubes. When this failed to relieve her symptoms (abdominal pain), she consulted two 'root doctors' (who gave her magical powders and candles to burn, and prayed over her), a 'sanctified woman' (who massaged her and prayed for her) and two local hospitals for X-rays and gastrointestinal tests to 'find out what is down there'. At one stage she was following the advice of all three folk healers simultaneously. As Scott points out, her contacts with doctors were not for curative purposes, but rather 'to check the effectiveness of the folk therapy' at each stage. Each of these healers may redefine the patient's problem in their own idiom, such as 'peptic ulcer' or 'witchcraft'. This simultaneous use of multiple forms of therapy is becoming increasingly common in most complex societies, especially in the presence of serious illness. Many people diagnosed as having cancer, for example, tend to change their behaviour and their diets, increase their intake of vitamins, pray more, join a self-help group, and consult with alternative or traditional healers[99] *in addition* to their biomedical treatment.

Ill people are at the centres of therapeutic *networks*, which are connected to all three sectors of the health-care system. Advice and treatment pass along the links in this network, beginning with advice from family, friends, neighbours and friends of friends, and then moving on to sacred or secular folk healers, or physicians. Even after advice is given it may be discussed and evaluated by other parts of the patient's network, in the light of their own knowledge or experience. As Stimson[100] has noted, a doctor's treatment is often evaluated 'in the light of his past performance, with what other people have experienced, and compared with what the person expected the doctor to do'. In this way ill people make choices, not only between different types of healer (popular, professional or folk), but also between diagnoses and advice that *makes sense* to them and those that do not. In the latter case the result may be non-compliance, or a shift to another part of the therapeutic network.

HEALTH CARE PLURALISM IN THE UNITED KINGDOM

In the UK, as in other complex industrial societies, there is a wide range of therapeutic options available for the alleviation and prevention of physical discomfort or emotional distress, and popular, folk and professional sectors of health-care can be identified. This section concentrates mainly on the popular and folk sectors. The professional sector has already been examined in detail by medical sociologists such as Stacey[101] and Levitt[102]. An overview of the three sectors of health care in the UK illustrates the full range of options available for the management of misfortune, including ill health.

THE POPULAR SECTOR

The two studies by Elliott-Binns,[103,104] from 1970 and 1985 quoted below, are among the few dealing in detail with lay therapeutic networks in the UK. Other studies have concentrated on the phenomenon of self-medication. For example, in Dunnell and Cartwright's[105] large survey in 1972, the use of self-prescribed medication was twice as common as the use of prescribed medicines. Self-medication was most commonly taken for temperature, headache, indigestion and sore throats. These, and other symptoms were common in the sample, but while 91 per cent of adults reported one or more abnormal symptoms during the previous 2 weeks, only 16 per cent of them had consulted a doctor for this. Self-medication was often used as an alternative to consulting the doctor, who was expected to deal with more serious conditions. The idea of using a particular self-prescribed patent medicine came from a number of sources, including: spouses (7 per cent), parents and grandparents (18 per cent), other relatives (5 per cent), friends (13 per cent) and the doctor (10 per cent). Fifty-seven per cent of the sample thought the local pharmacist a good source of health advice for many conditions. This is confirmed in Sharpe's study[106] in 1979 of a London pharmacy where, in a 10-day period, 72 requests for advice were received, especially for skin complaints, respiratory tract infections, dental problems, vomiting and diarrhoea. In an earlier study by Jefferys and colleagues[107] in a working-class housing estate, two-thirds of people interviewed were taking some self-prescribed medication, often in addition to a prescribed drug. Laxatives and aspirins were most commonly prescribed. Aspirin and other analgesics were used for many symptoms, including 'arthritis and anaemia, bronchitis and backache, menstrual disorders and menopausal symptoms, nerves and neuritis, influenza and insomnia, colds and catarrh, and of course for headaches and rheumatism'.

The hoarding and exchanging of medication, both patent and prescribed, is common in the UK. People who have been ill sometimes act as what Hindmarch[108] termed 'over-the-fence physicians', sharing their prescribed drugs with a friend, relative or neighbour with similar symptoms. Warburton[109] found that 68 per cent of young adults in his study in Reading admitted having received psychotropic drugs from friends or relatives. In his 1981 study in Leeds, Hindmarch also found that an average of 25.9 prescribed tablets or capsules *per person* were hoarded by people living in a selected street. Decisions whether to take prescribed drugs are also part of popular health culture, and lay evaluation of the drug as 'making sense' or not may, as Stimson[100] suggests, influence non-compliance. The rate of this phenomenon has been estimated by him at 30 per cent or more.

Elliot-Binns's second study in 1985[104] showed an increasing use of impersonal sources of health advice and information (books, magazines and the media). Since then, however, another impersonal source of medical advice – the *Internet* – is playing an ever-increasing role in people's lives, and in how they understand and deal with their own ill-health and that of their families. This important development is described in more detail in Chapter 13.

Few studies have been done on the actual efficacy of popular health care in the UK. Blaxter and Paterson,[110] in their 1980 study of working-class mothers in Aberdeen, Scotland, found that common children's illnesses (such as a discharging ear) were often ignored if they did not interfere with everyday functioning. However, in another study by Pattison and colleagues[111] the findings were very different, and it was found that mothers were able to recognize their babies' illnesses and seek medical help, even with their first children.

In the UK, a major group of individuals who provide health advice and care, are what one might term *voluntary aid workers* – often working for self-help groups (see below), or for various charitable organizations (such as the St John's Ambulance Service, the Red Cross, the Samaritans or Age Concern). In most cases these individuals receive some training from the organizations that they work with. Included here are the very large number of *counselors* now available – a number that has steadily increased since the 1990s. According to Árnason[112] about 2.5 million people in the UK now use counselling skills in the widest sense of the word, and this includes some 300 000 people who work as voluntary counsellors (plus 8000 who earn a living by counseling).

Self-help groups

An important component of the popular sector is the wide range of *self-help groups* that have blossomed in the UK since the Second World War. Like other parts of the popular sector, members' *experience*, not education, is important, especially experience of a specific misfortune. The total number of members of these groups is not known, though they number many thousands. One website *Self Help UK*[113] lists over 1000 groups loosely labelled 'self-help' in the UK or Eire, while another *Patient UK*[114] lists 1968 self-help or patient support groups. Overall, these groups can be classified on the basis of why people join them:

1 *Physical problems* (Migraine Trust, National Back Pain Association, Guillain–Barré Syndrome Support Group).
2 *Emotional problems* (National Phobics Society, Schizophrenia Association of Great Britain).

3 *Relatives* of those with physical, emotional or addiction problems (Association of Parents of Vaccine Damaged Children, Al-Anon, National Council for Carers and their Elderly Parents, Families Anonymous).

4 *Family problems* (Family Welfare Association, Parentline Plus).

5 *Addiction problems* (Alcoholics Anonymous, Gamblers Anonymous, Sexaholics Anonymous).

6 *Social problems*, including:

  a *Sexual non-conformity* (Lesbian and Gay Foundation, Lesbian Line, Gay Switchboards);

  b *One-parent families* (Families Need Fathers, Gingerbread, Single Parent Action Network);

  c *Life changes* (Pre-retirement Association, National Association of Widows);

  d *Social isolation* (Meet-a-Mum Association, Carers UK).

7 *Women's groups* (Women's Health Concern, Rape Crisis groups, Mothers' Union).

8 *Ethnic minority groups* (Ethiopian Health Support Network, Cypriot Advisory Service, Asian People's Disability Alliance, Organization of Blind African Caribbeans).

Most self-help groups have, as Levy[115] notes, one or more of the following aims or activities:

- information and referral
- counselling and advice
- public and professional education
- political and social activity
- fund-raising for research or services
- provision of therapeutic services, under professional guidance
- mutual supportive activities in small groups.

Many groups are 'communities of suffering', where *experience* of a type of emotional problem of misfortune is the credential for membership. For example, the National Phobics society website states that 'Our belief is that those who have experienced anxiety disorders are best placed to provide support to other sufferers because they are able to truly understand the impact these condi-

tions have on people's lives'.[116] In Levy's[115] study in 1982 of 71 self-help groups, 41 had membership reserved for people suffering a particular affliction, while in eight membership was mainly composed of relatives of those afflicted. Some groups overlap with the professional sector, like the Psoriasis Society; its 4000 members include sufferers and their relatives, doctors, nurses, and cosmetic and pharmaceutical companies.[117] Other groups are hostile to orthodox medicine, and have an antibureaucratic and antiprofessional stance.

Robinson and Henry[118] give a number of reasons for the growth of these groups in the popular sector, including the perceived failure of the existing medical and social services to meet people's needs, the recognition by members of the value of mutual help, and the role of the media in publicizing the extent of shared problems in the community. Other reasons might be the nostalgia for community (especially the caring community of the extended family) in an impersonal, industrialized world, as a coping mechanism for those with stigmatized conditions or marginal social status, and as a way of explaining and dealing with misfortune in a more personalized way.[119]

THE FOLK SECTOR

In the UK, as in other Western societies, this sector is relatively small and ill-defined. While local faith healers, gypsy fortune tellers, clairvoyants, psychic consultants, herbalists and 'wise women' still exist in many rural areas, the forms of diagnosis and healing characteristic of the folk sector are more likely to be found in urban areas, especially in alternative or complementary medicine. All estimates of the total number of consultations per year with CAM practitioners agree that the number is steadily rising.[120] One study, in 1981, estimated these consultations at 11.7–15.4 million consultations per year, and that about 1.5 million people (2.5 per cent of the total UK population) received some form of unconventional therapy during the course of a year, compared with the 72 per cent of the population that consulted their GP during a year.[120] Of the people consulting with CAM practitioners, 33 per cent were at the same time also receiving treatment from their medical practitioners.[120] As in non-Western societies, many CAM practitioners aim at a holistic view of the patient, which includes psychological, social, moral and physical dimensions, as well as an emphasis on health as balance. For example, a pamphlet from the National Institute of Medical Herbalists[121] states: 'The herbal practitioner regards disease as being a disturbance of the physiological and mental/emotional equilibrium which is the state of good health and, being aware of the forces of healing within the body, directs the treatment towards restoring that balance'. Similarly, from the Community Health Foundation:[122] 'Health is more than just the absence of pain or discomfort. Good health is a dynamic relationship between the individual, friends, family and the environment within which we live and work'.

Herbalism, faith healing and midwifery probably have the deepest roots in the UK. The first description of herbal remedies dates from 1260 AD, and numerous other 'herbals' have been published in the past 400 years. In 1636, for example, a herbal compiled by John Parkinson contained details of the medicinal use of 3800 plants.[123] Midwifery, another traditional form of health care, has been absorbed into the professional sector, especially since their compulsory registration under the 1902 Midwives' Act. Other forms of healing have been imported from abroad, such as acupuncture, homeopathy and osteopathy.

The folk sector includes both sacred and secular healers. An example of the former is the National Federation of Spiritual Healers (NFSH), who define spiritual healing as 'all forms of healing the sick in body, mind and spirit by means of the laying-on of hands or by either prayer or meditation whether or not in the actual presence of the patient'.[124] Since 1965, under an agreement with more than 1500 National Health Service hospitals, NFSH healer members may attend those patients in hospital who request their services. In addition, there are a number of Spiritualist Churches and healing circles in the UK that practise spiritual healing through prayer or the laying-on of hands; these include Christian Science Churches and some Afro-Caribbean Pentecostalist Churches. Christian healing is encouraged by the Christian Fellowship of Healing, the Churches' Council of Health and Healing, and the Guild of St Raphael.[125] Overall, many thousands of people practice spiritual healing and 'laying on of hands' in the UK. The two largest organizations of healers are the NFSH, founded in 1954, with 6000 members in the UK and others abroad,[126] and the Spiritualists' National Union with 368 affiliated spiritualist churches, with over 16 000 members.[127]

In contrast, an unknown number of *Wicca* or white magic groups or covens practise magical healing; writing in *Doctor* magazine 1981, de Jonge[128] claimed that there were 7000 'covens' in Britain, with a total membership of 91 000.

As a form of alternative healing, *homoeopathy* has a special position in the UK. The principles of homeopathy were first enunciated in Germany by Samuel Hahnemann in 1796, and the first homeopathic hospital in the UK was founded in London in 1849. There has been a long association between the British Royal Family and homoeopathy; in 1937 Sir John Weir was appointed homeopathic physician to King George VI, and this link with Royalty remains. In 1948 the homeopathic hospitals were incorporated into the National Health Service. There are now National Health Service (NHS) homeopathic hospitals in London, Liverpool, Bristol, Tunbridge Wells and Glasgow.[46,129] It was estimated that in 1971 there were about 383 available beds in homoeopathic hospitals, and 51 037 attendances at homeopathic medical outpatients clinics.[130] These hospitals are staffed by doctors qualified in orthodox medicine, who undertake postgraduate training in homoeopathy. In addition, in 1996 there were two professional associations for non-medically qualified homeopaths and 21 training schools.[129] Although it is based on different premises from orthodox medicine, homoeopathy in the UK enjoys greater legitimacy than other forms of alternative healing. Like other forms of CAM, it spans both folk and professional sectors of health care.

There is a two-way influence between these two sectors. Many orthodox doctors, for example, practise one or more forms of alternative healing. They are organized into collegial organizations such as the UK Homoeopathic Medical Association, the British Medical Acupuncture Society, and the British Society of Medical and Dental Hypnosis.[131] Similarly, alternative healers have been influenced, to a variable degree, by the training, organization, techniques, credentials and self-presentation of orthodox doctors, and are increasingly becoming 'professionalized' – forming professional organizations with an educational structure, and registers of accredited members. Some are organized on a collegial basis, like other British professions, for example, the British College of Acupuncture, the National Institute of Medical Herbalists, the Society of Homeopaths, and the General Council and Register of Osteopaths.[132] In 1979, the British Acupuncture Association offered a 2-year training course for a Licentiate, and a further year's study for a Bachelor's degree in acupuncture. It had 100 students in the UK, with 33 medically qualified and 420 non-medically qualified members on its register.[133] Over the last decade, pressure for professionalization has come not only from the healers themselves but also from the UK Government, the European Union, the medical profession and the consumers themselves.[131,134] The healers have responded in a variety of ways, from setting up their own professional groupings with voluntary self-regulation, such as the ones listed above, to seeking legal status and statutory regulation by the government.[135]

At the other end of the spectrum are the more individual forms of folk healing, including clairvoyants, astrologers, psychic healers, clairaudientes, palmists, Celtic mediums, Tarot readers, Gypsy fortune tellers and Irish seers, whose advertisements appear in the popular press, magazines, handouts and such publications as *Prediction, Horoscope* and *Old Moore's Almanack*. Many of these act as lay counsellors or psychotherapists: 'Do you have a health worry that you cannot get help on? Have you a personal or family worry you need advice on? Then maybe I can help you with both. I was born the 7th Son of a 7th Son', etc.[136] The majority of this group use some form of *divination*, using coins, dice, tea leaves, crystal balls, Tarot cards or palmistry to decipher supernatural and cosmic influences on the individual and reveal the causes of unhappiness, ill health or other misfortune. From the patient's perspective, this approach may have the advantage of placing responsibility for misfortune beyond the individual's control, where fate, bad luck, birth sign, or even the malevolence of another person, and not the patient's own behaviour, are the causes of misfortune. Some of these healers are also undergoing professionalization. For example, since it was founded in 1976, the British Astrological and Psychic Society has promoted a variety of esoteric, spiritual and New Age teachings, and its members offer a wide range of 'interpretive and divinatory arts'.[137] The forms of divination they offer include astrology, palmistry, numerology, aura readings, graphology, trance mediumship, I Ching, Tarot cards, clairvoyance, clairaudience, clairsentience and psychic art. It publishes a National Register of Consultants, has defined criteria for entry, has a Code of Ethics and Conduct, and offers courses and certificates in different forms of divination. Its booklet states that its 'consultants are competent in several disciplines and can move between them in order to fulfill a client's given needs'.[137]

Many ethnic minorities and immigrants in Britain continue to consult their own traditional healers, at least under certain circumstances. These include Muslim *hakims* and Hindu *vaids* from the Indian subcontinent (one estimate is that there are about 300 of them in the UK),[138] practitioners of traditional Chinese medicine (TCM) (including herbalism, acupuncture, and moxibustion), African *marabouts* and *obeah men*, and Caribbean *spiritual healers*. Newspapers for the South Asian, Caribbean and African communities, such as *Eastern Eye, Caribbean Times* and *The Voice*, all carry advertisements for a variety of spiritual healers and advisers, who deal with a range of personal problems, from relationships, health and financial worries to bad luck and witchcraft. Many of these healers ascribe their healing powers to the fact that they come from a 'healing family', often of many generations.

One fairly new group of healers – in the broadest sense of the word – are those involved primarily in improving their client's physical appearance, and thereby their psychological state. Throughout the UK there has been a proliferation of 'beauty clinics', staffed by 'beauty therapists'. Both the setting and atmosphere of these clinics is quasi-medical, with consultations, white coats, rows of bottles, complex machines and impressive diplomas on the wall. They are all part of a much wider phenomenon[–] the gradual 'medicalization' of all aspects of the human body, including its appearance.

Professional organizations of alternative healers

There are now many different professional bodies in the UK who practice and promote 'alternative', 'complementary' or 'holistic' forms of therapy. One of the largest is the Federation of Holistic Therapists who represent over 20 000 professional therapists, including practitioners of beauty therapy, electrolysis, aromatherapy, reflexology, and other forms of therapy. It publishes the journal *International Therapist*.[139]

In recent years, as there has been growing criticism of conventional medicine in some official quarters, so has there been a parallel increase in all forms of complementary and alternative medicine, and a burgeoning of organizations connected with it. Many of them aim to counter the skepticism of the medical establishment by increasing their research activities into these forms of therapy. For example, the Research Council for Complementary Medicine was founded in 1983 'to develop and extend the evidence base for complementary medicine in order to provide practitioners and their patients with information about the effectiveness of individual therapies and the treatment of specific conditions'.[140] The Institute for Complementary Medicine was founded in 1982 'to provide the public with information on Complementary Medicine'. It has initiated research 'to develop ways to control, regulate and research all the different disciplines and techniques in ways that protect the qualified practitioners and ensure safety of the general public', and administers the British Register of Complementary Practitioners (BRCP) which lists recognized complementary practitioners, and has 18 autonomous Divisions.[141] The British Holistic Medical Association, founded in 1983, aims 'To educate doctors, medical students, allied health professionals and members of the general public in the principles and practice of holistic medicine'.[142] It has both medical and lay members, and publishes the *Journal of Holistic Healthcare*. The British General Council of Complementary Medicine exists 'to advance the education in and the science and practice of complementary medicine for the benefit of the public'.[143]

There are no precise details about the total numbers of non-orthodox healers in the UK and the total number of consultations with them. In the early 1980s one major study, privately commissioned by the Threshold Foundation,[144] estimated that in 1980–1981 there were 7800 full- and part-time professional alternative practitioners in Britain, and about 20 000 men and women who practised spiritual and religious healing. There were also 2075 doctors who practised one or more alternative therapies although, with the exception of homoeopathy, their training was 'minimal'. The alternative healers (both medical and lay) included 758 acupuncturists, 540 chiropractors, 303 herbalists, 360 homeopaths, 630 hypnotherapists and 800 osteopaths. They also estimated that alternative practitioners spend, on average, eight times longer with their patients than do orthodox doctors. (First consultations in traditional acupuncture and homeopathy can take up to 2 hours each). Many of these practitioners practised more than one form of therapy. In a study in 1984 of 411 practitioners, 51 per cent practised a second therapy and 25 per cent a third.[144]

In 1989, The Institute for Complementary Medicine[145] estimated that there were about 15 000 alternative practitioners in the UK in professional practice. They defined a professional 'practitioner' here as an individual who is 'in full time practice, who is a member of a professional organization with a code of ethics and practice and a disciplinary committee to enforce them, and who is covered by personal indemnity and a third party liability'. On this basis, their figures included 7000 spiritual healers, 1500 osteopaths, 1500 acupuncturists, 1000 massage practitioners, 500 hypnotherapists, 350 nutritionists, 350 chiropractors, 300 reflexologists and 250 aromatherapists.

More recently, in 1995, Fulder[129] estimated that there were about 50 000 alternative practitioners in the UK (about 60 per cent more than the total number of general practitioners). They included 3039 osteopaths, 3000 acupuncturists, 1200 homeopaths, 900 chiropracters, 750 naturopaths, 600 herbalists and 219 radionics practitioners. Walker and Budd[135] reported that one of the fastest growing complementary therapies in the UK is aromatherapy, and that the number of registered therapists has risen from 2500 in 1991 to 6000 in 2000.

Training schools and professional associations for non-medically qualified healers continue to proliferate. For example, by 1996 the (non-medically qualified) homoeopaths had two professional associations and 21 training schools, while the reflexologists had 13 professional organizations and over 100 schools.[131]

In 1993 The British Medical Association published a detailed report into alternative medicine in the UK,[146] and their conclusions were cautiously positive: 'It is clear that there are many encouraging initiatives currently taking place in the field of non-conventional therapy, and it is to be hoped that good practice can be extrapolated for general use'. However, they recommended that, before making use of it, potential clients should enquire:

1 Whether the therapist is registered with a professional organization.
2 Whether that body has a public register of members, a code of practice, effective disciplinary procedures and sanctions and a complaints mechanism.
3 About the type of qualifications the therapist has, and where they were obtained.
4 How long he or she has been practising.
5 Whether the therapist is covered by any form of malpractice insurance.

By virtue of the Osteopaths Act of 2000 and the Chiropracters Act of 2001, osteopathy and chiropractic finally joined the ranks of recognized health care and paramedical professions for the first time,[135] just as the pharmacists had done in 1852 and 1868, the dentists in 1878, and the midwives in 1902. In 1993, the UK Parliament set up the General Osteopathic Council to regulate the profession, and set up a single register of practitioners, while a General Chiropractic Council was set up in 1994.[135]

However, not all alternative healers want to become 'professions', under the direct or indirect control of the government or the medical system. Many are ideologically opposed to all aspects of the medical model and what they see as its limitations and dangers; thus they see themselves as truly *alternative*, rather than complementary, to it. Nevertheless, many forms of alternative medicine in the UK besides osteopathy and chiropractic – especially herbalism, acupuncture and aromatherapy – are gradually undergoing the same process of professionalization as is happening to traditional folk healers in parts of the developing world.[27, 131,134]

Consultations with CAM practitioners

Looked at in perspective, consultations with CAM practitioners in the UK often have certain features in common, when compared with rushed consultations with an NHS medical practitioner. Many (though not all) of these features were once part of 'old-style' medical practice, especially in rural areas. They include:

- Consultations generally last longer, giving the clients more time to explore their 'illness' as well as their 'disease'
- Consultations are often more tactile, sometimes involving massage, or physical manipulation
- Consultations are often more 'holistic', in the sense of placing the individual's suffering in the wider social, psychological or spiritual context of their lives
- Consultations often have a 'religious' or mystical element (sometimes borrowed from Eastern religions) and do not just focus on physical abnormalities
- Treatments usually do not penetrate body boundaries, with the sole exception of acupuncture (the growing acceptability of acupuncture may well be due to familiarity with injections, as a common form of treatment)
- Consultations and treatment are paid for, since most CAM in the UK is in the private sector, and not covered by the NHS. This may give clients a greater feeling of control over the consultation, and the choice of practitioner

THE PROFESSIONAL SECTOR

This includes the wide range of medical and paramedical professionals, each with their own perceptions of ill health, forms of treatment, defined areas of competence, internal hierarchy, technical jargon and professional organizations. In 1980 the Office of Health Economics[147] estimated the numbers of all health professionals within the NHS as 23 674 general practitioners, 31 421 hospital medical staff, 301 081 hospital nursing staff, 17 375 hospital midwives, 32 990 community health nurses and 2949 community health midwives. In 1981 the community nurses included 9244 health visitors.[148] However, by 2005 the total number of nurses had risen to 672, 897 (including 33 000 working as midwives),[149] over 50 per cent of the total staff employed by the NHS.[150] Of these nurses, only 10.73 per cent were male.[149] In addition there are a large number of chiropodists, physiothera-

pists, radiographers, occupational therapists, pharmacists and hospital technicians. Each of these categories offers some form of defined professional care, but they may also be called upon for informal advice about illness as part of the popular sector.

Despite its large size, it has been estimated[151] that about 75 per cent of abnormal symptoms are treated *outside* the professional sector – which sees only the tip of the 'iceberg of illness' – and the rest are dealt with in the popular and folk sectors of health care.

In the UK, there are two complementary forms of professional medical care, the National Health Service and private medical care, though there is an overlap of personnel between the two.

The National Health Service

Since 1948 the NHS has offered free and unrestricted access to health care in the UK, at both the general practitioner and hospital levels. These two forms of medical care have different genealogies and different perspectives on ill health. The precursors of the general practitioners were specialized tradesmen called apothecaries. From 1617 they were licensed only to sell drugs prescribed by physicians. By 1703 they were entitled to see patients and prescribe for them. They became the GPs of the poor and middle classes. Physicians had a higher status initially than surgeons or apothecaries, and for centuries were the only 'real' doctors. Both physicians and surgeons enhanced their position during the growth of the hospital sector, which began in about 1700. To some extent the split and difference in status between GP and hospital medicine still persists, and is reflected in the allocation of resources. In England and Wales in 1972, for example, more than half the NHS budget was spent on the hospital sector, even though only 2.3 per cent of patients were actually cared for as hospital inpatients.[152] The NHS remains one of the largest employers in the country – and in the world – with a total workforce in 2004 of 1.3 million, including 117 036 doctors.[150]

The hospital sector

Many of the organizational and cultural aspects of hospitals have already been described, especially that of specialization. In 1974, according to Levitt,[153] there were 42 recognized clinical specialties within the NHS hospital service, though the number has increased considerably since then, with the addition of various subspecialties. There are also numerous specialty hospitals, such as eye, ear, nose and throat (ENT), heart or maternity hospitals. The hospital is the place where 99 per cent of people in the UK are born,[154] and most will die. Between those two points, many people associate it with the more severe forms of ill health that cannot be dealt with by GPs or by the popular or folk sectors. As in other Western societies, the emphasis is on the individual patient as a case or problem to be solved in as short a time as possible and with maximum efficiency. To a large extent, the social, familial, religious and economic aspects of the patient's life are invisible to the hospital staff, though attempts are made to gather this information via social workers. The emphasis is mainly on the identification and treatment of physical disease, though this is less true of psychiatric hospitals. Looked at in perspective, the hospital service deals mostly with acute, severe or sometimes life-threatening episodes of ill health, as well as birth or death. It is less orientated towards dealing with the subjective meanings associated with illness, which are usually dealt with in the popular or folk sectors, or by ministers of religion. Overall, in the period 1997–98 a total of 52 per cent of NHS gross expenditure was spent on hospital services, while only 10 per cent was spent on community health services, and 8 per cent on general medical services (general practice).[155]

The general practitioner service

Unlike the USA, this area of health care is largely separated from hospital medicine, and this situation has existed for some time. For example, in 1976 of the 482 782 hospital beds allocated in England, Scotland and Wales, only 13 665 (2.8 per cent) were 'general practitioner beds', and 5406 of these were obstetric beds.[156] In 1978, in England and Wales, there were only 350 GP-run cottage hospitals, with an average of 20–40 beds each.[157] While GPs can visit the wards and discuss management of their patients with the hospital medical staff, most of the responsibility for medical care rests with the hospital.

Although in 1976 each GP had, according to Levitt,[158] an average of 2347 patients on his or her list, this number has now dropped to about 1700.[159] In 2004 there were a total of 41 574 GPs in the UK, a 14.6 per cent increase since 1997.[159] Not all of these GPs work full-time, and the full-time equivalent (FTE) of this number is 33 915 GPs. The proportion of female GPs in the UK has also increased steadily from 30.35 per cent in 1997 to 36.67 per cent in 2004.[159]

General practice medicine is home- and community-based, and social, psychological and familial factors are considered relevant in making a diagnosis. According to Harris,[160] 'all diagnoses have a social component, whether or not there are social problems' and 'in general practice it is easy to appreciate how a patient's illness and social circumstances are related, because the social circumstances are visible'. Similarly, Hunt[161] believes that GPs should 'put care of the patient's mind before that of his body', and 'the family doctor's awareness of what patients think and feel is vitally important for the whole of his or her work'. Unlike most hospital doctors, the British GP is often a familiar figure in the community. Most live locally, take part in local community activities, dress in 'civilian' clothes and use everyday language in their consultations (Figure 4.3). As well as caring for ill people, they are associated with many of the natural milestones of life: they do antenatal and postnatal examinations, perform check-ups on infants, give immunizations and contraceptive advice, carry out cervical smears, deal with marital and school problems, and counsel bereaved families. Unlike hospital doctors (and most folk healers) they make home visits, and deal with more than one generation of a family. Unlike the hospital sector, the illnesses they deal with tend to be relatively minor; in one 1971 study of the morbidity of 2500 patients in an NHS family practice in one year, 1365 had minor illnesses, 588 chronic illness, and only 288 major illness.[162] Although consultations with GPs are usually quite short (one study put them at 5–6 minutes, on average),[163] patients may be called back for repeated consultations or follow-up as often as is necessary.

In the 1970s, according to Levitt,[162] the GP was the first point of contact for about 90 per cent of those who sought professional medical help under the NHS. Since then, however, while the NHS GP still remains the most common first point of contact for patients, more and more patients are tending to bypass them by going directly to the Accident and Emergency (Casualty) departments of their local hospital, telephoning NHS Direct (see Chapter 18), getting health information from the Internet or from other people, or paying for treatment from 'alternative' practitioners such as osteopaths chiropractors, massage therapists, or psychotherapists.

Increasingly, most NHS GPs now work as part of 'primary health-care teams';[164] these usually include receptionists, practice nurses and counsellors employed directly by the GP, as well as health visitors, district nurses, community psychiatric nurses, community midwives and social workers employed by the NHS. General practitioners, in association with their primary health-care team, share some of the attributes of the folk sector, particularly the emphasis on 'illness' (see Chapter 5) – that is, the social, psychological and moral dimensions of ill health – and on the normal milestones of human life. From 2000 onwards, GPs, nurses, dentists, hospitals, walk-in centres, and other aspects of primary health-care have all been incorporated into large regional *Primary Care Trusts* (PCTs): organizations responsible for planning and commissioning health care services for their local populations – ranging from 50 000 to 250 000 – and for integrating medical and social care.[165]

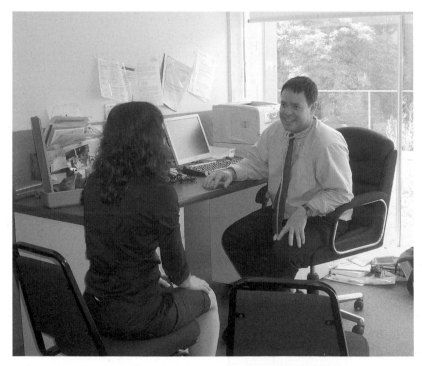

Figure 4.3 A National Health Service general practitioner and his patient in London, UK. (Source: © S Rankin. Reproduced with permission.)

The nursing service

Nurses and midwives form the largest professional group within the NHS. As noted above, in 1990 they comprised over 50 per cent of its total personnel.[150] The majority of the nursing service is female, while the majority of doctors are male. However, about 10 per cent of the nursing staff in NHS hospitals are now male (the percentage is even higher in psychiatric hospitals), but very few male nurses work in the community.[166] In 2005, of the total of 672 897 nurses registered in the UK, 10.7 per cent were male and the percentage of men in nursing has not risen much in the last decade.[149] The vast majority of midwives are female, and in 2003 out of a total of 33 000 midwives only 102 of them were male.[167] Most nurses work in the hospital sector, the remainder in the community. Within the hospitals, nurses spend many more hours in direct patient care than any of the medical hierarchy, and yet have a lower income and lower prestige than doctors

Like the medical staff, the nurses are organized into their own professional hierarchies. In many UK hospitals, this hierarchy ranges from Director of Nursing down through the various grades of Senior Nurse Manager, Clinical Nurse Specialist, Ward Sister/Ward Manager, Staff Nurse, Enrolled Nurse and Nursing Auxiliary/Health Care Assistant. Many hospital nurses specialize in different areas of care, such as ophthalmics, orthopaedics, accident and emergency, coronary or intensive care, and have extra qualifications in addition to their basic training. Various specialist nurses – Clinical Nurse Specialists – have a liaison role between the hospital and the community; for example, those working in palliative care, or with diabetic or stoma patients or as incontinence advisers. Within the community some nurses, also with extra qualifications, work as District Nurses, others as Community Midwives, Health Visitors, School Nurses, Practice Nurses (working within a GP practice), or as hospital-based Community Psychiatric Nurses. Unlike in the USA, the emerging and important role of Nurse Practitioners is not yet formally recognized in terms of a specific qualification. Despite this they now work in a variety of contexts, in some cases carrying out tasks previously dealt with by doctors.

Some of the features of the nursing profession are described further in Chapter 6.

Private medical care

This form of health care preceded the NHS, and now coexists with it. It grew rapidly from the late 1970s to the early 1990s, encouraged by the government of the time. In 1971 only 2.1 million in the UK were covered by private health insurance; by 1990 it had tripled to 6.7 million (almost 12 per cent of the UK population),[168] but by 1999 it had stabilized at about 11 per cent of the total population.[169] The initial increase resulted partly from cutbacks in the NHS that reduced the number of hospital beds and increased waiting lists for operations and outpatient appointments (by 1990 there were 710 300 people, or 1 per cent of the UK population, on waiting lists for inpatient admissions to NHS hospitals).[170] However, for poorer people, private health care has long been an unaffordable luxury: in England in 1987, for example, 27 per cent of those in professional occupational groups but only 1 per cent of unskilled manual labourers, were covered by private medical insurance.[168]

Today there is a considerable overlap in personnel between private and public medical care, though some doctors practise private medicine only. There are several private hospitals and clinics, and a number of large health funds. Also, with the exception of homoeopathy and, occasionally, acupuncture, all forms of alternative or folk healing are in the private sector. From some patients' perspective, private medicine offers more control over time and choice of treatment when they are ill. Consultation times are longer in the private sector, and this provides more time for explanations of the diagnosis, aetiology, prognosis and treatment of their condition. There are also shorter waiting lists for consultations with specialists or for surgical operations, and the patient has a choice of specialist and of hospital. Control over time and choice when ill is largely confined to those with an income sufficient to afford private health insurance, or those who work for large organizations that provide their employees with such insurance.

The NHS and private sectors are not 'watertight'; as with other areas of the health-care system there is a considerable flow of ill people between them, and many doctors work within both systems.

THE HEALTH–CARE SYSTEM IN THE UK

To view the UK health-care system in perspective, most of the available sources of health care or advice are listed in Table 4.3.

'Healer' in Table 4.3 refers to all those who, either formally or informally, offer advice and care for those suffering from physical discomfort and/or psychological distress, or who

Table 4.3 Professional, folk and popular healers in the UK

Hospital doctors (NHS)	Chinese acupuncturists and herbalists
General practitioners (NHS)	West Indian healing churches
Private doctors (hospital or GP)	African *marabouts* and *obeah men*
Nurses (hospital, GP, school or community)	Healing churches and cults
Midwives	Christain healing guilds
Health visitors	Spiritualist churches and healers
Social workers	Church counselling services
Physiotherapists	Hospital and other chaplains
Occupational therapists	Probation officers
Pharmacists	Citizens' Advice Bureaux
Dieticians	Complementary and alternative healers (lay and
Opticians	medical)
Dentists	Acupuncture
Hospital technicians	Homeopathy
Nursing auxiliaries	Osteopathy
Medical receptionists	Chiropractic
Local authority health clinics	Radionics
Clinical psychologists and psychoanalysts	Herbalism
Counsellors (marriage, child guidance, pregnancy,	Spiritual healing
contraception)	Hypnotherapy
Alternative psychotherapists (Gestalt, bioenergetics,	Naturopathy
primal therapy, etc.)	Massage etc.
Group therapists	Diviners
Samaritans and other 'phone-in' counsellors	Astrologers
Self-help groups	Tarot readers
Yoga and meditation groups	Clairvoyants
Health food shops salespeople	Clairaudientes
Beauty therapists	Mediums
Media healers (advice columnists in newspapers and	Psychic consultants
magazines, TV and radio doctors)	Palmists
NHS Direct (for telephone advice)	Fortune tellers, etc.
Ethnic minority healers	Lay health advisers (family, friends, neighbours,
Muslim *hakims*	acquaintances, voluntary or charitable workers,
Hindu *vaids*	salespeople, hairdressers, etc.)

GP, general practitioner; NHS, National Health Service.

advise on how to maintain health and a feeling of wellbeing. This list therefore spans all three sectors of health care in Britain: popular, folk and professional.

Case study: sources of lay health advice in Northampton, UK

Elliott-Binns[103] in 1970 studied 1000 patients attending a general practice in Northampton, UK. The patients were asked whether they had previously received any advice or treatment for their symptoms. The source, type and soundness of the advice were noted, as well as whether the patient had accepted it. It was found that 96 per cent of the patients had received some advice or treatment before consulting their GP. Each patient had had an average of 2.3 sources of advice, or 1.8 excluding self-treatment; that is, 2285 sources of which 1764 were outside sources and 521 self-advice. Thirty-five patients received advice from five or more sources; one boy with acne received it from 11 sources. The outside sources of advice for the sample were: friend, 499; spouse, 466; relative, 387; magazines or books, 162; pharmacists, 108; nurses giving informal advice, 102; and nurses giving professional advice, 52. Among relatives and friends, wives' advice was evaluated as being among the best and that from mothers and mothers-in-law the worst. Male relatives usually said 'go to the doctor', without offering practical advice, and rarely gave advice to other men. Advice from impersonal sources, such as women's magazines, home doctor books, newspapers and television was evaluated as the least sound. Pharmacists, consulted by 11 per cent of the sample, gave the soundest advice. Home remedies accounted for 15 per cent of all advice, especially from friends, relatives and parents.

Overall, the best advice given was for respiratory complaints and the worst for psychiatric illness. One example of the patient sample was a village shopkeeper with a persistent cough. She received advice from her husband, an ex-hospital matron, a doctor's receptionist and five customers, three of whom recommended a patent remedy 'Golden Syrup', one a boiled onion gruel and one the application of a hot brick to the chest. One middle-aged widower had come to see the doctor complaining of backache. He had consulted no one because he 'had no friends and anyway if I got some ointment there's no one to rub it in'.

Elliott-Binns[104] repeated this study 15 years later, on 500 patients in the same practice in Northampton. Surprisingly, the pattern of self-care and lay health advice had remained largely unchanged; 55.4 per cent of patients treated themselves before going to the doctor, compared with 52.0 per cent in 1970. The only significant changes were an increase in impersonal sources of advice on health, such as home doctor books and television, and a decline in the use of traditional home remedies (although they still accounted for 11.2 per cent of health advice). In addition, the use of advice from pharmacists increased from 10.8 per cent in 1970 to 16.4 per cent in 1985. Overall the study suggested that, in UK, self-care still remains the chief source of health care for the average patient.

Since Elliott-Binns two studies were published,[103,104] the major developments in popular health-care in the UK have been the public's increasing recourse to *impersonal* sources of health advice and information, including telemedicine (such as NHS Direct) for medical advice, and the Internet for medical information. Both these developments are discussed in more detail in Chapter 13.

KEY REFERENCES

2 Kleinman, A. (1980). *Patients and Healers in the Context of Culture*. Berkeley: University of California Press, pp. 49–70.

21 Lewis, I. M. (1971). *Ecstatic Religion*. London: Penguin, pp. 49–57.

30 World Health Organization (1978). *The Promotion and Development of Traditional Medicine*. WHO Tech. Rep. Ser. No. 622. WHO.

43 Frank, R. and Ecks, S. (2004) Towards an ethnography of Indian Homeopathy. *Anthropology and Medicine* 11(3), 307–26.

46 Fisher, P. and Ward, A. (1994) Complementary medicine in Europe. *Br. Med. J.* 309, 107–111.

51 Kaptchuk, T.J. & Eisenberg, D.M. (2001) Varieties of healing. 1: Medical pluralism in the United States. *Ann. Intern. Med.* 135, 189–95.

52 Kaptchuk, T.J. and Eisenberg, D.M. (2001) Varieties of healing. 2: A taxonomy of unconventional healing practices. *Ann. Intern. Med.* 135, 196–204.

73 Konner, M. (1993). *The Trouble with Medicine*. London: BBC Books, pp. 22–47.

81 Davis-Floyd, R.E. (1992). *Birth as an American Rite of Passage*. Berkeley: University of California Press.

86 Helman, C.G. (1985). Disease and pseudo-disease: a case history of pseudoangina. In: *Physicians of Western Medicine* (Hahn, R. A. and Gaines, A.D. eds). Dordercht: Reidel, pp. 293–331.

119 British Medical Association (1993). *Complementary Medicine: New Approaches to Good Practice*. London: British Medical Association, pp. 28–30.

150 Department of Health (2004) *Staff in the NHS 2004*. London: Department of Health. http://www.dh.gov.uk/assetRoot/04/10/67/08/0410 6708.pdf (Accessed on 11 August 2005).

See http://www.culturehealthandillness.com for the full list of references for this chapter.

RECOMMENDED READING

Sectors of health care

Kleinman, A. (1980). *Patients and Healers in the Context of Culture*, Chapters 2 and 3. Berkely: University of California Press.

Folk and popular sectors

Eisenberg, D. *et al.* (1993). Unconventional medicine in the United States. *N. Engl. J. Med.*, 328, 246–52.

Ernst, E. (1996) *Complementary Medicine*. Oxford: Butterworth Heinemann.

Finkler, K. (1994). Sacred healing and biomedicine compared. *Med. Anthrop. Q. (New Ser.)*, 8, 178–97.

Fulder, S. (1996) *Handbook of Complementary Medicine*, 3rd edn. Oxford: Oxford University Press.

McGuire, M. B. (1988). *Ritual Healing in Suburban America*. Piscataway: Rutgers University Press.

O'Connor, B. B. (1995). *Healing Traditions*. Philadelphia: University of Pennsylvania Press.

World Health Organization (2002) *WHO Traditional Medicine Strategy 2002–2005*. WHO.

RECOMMENDED WEBSITES

National Center for Alternative and Complementary Medicine (National Institutes of Health): http://nccam.nih.gov

Self Help UK (online database of over 1000 self-help groups and support groups in the UK): http://www.self-help.org.uk

Self-Help Group Sourcebook Online (USA): http://mentalhelp.net/selfhelp

World Health Statistics 2005 (World Health Organization): http://www3.who.int/statistics

5 Doctor–patient interactions

Doctors and their patients, even if they come from the same social and cultural background, view ill health in very different ways. Their perspectives are based on very different premises, employ a different system of proof, and assess the efficacy of treatment in a different way. Each has its strengths, as well as its weaknesses. The problem is how to ensure some *communication* between them in the clinical encounter between doctor and patient. In order to illustrate this problem, the differences between medical and lay views of ill health – between, that is, 'disease' and 'illness' – will be described in some detail.

'DISEASE' – THE DOCTOR'S PERSPECTIVE

As described in the previous chapter, those who practice modern scientific medicine form a group apart, with their own values, theories of disease, rules of behaviour and organization into a hierarchy of specialized roles. The medical profession can be seen as a healing 'subculture', with its own particular world view. In the process of medical education, students undergo a form of *enculturation* whereby they gradually acquire a perspective on ill health that will last throughout their professional life. They also acquire a high social status, high earning power and the socially legitimized role of healer, which carries with it certain rights

and obligations. Some of the basic premises of this medical perspective are:

1 Humanitarian outlook.
2 Scientific rationality.
3 The emphasis on objective, numerical measurement.
4 The emphasis on physicochemical data.
5 Mind–body dualism.
6 The view of diseases as entities.
7 Reductionism.
8 The emphasis on the individual patient, rather than on the family or community.

Since ancient times, medicine's core approach has been *humanitarian*: that is, its main concern has been to treat illness, improve human welfare, and alleviate human suffering and pain, by all the means at its disposal. In order to achieve this, modern medicine is based on *scientific rationality*, whereby all its assumptions and hypotheses must be capable of being tested and verified under objective, empirical and controlled conditions. Phenomena relating to health and sickness only then become 'real' when they can be *objectively* observed and measured under these conditions. Once they have been observed, and often quantified, they become clinical 'facts', the cause and effect of which must then be discovered. All 'facts' have a cause, and the task of a clinician is to discover the logical chain of causal influences that led up to this particular fact. For example, iron-deficiency anaemia may result from loss of blood, which may be the result of a bleeding stomach tumour, which may have been caused by certain carcinogens in the diet. Where a specific causal influence cannot be isolated, the clinical fact is labelled 'idiopathic' – that is, it *has* got a cause, but that cause has yet to be discovered. Where a phenomenon cannot be objectively observed or measured, for example a person's beliefs about what caused an illness, it is somehow less 'real' than, say, the level of the patient's blood pressure or white cell count. Because blood pressure and white cell count can be measured and agreed upon by several observers, they form the sorts of clinical 'facts' upon which diagnosis and treatment will be based.

These 'facts', therefore, arise from a *consensus* among the observers, whose measurements are carried out in accordance with certain agreed guidelines. The assumptions underlying these guidelines that determine which phenomena are to be looked for, and how they are to be verified and measured provide what is termed a conceptual *model*. As Eisenberg[1] points out, models 'are ways of constructing reality, of imposing meaning on the chaos of the phenomenal world' and 'once in place, models act to generate their own verification by excluding phenomena outside the frame of reference the user employs'. The model of modern medicine is mainly directed towards discovering and quantifying physicochemical information about the patient, rather than less measurable social and emotional factors. According to Kleinman and colleagues,[2] the modern Western doctor's view of clinical reality 'assumes that biologic concerns are more basic, "real", clinically significant, and interesting than psychological and sociocultural issues'.

This emphasis on physiological facts means that a doctor confronted with a patient's symptoms tries first of all to relate these to some underlying physical process. For example, if a patient complains of a certain type of chest pain, the doctor's approach is likely to involve a number of examinations or tests to try to identify the physical cause of the pain – perhaps coronary heart disease. If no physical cause can be found after exhaustive investigation the symptom might be labelled 'psychogenic' or 'psychosomatic', but this diagnosis is usually only made by excluding a physical cause. Subjective symptoms, therefore, become more 'real' when they can be explained by objective, physical changes. As the Goods[3] describe it: 'Symptoms achieve their *meaning* in relation to physiological states, which are interpreted as the referents of the symptoms. Somatic lesions or dysfunctions produce discomfort and behavioural changes, communicated in a patient's complaints. The critical task of the physician is to "decode" a patient's discourse by relating symptoms to their biological referents in order to diagnose a disease entity'. These somatic or biological referents are discovered by the doctor's examination and sometimes by the use of specialized tests, often using diagnostic technology.

As described in the previous chapter, Feinstein[4] has pointed out the shift in recent years in how doctors collect information about underlying disease processes. The traditional method was by listening to the patient's symptoms and how they developed (the history), and then searching for objective physical signs (the examination). Increasingly, though, modern medicine has come to rely on diagnostic technology to collect and measure clinical facts. This implies a shift from the *subjective* (the patient's subjective symptoms, the physician's subjective interpretation of the physical signs) towards the notionally *objective* forms of diagnosis. The underlying pathological processes are now firmly identified by blood tests, X-rays, scans and other investigations, usually carried out in specialized laboratories or clinics (see Chapter 4). One result of this is the increasing use of *numerical* definitions of health and disease. Health or normality are defined by reference to certain physical and biochemical parameters, such as weight, height, circumference, blood count, haemoglobin level, levels of electrolytes or hormones, blood pressure, heart rate, respiratory rate, heart size or visual acuity. For each measurement there is a numerical range – the 'normal value' – within which the individual is considered normal and 'healthy'. Above or below this range is 'abnormal', and indicates the presence of 'disease'. Disease, then, is seen as a deviation from these normal values, accompanied by abnormalities in the structure or function of body organs or systems. For example, lower than the normal value of thyroid hormone in the blood is *hypo*thyroidism, above it is *hyper*thyroidism; between the two the thyroid is functioning normally.

Diseases

The medical definition of ill health, therefore, is largely based on objectively demonstrable physical changes in the body's structure or function, which can be quantified by reference to 'normal' physiological measurements. These abnormal changes, or *diseases*, are seen as 'entities', each with their own unique 'personality' of symptoms and signs. Each disease's personality is made up of a characteristic cause, clinical picture (symptoms and signs), results of hospital investigations, natural history, prognosis and appropriate treatment. For example, tuberculosis is known to be caused by a particular bacillus, to reveal itself by certain characteristic symptoms, to display certain physical signs on examination, to show up in a particular way on chest radiographs and sputum tests, and to have a likely natural history, depending on whether it is treated or not. As Fabrega and Silver[5] point out, the medical perspective assumes that diseases are 'universal in form, progress, and content', and that they have a recurring identity; that is, it is assumed that tuberculosis will be the same disease in whatever culture or society it appears. It will always have the same cause, clinical picture, treatment, and so on. However, this perspective does not include the social, cultural and psychological dimensions of ill health, and the context in which it appears, which determine the *meaning* of the disease for the individual patients and those around them. Because medicine focuses more on the physical dimensions of illness, factors such as the personality, religious belief, culture and socio-economic status of the patient are often considered largely irrelevant in making the diagnosis or prescribing treatment. Engel[6] sees this approach as further evidence of 'mind–body dualism', a medical way of thinking that focuses on identifying physical abnormalities while often ignoring 'the patient and his attributes as a person, a human being'. Reducing him, that is, to a set of abnormal physiological parameters. This conceptual dualism can be traced back at least to Descartes in the seventeenth century, who divided man into 'body' (to be studied only by science), and 'mind' or 'soul' (to be studied by philosophy and religion). In more recent times, 'mind' has been handed over to psychiatrists and behavioural scientists to study (rather than priests), while 'body' – seen increasingly as an animated machine – has been handed over to medical science and its diagnostic technology. Thus, in modern medicine the basic dualism still remains.

Reductionism

A further point is that modern medicine is often very reductionist in its approach. With the exception of the specialties of public health and family medicine, its focus is mainly on the individual patient, rather than on their families, communities or wider society. In some cases, that focus has moved beyond the individual, to concentrate instead on a particular diseased organ, system, group of cells or region within their body. This development has been made possible by advances in equipment and diagnostic technology, which can now reveal changes at the cellular, biochemical or even molecular levels, and can exactly localize the site of pathology. In recent years, there has also been a growing emphasis on the human genome (see Chapter 14), and on genetic abnormalities as indicators, or predictors of hereditary diseases. As mentioned in the previous chapter, advances in diagnostic technology have led to the development of a new group of 'patients' produced by that technology, such as X-ray plates, scans, printouts of blood test results or the strips of paper from an electrocardiogram. The development of these 'paper patients' as a growing feature of clinical consultations, case conferences and hospital grand

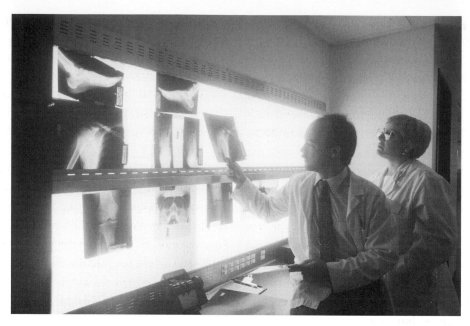

Figure 5.1 Advances in diagnostic technology have helped shift medicine towards an increased focus on *physical* abnormalities – rather than on the patient's symptoms, their psychological state, or their social and cultural background. (Source: © Corbis MED 028. Reproduced with permission.)

rounds is a further step towards medical reductionism. Furthermore, many doctors now diagnose and treat abnormalities of only a small part of the human body. Their professional aim is, in a sense, to know more and more about less and less (and often this results in knowing less and less about more and more). In modern medicine these hyper-specialists tend to have a higher status and a higher income than many generalists, such as general practitioners. In addition, those specialists, who are publicly seen to 'cure', have a higher status than those who merely 'care'. Treating a small area of the body in a relatively short period of time and with a clearly defined outcome has a much higher status than dealing with those conditions where no short-term cure is evident or even possible. Thus surgeons generally have a higher status than doctors working in geriatrics, psychiatry, physical disability, terminal illness, chronic disease or preventive medicine. Even within surgery there is a hierarchy of prestige, depending on the symbolic value our society gives to different parts of the body. This applies especially to the brain and the heart, so that brain surgeons and heart surgeons

have a much higher prestige than, say, rectal or gynecological surgeons.

THE RANGE OF MEDICAL MODELS

The medical model should not, therefore, be seen as homogeneous and consistent. In understanding doctor–patient interactions, one should always ask: '*which* doctor?', or perhaps 'which *type* of doctor?' There is really no such thing as a uniform 'Western' or 'scientific' medicine; as illustrated in Chapter 4. Although it is now international, there are enormous variations in how Western medicine is practiced in different parts of the world. This applies in different Western industrialized countries, and even within those countries themselves. Furthermore, the medical model is always to a large extent culture-bound, and varies greatly, depending on the context in which it appears. Even within the same society, huge differences in perspective exist between different branches of medicine and the different specialties – between, say, the perspectives of surgeons,[7] psychiatrists, epidemiologists, general practitioners and public health specialists. In some cases, their approach to a particular case may be quite incompatible: an example of a professional 'culture-clash'. They may concentrate on different aspects of the patient's condition, but ignore others. Some may focus only on a small area of the body, others mainly on the patient's state of mind, or on relationships with their families and communities. This type of clash of perspectives is often seen also in the relationships between doctors and nurses.

When a particular doctor trained in modern scientific medicine makes a diagnosis, he or she usually employs a number of *different* models or perspectives, each of which looks at the problem in a particular way. As the Goods[3] note, 'any physician or medical discipline has a repertoire of interpretative models – biochemical, immunological, viral, genetic, environmental, psychodynamic, family interactionist and so on', each with its own unique perspective on the disease. In some cases these perspectives, or models, might be very different from one another. In psychiatry, for example, Eisenberg[1] points out that 'multiple and manifestly contradictory models' are used by different psychiatrists in explaining the psychoses. These include:

1 The *organic* model, which emphasizes physical and biochemical changes in the brain.
2 The *psychodynamic* model, which concentrates on developmental and experiential factors.
3 The *behavioural* model, where psychosis is maintained by environmental contingencies.
4 The *social* model, with its emphasis on disorders in role performance.

Whatever specialty they choose to work in, it should be noted that physicians themselves are also part of the 'folk' world for most of their lives – both before and after graduating from medical school. Both as individuals and as members of a particular family, community, religion or social class, they bring with them a specific set of ideas, assumptions, experiences, prejudices and inherited folklore, and this can greatly influence their medical practice. When they impose (often unconsciously) their own cultural values, assumptions and expectations on their patients, that phenomenon – using psychoanalytic imagery – could be seen as an example of what I would term *cultural counter-transference*.

All medical and psychiatric models tend to change over time as new concepts are developed and new discoveries are made. Disease entities such as hypertension, cancer or coronary heart disease are continuously being re-examined or reworked as new theories of aetiology are advanced and new techniques of diagnosis and treatment are invented. The different models used by clinicians in different specialties also means that they might perceive and diagnose the *same* episode of ill health in very different ways, if an ill person consults with each of them over a period of time.

MEDICINE AS A SYSTEM OF MORALITY

A final issue is that, with the decline in organized religion in many Western societies, the moral concerns of the contemporary age are increasingly being expressed in medical rather than religious terms. Medicine has always been more than a system of scientific ideas and practices; it has also been a *symbolic* system, expressing some of the basic underlying values, beliefs and moral concerns of the wider society. In a more secularized age, religious ideas of sin or immorality often seem to be replaced by ideas of health and disease. Today, medical metaphors have become part of the daily discourse, for example a 'sick society', an 'epidemic of crime', an 'ailing economy', 'the plague of terrorism'. Whereas a few generations ago religion spoke out against a 'sinful life', medicine now condemns the 'unhealthy lifestyle', but the punishments occur in this world, rather than in the world to come. The ancient Deadly Sins of 'gluttony' and 'sloth' have been reconceptualized as 'overeating' and 'lack of exercise'. Because so much moral discourse is now couched in medical terms, the definitions of certain behaviours – alcoholism, illegitimacy, truancy, drug abuse and criminality – have shifted from being bad or sinful to being in some way in the domain of medicine or psychiatry.

A related phenomenon in most industrialized societies is the growth of the *insurance* industry. While it penalizes those of its clients who have an unhealthy lifestyle (who smoke or drink, for example), it compensates individuals for unexpected illness, accident or other misfortune – events that, in previous generations (and elsewhere in the world), were dealt with by the religious system. Arguably, in those societies where organized religion is weak, the insurance industry (like the medical system itself) provides some people with a rational, secularized way of responding to misfortune and of diminishing its effects. However, both approaches focus much less on moral responsibility than does religion; despite medicine's enhanced social role, its main focus is still on the *consequences* of illness, accident or misfortune, rather than on their cause.

Despite these changes in the social and symbolic role of medicine in modern society, and variations within the medical model itself, its predominant approach in clinical practice still remains the search for *physical* evidence of disease or dysfunction and the use of physical treatments (such as drugs, surgery, or radiation) in correcting these underlying abnormalities.

'ILLNESS' – THE PATIENT'S PERSPECTIVE

Cassell[8] uses the word 'illness' to represent 'what the patient feels when he goes to the doctor', and 'disease' for 'what he has on the way home from the doctor's office'. He concludes: 'Disease, then, is something an organ has; illness is something a man has'. *Illness* is the subjective response of an individual and of those around him to his being unwell – particularly how he and they interpret the origin and significance of this event, how it affects his behaviour and his relationship with other people, and the various steps he takes to remedy the situation. It not only includes his experience of ill health, but also the *meaning* he gives to that experience. For example, people who suddenly fall ill might ask themselves 'why has it hap-

pened to *me*?', 'why *now*?', 'have I done anything wrong to deserve this?' or even, in some societies, 'has anyone *caused* me to be ill?'. Both the meaning given to the symptoms and their emotional response to them are influenced by their own background and personality, as well as the cultural, social and economic context in which the symptoms appear. In other words, the same 'disease' (such as tuberculosis) or symptom (such as pain) may be interpreted completely differently by two individuals from different cultures or social backgrounds and in different contexts. This will also affect their subsequent behaviour, and the sorts of treatment they will seek out.

The patient's perspective on ill health is usually part of a much wider conceptual model used to explain misfortune in general; within this model, illness is only a specialized form of adversity. For example, in many societies *all* forms of misfortune are ascribed to the same range of causes; a high fever, a crop failure, the theft of one's property or a roof collapsing might all be blamed on witchcraft or on divine punishment for some moral transgression. In the last case, they may cause similar emotions of shame or guilt and call for similar types of treatment, such as prayer or penitence. 'Illness' therefore often shares the psychological, moral and social dimensions associated with other forms of adversity, within a particular culture. It is a wider though more diffuse concept than 'disease' and should be taken into account in understanding how people interpret their ill health and suffering, and how they respond to it.

BECOMING ILL AND DEFINITIONS OF 'HEALTH'

Definitions of what constitutes both 'health' and 'illness' vary between individuals, families, cultural groups and social classes. In most cases, *health* is seen as much more than just an absence of unpleasant physical symptoms. The World Health Organization (WHO),[9] for example, defined it in 1946 as 'a state of complete physical, mental and social well-being and not merely the absence of disease or infirmity'. 'Health' is really a *multi-dimensional* and holistic concept, which includes physical health, psychological health, social health, and spiritual health. A disturbance of any one of these, such as a major conflict with a spouse or close relative, unsettling dreams, or a sense of being 'bewitched, may be seen as a form of 'illness', especially if it interferes with daily life and activities. That is because in many non-industrialized societies, health is conceived of as a balanced *relationship* between people, between people and nature, and between people and the supernatural world. It is also seen as an internal balance, both physical and emotional. A disturbance of any of these dimensions proves that one is not 'healthy', especially as this imbalance may manifest itself by physical or emotional symptoms. Among Western communities, definitions of health tend to be rather less all-embracing, owing to Western biomedicine's over-emphasis on physical abnormalities *within* the body, but they almost always include some physical, psychological and behavioural aspects. In modern discourse, some traces of the 'balance' idea still remains, in phrases such as 'a well-balanced person', 'to be mentally unbalanced', 'to eat a balanced diet' and 'everything in proportion'.

Definitions of 'health' also vary between social classes. For example, Fox[10] quotes a classic 1960s study of 'Regionville', a town in upper New York State where members of the highest socio-economic class usually reported a persistent backache to their physician as an abnormal symptom, while members of the poorer socioeconomic class regarded it as 'an inevitable and innocuous part of life and thus as inappropriate for referral to a doctor'. Similarly, in Blaxter and Paterson's 1981 study[11] in Aberdeen, Scotland, working-class mothers did not define their children as ill, even if they had abnormal physical symptoms, provided that they continued to walk around and play normally. This functional definition of health, common among poorer people, is probably based on the (economic) need to keep working regardless of what they feel, as well as on low expectations of medical care. These lay definitions of health can

obviously differ from those of the medical profession, as will be described.

On an individual level, the process of defining oneself as being 'ill' can be based on one's own perceptions, on the perceptions of others, or on both. Defining oneself as being ill usually follows a number of subjective experiences including:

- perceived changes in bodily appearance, such as loss of weight, changes in skin colour, or hair falling out
- changes in regular bodily functions, such as urinary frequency, heavy menstrual periods, irregular heart beats
- unusual bodily emissions, such as blood in the urine, sputum or stools
- changes in the functions of limbs, such as paralysis, clumsiness or tremor
- changes in the five major senses, such as deafness, blindness, lack of smell, numbness or loss of taste sensation
- unpleasant physical symptoms, such as pain, headache, abdominal discomfort, fever or shivering
- excessive or unusual emotional states, such as anxiety, depression, guilt, nightmares or exaggerated fears
- behavioural changes in relation to others, such as marital or work disharmony
- certain spiritual experiences such as visions or dreams, or the sense of having being punished by the deity, or of being bewitched, or 'possessed' by a malevolent spirit

Most people experience some of these abnormal changes in their daily lives, though usually in a mild form, and this has been demonstrated in several studies. In Dunnell and Cartwright's study[12] in 1972, 91 per cent of a sample of adults had experienced one or more abnormal symptoms in the 2 weeks preceding the study (while only 16 per cent had consulted a doctor during this time). Having one or more abnormal changes of symptoms may therefore not be enough to label oneself as being 'ill'. For example, in Apple's study[13] of middle-class Americans, abnormal symptoms were only considered an illness if they interfered with the usual daily activities, were recent in onset and were ambiguous – that is, difficult for a layman to diagnose.

Other people can also define one as being ill, even in the absence of abnormal subjective experience, by statements such as 'You look pale today, you must be ill' or 'You've been acting very strangely recently'. In the absence of behavioural changes, cultures vary as to whether a particular form of behaviour is defined as illness or not. In Guttmacher and Elinson's[14] 1971 study, different social and ethnic groups in New York City were asked whether certain types of socially deviant behaviour (such as transvestism, homosexuality or getting into fights) were evidence of illness. The Puerto Rican group was found to be less likely to describe these as illness than other groups such as Irish, Italian, Jewish or Black. In most cases, though, a person is defined as being 'ill' when there is agreement between his perceptions of impaired wellbeing and the perceptions of those around him. In that sense, becoming ill is always a *social* process that involves other people in addition to the patient. Their cooperation is needed in order for him to adopt the rights and benefits of the 'sick role' – that is, of the socially acceptable role of an 'ill person'. People who are so defined are temporarily able to avoid their obligations towards the social groups to which they belong, such as family, friends, work-mates or religious groups. At the same time, these groups often feel obligated to care for their sick members while they are ill. The sick role therefore provides, as Fox[10] pointed out, 'a semi-legitimate channel of withdrawal from adult responsibilities and a basis of eligibility for care by others'. In most cases this role is most potent when validated by a doctor or some other health professional. This care usually takes place within the popular sector of health care, and especially within the family, where the patient's symptoms are discussed and evaluated and decisions made about whether they are ill or not and, if so, how they should be treated.

The process of 'becoming ill' involves, therefore, both subjective experiences of physical or emotional changes and, except in the very isolated, the confirmation of these changes by other people. In order for this confirmation to take place there must be a *consensus* among all concerned about what constitutes health and abnormal symptoms and signs. There must also be a standardized way in which an ill person can draw attention to these abnormal changes so as to mobilize care and support. According to Lewis,[15] 'in every society there are some conventions about how people should behave when they are ill... in most illness there is some interplay of voluntary and involuntary responses in the expression of illness. The patient has some control of the way in which he shows his illness and what he does about it'.

Both the presentation of illness and others' response to it are largely determined by socio-cultural factors. Each culture (and to some extent each gender, social class, region and even family) has its own *language of distress*, which bridges the gap between subjective experiences of impaired wellbeing and social acknowledgement of them. Cultural factors determine *which* symptoms or signs are perceived of as abnormal; they also help *shape* these diffuse emotional and physical changes into a pattern that is recognizable to both the sufferer and those around him. The resultant pattern of symptoms and signs may be termed an 'illness entity', and represents the first stage of becoming ill.

THE EXPLANATORY MODEL

Kleinman[16] has suggested a way of looking at the process by which illness is patterned, interpreted and treated, which he terms the *Explanatory Model* (EM). Although there are limitations to this model, it can be useful on occasion. The EM is defined as 'the notions about an episode of sickness and its treatment that are employed by all those engaged in the clinical process'. Explanatory models are held by both patients and practitioners, and they 'offer explanations of sickness and treatment to guide choices among available therapies and therapists and to cast personal and social meaning on the experience of sickness'. In particular, they provide explanations for five aspects of illness:

1 The aetiology or cause of the condition.
2 The timing and mode of onset of symptoms.
3 The pathophysiological processes involved.
4 The natural history and severity of the illness.
5 The appropriate treatments for the condition.

These models are marshalled in response to a particular episode of illness, and are not identical to the general beliefs about illness that are held by that society. According to Kleinman, lay EMs tend to be 'idiosyncratic and changeable, and to be heavily influenced by both personality and cultural factors. They are partly conscious and partly outside of awareness, and are characterized by vagueness, multiplicity of meanings, frequent changes, and lack of sharp boundaries between ideas and experience'. He contrasts this with physicians' EMs, which are also marshalled to deal with a particular illness episode but are mostly based on 'single causal trains of scientific logic'. Explanatory models, therefore, are used by individuals to explain, organize and manage particular episodes of impaired wellbeing. Consultations with a doctor are actually transactions between lay and medical EMs of a particular illness.[17]

Another way of looking at lay explanations of ill health is to examine the sorts of questions that people may ask themselves when they perceive themselves as being ill[17] (or when they suffer from any other misfortune), and how they weave the answers to these questions into the story or *narrative* of their ill health. These questions include:

1 *What has happened?* This includes organizing the symptoms and signs into a recognizable pattern, and giving it a name or identity.
2 *Why has it happened?* This explains the aetiology or cause of the condition.
3 *Why has it happened to me?* This tries to relate the illness to aspects of the patient, such as behaviour, diet, body build, personality or heredity.

4 *Why now?* This concerns the timing of the illness and its mode of onset, sudden or slow.
5 *What would happen to me if nothing were done about it?* This considers its likely course, outcome, prognosis and dangers.
6 *What are its likely effects on other people (family, friends, employers, workmates) if nothing is done about it?* This includes loss of income or of employment, or a strain on family relationships.
7 *What should I do about it – or to whom should I turn for further help?* This includes strategies for treating the condition, including self-medication, consultation with friends or family, or going to see a doctor.

For example, someone suffering from a 'head cold' might answer these questions as: 'I've picked up a cold. It's because I went out into the rain on a cold day, directly after a hot bath, when I was feeling low. If I leave it, it may go down to my chest and make me more ill. Then I might have to stay at home for a long time, and lose a lot of money. I'd better go see the doctor, and get some medicine for it'. Before these questions can be asked or answered, the patients must see their symptoms or signs – such as muscular aches, shivering or a runny nose – as 'abnormal', before grouping them into the recognizable pattern of 'a cold'. This implies a fairly widespread belief in the patient's community about what 'a cold' is and how it can be recognized, although the EM of a particular cold is likely to have personal, idiosyncratic elements. Where many people in a culture or community agree about a pattern of symptoms and signs, and its origin, significance and treatment, it becomes an 'illness entity' or *folk illness*, with a recurring identity. This identity is more loosely defined than medical 'diseases', and is greatly influenced by the socio-cultural context in which it appears.

The context of explanatory models

Explanatory models, however, do not ever exist in isolation. They are not concrete, unchanging 'things' that are somehow separate from the unique circumstances of a particular human life. Unlike some biomedical tests, they are not a type of 'diagnostic test' of someone's worldview, or psychological condition, but only a reflection of how, at that particular moment in time, they explain what has happened to them, and how it should be dealt with. Furthermore, EMs can only be fully understood by examining the specific *context* in which they are employed, since this usually has a major influence upon them.

Because EMs are strongly shaped by context, explanations for the *same* illness event may vary, depending on when and where they are given, by whom, and to whom. Ill people may give different explanations for their illness to themselves, to their family, and to their doctor. In turn, each of these parties may view the illness in a completely different way. The wider context of an EM also includes the social and economic organization and dominant ideology (or religion) of the society in which a particular individual got ill, and in which they consulted a doctor or other health professional. It can depend also on the particular social and economic circumstances of someone's life at that time. For example, an ill person's assessment of how serious an illness is (and how it will affect their life) may depend not only on their explanation of the origin of their condition, but also on whether they are able to afford to miss work, whether they can afford private health insurance, and whether the state will provide them with free health care and disability payments while they remain unfit to work. A broken leg will have different economic implications for a manual labourer or farm worker than for a computer programmer, and their EMs of the same condition will thus be very different. The social and economic context will also influence the types of treatment that patients can afford for their illness, and whether these take place mainly in the popular, folk or professional sectors. Finally, the gender, age group and stage of the life cycle of different individuals will greatly influence the EMs that they employ: those of children, the elderly, new mothers and family bread-winners are all likely to be very different from one another.

The ways that lay and medical EMs interact in the clinical consultation are influenced not only by the physical context in which they occur (such as a hospital ward, or doctor's office),[18] but also by the social class, gender and age of the two parties involved. The *power* invested in clinicians by virtue of their background and training (as well as gender or social class) may allow them to mould the patient's EM to make it fit into the medical model of disease, rather than allowing the patient's own perspective on illness to emerge.

FOLK ILLNESSES

As mentioned above, folk illnesses can be regarded as EMs *shared* by a group of people. Rubel[19] has defined them as 'syndromes from which members of a particular group claim to suffer and for which their culture provides an aetiology, a diagnosis, preventive measures and regimens of healing'. Anthropologists have described dozens of these folk illnesses from around the world, each with its own unique configuration of symptoms, signs and behavioural changes. Some examples are: *susto* throughout Latin America; *amok* in Malaysia; *windigo* in north-eastern America; *narahatiye qalb* ('heart distress') in Iran; *dil ghirda hai* ('sinking heart') in the Punjab, India; *koro* in China; *brain fag* in parts of Africa; *tabanka* in Trinidad; *nervios* in much of Latin America; *vapid unmada* in Sri Lanka; *crise de foie* in France; *high blood* in the USA; and *colds* and *chills* in much of the English-speaking world. Each of these is a 'culture-bound syndrome' (see Chapter 10) in the sense that it is a unique disorder, recognized mainly by members of a particular culture, and treated by them in a culturally specific way. One is dealing with a culture-bound folk illness when, as Rubel puts it, 'symptoms regularly cohere in any specified population, and members of that population respond to such manifestations in similarly patterned ways'.

Folk illnesses are more than specific clusterings of symptoms and physical signs. They also have a range of *symbolic* meanings – moral, social or psychological – for those that suffer from them. In some cases they link the suffering of the individual to changes in the natural environment, or to the workings of supernatural forces. In other cases, the clinical picture of the illness is a way of expressing, in a culturally standardized way, that the sufferer is involved in social conflicts, such as disharmony with family, friends or neighbours.

The following case studies are two examples of folk-illness, described by anthropologists.

Case study: 'Heart distress' in Maragheh, Iran

Good[20] in 1977 described an example of this type of folk illness, *narahatiye qalb* or 'heart distress' in Maragheh, Iran. This is a complex folk illness that usually manifests itself in physical symptoms, such as trembling, fluttering or pounding of the heart, and feelings of anxiety or unhappiness, also associated with the heart ('my heart is uneasy'). This illness is 'a complex which includes and links together both physical sensations of abnormality in the heartbeat and feelings of anxiety, sadness, or anger'. The abnormal heartbeat is linked both to unpleasant affective states and to experiences of social stress. It is more frequent among Iranian women, and expresses some of the strains and conflicts of their lives. 'Heart distress' often follows quarrels or conflict within the family, the deaths of close relatives, pregnancy, childbirth, infertility and the use of the contraceptive pill (which is seen as a threat to fertility and lactation). It is primarily a self-labelled folk illness that expresses a wide range of physical, psychological and social problems at the same time. The label 'heart distress' is an image that draws together a network of symbols, situations, motives, feelings and stresses that are rooted in the structural setting in which the people of Maragheh live. The basic presentation of this illness, however, is in the form of common physical symptoms associated with the heart.

Case study: 'Sinking heart' among Punjabis in Bedford, UK

Krause[21] in 1989 described a similar syndrome among both Hindu and Sikh Punjabis living in Bedford, England. The image of *dil ghirda hai* ('sinking heart') links together physical sensation, emotions and certain social experiences into one illness complex, which has specific meanings for the community. 'Sinking heart' – certain physical sensations in the chest – can happen repeatedly to the same individual, and may eventually result in heart 'weakness', heart attacks or even death. Among its many causes are: excessive heat from food or climate or from excessive emotions (such as anger) that make the body 'hot'; other emotional states such as shame, pride, arrogance or worry about one's fate, which are all seen as evidence of self-centredness; and hunger, exhaustion, old age and poverty, which all make people 'weak' and therefore unable to fulfil their moral obligations and may in turn result in worry and sadness. 'Sinking heart' is thus especially linked to 'a profound fear of social failure', and to cultural values that stress the importance of carrying out social obligations, being able to control one's personal emotions, being altruistic and not too worried and self-absorbed and, for men, being able to control the sexuality of their female relatives. Failure in any of these – for example, being unable to prevent the disrespectful and promiscuous behaviour of one's daughters – may result in a loss of *izzat* (honour or respect) in the community, and in *dil ghirda hai*. Like many folk illnesses, therefore, the syndrome blends together physical, emotional and social experiences into a single image or metaphor.

Somatization

A feature of many folk illnesses is that of somatization (see Chapter 10), which Kleinman[22] defines as 'the substitution of somatic preoccupation for dysphoric affect in the form of complaints of physical symptoms and even illness'. That is, unpleasant emotional states (such as depression) or the experience of various social stresses is mainly expressed in the form of physical symptoms. In Taiwan, for example, Kleinman[22] describes how depression is commonly presented in the form of physical symptoms and signs. In Taiwanese culture mental illness is heavily stigmatized, as is the use of psychotherapy, and therefore stress from family problems or financial difficulties is often expressed by physical symptoms. Although these symptoms do not necessarily appear in a standardized form, they are more easily recognized by Chinese folk healers (who are more familiar with this mode of presenting personal problems and conflicts) than by Western-trained physicians.

Folk illnesses can be 'learnt', in the sense that a child growing up in a particular culture learns how to respond to, and express, a range of physical or emotional symptoms or social stresses in a culturally patterned way. Children see relatives or friends suffering from a condition and gradually learn to identify its characteristic features, both in themselves and in others. Frankenberg[23] notes how people's experience of a particular form of ill health is also shaped by much wider cultural and social forces, such as television, advertisements, newspapers and novels (and, increasingly, the Internet), as well as by the dominant ideology and social structure of the society in which they live.

A health professional working in any culture or society should therefore be aware how folk illnesses are generated, how they are acquired and displayed, and how this may affect patients' behaviour and the diagnosis of ill health.

METAPHORS OF ILLNESS

In most of the industrialized world a large number of folk illnesses still persist, many of them largely untouched by the medical model and still rooted in traditional folklore. In addition, certain serious and life-threatening diseases, such as cancer, heart disease or acquired immune deficiency syndrome (AIDS), have also become folk illnesses, though of a particular and powerful type. Often these conditions are linked in the public imagination with traditional beliefs about the moral nature of health, illness and human suffering. These diseases (especially those that are difficult to treat, explain, predict or control) come to symbolize many of the more general anxieties that some people have, such as a fear of the breakdown of ordered society, of invasion or of divine punishment. In the minds of many of the population these diseases become more than just a clinical condition; they become *metaphors* for many of the terrors of daily life. Some of the metaphors associated with AIDS, at least in the early years of the epidemic, are described in Chapter 16.

Metaphors of cancer

Susan Sontag[24] has described how, historically, certain serious diseases, especially those whose origin was not understood and whose treatment was not very successful, became metaphors for all that was 'unnatural' and socially or morally wrong with society. In the Middle Ages, epidemic diseases such as plague were metaphors for social disorder and the breakdown of the religious and moral order. In the last two centuries, syphilis, tuberculosis and cancer have all been used as contemporary metaphors for evil. In the twentieth century in particular, cancer has been described (in the media, literature and popular discourse) as if it were a type of unrestrained and chaotic evil force, unique to the modern world, and which is composed of 'primitive', 'atavistic', 'chaotic' and 'energetic' cells that behave completely without inhibitions and always destroy the natural order of the body (and of society). According to Sontag, a result of this moral model of cancer is that, for many sufferers, the disease is 'often experienced as a form of demonic possession – tumours are "malignant" or "benign", like forces – and many terrified cancer patients are disposed to seek out faith healers, to be exorcised'. In the media too, crime, terrorism, drug abuse, strikes, immigration and even political dissent have all been described as 'a cancer', a demonic force gradually destroying the very fabric of society. One result of this, as Lupton[25] notes, is the widespread use of 'invasion', 'battle' and 'war' metaphors in cancer treatment. An example of this was President Nixon's declaration in 1971 of a 'War on Cancer'.

Metaphors, as Kirmayer[26] notes, are creative of meaning. Their use 'involves a process of discovery or invention'. They are, in a sense, *new* ways of viewing and experiencing the world we live in. In the case of serious conditions such as cancer, these metaphors carry with them a range of symbolic associations that can have serious effects both on how sufferers perceive their own condition, and how other people behave towards them. For example, Peters-Golden[27] described how the stigma associated with breast cancer can cause other people to avoid the sick person and withdraw their social support from her. In her study in the USA of 100 women with breast cancer, 72 per cent of the sample said that other people treated them differently after they knew the diagnosis; 52 per cent found they were avoided or feared, 14 per cent felt they were pitied and only 3 per cent thought people were nicer to them than they had previously been. One reason for this may be the fear that cancer is, in some way, 'contagious'. Similarly, Herzlich and Pierret[28], in their study of French illness beliefs, also found evidence for this. For example, one woman with breast cancer asked her doctor whether it was 'contagious', and whether she could cause any harm to her daughter by sharing her plate.

Similarly, Gordon's study[29] in Italy found that many women described breast cancer as an epidemic or a 'plague' – a malevolent force that somehow invaded them from outside. To one woman 'it is a thing in the air… It plants itself in a part of the body, then begins to eat the whole person', to another 'I see it as something that comes from outside that disturbs something perfect that is inside of me…'. Others saw it as 'an animal', 'a beast' or 'a monster' that invades and then devours the woman's body. Seeing cancer as something originating outside the body – an idea that draws on more ancient imagery of the plague, or of possession by malevolent spirits – inevitably reinforces the sense of it being dangerous, or contagious, to those in contact with one of its victims.

Hunt's study[30] in southern Mexico showed further how women with cancer struggled to deny this sense that the disease was arbitrary. To try to restore the 'sense of a general orderliness to life', they blamed it on previous events in their personal lives. These included emotional upsets, worrying too much, improper sexual behaviour, infidelity by a spouse, failure to reproduce, or a physical blow (*golpe*) to the body, as well as environmental pollution. Thus, 'the illness did not just happen, it happened for a reason'. Similar findings have been reported in the USA by Chavez and colleagues,[31] among Mexican and Salvadorean immigrants. These lay explanations for cancer may imply, therefore, that the disease has a moral element, and that responsible behaviour can somehow avert it.

Metaphors for cancer are not static, however, and may change considerably over time. Also, different types of cancer seem to attract different types of metaphor, depending on the part of the body affected, the duration of the condition, and the speed of onset.

Comparison of illness metaphors

Weiss[32], in a study in Israel, compared the metaphors used for cancer, AIDS and heart disease. Cancer metaphors were those of flux and transformation, of the destruction of boundaries both within the body and beyond it. As in the examples above, the disease was described as an alien 'thing' – an 'amoeba', 'octopus', 'spider', 'worm' or 'parasite' – that 'eats up' the victim's body from within ('Cancer eats up your body… It eats whatever it comes across. It has an open mouth with teeth and it bites off everything'). Yet although it was alien, it somehow originated within the person. In contrast, AIDS (see Chapter 16) was not seen as an isolated 'thing', but an all-embracing part of the self ('it's his whole body that's infected, not a single discernible organ of it'). Unlike cancer, it was seen as originating completely outside the individual ('AIDS attacks you from without… Cancer, from within'), and was linked to notions of outside pollution. Metaphors of both cancer and AIDS suggested 'an entity beyond culture'; a sense of something that belongs 'outside' yet somehow has become incorporated 'inside' both body and self (and society) and is now destroying it. Conversely, the metaphors for heart disease were much less dramatic. They described it in less symbolic but more familiar and mechanical terms. It was seen as essentially 'a problem in plumbing', and heart attacks as simply a 'pump' that suddenly fails.

A fuller discussion of the metaphors associated with human immunodeficiency virus (HIV) and AIDS, is given in Chapter 16.

All these illness metaphors are not just phenomena of language. They are also, in a sense, *embodied* or internalized by those that use them. They become part of the way that individuals experience events – both within their own bodies and beyond it – and the meanings that they give to those experiences. Metaphors often come into play at times of vulnerability caused by illness, pain, anxiety or other forms of suffering. Such metaphors are often a feature, as Becker[33] noted, of 'disrupted lives' – of sudden, traumatic events that interrupt the normal flow of human events. Under these circumstances, therefore, some of the metaphors of severe illness may well contribute towards the *nocebo* effect (see Chapter 8), with damaging consequences for the physical or mental health of the person concerned, as well for as those around them.[34]

Therefore, as the examples of cancer, AIDS and other conditions illustrate, under some circumstances certain serious medical *diseases* can also become forms of *folk illness*, and this can seriously impair the recognition, diagnosis, management and control of these conditions.

LAY THEORIES OF ILLNESS CAUSATION

As noted above, lay theories about illness are part of wider concepts about the origin of misfortune in general. They are also based on beliefs about the structure and function of the body and the ways in which it can malfunction. Even if based on scientifically incorrect premises, these lay models frequently have an internal logic and consistency, which often helps the victim of illness 'make sense' of what has happened and why. In most cultures they are part of a complex body of inherited folklore, which is increasingly influenced – especially in industrialized countries – by concepts borrowed from the media, the Internet and the medical model.

In general, lay theories of illness place the aetiology or causation of ill health in one of the following sites, or in combinations of them:

1 Within the individual.
2 In the natural world.
3 In the social world.
4 In the supernatural world.

This is illustrated in Figure 5.2. In many cases, illness is ascribed to combinations of two or more causes, or to interactions between these various worlds.

As a very broad generalization, social and supernatural aetiologies tend to be a feature of some communities in the non-industrialized world (especially those in rural areas), while natural or patient-centred explanations of illness are more common in the Western industrialized world, though the division is by no means absolute. For example, Chrisman[35] described eight groups of lay aetiologies that are most commonly reported among patients in the USA. They are:

1 Debilitation.
2 Degeneration.
3 Invasion.

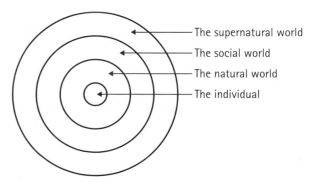

Figure 5.2 Sites of illness aetiology.

4 Imbalance.
5 Stress.
6 Mechanical causes.
7 Environmental irritants.
8 Hereditary proneness.

As in other Western countries, most of these aetiologies are patient-centred and do not invoke either supernatural or social explanations of why people get ill.[36] In practice, these aetiologies tend to overlap, since many lay explanations for illness are *multicausal*. For example, a person might blame their illness on 'stress' at work, which has caused some 'imbalance' in their life, resulting in weakness ('debilitation') and 'reduced resistance, and therefore making them more prone to 'invasion' by a virus or other microbe.

The lay concept of 'stress' is discussed in Chapter 11, the notion of 'hereditary proneness' in Chapter 14, while the other lay aetiologies will be discussed in more detail below.

The individual

Lay theories that locate the origin of ill health within the individual deal mainly with malfunctions within the body, sometimes related to changes in diet or behaviour. Here the *responsibility* for illness falls mainly (though not completely) on the patients themselves.[36] This belief is especially common in the Western world (where it is often encouraged by government health education campaigns), and where ill health is increasingly blamed on not taking care of one's diet, dress, hygiene, lifestyle, relationships, sexual behaviour, smoking and drinking habits, and physical exercise. Ill health is therefore evidence of such carelessness, and the sufferer should feel guilty for causing it. This applies especially to stigmatized conditions such as obesity, alcoholism, sexually transmitted diseases and, as mentioned earlier, to some extent to AIDS. Other more common conditions are also ascribed to incorrect behaviour; in the UK, colds and chills can be caused by 'doing something abnormal' such as 'going outdoors when you have a fever', 'sitting in a draught after a hot bath', or 'walking barefoot on a cold floor'. Wrong diet can also cause ill health; for example, as described in Chapter 2, 'low blood' and low blood pressure in the southern USA are thought to result from eating too many acid or astringent foods, such as lemons, vinegar, pickles, olives and sauerkraut, while 'high blood' results from eating too much rich food, especially red meat.[37] In another study,[38] one-quarter of the women interviewed believed one should eat differently during menstruation so as to avoid causing ill health. For example, sweets were said to keep the menstrual flow 'going longer', while other foods caused it to stop, resulting in menstrual cramps, sterility, strokes or 'quick TB'. Similar dietary prohibitions applied to pregnant women. Other examples of personal responsibility for ill health are some traumatic injuries (also ascribed to carelessness), or injuries that are clearly self-inflicted, such as unsuccessful attempts at suicide. Finally, one's moods, feelings and emotional state can be blamed for ill health, and the responsibility of the individual is to avoid worry, sadness and despair[28] and cultivate feelings of happiness and contentment. As one French woman put it, 'I have the impression it is because I am happy that I am no longer ill'.[28]

Whether people perceive ill health as resulting from their own behaviour, diet or emotions depends on a number of factors. Pill and Stott[39] in their 1982 study of 41 working-class mothers in Cardiff, UK, found that the extent to which people believed their health was determined by their own actions (as opposed to luck, chance or powerful external forces) correlated with socioeconomic variables such as education and home ownership. Those people who had most economic *control* over their own lives accepted more responsibility for ill health causation than those who perceived themselves as socially and economically powerless. In this latter group, illness was believed to result from external forces over which the victim had no control, and for which he or she felt no responsibility.

Other aetiological factors are believed to lie within the body but to be outside the victim's conscious control. This includes notions of personal

135

vulnerability – psychological, physical or hereditary. Personality factors include the 'type of person one is', especially if overanxious or easily worried. In Pill and Stott's study,[39] this is illustrated in quotes like: 'Well, I think something you bring on yourself, like nerves or anything like that, it's partly down to you, I would think – to what sort of person you are. Like I'm a little bit highly strung, you know'. Physical vulnerability is based on lay notions of *resistance* and *weakness*. Some people in the sample were believed to be more resistant to illness than others ('I think some people have a better body resistance than somebody else. I don't really know why – whether it's to do with the blood grouping').[39] This resistance could be strengthened by proper diet, clothing, tonics and so on, but was often seen as being inherited and constitutional ('Some people are born resistant to colds and things'). Similarly 'weakness' can be inherited or acquired; in the UK, some 'weaknesses' are thought to 'run in families' ('all our family have weak chests'), but people who have been severely penetrated by environmental cold may also retain a permanent weakness or gap in their defences in that part of their body ('a weakness of the chest'). Similarly, in Chrisman's[35] classification, *debilitation* – a weakness of the body which results from overworking, being 'run down', a chronic disease or a 'weak spot' in the body – was a common lay aetiology. There was also *hereditary proneness*, which is the genetic transmission of a particular illness, quality or trait, which includes 'weakness' (see Chapter 14). In addition he describes *degeneration* in the structure or function of body tissues or organs, such as occurs in the process of aging, and *invasion*, which in the USA spans the 'individual' and 'natural' zones of aetiology. Here, illness is caused either by external invasion by a 'germ' or other object, or internal spread from an existing problem such as cancer. The other common 'individual' aetiologies are: *imbalance*, perceived as a state of disequilibrium (excess or depletion) within the body, such as 'vitamin deficiency' or 'a lack in the blood'. Imbalance may also result from eating the wrong

foods, and in the wrong proportions, especially in a culture with a 'hot-cold' classification of foodstuffs (Chapter 3); and *mechanical causes* include abnormal functioning of organs or systems ('bad circulation'), damage to parts of the body such as a fracture or wound, 'blockage' of internal organs or blood vessels, and 'pressure' inside organs or parts of the body.

Explanations for ill health that are individual-centred are thus important in determining whether people take responsibility for their health, or whether they see the origin and curing of ill health as lying largely outside their own control.

The natural world

This includes aspects of the natural environment, both living and inanimate, which are thought to cause ill health. Common in this group are climatic conditions such as excess cold, heat, sunlight, wind, rain, snow or dampness. In the UK, for example, areas of environmental cold are believed to cause colds or chills if allowed to penetrate the boundary of skin; cold draughts on the back cause a 'chill on the kidneys', cold rain on the head causes 'a head cold'. In Morocco, excess environmental heat (as in sun-stroke) can enter the body and expand the blood vessels to cause a fullness and throbbing in the head – 'the blood has risen to my head', and, as in the UK, cold air, cold draught and getting wet are thought of as the cause of 'colds' (*berd*) or 'chills' (*bruda*).[40] Other climatic conditions include natural disasters such as cyclones, tornadoes or severe storms.

The supposed influences on health of the moon, sun and planetary bodies, which is a common feature of societies where astrology is practised, could be included here – and astrological birth signs can also be seen as a form of hereditary proneness to health or illness. Other 'natural' aetiologies include injuries caused by animals or birds and, at least in the Western world, infections caused by microorganisms. In the UK, infectious 'fevers' are commonly ascribed to penetration of the body by living entities called, interchangeably, 'germs', 'bugs' or 'viruses', which are commonly thought of as being 'insect-like' ('a tummy bug'). In some cases, as noted above, cancer is conceived of as invasion of the body by an external living entity, which then grows and 'eats up' the body from within. Parasitic infestations, such as round- or threadworms, also form part of this group, as do accidental injuries. In Chrisman's classification, *environmental irritants* such as allergens, pollens, poisons, food additives, smoke, fumes and other forms of pollution were commonly ascribed causes of illness in the USA. In France, Herzlich and Pierret[28] found that the 'air, climate and seasons' were all blamed for causing ill health, and that modern notions of environmental pollution were, in many cases, a return to more traditional theories of *miasmas*, or 'dirty air', as a cause of disease.

The social world

Blaming other people for one's ill health is a common feature of smaller-scale societies, where interpersonal conflicts are frequent. In some non-industrialized societies, the commonest forms of these are witchcraft, sorcery and the 'evil eye'. In all three, illness (and other forms of misfortune) is ascribed to interpersonal malevolence, whether conscious or unconscious. In *witchcraft* beliefs, which are particularly common in Africa and the Caribbean, certain people (usually women) are believed to possess a mystical power to harm others. As Landy[41] points out, this power is usually an intrinsic one, and is inherited either genetically or by membership of a particular kinship group. Witches are usually 'different' from other people, either in appearance or behaviour; often they are ugly, disabled or socially isolated. They are usually the deviants or outcasts of a society, on whom all the negative, frightening aspects of the culture are projected. Their malevolent power, however, is often unconsciously practised, and not all 'witches' are observably deviant.

Anthropologists have pointed out that witchcraft accusations are more common at times of social change, uncertainty and social conflict. Competing factions within a society, for example, may accuse each other of causing their misfortunes

by practising witchcraft. Under these circumstances, the identity of the witch may need to be exposed in divinatory ritual and its negative effect exorcised. Witchcraft beliefs were common in Europe in the Middle Ages; in England, illness was often ascribed to a witch's *maleficium*, and thousands of women were condemned as witches in the sixteenth and seventeenth centuries. This belief system has largely disappeared, but traces of interpersonal conflicts causing ill health still persist in the language – 'He broke her heart' or 'She caused him much pain' – and in modern psychiatric concepts such as the 'schizophrenogenic mother'.

Sorcery, defined by Landy[45] as 'the power to manipulate and alter natural and supernatural events with the proper magical knowledge and performance of ritual', is different from witchcraft. It is also extremely common in some non-Western societies. The sorcerer exerts his or her power consciously, usually for reasons of envy or malice. He causes illness by certain spells, potions or rituals. For example, in a 1976 study[42] of health beliefs among low-income African-Americans, ill health was often ascribed to sorcery, known variously as 'voodoo', 'hoodoo', 'crossing up', 'fixing', 'hexing' or 'witchcraft'. Sorcery is often practised among the social world of friends, family or neighbours, and is often based on envy; as one of Snow's informants declared 'Put on a few little clothes and some people get begrudged-hearted'. The daughter of another informant had been 'killed by sorcery' practised by her in-laws, who were jealous of her pretty face, attentive husband and nice home'. In other cases sorcery was used to control the behaviour of others, such as a wife using spells to prevent her husband leaving her. Illnesses that were ascribed to sorcery included a range of gastrointestinal conditions, as well as general changes such as anorexia or weight loss. Sorcery beliefs of this type usually occur in groups whose lives are characterized by poverty, insecurity, danger, apprehension and a feeling of inadequacy and powerlessness.

The *evil eye* as a cause of illness has been reported throughout Europe, the Middle East and

North Africa. In Italy it is the *mal occhia*, in Hispanic cultures it is *mal de ojo*, in Greece the *mati*, in Turkey the *nazar*, in Arabic cultures the *ayn*, in Hebrew the *ayin ha-rah*, and in Iran the *cašm-e šur*. It is also known as 'the narrow eye', 'the bad eye', 'the wounding eye' or simply as 'the look'. Spooner[43] describes how it is found in the Middle East among all the communities there, whether Islamic, Jewish, Christian or Zoroastrian. He defines the main features of the evil eye as 'it relates to the fear of envy in the eye of the beholder, and [that] its influence is avoided or counteracted by means of devices calculated to distract its attention, and by practices of sympathetic magic. Jealousy can kill via a look'. It can also cause several types of ill health. The possessor of the evil eye usually harms unintentionally, is often unaware of his or her powers and is unable to control them. In their study of Yemen, the Underwoods[44] point out that such a person 'is usually either a stranger or a local person whose social activity, appearance, attitudes or behaviour is to some degree unorthodox or different', especially a person who 'stares' rather than speaks. In this type of society, therefore, a tourist or health worker from overseas might be thought of as a source of illness, whatever their good intentions, especially if they were seen staring at a child and complimenting its appearance just before it got ill.

The social aetiology of illness also includes physical injuries, such as poisoning or battle wounds, inflicted by other people. In many non-industrialized societies, though, other people usually cause illness by magical means, such as witchcraft, sorcery or the evil eye. In Western society, lay notions of *stress* (see Chapter 11) often play the same role, placing the origin of ill health within other people – for example, blaming illness on spouses, children, family, friends, employers or workmates; 'I usually get a migraine if I have a row with the family' or 'I get ill whenever my boss gives me stress'. Infections can also be blamed on other people, as in 'He gave me his cold' or 'I caught his germ', or in the case of sexually transmitted diseases. It could also be argued that overuse of *litiga-tion*, especially in the USA, is analogous to witchcraft accusations, since it displaces the blame for accidents, suffering or misfortune away from oneself and onto the malevolence or carelessness of other people.

In general, though, the widespread blaming of other individuals for one's own ill health is generally more commonly a feature of smaller and preindustrialized societies, mainly in rural areas rather than in more urban, Western societies. However, it should be noted that very similar beliefs are found in many different settings, in many different parts of the world, both rich and poor.

The supernatural world

Here illness is ascribed to the direct actions of supernatural entities, such as *gods*, *spirits* or *ancestral shades*. In the study by Snow[42] quoted above, illness was often described as a 'reminder' from God for some behavioural lapse, such as neglecting to go to Church regularly, not saying one's prayers or not thanking God for daily blessings. Illness was a *whuppin*, a divine punishment for sinful behaviour. On this basis, neither home remedies nor a physician were considered useful in treating the condition. A cure involves acknowledgment of sin, sorrow for having committed it, and a vow to improve one's behaviour. Here, as described by Snow,[42] 'Prayer and repentance, not penicillin, cure sin'. Similar approaches that link ill health to divine disapproval of one's behaviour have also been described among middle-class suburban Americans.

In other societies, illness is ascribed to invasion by capricious, malevolent spirits. These have been described by Lewis[45] in some African communities, where 'disease-bearing spirits' strike unexpectedly, causing a variety of symptoms in their victims. Their invasion is unrelated to the individual's behaviour, and he or she is therefore considered blameless and worthy of sympathetic help from others. Like germs or viruses in the Western world, these pathogenic spirits reveal their identity by the particular symptoms they cause, and can only be treated by driving them out of the body. A similar form of spirit possession – the *jinn* or *ginn* – is common in the Islamic world. In the Underwoods' description,[44] they are ubiquitous and capricious spirits that are 'semihuman rather than supernatural', and can also cause ill health. Another form of 'spirit possession', described by Lewis,[45] occurs when individuals are invaded and made ill by the spirits of their ancestors whom they have offended. This happens when the victim is guilty of immoral, blasphemous or antisocial behaviour. Diagnosis takes place in a divinatory séance, where illness is seen as punishment for these transgressions, and the moral values of the group are reaffirmed. While such supernatural explanations for illness as divine punishment or spirit possession are less common in the industrialized world, the main equivalent is blaming ill health on bad luck, fate, the stars, or 'an act of God'. However, among many Western religious communities illness is blamed on moral error, on not thinking or acting in a spiritual enough way. As one American Christian Scientist explained to McGuire:[46] 'The medical way they don't heal anyone. They just don't heal, because our sense of it is if someone is ill, it's a product of his thinking. And [doctors] don't correct thinking'.

In most cases, as noted above, these lay theories of illness aetiology (like medical explanations) are *multicausal* – that is, they postulate several causes acting together. This means that individual, natural, social and supernatural causes are not mutually exclusive but are usually linked together in a particular case. For example, careless or immoral behaviour may predispose to natural illnesses, divine anger or spirit possession, or an ostentatious lifestyle may attract sorcery or the evil eye. In a study in Emilia-Romagna, Italy, for example, Whitaker[47] found that, in understanding what caused ill-health, people used a combination of traditional models and modern scientific theory: the body was seen as vulnerable to 'germs', but most especially when it was not 'in balance', in terms of the symbolic qualities of 'hot' and 'cold'.

In understanding any specific type of illness, lay EMs within a community often vary in how they explain its aetiology; Blaxter's[48] study of working-class women in Aberdeen, UK, for example, found variation in how some common conditions were explained. Of the 30 working-class women interviewed, eight attributed bronchitis to environmental factors, two attributed it to behaviour, four to heredity, three to 'susceptibility', 10 to being secondary to other conditions and three as the consequence of pregnancy or childbirth. While these were seen as discrete categories in this study, most EMs see illness as multicausal, with elements of several types of aetiology involved in a particular episode of ill health.

CLASSIFICATION OF ILLNESS AETIOLOGIES

Foster and Anderson[49] proposed an alternative way of classifying lay illness aetiologies, especially in non-Western societies. They differentiate between *personalistic* and *naturalistic* systems. In the former, illness is caused by the purposeful active intervention of an agent, such as a supernatural being (a god), a non-human being (ghost, ancestral spirit or capricious spirits) or human being (witch or sorcerer). One could also include modern notions of 'germs' in this category, especially those causing 'fevers'. In naturalistic systems, illness is explained in impersonal, systemic terms. It can be caused by natural forces or conditions such as cold, wind or damp, or by disequilibrium within the individual or the social environment. Included in this 'disequilibrium' group are systems of illness explanation such as humoral or 'hot–cold' systems in Latin America, Ayurvedic medicine in India, and the Yin–Yang system of traditional Chinese medicine. The 'colds' and 'chills' caused by environmental cold could also be included here.

Young[50] classified belief systems about ill health as either *externalizing* or *internalizing*. Externalizing belief systems concentrate mainly on the aetiology of the illness, which is believed to arise *outside* the sick person's body, especially in their social world. Thus, in trying to identify a cause for the individual's illness, people closely examine the circumstances and social events of his life before he fell ill – such as tracing the cause of an illness from a grudge between two people, which led to feelings of resentment, then to some pathogenic act (such as witchcraft or sorcery), which then led on to the illness itself. Many of the lay models of illness aetiology from different parts of the world and described in this chapter can therefore be described as externalizing types of explanations.

In contrast, internalizing belief systems concentrate less on aetiological explanations and more on events that occur (and arise) *inside* the individual's body, and they always emphasize physiological and pathological processes as explanations for how and why some people get ill. This is the perspective of the modern scientific medical model. Its strength lies in its detailed perception of physiological events within the individual body, but its weakness lies in ignoring the social and psychological events that preceded the onset of symptoms – while the reverse is true of the externalizing systems.

Narratives of illness and misfortune

A feature of externalizing explanations for ill health is that they often take the form of a *narrative* or story about how and why that person got ill[51]. In each case the story is presented in a specific *language of distress*, either verbal or non-verbal. A verbal story might include events from the sufferer's life and even events that preceded their birth, such as 'I inherited my weak chest from my father's family'. As Brody[52] pointed out, telling such 'stories of sickness' is a way of giving *meaning* to the experience of ill health, of placing it in the context of the individual's life history. It also relates it to the wider themes of the culture and society in which they live. A narrative is thus a basic way of organizing an experience, especially a traumatic one; of 'making sense of it', and giving it meaning.

Narratives of personal suffering are not only personal. They also draw on the repertoire of language, idiom, metaphors, imagery, myths and leg-

ends provided by the culture in which that suffering took place.[51] In that sense they are usually *culture-bound* to some extent – that is, the way people tell the story of their suffering in one culture may be very different from how they tell it in another. Narratives are thus, as Becker[53] describes them, 'cultural documents'. She points out that they come into being at times of unexpected disruption in the flow of everyday life. This implies a concept of an earlier state of 'normality', which may in turn be defined largely in cultural terms. At times of illness or misfortune, therefore, narratives are usually highly personal stories, but expressed in a culturally specific way.

Many narratives are created with the help of other people – with the members of a family, for example, or of a healing cult or a self-help group. In particular, healers of every sort take a major role in helping to construct their clients' narratives. Helping to reveal and then to shape these narratives of misfortune is characteristic not only of medical care but also of most forms of symbolic healing, from shamanism to psychoanalysis (see Chapter 10), and of most religious traditions. In each case, the healer aims to impose a sense of coherent order on the chaos of the patient's symptoms and feelings. Usually, this places individual suffering in a much wider context of time and place, and employs cultural, religious or scientific concepts of cause and effect. In many cases, the new form of the narrative is negotiated between healer and client during the consultation. This shared, syncretic creation is then carried back home, as a sort of 'gift' from the healer to the client. In terms of symbolic healing, the healer's explanation of what has happened and why is often more important to clients than the herbs, prescriptions or other forms of physical treatment that they have been given.

Western medicine is unique in the type of narrative structure that it seeks to impose on its patients. Usually this takes a *linear* form, in keeping with pervasive Western notions of monochronic time (see Chapter 2). This seeks to organize a patient's story – their history – into a linear form, with a clear beginning for events, a sense of duration and an ending at the present time. Questions such as 'When did the pain begin?', 'What happened next?', 'Where did it move to then?', 'What did you do then?' and 'What has happened since I gave you the medicine?' all impose such a linear narrative form, sometimes inappropriately, on patients' experience. Patients who fail to produce a clear oral history are often branded a 'poor historian'. In Western medicine, the doctor's narrative of the patient's experience now takes a standardized form, found in every medical journal, where it is known as the 'case history'.

Unlike in many traditional societies, the patient in Western medicine, as in psychoanalysis, does most of the talking, with the healer asking only the occasional question for clarification. In traditional healing systems, however, the situation is often reversed. The patient offers the healer only a small amount of information – their date and time of birth, for example, or the content of a particular dream – and the healer does most of the talking. In these systems, therefore, the sign of a good healer is one who quickly 'knows' the diagnosis, sometimes with the aid of divination. Their diagnosis is made without having to ask numerous questions, or eliciting a lengthy narrative from the client. To people from these communities, therefore, the sign of a good doctor may be someone who asks very *few* questions – since they should already sense or 'know' the diagnosis by other means.

Non-verbal narratives

Many narratives of suffering are *non-verbal*. Personal suffering may be acted out in terms of a specific pattern of behaviour – for example, withdrawal, silence, self-neglect, changes in clothing, fasting, substance abuse or even violence – over a period of time. Often this performance aspect of narrative is played out more as a mime than as a spoken play. It may take the form of behaviour changes, such as too-frequent consultations with a doctor, constantly missing medical appointments, losing prescriptions, or always taking the wrong

dose of medication – all of which can only be 'decoded' over time. In some societies narratives are commonly acted out in the form of a standardized, sometimes very theatrical 'culture-bound syndrome' (see Chapter 10), its meaning clearly understood by other members of the group, but often not by outsiders. In clinical and psychotherapeutic practice, narratives often take the form of particular patterns of physical symptoms revealed over time – especially in the case of *somatization* found in some psychosomatic disorders. In many cultures depression, too, presents mainly as somatic symptoms, rather than as the emotional states of sadness or despair. Part of the task of the clinician then is to understand both the personal and the cultural meanings hidden within these patterns of symptoms. That is, to decode the somatic language in which the narrative of illness may be couched.

Thus, whatever the form they appear in, whether verbal or non-verbal, understanding narratives is an intrinsic part of understanding the nature of human suffering and the many dimensions of illness.

In the following case studies, two folk illnesses, one from the USA and one from the UK, are briefly described. In both cases the folk illness is a cluster of symptoms and signs that are subject to individual and contextual variations, including changes over time.

Case study: 'hyper-tension' in Seattle, USA

Blumhagen's study[54] in 1980, carried out in Seattle at the Veterans' Administration Medical Center, was on patients suffering from hypertension. He discovered a lay EM (explanatory model), held by many of the patients about their condition, termed 'hypertension'. The majority saw their condition as arising from stress or tension in their daily lives – hence hyper-*tension*. In 49 per cent of the sample, chronic external stresses such as overwork, unemployment, 'life's stresses and strains' and certain occupations were blamed for the condition;

14 per cent blamed chronic internal stress, such as psychological, interpersonal or family problems. Fifty-six per cent of the total sample thought that the condition could be precipitated by acute stress, such as anxiety, excitement or anger. In this model, 'hypertension' is characterized by subjective symptoms such as nervousness, fear, anxiety, worry, anger, upset, tenseness, overactivity, exhaustion and excitement. It is brought on by stress, which makes the individual susceptible to becoming 'hyper-tense'. In many cases, patients did not perceive that 'hyper-tension' was the same as high blood pressure, since their model emphasized the psychosocial origin and manifestations of the condition. A smaller number saw 'hyper-tension' as resulting from hereditary or physical factors, such as excess salt, water or fatty foods. Overall, though, 72 per cent believed that hypertension is 'a physical reflection of past social and environmental stressors, which are exacerbated by current stressful situations', and this allowed them to withdraw from familial, social or work obligations – which they saw as sources of tension. They also labelled themselves as 'hyper-tense', even in the absence of medical evidence for hypertension.

Case study: 'colds', 'chills' and 'fevers' in London, UK

The author's own research,[55,56] dealt with a set of commonly held beliefs about 'colds', 'chills' and 'fevers' held by people living in a London suburb, and how these have changed from the 1970s to the present day. In the late 1970s, 'Nature' was seen as a potential cause of disease. 'Colds' and 'chills' were caused by the penetration of the natural environment (particularly areas of cold or damp) across the boundary of skin and into the human body. In general, damp or rain (cold/wet environments) caused cold/wet conditions in the body, such as a 'runny nose' or a 'cold in the head', while cold winds or draughts (cold/dry environments) caused cold/dry conditions, such as a feeling of cold, shivering and muscular aches. Once they entered the body, these cold forces could move from place to place – from a 'head cold', for example, to a 'chest cold'. 'Chills' occurred mainly below the belt ('a bladder chill', 'a chill on the kidneys', 'a stomach chill'), and colds above it ('a head cold', 'a cold in the sinuses', 'a cold in the chest'). These conditions were caused by careless behaviour, by putting oneself in a position of risk vis-à-vis the natural environment – for example, by 'walking barefoot on a cold floor', 'washing your hair when you don't feel well' or 'sitting in a draught after a hot bath'. Temperatures intermediate between hot and cold; where the former gave way to the latter, such as going outdoors after a hot bath, or autumn, where hot summer is giving way to cold winter, were specially conducive to 'catching cold'. Because colds and chills were brought about primarily by one's own behaviour, they provoked little sympathy among other people; individuals were often expected to treat themselves by rest in a warm bed, eating warm food ('feed a cold, starve a fever') and drinking hot drinks.

By contrast, 'fevers' were caused by invisible beings called 'germs', 'bugs' or 'viruses', which penetrate the body through its orifices (mouth, nose, ears, anus, urethra and nostrils) and then cause a raised temperature and other symptoms. The causative agents were conceived of as unseen, amoral, malign entities, which existed in and among people, and which traveled between people through the air. Germ infection was therefore an inherent risk of all social relationships. Some of these germs, such as 'tummy bugs', were thought of as almost insect-like, though of a very small size. Germs also had 'personalities' of symptoms and signs, which revealed themselves over time ('I've got that germ, doctor, you know – the one that gives you the dry cough and the watery eyes'). Unlike with colds, the victims of a fever were blameless, and could mobilize a caring community around themselves. The germs responsible for these conditions could be flushed out by fluids (such as cough medicines), starved out by avoiding food or killed in the body by antibiotics, though in the latter case no differentiation is made between 'viruses' and 'germs'. These lay beliefs about the colds/chills/fevers range of illnesses could thus affect behaviour, self-medication and attitudes towards medical treatment in both adults and children.

Since the 1970s, the model has changed considerably.[56] Although in 2003 these beliefs were still held among many older people, there has been a significant shift in how younger people explain these minor respiratory infections. The two sets of opposites in the original 'feed a cold, starve a fever model' – colds, Nature, and self-blame on one side and fevers, social relationships ('Society') and innocence on the other – have now synthesized into a single, composite model. Now Nature is seen not as a source of infection, but as a positive, health-giving force – and one that is under threat from our modern, industrialized lifestyle. This shift is evident in the new vocabulary of 'natural' or 'organic' as positive qualities, especially in foods and in types of healing. It is now Society – that is, other people – that is now seen as potentially dangerous to the individual, and as a source of ill-health. Blaming illness on 'germs' from other people, rather than on the natural world, has now spread to cover almost all the common colds and chills (as well as fevers), as well as many other conditions. The effect of this shift is to make the ill people feel less guilty for their illness, and see themselves instead as the blameless victim of some external force. This shift in perception also matches several other ways that young people now increasingly blame their misfortunes on others, such as their parents, their teachers, their spouses, their employers, or the state. 'Colds' and 'chills' have thus become a much more *social* concept, an image which seems to express an underlying anxiety about the dangers inherent in all human relationships – especially in the over-crowded cities, apartment blocks, trains and subways of modern life.

Furthermore, this metaphor of invisible 'infection' from others causing illness and misfortune is increasingly used to explain many of the *other* aspects of modern life over which people feel they have no control (a cultural phenomenon I call 'germism').[57] Civil unrest, crime, inflation, terrorism, divorce are now often described in the media as reaching 'epidemic proportions', as if they were somehow caused by invisible, capricious pathogens, outside of their victims' control. Despite all the modern emphasis on individuality and autonomy, this passive model of misfortune seems often to apply at the individual level as well.[58]

CHILDREN'S PERCEPTION OF ILLNESS

Within any community, different groups – depending on age, gender, education, ethnicity, religion and social position – often have very different perceptions of illness. Recent research has focused on *children* and on how they perceive and experience illness and medical care.

The research suggests that, despite their age, children *do* have their own unique understandings of illness, what causes it and how it should be treated. Like adults, they speculate about why and how it has happened to them, and why at that particular time. Their EMs are usually a blend of ideas derived from personal experience and family influences, from school and the media. In most cases these perceptions of illness duplicate those of adults, but sometimes they are very different.

In Europe, a considerable amount of data on the subject has come from a large multinational study carried out between 1990 and 1993 on children aged 7–12 years, and funded by the European Union. Known as the COMAC Childhood and Medicines Project,[59,60] it examined children's experience of illness and medicines in nine European countries. The research methods included a drawing-interview, where the children were each asked to make a drawing of the last time that they were ill and then interviewed about the content and meaning of the drawing. The results showed interesting differences, but many similarities, between the different countries.

The most common symptoms described by the children were those associated with fever, headache, dizziness or rash. Their drawings portrayed themselves as the central figure in the drama of illness, often surrounded by familiar persons or objects. Trakas[61] pointed out that their drawings often give a sense of isolation or loneliness, or of boredom, anxiety or sadness. They show a solitary figure lying in bed, 'entirely alone, seemingly passively waiting for "something" to change their state'.[61] Unlike adults, however, the children's experience of illness was not all bad. Although they described a series of negative sensations (such as pain, or fever) associated with the illness, they also described many positive experiences (such as watching television or videos, getting sweets and toys, having visitors and getting a lot of attention). While visitors were generally welcome, too many caused anxiety, as they were seen as a sign that the illness was serious. In almost all cases, the children emphasized the key role of their mother as the main caregiver. In Botsis and Trakas's study[62] in Athens, Greece, for example, their mothers were drawn 'serving hot tea, asking if juice was wanted, holding thermometers in their hand, and bringing flowers'. In contrast, fathers were hardly ever portrayed (a similar finding to the Spanish study). However, the doctor – whether male or female – was a prominent figure in many of the drawings.

Like adults, the children theorized about why they got ill. Illness was seen as something sudden and unexpected, that 'just happens', often without any reason. Their explanations for its origin – often complex and multicausal – showed how many cultural models (such as the germ theory) they had already absorbed from the adult world around them. These included concepts of the role of 'germs', contagion, cold weather, diet, and their own lifestyle or behaviour. Social causes were only occasionally mentioned, although one girl in Athens speculated that she had got stomach ache because of a spoiled cheese pie given to her by an aunt who disliked her mother. Unlike adults, though, the children usually did not ascribe their illness to supernatural, religious or similar causes.[63]

Climate and the weather were often blamed for causing illness. In their study of 100 children in Spain (Madrid and Tenerife), Aramburuzabala and colleagues[64] found that cold weather was frequently seen as a cause of illness – especially after doing 'something wrong', such as 'walking without my shoes'. Ideas of contagion were also common, and terms such as 'germs' and 'viruses', and 'picking up a germ' were freely used: 'Someone coughs and he gives me his germs; when you breathe, germs get into your body through your nose and mouth; germs are little animals that get inside and make you sick ... colds and things like that'.

In Finland[63], the 7–10-year-olds interviewed in Jyväskylä also revealed how far they had adopted the adult microbiological model, often blaming their illness on contagion by invisible entities called 'bacteria', 'viruses' or 'bugs' – terms that they used interchangeably. One child described bacteria as 'such little things that we people do not see as they are too small'. Like other European children, they also related illness to their own behaviour ('staying too long out in the cold') as well as climatic conditions (cold, damp, rain, snow). Although illness was seen as an interruption in their normal social relationships, it also brought them closer to their parents and got them more attention.

In Holland (Amsterdam and Groningen), Gerrits and colleagues[65] also found close agreement between the views of schoolchildren and those of their parents. Both shared an emphasis on body temperature and the central role of fever in defining whether a child was ill or not and whether to call the doctor. However, the parents differed among themselves in what level was dangerous, the range varying between 38.5°C and 41°C (101.3–105.8°F).

Overall, Vaskilampi and colleagues[63] pointed out that the children's view of health is a holistic, multidimensional one, incorporating physical, psychological and social elements in it. For this reason they tended to see illness in functional terms: as not being able to *do* things.

The COMAC study revealed that childrens' attitudes to *medication*, both prescribed and over-the-counter, varies quite widely, although usually it is quite positive. As one Spanish child put it, 'Medicine advances and kills the microbes, which are bacteria. You get the bacteria and it harms your body; the medicine kills them'. The researchers believed that this attitude matches what, in their view, is the overuse of medication in many Spanish households.[64] Elsewhere in Europe, and especially in Holland,[65] some children were more sceptical about medication than their parents. Some thought taking medicines was less important for their recovery than resting, while others were afraid of their side effects ('A lot of medicines are not right. Something gets better, but at the same moment something else gets worse').

Reviewing the COMAC study, van der Geest[66] noted four themes common to most of the European studies:

1 Children's experiences of illness are expressed by how they describe the medicines they were prescribed. For example, they remember a sweet taste if their experience of illness was positive (such as being pampered and spoilt), but a bitter taste if they were bored and lonely.
2 In many of their accounts of their illness, children never mentioned that they were given medicines. Other aspects of treatment, such as rest and attention, are more important to them. Usually they see illness in *social* terms; as a time when they enjoy special care and attention from other people. Thus, unlike adults, they often welcome the increased dependency of ill health, which gets them more care than they are usually entitled to.
3 In illness, medicines communicate to children the powers that adults hold over them. As sub-

stances forbidden to children, except with adult supervision, they are ways of representing the boundary between child and grown-up – symbols of power and adulthood.
4 The thermometer, as a ritual symbolic object, plays an important part in marking the boundary between health and illness.

Other recent studies have indicated that a major difference between adults and children lies in the perception of *time*, since both experience life within very different timeframes. James and colleagues,[67] and others, have pointed out the many ways that adults impose their own timeframes on children and how, in the home, the temporal rhythms of the child are dictated by family routines, which impose mealtimes and bedtimes on them. Beyond that, there is also the annual cycle of birthdays, major family events, vacations, and national and religious festivals. Later on, numerous other rhythms will impose themselves on the child, often against his or her will. These include the cycle of childhood vaccinations, and then of school timetables, with their rigid control by linear (or monochronic)[68] clock time (see Chapter 2). Also, children's notions of the future and the past are very different from those of adults. One reason why health-promotion campaigns about not smoking, drinking or practising safe sex often have very little impact is because children's ideas of 'distant time' (when these 'bad behaviours' will begin to affect then) are so blurred that they have such little reality for them. Telling a child or adolescent that in 30 or 40 years' time they will develop lung cancer from smoking, or liver damage from alcohol abuse, is a meaningless concept, since they have not lived '30 or 40 years', and have no experience of what that feels like.

Illness therefore highlights these differences in the perception of time. Parents (and doctors) see illness in discrete timeframes, which they use as a way of measuring its danger and severity. These notions determine when to call the doctor if there is no improvement: 'take this aspirin, and let's see if you feel better in half an hour'. Conversely, 'young children's conception of sickness is … primarily an experience without time limits; whether it is of short or long duration, it is the event of sickness itself, with its associated dramas, which is important'.[67] Because illness has an immediate effect, the child wants immediate relief. In some ways, this experience of illness time is similar to Hall's model[68] of 'polychronic' time (see Chapter 2), where time is experienced not in a linear monochronic way, but as a special point at which events and relationships converge.

Finally, other research indicates that children's perceptions of their doctors can be based on very idiosyncratic criteria. For example, one British study[69] found that children saw formally dressed paediatricians as competent but not friendly, but casually dressed paediatricians as friendly but not competent.

These and other studies therefore indicate that doctors and parents should acknowledge and respect children's views of their illness, even if these views are sometimes 'unexpected and amazing'.[61] Like adults, their ideas often have a very clear internal logic, even if they are not scientific. The studies indicate that, in general, children *are* able to recognize abnormal symptoms and understand much of what their doctors say to them. Children – even younger children – are not merely passive spectators of their own ill health. Where appropriate, it is important to give them explanations that make sense to them, in terms of their own unique frame of reference. As Trakas[61] concludes, 'Children who are able to communicate with their health-care providers will grow into adults who can do the same'.

THE DOCTOR–PATIENT CONSULTATION

Against this background of medical beliefs about disease, and lay beliefs about illness, three aspects of the doctor–patient interaction can be viewed:

1 Why do people decide (or not decide) to consult a doctor when ill?
2 What happens during the consultation?
3 What happens after the consultation?

REASONS FOR CONSULTING, OR NOT CONSULTING, A DOCTOR

Several studies have examined the reasons why some ill people consult a doctor while others with the same complaint do not. Often this is because people simply cannot afford to pay for medical care, or because medical care is not available to them. However, even when they *can* afford it there is often little correlation between the severity of a physical illness and the decision to seek medical help. In some cases this delay can have serious consequences for the person's health. Other studies have shown that abnormal symptoms are common in the population, but that only a small percentage of them are brought to the attention of doctors. There are therefore a number of *non*-physiological factors that influence what Zola[70] terms the 'pathways to the doctor'. These include:

1 The availability of medical care.
2 Whether the patient can afford it.
3 The failure or success of treatments within the popular or folk sectors.
4 How the patient perceives the problem.
5 How others around him or her perceive the problem.

Obviously the sparse availability of medical care in many parts of the world, and the inability to pay for what care there is (or for medications, special diets, or transport to a clinic), are crucial in determining whether people consult a doctor or not; as is the failure of non-medical care to cure or reassure the individual patient. In this section, however, only the last two points, and the relationship between them, will be discussed.

The process of becoming 'ill' has already been described, particularly the definition of some symptoms as abnormal by patients and their families. Zola[70] has pointed out that this definition depends on how common the symptom is in their society, and whether it fits with the major values of that society or group. A symptom that is very common may be considered normal (though not necessarily good or desirable) and therefore be accepted fatalistically; for example, Zola found that tiredness is often considered to be normal, even though it is sometimes a feature of severe illness.[70] In the study of 'Regionville' mentioned previously, backache was considered to be a normal part of life, at least by the lower socio-economic groups. The second point is that symptoms and signs must *fit* with society's view of what constitutes illness in order to gain sympathetic attention, and for treatment to be arranged. The same symptom or sign might be interpreted differently, therefore, by different groups of individuals, as illness in one or as normal in another. In both cases, the definition of ill health depends on the underlying concept of health, which, as noted earlier, often includes social, behavioural or emotional elements.

Zola[71] has also examined how this wider definition of health affects patients' decisions to consult a doctor. In the mid-1960s he interviewed more than 200 American patients from three ethnic groups – Irish-Americans, Italian-Americans and Anglo-Saxon Protestant Americans – attending outpatient clinics in two Boston hospitals. The study aimed to find out why they had decided to consult a doctor, and how they communicated their distress to him. It was found that there were two ways of perceiving and communicating one's bodily complaints: either 'restricting' or 'generalizing' them. The first was typical of the Irish, the second of the Italians. The Irish focused on a specific physical dysfunction (such as poor eyesight or ptosis), and restricted its effect to their physical functioning. The Italians displayed many more symptoms, and a more 'global malfunctioning' of many aspects of their body, appearance, energy level, emotions, and so on. In their perception, the physical symptoms (such as poor eyesight) interfered with their general mode of living, their social relationships and their occupations.

On this basis, Zola[71] was able to identify five non-physiological 'triggers' to the decision to seek medical aid:

1 An interpersonal crisis.
2 Perceived interference with personal relationships.
3 'Sanctioning'; that is, one individual taking primary responsibility for the decision to seek medical aid for someone else (the patient).
4 Perceived interference with work or physical functioning.
5 The setting of external time criteria ('If it isn't better in three days ... then I'll take care of it').

The first two patterns draw attention to the symptom, by signifying that there is 'something wrong' in the patients' daily lives; this pattern was common among the Italians. The third pattern was common among the Irish, and illustrates the social dimensions of illness ('Well I tend to let things go but not my wife, so on the first day of my vacation my wife said, "Why don't you come, why don't you take care of it now?" So I did'). The functional definition (the fourth pattern) of health was common among both Irish and Anglo-Saxon groups (cf. Blaxter and Paterson).[11] The fifth pattern was common among all the groups, and echoes the adult perception of time described above.

This study illustrates that decisions to consult a doctor may be related to socio-cultural factors, such as wider definitions of health, rather than to an illness's severity. Zola noted that in any community unexplained epidemiological differences may result from the differential occurrence of these factors, which reflect the 'selectivity and attention which get people and their episodes into medical statistics, rather than to any true difference in the prevalence and incidence of a particular problem or disorder' (see Chapter 15).

Apple[13] pointed out the dangers of defining a symptom as illness only when it interferes with usual activities and is of fairly recent onset. It means that more chronic, insidious conditions, such as heart disease, hypertension, cancer or HIV infection, may not be defined as abnormal, provided that one can carry on with daily life. Other reasons for the delay in seeking medical advice have been studied at the Massachusetts General Hospital in Boston: Hackett and colleagues[72] examined the delay between the first sign or symptom of cancer and the search for medical help in 563 patients. Only 33.7 per cent were 'early responders' and consulted within the first 4 weeks, while two-thirds waited over a month; 8 per cent of the sample avoided medical help until they could no longer function independently, and only then did they 'yield to family or community pressure and receive medical help'. The role of emotional factors was important: people who worried more about cancer tended to delay seeking help more than non-worriers, and it was hypothesized that the reason for the delay might be to avoid hearing a fatal diagnosis. The label given to the illness also affected the delay; labelling it candidly as 'cancer' led to a quicker response. In general, patients from higher socio-economic levels delayed a shorter time than those from poorer classes, although 'there is little evidence that cancer education programmes *per se* can be credited for this difference'. In a similar study, Olin and Hackett[73] studied 32 patients with acute myocardial infarction; most had explained away their chest pain as resulting from less serious conditions, such as indigestion, lung trouble, pneumonia or ulcer, despite the fact that they were familiar with the symptoms of coronary heart disease. The immediate response was denial, which was 'the consequence of an emotional crisis induced by chest pain and the menacing associations it evokes'. In the majority of cases, only increasing incapacity or the persuasion of family or friends led them to seek medical help.

Whether medical care is utilized – provided, of course, that it is available and affordable – depends also on the perceived *cause* of the condition and whether it is believed to originate in the individual, or in the natural, social or supernatural worlds. Some groups consider medicine is better at treating symptoms than eliminating the cause, especially if it is supernatural. In a study[74] of five ethnic groups in Miami, for example,

patients sought symptomatic relief from a medical doctor but expected a folk healer to explain the cause in culturally familiar terms (such as witchcraft), and then to treat it by mystical means.

In all the above cases, a number of non-physiological factors (social, cultural and emotional) influence whether ill people or their families seek medical help or not. These factors also influence how this illness is presented in the doctor–patient consultation.

THE PRESENTATION OF ILLNESS

The way in which different individuals, social and cultural groups, use different *languages of distress* in communicating their suffering to others, including to doctors, has been described earlier. A clinician who is unable to decode this language, which may be verbal or non-verbal, somatic or psychological, is in danger of making the wrong diagnosis and providing the wrong sort of treatment. For example, in Zola's study in 1966,[71] the Italian-Americans presented their illness in a more voluble, emotional and dramatic way, complaining of many more symptoms, and stressing its effect on their social circumstances. In contrast, the Irish tended to underplay their symptoms. Where no organic disease was found, the physicians tended to diagnose the Italians as having neurotic or psychological conditions, such as tension headaches, functional problems or personality disorders, while the Irish were given a neutral diagnosis such as 'nothing found on tests', without being labelled neurotic. At the same time, the Irish stoicism in the presentation of illness could lead to more serious conditions being missed. In an early paper by Zborowski,[75] the findings were similar: in his study of responses to pain by Irish-American, Italian-American and Jewish-American patients in New York he found that the more emotional the language of distress, the more likely the patient was to be wrongly labelled as 'neurotic' or 'overemotional'.

The presentation of illness may also be learned from doctors, as well as from the media, especially by patients with chronic diseases. They learn to display the typical clinical picture that the doctors are looking for. In the author's study[76], a man who was mistakenly diagnosed as having angina from 'heart trouble' developed psychosomatic chest pain, and this gradually came to resemble 'real' angina the more contact he had with clinicians, especially cardiologists. This 'symptom choice', in the absence of physical disease, has been described by Mechanic[77] in the case of 'medical students' disease', a form of hypochondria believed to afflict up to 70 per cent of medical students. As they learn about the various diseases, they frequently imagine they are suffering from them and even develop their typical symptoms and signs. This is because the stressful conditions of medical school cause many transient symptoms in the students, and those 'diffuse and ambiguous symptoms regarded as normal in the past may be reconceptualized within the context of newly acquired knowledge of disease'. This may influence the patterning and presentation of their symptomatology. This, then, is an example of the language of distress acquired from the medical profession – a situation that is becoming increasingly common as people become more knowledgeable about health issues.

PROBLEMS OF THE DOCTOR–PATIENT CONSULTATION

The clinical consultation, as Kleinman[16] has noted, is a transaction between lay and professional EMs. It is also, however, a transaction between two parties separated by differences in *power*, both social and symbolic. This power differential may be based on social class, ethnicity, age or gender, and is a crucial influence on any consultation.

Although the consultation is characterized by ritual and symbolic elements, its manifest functions are:

1 The presentation of 'illness' by the patient, both verbally and non-verbally.

2 The translation of these diffuse symptoms or signs into the named pathological entities of medicine; that is, converting 'illness' into 'disease'.

3 The prescription of a treatment regimen that is acceptable to both doctor and patient.

Some of its more latent functions, especially in relation to social control, have already been discussed in the previous chapter. In order for the consultation to be a success, there must be a *consensus* between the two parties about the cause, diagnostic label, physiological processes involved, prognosis and optimal treatment for the condition. The search for a consensus – an agreed interpretation of the patient's condition – has been called 'negotiation' by Stimson and Webb.[78] In this process, each tries to influence the other regarding the outcome of the consultation – the diagnosis given and the treatment prescribed. Patients may try to reduce the seriousness of a diagnosis, or the severity of a treatment regimen, for example. In particular, they may strive for diagnoses and treatments that make sense to them in terms of their lay view of ill health, such as the appeal for 'tonics' or vitamins in the UK, which have deep roots in traditional medicine. The consultation is also a social process, whereby the ill person acquires the social role of patient, with all the rights and obligations that this entails. It should always be remembered, however, that achieving a consensus between doctor and patient is no guarantee in itself that the diagnosis will be correct, or that the treatment offered will be effective.

Within the consultation, one can isolate a number of recurring problems that interfere with the development of consensus. These problems, many of which have already been described, include the following.

Differences in the definition of 'the patient'

Western medicine tends to focuses increasingly on the *individual* patient[36] (or even on an individual organ or body system), but it may be the family, the community or even the wider society that are pathological, and not the individual. An inappropriate focus only on the individual and his or her symptoms, while ignoring wider familial, social and economic issues, may make both a consensus and a solution to the problem difficult to achieve. Modern family therapy thus emphasizes the role of the family in causing, and maintaining, certain types of mental or behavioral disorders in children, and therefore that for a solution to this problem the family, as well as the child, also has to undergo treatment.

Misinterpretation of patients' 'languages of distress'

These are clearly illustrated in the studies of Zola,[71] Apple[13], Mechanic[77] and Zborowski[75], and in the case of many of the 'culture-bound syndromes'. This phenomenon is more likely if the doctor and patient come from different cultural or religious backgrounds, or socio-economic classes, though it can also arise if doctor and patient are of different age groups or gender. A common example is the misinterpretation of somatization (see Chapters 7 and 10) as evidence of physical disease, or hypochondria, or of an absence of psychological 'insight'.

Incompatibility of explanatory models

Medical and lay models may differ greatly in how they interpret a particular illness episode, especially its cause, diagnosis and appropriate treatment. For one thing, they are often based on different understandings of the structure and function of the body. For example, many Western-trained doctors working in a rural setting in the non-industrialized world may have difficulty in understanding supernatural and interpersonal explanations of ill health, or definitions of good health as moral or social 'balance'. The sometimes limited disease perspective of modern medicine, with its emphasis on quantifiable physical data, may ignore the many dimensions of meaning – psychological, moral or social – that characterize the illness perspective of the patient and those around him or her. Thus the doctor, who concentrates only on diagnosing and treating physical dysfunction,

may not take emotional states such as guilt, shame, remorse or fear on the patient's part into account.

Disease without illness

This is an increasingly common phenomenon in modern medicine, with its emphasis on the use of diagnostic technology (see Chapter 4). Physical abnormalities of the body are found, often at the biochemical or cellular levels, but the patient does not feel ill. Examples of this are hypertension, raised blood cholesterol, cervical carcinoma *in situ*, or HIV infection, which are found on routine health screening programmes. People who are asymptomatic may not make use of these programmes, or may refuse treatment if an abnormality is found ('But I don't *feel* unwell'). This may also explain much of the reported non-compliance with prescribed medication; for example, a person prescribed a 1-week course of antibiotics may stop taking them after 2 or 3 days because they feel much better.

Illness without disease

Here the person feels that 'something is wrong' in their life – physically, emotionally, socially or even spiritually – but despite their subjective state they are told, after a physical examination and tests, that 'there is nothing wrong with you'. However, in many cases they continue to feel unwell or unhappy. Many of these people can be called the 'worried well'. Also included here are the many unpleasant emotions or physical sensations for which no physical cause can be found, many of them arising from the difficulties and strains of everyday life: the various 'psychosomatic' disorders (such as irritable colon, spasmodic torticollis, hyperventilation syndrome or Da Costa's syndrome); hypochondria (such as 'medical students' disease'); and the wide range of folk illnesses (such as 'spirit possession', *susto* or 'high blood'). In each of these cases the illness plays an important part in the patient's life and in the lives of their family, and reassurance that nothing is wrong physically may not be enough to treat it, as illustrated in the following case history.

Case study: illness without disease, London, UK

Balint[79] described the case of Mr U, aged 35 years, a skilled workman who was partly disabled as a result of having contracted polio in childhood. Nevertheless, he had managed to work, 'over-compensating his physical shortcomings by high efficiency'. One day he received a severe electric shock at work and was knocked unconscious; no organic damage was found at the hospital, and he was discharged. He then consulted his family doctor for pains in all parts of his body, which were getting worse and worse, and he 'thought that something had happened to him through the electric shock'. Despite exhaustive tests, no physical abnormality was found, but Mr U still experienced his symptoms: 'They seem to think I am imagining things: I know what I've got'. He still definitely felt ill and wanted to know what condition he could have causing all these pains. Despite more hospital tests that were negative, he still felt himself to be ill. In Balint's view, he was 'proposing an illness' to the doctor, but this was consistently rejected; the doctor's emphasis was not on the patient's pains, anxieties, fears and hopes for sympathy and understanding, but on the exclusion of an underlying physical abnormality.

Problems of terminology

Clinical consultations are usually conducted in a mixture of everyday language and medical jargon. However, the language of medicine itself has become more and more technical and esoteric over the past century or so,[80] and increasingly incomprehensible to the lay public. Where medical terms *are* used by either party, there is often a danger of mutual misunderstanding; the same term, for example, may have entirely different meanings for doctor and patient. In a study in 1970, Boyle[81] found that doctors and patients interpreted common medical terms such as stomach, heartburn, palpitations, flatulence or lungs in very different ways. The marked variations between the two groups could have important clinical implications, especially since many consultations include questions such as, 'Do you have pain in your stomach?' (which 58.8 per cent of the patients thought occupied their entire abdominal cavity). Similarly, a study by Pearson and Dudley[82] also showed major misunderstandings of terms such as gallbladder, stomach or liver. They pointed out that patients awaiting cholecystectomy could become extremely anxious if (like some of the sample) they believed that the gall-*bladder* was concerned with the storage of urine. Blumhagen's study[54] on lay beliefs about the meaning of 'hyper-tension' also found them to be different from medical definitions of hypertension. In the study of lay beliefs about 'germs' and 'viruses' quoted above, these bore little relation to their description in microbiology; both were considered vulnerable to antibiotics, and these drugs were demanded even if the diagnosis was of a 'viral infection'. The use of the same terminology by doctor and patient is *not*, therefore, a guarantee of mutual understanding as the terms, and their significance, may be conceptualized by both parties in entirely different ways.

Patients' use of specialized folk terminology may also confuse the clinician: statements such as 'I have been hexed' or 'a spirit has made me ill' may be incomprehensible to doctors unless they are aware of lay theories of illness causation. The same applies to self-labelled folk illnesses such as *susto*, 'heart distress' or 'brain fag', especially where the clinician comes from a different social or cultural background.

Questions in the consultation that are designed to uncover emotional distress may also involve problems of terminology. For example, Leff,[83] in a study in London, compared psychiatrists' and patients' concepts of unpleasant emotions. It was found that the psychiatrists clearly differentiated between anxiety, depression and irritability as discrete types of emotional distress, while the patients saw them as closely overlapping. To the patients, somatic symptoms such as palpitations, excessive perspiration or shakiness were considered to be as characteristic of 'depression' as of 'anxiety'. This would clearly influence how patients responded to specific questions such as, 'Do you feel depressed?' or 'Do you feel anxious?' Again, ignorance of how patients conceptualize and label ill health can lead to misinterpretation of symptoms during the consultation.

Problems of treatment

In order for medical treatment to be acceptable to patients, it must make sense in terms of their EMs. Consensus here about the form and purpose of treatment is as important as consensus about the diagnosis. This is particularly important if the treatment involves unpleasant physical sensations or side-effects, where it induces, in effect, a form of temporary 'illness'. This is the case in surgery, injections, radiotherapy, chemotherapy and certain diagnostic tests such as biopsies and sigmoidoscopy. Prescribed medication may not be taken if it is perceived to cause illness or, as in the case of asymptomatic hypertension, if the patient does not feel at all ill. A medication may also not be taken if relatives or friends have previously had side-effects from it. Another problem, mentioned elsewhere, is that the use of self-prescribed medicines is common in combination with the use of prescribed drugs; people may use both in ways that make sense to them in terms of their own view of ill health. The phenomenon of *non-compliance* has been estimated, in the UK, as 30 per cent or more.[84] In one UK study by Waters and colleagues[85] in 1976, out of 1611 prescriptions issued by general practitioners, 7 per cent were not even presented to pharmacists. The misuse of prescribed medication, based on specific lay beliefs, has been described by Harwood[86] among a group of Puerto Ricans in New York City (see Chapter 3). They divided all illnesses, foods and medicines into three groups: hot, cold and (sometimes) cool. Penicillin was regarded as a 'hot' drug, and was appropriate for prophylactic treatment in rheumatic heart disease (a 'cold' ill-

ness). If, however, an individual had diarrhoea or constipation ('hot' conditions), they would immediately break off penicillin treatment. In pregnancy, 'hot' foods or medications were also avoided in case they caused 'hot' illnesses, such as rashes or red skin, in the baby; because iron supplements or vitamins were 'hot', they might also be refused. Similar avoidance of certain foods or medicines classified as 'hot' have been found in many other communities elsewhere in the world.

The *success* of a treatment or medication is often evaluated very differently by doctors and their patients. The disappearance of an identifiable physical disease may not be accompanied by the disappearance of illness, though this situation can be reversed. For example, Cay and colleagues[87] examined patients' assessment of the results of surgery for peptic ulcers and compared these with the assessments of their surgeons, and found marked discrepancies between the two. Doctor-determined criteria of success, such as acid reduction, absence of diarrhoea, freedom from recurrence or completeness of antrectomy or vagotomy, differed from those of patients, who used quality of life criteria such as the effect on family life, social life, work, sex and sleeping habits. A successful operation in the eyes of the surgeon was sometimes seen as a failure by the patient, especially if it had interfered with any of these aspects of quality of life. That is, 'a bad result … is determined more by psychosocial than physical evidence of failure'. Conversely, operations that the surgeons regarded as failures – owing to residual symptoms of diarrhoea, for example – were regarded as a success by patients, and the residual symptoms 'a price worth paying' for the absence of severe and unpredictable ulcer symptoms. In both cases an underlying functional definition of health can be hypothesized, against which the success of the operation was judged.

The role of context

A final but very important source of problems in the doctor–patient consultation is the role played by the *context* of the consultation itself. There are two aspects to this context, both of which play a crucial role in the doctor–patient relationship:

1 An *internal context* of the prior experience, expectations, cultural assumptions, explanatory models and prejudices (based on social, gender, religious or racial criteria) that each party brings to the clinical encounter.[88]
2 An *external context*, which includes the actual setting in which the encounter takes place (such as a hospital, clinic or doctor's office) and the wider social influences acting upon the two parties. These include the dominant ideology, religion and economic system of the society, as well as its divisions and social inequalities based on class, gender or ethnicity. All of these factors help to define who has power in the consultation and who does not. Of key importance here is the role of economic and social inequalities – particularly the differences in power between doctor and patient.

The sum of these two types of contexts can greatly influence the types of communication possible between doctor and patient, for they help to determine what is said in the consultation, how it is said, and how it is heard and interpreted.

THE DOCTOR–PATIENT RELATIONSHIP: STRATEGIES FOR IMPROVEMENT

This chapter has outlined some of the potential differences in medical and lay perspectives on ill health – between models of disease and those of illness – and some of the problems that this raises in the consultation. Six main strategies can be suggested to deal with these problems:

1 Understanding illness.
2 Improving communication.
3 Increasing reflexivity.
4 Treating illness *and* disease.
5 Respecting diversity.
6 Assessing the role of context.

UNDERSTANDING 'ILLNESS'

As well as searching for disease, the clinician should try to discover how patients and those around them view the origin, significance and prognosis of the condition, and also how it affects other aspects of their lives – such as their income or social relationships. The patient's emotional reactions to ill health (such as guilt, fear, shame, anger or uncertainty) are all as relevant to the clinical encounter as physiological data, and sometimes more so. The patient's EM of their ill health, and those of their family, should be elicited by obtaining answers to the seven questions listed in the The Explanatory Model section earlier in this chapter. Information should also be gathered about the patients' cultural, religious and social background, their economic status, previous experience of ill health and hopes and fears, and, if possible, their view of misfortune in general, in order to put their explanations for ill health in a wider context.

IMPROVING COMMUNICATION

The clinician should acquire knowledge of the specific language of distress used by the patient, especially the presentation of culturally specific folk illnesses. There should also be an awareness of the problems of terminology mentioned above, especially the misinterpretation of medical terms. The clinician's diagnosis and treatment must *make sense* to the patients, in terms of their lay view of ill health, and should acknowledge and respect the patients' experience and interpretation of their own condition. As stated by Mechanic[77], 'The efficacy of the doctor's interpretations of his patient's problems will depend on the extent to which they are credible in terms of the patient's experience and the extent to which he anticipates the patient's experiences and… the patient's reactions to symptoms and treatment'. However, as noted earlier, while good communication is essential, it does not in itself guarantee good medical care.

INCREASING REFLEXIVITY

Successful doctor–patient communication is not really possible without a heightened sense of self-awareness (or "reflexivity'),[89] on the doctor's part, in all clinical encounters. Whether in making a diagnosis or prescribing treatment, the clinician should always reflect on the role of his or her *own* social and personal background, especially culture, economic status, gender, religion, education, experiences, prejudices and professional power – in either improving or diminishing both communication with patients and effective health care. That is, they should be aware of, and where possible diminish, the possibility of *cultural counter-transference*. Doctors are not only the standardized products of medical schools and their disease perspective, their perceptions are personal, idiosyncratic and cultural as well as professional. For this reason it is important to emphasize that one cannot really understand other people's inner motivations and beliefs without, to some extent, understanding one's own.

TREATING ILLNESS AND DISEASE

Medical treatment should never deal solely with physical abnormalities or malfunctions. The many dimensions of illness – emotional, social, behavioural, religious – should also be treated by adequate explanation and reassurance in terms that make sense to the patients and those around them. Where necessary, treatment may have to be shared with a psychotherapist, counsellor, priest, alternative practitioner, social worker, self-help group, community organization, housing or employment agency or even, in some settings, with a culturally sanctioned folk healer. In this way *all* dimensions of the patient's illness can be treated, as well as any physical disease.

RESPECTING DIVERSITY

Clinicians need to acknowledge that the Western medical model of ill health is not the only valid one available. They have to recognize that there are many other ways, world-wide, of interpreting human suffering, and many different ways of relieving it. Furthermore, some of these have distinct advantages over the biomedical model, although others do not. This should imply a respect for the diversity of health beliefs and practices found in different countries, communities and individuals. It also involves seeing biomedicine in proportion – as just one part (albeit a very successful and important part) of a world-wide system of pluralistic health care.

ASSESSING THE ROLE OF CONTEXT

In order to understand any doctor–patient interaction, the role of both the internal and external *contexts* described above should always be assessed. It is particularly important to understand those external contexts – such as social and economic factors (including poverty, discrimination, deprivation, racism, unemployment, overcrowding and gender roles) and environmental factors (such as pollution, overpopulation, shortage of health-care facilities and contaminated water supplies) – that may contribute to the origin, presentation and prognosis of ill health. A consideration of context also helps the clinician to decide who is the real patient, and whether the focus of diagnosis and treatment should be on sick individuals, their family, their community, or the wider society in which they live.

KEY REFERENCES

3 Good, B. J. and Good, M. D. (1981). The meaning of symptoms: a cultural hermeneutic model for clinical practice. In: *The Relevance of Social Science for Medicine* (Eisenberg, L. and Kleinman, A.eds). Dordrech: Reidel, pp. 165–96.

8 Cassell, F.J. (1976). *The Healer's Art: A New Approach to the Doctor–Patient Relationship*. Philadelphia: Lippincott, pp. 47–83.

16 Kleinman, A. (1980). *Patients and Healers in the Context of Culture*. Berkeley: University of California Press, pp. 104–18.

19 Rubel, A.J. (1977). The epidemiology of a folk illness: *Susto* in Hispanic America. In: *Culture, Disease and Healing: Studies in Medical Anthropology* (D. Landy, ed.). London: Macmillan, pp. 119–28.

21 Krause, I. B. (1989). Sinking heart: a Punjabi communication of distress. *Soc. Sci. Med.*, 29, 563–75.

24 Sontag, S. (2001). *Illness as Metaphor and AIDS and its Metaphors*. London: Picador.

32 Weiss, M. (1997). Signifying the pandemics: metaphors of AIDS, cancer, and heart disease. *Med. Anthropol. Q. (New Series)* 11, 456–76.

43 Spooner, B. (1970). The evil eye in the Middle East. In: *Witchcraft Confessions and Accusations* (Douglas, M. ed.). London: Tavistock, pp. 311–19.

46 McGuire, M.B. (1988). *Ritual Healing in Suburban America*. Piscataway: Rutgers University Press, p. 83.

67 James, A., Jenks, C. and Prout, A. (1998). *Theorizing Childhood*. Cambridge: Polity Press, pp. 77–9.

88 Hall, E. T. (1977). *Beyond Culture*. Grantham: Anchor Books, pp. 85–103.

See http://www.culturehealthandillness.com for the full list of references for this chapter.

RECOMMENDED READING

Disease versus illness

Kleinman, A. (1980). *Patients and Healers in the Context of Culture*. Berkeley: University of California Press.

Lock, M. and Gordon, D. (eds) (1988) *Biomedicine Examined*. Dordrecht: Kluwer.

Lay health beliefs

Currer, C. and Stacey, M. (eds) (1986). *Concepts of Health, Illness and Disease*. Oxford: Berg Publishers.

Snow, L. F. (1993). *Walkin' over Medicine*. Boulder: Westview Press.

Narratives of illness

Becker, G. (1997). *Disrupted Lives*. Berkeley: University of California Press.

Brody, Howard (2003) *Stories of Sickness*, 2nd edn. Oxford: Oxford University Press.

Kleinman, A. (1988). *The Illness Narratives*. New York: Basic Books.

6

Gender and reproduction

All human societies divide their populations into two social categories, which they call 'male' and 'female'. Each of these categories is based on a series of assumptions – drawn from the culture in which they occur – about the different attributes, beliefs and behaviours characteristic of the individuals included within that category.

Although this binary division of humanity into two genders is universal, on closer examination it is clearly a rather more complex phenomenon, with many variations reported in how male and female behaviour is defined in different cultural groups. To illustrate this point, the following chapter will examine two separate, though interrelated, subjects: anthropological research into gender, and its relationship to health and health care; and pregnancy and childbirth in a cross-cultural perspective.

GENDER

THE 'NATURE' VERSUS 'NURTURE' CONTROVERSY

One of the basic debates of social thought, especially for the past century or so, has been the nature *versus* nurture controversy – which in anthropology has been the debate between the ideas of 'nature' and those of 'culture'. In summary, this nature/nurture debate centred on whether human behaviour and the human mind (including its intelligence and person-

ality), as well as perceived differences between human groups (such as ethnic or religious groups, social classes or genders), were all the result of *nature* or of *nurture*. 'Nature' was conceptualized as rooted in biology, and as something fixed, universal and immutable, while 'nurture' was seen as the influence of the environment (both social and cultural), and was therefore more changeable and more dependent on local contexts. This conceptual division had all sorts of political and social implications; taking the strict nature line, for example, could mean that one group of people (or another gender) was regarded as biologically inferior to another, and that this could never be altered, no matter what environmental influences were brought to bear upon them. Within the last century this approach has often been used as a justification for the persecution, colonization or exploitation of various groups of people in different parts of the world.

Today, this type of debate has largely receded, at least in academic circles, and most anthropologists would reject both extreme biological determinism *and* extreme environmental determinism. In explaining human behaviour they would look instead at the complex *interaction* (within a specific environment) between culture, ecology and social structure, and the psychobiological nature of human beings.[1]

The echoes of the nature/nurture debate still remain in contemporary discussions of gender. Here gender is often described as if it were the result of either nature *or* of culture (that is, of nurture). Feminist anthropologists[2] have pointed out that, in Western thought in particular, women and their sexuality have often been seen as less 'cultural' than men, and equated with 'nature' (uncontrolled, dangerous, polluting) rather than with the 'culture' (controlled, creative, ordered) of the male world. They have argued that this conceptual division of nature from culture (and the implied opposition between the two) is in itself artificial, a false dichotomy that represents a specifically Western and culture-bound way of looking at human behaviour. Furthermore, this way of thinking, and the conceptual division of the world into these two value-laden categories, is not found to the same extent elsewhere in the world.

They have also pointed out the social implications of this division, for in Western thought culture is usually seen as being superior to, and more human than, nature. At its most extreme – especially in the nineteenth century – this model provided a justification for the superiority of men, since it saw female nature as something to be conquered, transformed and then made productive by the forces of male culture.

In looking at sexual identity, though, it is reasonable to say that both biological *and* environmental influences play some part in the definition of any individual's gender. In all societies, men and women have different body shapes and different physiological cycles; women menstruate, become pregnant, give birth and lactate, while men do not. There are also emotional and behavioural differences between the two. However, it is the *cultural meanings* that are given to those physiological, psychological and social phenomena, and how these in turn influence people's behaviour and even the social, political and economic system of the society, that is of chief interest to the modern anthropologist.

COMPONENTS OF GENDER

The 'gender' of a particular individual can best be understood as the result of a complex combination of a number of elements. These include:

1 *Genetic gender*, based on genotype and the combinations of the two sex chromosomes, X and Y (XX = female and XY = male).
2 *Somatic gender*, based on phenotype (especially physical appearance) and the development of secondary sex characteristics (external genitalia, breasts, voice and distribution of body fat and hair).
3 *Psychological gender*, based on the person's own self-perception and behaviour.
4 *Social gender*, based on the wider cultural categories of male and female, which define how individuals are perceived by society, how they must look, think, feel, dress, act and perceive the world that they live in.

However, at each of these levels there are areas of anomaly and ambiguity in this neat binary division of humankind. At the genetic level, for example, the division of the population into either XX or XY can be altered where certain abnormalities of the sex chromosomes occur, such as in Turner's syndrome (XO), Klinefelter's syndrome (XXY), Y polysomy (XYY) or even true hermaphroditism (XX/XY).[3] At the somatic level, abnormalities of hormonal development can lead to secondary sex characteristics that are at variance with genetic gender. Examples include both male and female *pseudohermaphroditism*, where an individual has the genetic constitution and gonads of one sex but the external genitalia of the other.[3] People may also have both genotype and phenotype of a biological male, be defined as male by the wider society, and yet behave, dress and perceive themselves as essentially *female* – as in the case of some transsexuals.

Of all aspects of gender identity, 'social gender' is the most flexible one and that most influenced by social and cultural environment. Anthropologists who have studied the two categories of male and female in many societies throughout the world have found a great many variations in the scope and content of each of these categories. That is, they have found that behaviour considered appropriately 'male' (or 'female') in one group may often be considered more 'female' (or 'male') in another.

GENDER CULTURES

Until comparatively recently, most of the fieldwork carried out by male anthropologists paid little attention to the 'women's worlds' of the societies that they studied.[4] Where the male and female worlds were very separate, they had virtually no access to the inner secrets of the women's worlds, especially to their beliefs and practices relating to sexuality, pregnancy, childbirth and menstruation. In recent years, however, a large number of ethnographies have been done, especially by female anthropologists, which have corrected this earlier imbalance. One of the features of this new wave of research is to highlight the role of 'nurture', or social and cultural influences, on the definitions of gender in human societies.

In all societies, the division of the social world into 'male' and 'female' categories means that boys and girls are socialized in very different ways. They are educated to have different expectations of life and to develop emotionally and intellectually in particular ways, and are subject in their daily lives to different norms of dress and behaviour. Whatever the contribution of biology to human behaviour, it is clear that *culture* also contributes a set of guidelines, both explicit and implicit, that are acquired from infancy onwards, and tell the individual how to perceive, think, feel and act as either a male or a female member of that society.

These two sets of guidelines within a particular society can be described as the *gender cultures* of that society. In some parts of the world, especially in less industrialized countries, these gender cultures may be so different from one another that men and women in that society could be described as living like 'two nations under one flag'.

As an example of this, in many societies in New Guinea, men's and women's worlds are so polarized that they actually live in separate houses in different parts of the village and, in Keesing's[5] words, 'have sexual relations infrequently in an atmosphere of tension and danger'. In some of these societies, where homosexuality is institutionalized, this adds further to the polarization of the two sexes.

In another example, Goddard[6] in 1987 described the different male and female worlds in the city of Naples, Italy, especially in relation to sexual behaviour and to the cultural values of honour and shame. As in other Mediterranean societies, very different norms (and a moral double standard) operated for each of the sexes. For example, healthy, 'normal' men were expected to have many premarital and extramarital affairs as proof of their masculinity, while women were barred from either. Men were expected actively to defend their own and their family's honour, while women's honour lay in preserving their purity and chastity. Men's honour could be damaged (and be replaced by shame) if the honour of their womenfolk was compromised in any way. However, as in other cultures, there was an ambivalence in the men's attitudes towards women – in this Mediterranean community they were seen as 'either dangerously vulnerable or eminently available and seducible'. Dunk[7] in 1989 described a similar picture among Greek villagers living in Montreal, Canada. Despite local variations, there was a general assumption in rural Greece that men's role is to protect the family honour through their self-respect or sense of honour (*philotimo*), while women's sexual modesty or shame (*dropi*) must be protected through their carefully controlled behaviour. In order to protect their *dropi*, women were expected to exert considerable self-control both in private and in public. Family honour and social worth were particularly important and were constantly being scrutinized by other families. Shepherd[8] in 1982 described a similar division of norms among Muslim Swahilis in Mombasa, Kenya. Women were thought of (by men) to be 'sexually enthusiastic and sexually irresponsible, given the opportunity'. They were expected to be dependent on men, but at the same time the men also feared the polluting power of their menstrual blood. However, men were expected to support – and therefore control – both women and children. This control was considered most effective when exerted over the virginity of their unmarried daughters, but less effective when dealing with the faithfulness of their wives. For a young girl in that community, marriage and its consummation were 'the only pathway to female adulthood'.

In each of these cases quoted above, as elsewhere in the world, the division of human society into two gender cultures is one of the most basic elements of social structure, and an important part of the symbolic system of any particular society. However, part of this binary structure expresses the ambivalence with which some men regard the women of their community; at times as nurturant mothers or healers (see Chapter 4), and at other times as malevolent 'witches' (see Chapter 5) or as dangerous sources of menstrual pollution (see Chapter 2).

Variations in gender cultures

Gender roles, however, are by no means completely rigid, and they can often change and develop, especially under the influence of urbanization and industrialization. In industrial societies, as the Embers[9] have noted, 'when machines replace human strength and when women can assign child care to others, strict division of labour by sex begins to disappear'.

Although there are always certain constancies cross-culturally in the gender divisions of labour,[4,9] there is also considerable evidence from anthropological research of the wide variation in gender cultures in different parts of the world. That is, what may be seen as typical of the behaviour of one gender in a particular society may not be regarded as such in the next. For example, in some societies women have only a domestic role and are restricted to the home and never allowed to work outside it (such as the *purdah* system in many Islamic societies[9]), while in other societies women play a major role in the wider economic system. In some industrial societies they are major wage earners – in the USA, for example, more than 50 per cent of married women now work outside the home,[9] while in many peasant societies, in addition to their domestic role, women are involved in the raising of livestock, the planting, cultivation, harvesting and marketing of crops and the production of clothes, pottery and various handicrafts for market.

Some anthropologists have suggested that the subordination of women (especially their relegation to the domestic rather than the public sphere of life) is a universal phenomenon, and common to all human societies.[10] However, other anthropologists have argued against this concept, and have pointed out that the situation is much more complex and that each case must be evaluated differently. For one thing, in all societies men envy the biological powers of women to create life, bring it to birth and sustain it with breast milk,[4] especially as this power is reinforced by the rites and religions of almost all societies. Furthermore, in many traditional societies, women – especially older married women with children – wield great personal, symbolic and economic power, have considerable autonomy and are sometimes key power brokers within that society. As Keesing[4] points out, 'women's power exercised behind the scenes may in some sense be more genuine than men's power enacted on centre stage', which in turn may merely be 'empty posturing and pageantry'.

Later in this chapter some of the relationships between the various gender cultures and health will be described, for, if the role of physiological differences between the sexes is excluded, it is possible to see how each of the two gender cultures may (depending on the context) be either *protective* of health or *pathogenic*. That is, the beliefs and behaviours characteristic of a particular gender culture may contribute to the cause, presentation and recognition of various forms of ill health.

Gender cultures and sexual behaviour

Although gender cultures lay down norms of sexual behaviour for each of the sexes, there are many variations cross-culturally in what those norms are. For example, ethnographic studies indicate that there is much variation between societies in the degree of heterosexual activity permitted before marriage, outside of marriage and even within marriage itself.

As an example of this, studies quoted by the Embers[9] indicate that extramarital sex occurs in many societies; in an estimated 69 per cent of the world's societies the men commonly have extramarital sex, and in about 57 per cent the women commonly do so. Significantly, while 54 per cent of societies say they allow extramarital sex for men, only 11 per cent say they allow it for women.

Patterns of sexual behaviour are important in the transmission of several diseases. Where promiscuity and extramarital sex is common within a society, there is a greater likelihood of the spread of sexually transmitted diseases, such as gonorrhoea, syphilis, herpes genitalis and acquired immune deficiency syndrome (AIDS), as well as of hepatitis B and possibly cervical cancer (see Chapter 15). A strict 'double standard' of extramarital sexual behaviour, especially with frequent recourse to prostitutes, may also contribute to the persistence and spread of these diseases. In this case, the prostitutes may act as the 'reservoirs' of the infection within the community. The recent AIDS epidemic has led to an increased emphasis by health education authorities on the importance of limiting promiscuous sexual behaviour among both heterosexuals and homosexuals. The practice of anal intercourse among adolescent heterosexuals in some societies,[11] as a way of preserving female virginity, is also relevant to the spread of this disease.

Membership of a particular gender culture does not always coincide with sexual behaviour. For example, there are vast variations world-wide in whether societies are tolerant of some forms of sexual behaviour, such as homosexuality (both male and female), that transgress the usual norms of a gender culture. In some societies homosexuality is completely forbidden, but in others it is accepted or limited to certain times and to certain individuals. Among the Etoro people of New Guinea, for example, heterosexuality was prohib-

ited for as many as 260 days a year, while homosexuality 'is not prohibited at any time and is believed to make crops flourish and boys become strong'.[9] Shepherd[8] has described male and female homosexuality among the Swahili in Mombassa, Kenya, where the rigid gender boundaries were often transgressed by the institution of homosexuality and transvestism. Both male and female homosexuality were common and were tacitly tolerated. Homosexuality among teenage boys was particularly common, though most of them would later have heterosexual relations and eventually get married. She points out that this homosexual behaviour does not weaken the rigid conceptual divisions between men and women since, whatever their sexual practices, 'their biological *sex* is much more important than their *behaviour* as a determinant of gender' (italics in original). She contrasts this with the modern UK and USA, where behaviour is more important in defining one's gender, and male behaviour that transgresses gender rules is often described as 'womanish' or effeminate.

Caplan[12] has argued that where desire for fertility and childbearing is high, sexuality and fertility are hardly separated from each other conceptually and, as described above, it is the *biological* sex of individuals that is most important in defining their gender, whatever their sexual behaviour. Where the desire for many children is less (as in the modern, urban Western world) and where contraception is more easily available, sex becomes gradually divorced from fertility, and sexual practices that do not lead to pregnancy (such as homosexuality) are more tolerated; gender in these modern societies is therefore defined less by biological criteria and more by social and sexual behaviour. It has also been suggested[9] that societies more tolerant of homosexuality are those with population pressure – that is, too many people for their resources – and where an increase in population from heterosexual sex is therefore less desirable.

Gender cultures and health care

As described earlier in this book, in almost every culture most primary health care takes place within the family, and in the *popular* sector the main providers of health care are usually women – often mothers and grandmothers. Also, within the popular sector, women often organize themselves into *healing* cults, circles or churches, which act as either self-help groups for their members (such as the *Dertlesmek* or 'sharing of sorrow' groups described by Devisch and Gailly[13] among Turkish immigrants to Belgium) or as groups that combine self-help with the healing of outsiders (such as the *zar* possession cults in Africa, described by Lewis,[14] or the churches and cults practising ritual healing in the middle-class suburbs of the USA).[15] Within the *folk* sector, women have always played a central role, from the village 'wise woman' and the several types of female medium or spiritual healer in the UK to the many female folk healers in the non-industrialized world and the traditional birth attendants (TBAs) that still provide the majority of the obstetric care in those countries.

Within the *professional* sector of modern medicine, however, while the majority of health-care professionals (nurses and midwives) are still female, the higher-paid and higher-prestige jobs are usually held by male physicians. As described in Chapter 4, the medical profession is always, to some extent, an expression of the dominant social ideology and economic system of that society, including its division into social strata and its sexual division of labour. Thus medicine, until quite recently, was a predominantly male profession in most Western countries. For example, in the UK in 1901 there were only 212 female doctors out of a total of 36 000 registered medical practitioners.[16] Medicine remained a predominantly male profession until the 1970s, since when more women have been admitted into medical schools. By 1985 about 23 per cent of all UK-registered medical practitioners were women.[17] Within the National Health Service (NHS) in the UK about 75 per cent of personnel are women, but these are mostly found in its lower echelons, as nurses, ancillary workers, caterers and cleaners.[17] Most of the administrators and most of the doctors are male. For example, in 1981, 89 per cent of hospital consultants (special-ists) and 75 per cent of junior hospital doctors were male.[18] In general practice/family medicine the picture is very different, with a higher proportion of female doctors. Figures from England and Wales in 1983 showed that only 17.4 per cent of general practitioners were female (many of whom worked part-time), while 82.6 per cent were male. However, by 2004 the proportion of female GPs in the whole of the UK had more than doubled to 36.6 per cent of the total.[19]

On the other side of the Atlantic, the majority of doctors in the USA are also male: in 2002 out of a total of 813 770 physicians in the country, about 76 per cent were men and 24 per cent women.[20]

The nursing profession

Nursing is predominately a female profession. For example, in the USA in 2000 there were 2 694 540 registered nurses (RNs), of whom only 146 902 (5.5 per cent) were men.[21] However, this proportion is steadily growing, and the number of men in the profession has grown at a faster rate than the total RN population itself.

From an international perspective, there is a wide variation in the numbers of nurses available to the population in different parts of the world. As mentioned in Chapter 4, the World Health Organization (WHO) *World Health Statistics* for 2005,[22] based on data collected from 1997–2003, indicate huge variations in the worldwide availability of nurses and midwives, and in the proportion of nurses and midwives to doctors. To illustrate this, the figures from selected countries are shown in Table 6.1. These data clearly indicate that in many countries in the world, especially poorer countries, nurses carry the main burden of providing health care for the population.

In the UK, the nursing profession (including midwives) is the single largest group of health professionals within the NHS, and in 1990 made up over 50 per cent of its total personnel.[23] In 2005 there were 672 897 nurses registered in the UK.[24] Despite the fact that over 90 per cent of nursing staff in the UK are female, there is a disproportionately high number of men (30–40 per cent) in

Table 6.1 Relation of nurses and midwives to population, and to numbers of physicians, in selected countries

Country	Nurses and midwives per 10 000 population	Ratio of nurses and midwives to physicians
Malawi	2.2	22.6
Tanzania	3.7	16.2
India	7.9	1.3
China	9.6	0.6
Jamaica	16.5	1.9
United Kingdom	54.0	2.5
Philippines	61.4	5.3
Japan	86.3	4.3
United States of America	97.2	3.5

World Health Organization (2005).[22]

senior nursing management positions.[25] The overall percentage of men in nursing in the UK has not risen much in the last decade; it was 9.01 in 1995 and 10.7 in 2005.[24] Midwifery in particular remains almost entirely a female occupation: in 2003 out of a total of 33 000 midwives, only 102 were male.[26]

Most nurses work within the hospital sector where, like most other institutions in Western society, many of the basic gender divisions of the wider culture are recreated. Gamarnikow[27] has argued that the relation of doctors to nurses still mirrors the gender divisions of the Victorian family, in the days when Florence Nightingale developed her model of nursing. This means that, within the hospital structure, the equation is still doctor = father, nurse = mother and patient = child. In terms of power relationships in the provision of health care, the nurse's sphere is separate but still subordinate to that of the male doctor. This view is supported by some of the family-imagery still used in the UK hospital structure, where the various ranks of the nursing profession were, until very recently, designated in some hospitals as either 'nurses', 'sisters' or 'matrons'.

Also, a nurse's job, like that of the mother of a young infant, is more tactile, and involves intimate contact with the patient's body (particularly with

its surface) and with its various waste products. According to van Dongen and Elema,[28] in their study of nurses in the Netherlands, 'Nursing and the way nurses touch and react to touch are linked with ideas and values of caring, with the importance of empathy and human love, and with the value of human relationships in our society'. Conversely, doctors, spend relatively little time in the company of patients and have virtually no prolonged contact with the patient's body or their bodily wastes, and their specialized knowledge is mainly of the inner biological secrets and workings of their patients' bodies. Because gender divisions of labour within the medical profession continue to persist, despite major social changes this century, two anomalous types of health professionals are gradually becoming more common: the ambiguous roles of the 'male nurse' and the 'lady doctor'.

Shifts in nursing culture

Stacey[16] has described how the nursing profession in the UK grew out of religious orders and how, when hospitals were established in the eighteenth and nineteenth centuries, nurses were incorporated largely to do the domestic work and watch over the sick. From the nineteenth century onwards nursing gradually emerged as a profession in its own right, but still remained subordinate to the medical profession. The College of Nursing was founded in 1916, a Register of nurses was established in 1918, and the 1943 Nurses' Act established a Roll of nurses in addition to the Register. Since then, training within the nursing profession has become increasingly specialized, and in both Europe and the USA many nurses now have postgraduate training within a range of specialties and subspecialties. In the USA, the numbers of nurses who acquired higher college degrees rose dramatically between 1980 and 2000: from 17 per cent to 29 per cent with baccalaureate degrees, and from 5 per cent to 10 per cent with masters degrees or doctorates.[21] Nursing is now well established as an independent health profession in its own right.

Case study: advertisements in medical and nursing journals in the USA

Krantzler[29] in the mid-1980s analysed advertisements in medical and nursing journals in the USA. She pointed out how these adverts had shown a gradual reduction of the traditional medical symbols used by doctors (such as the white coat and stethoscope). Instead, this symbolic display of science-in-action was now more frequently seen in nursing journals, and it was nurses who were now more frequently shown using the healing symbols previously associated only with physicians. In many of the adverts they were still associated with the older key symbols of nursing – the white uniform and cap – but, increasingly, these adverts suggested that nursing symbols and behaviour had come to mimic those of physicians. She speculated that this 'reflects the desire not merely for respectability but for professional status'. In these nursing adverts, male physicians now tend to be peripheral and 'nurses are shown alone, with other nurses or with patients'. She noted that in the USA, this 'direct relationship with a client, unmitigated by a third party, is an important symbol of professionalization'.

Littlewood[30] has suggested that, although nursing education still takes place mainly within a biomedical framework, nurses are much better placed than physicians to understand and to deal with the problems of 'illness' as well as 'disease' (see Chapter 5). She notes the crucial role of nursing in assessing and managing chronic illnesses, disability, pregnancy and the health problems of the elderly. In each of these cases, the 'quick fix' of the medical model is either inappropriate or of little benefit. In the case of the chronically sick and disabled, who in this society are marginal people 'with discredited social identities', nursing can have a major impact on the quality of life and in understanding the meanings patients give to their life and suffering. She therefore sees the nurse as the health professional best placed to 'negotiate between the goals of the doctor … and the goals of the patient'.

More recently, Sandelowski[31] points out that new technological innovations, such as 'tele-nursing' (see Chapter 13) are now challenging the traditional role of nurses. She notes that nursing was always characterized by 'body work': by the nurse's 'bodily presence' in touching, holding, dressing, cleaning, or feeding the ill body of the patient, as well as providing them with personal, emotional support. This unique characteristic of care is what distinguished them from the more detached behaviour of doctors. It was a source of professional pride, and provided them with a 'sense of self, self-esteem, and agency, and a way to differentiate them from other health care advisers.' In recent years, however, many nurses have been turning to technology in their practices – using telephone consultations, telemetry, or video-monitoring, as well as delegating 'body work' to ancillary personnel. Although this trend has often increased their status and income, it has also eroded much of the traditional 'essence of nursing': the more intimate, engaged, physical care of ill people.

MEDICALIZATION

In recent years the concept of *medicalization* has

been put forward by critics of modern medicine, such as Illich[32], as well as by many medical sociologists. Gabe and Calnan[33] define medicalization as 'the way in which the jurisdiction of modern medicine has expanded in recent years and now encompasses many problems that formerly were not defined as medical entities'. These include a wide variety of phenomena, such as many of the normal phases of the female life cycle (menstruation, pregnancy, childbirth and menopause) as well as old age, unhappiness, loneliness and social isolation, and the results of wider social problems such as poverty or unemployment.

There are many explanations for medicalization. Many medical sociologists have argued that modern medicine is increasingly used as an agent of social control (especially over the lives of women),[34] making them dependent on the medical profession and on its links with the pharmaceutical and other industries.[35] It has also been seen as a way of controlling socially deviant behaviour, by defining those who do not conform to social norms as 'ill' or 'mad' rather than as 'evil' and 'bad'. Perhaps most importantly, the decline of a religious world-view and the gradual replacement with health as a moral model of the universe have meant the spread of medical explanations into areas of life and its misfortunes which it was never designed to deal with. Nowadays, as described in Chapter 5, the notion of the unhealthy lifestyle resulting in ill health has replaced the earlier religious concepts of sinful behaviour leading to divine retribution. This process has probably been aided by the undoubted successes of technology and science (including medical science) in improving the expectation and quality of life in many ways. Medicalization is probably also more likely if the body is conceptualized as a 'machine', and one that is only viewed stripped of its social and cultural context (see Chapter 2). A final possible reason for the growth of medicalization was suggested earlier, in the discussion of the nature/nurture controversy. If some men still see women and their physiology as representative of nature – that which is uncontrolled, unpredictable

and dangerously polluting – then medical rituals and medical technology become a way of taming the uncontrolled (especially in the age of feminism) and making it more 'cultural' in the process.

In describing cases which some sociologists and anthropologists have cited as examples of medicalization, this section will focus on:

1 Aspects of the life stresses of women, and their relation to psychotropic drug prescribing.
2 Aspects of the female physiology and life cycle, such as menstruation, menopause and, later in this chapter, childbirth.

WOMEN AND PSYCHOTROPIC DRUG PRESCRIBING

The widespread use of psychotropic drugs in the industrialized world as a solution to personal and social problems will be discussed in Chapter 9. However, studies in several Western countries have all indicated that *women* are prescribed psychotropics roughly twice as often as men.[35] The reasons why doctors prescribe more of these drugs for women than for men are complex, but they include the influence of the advertisements from the pharmaceutical industry, promoting these drugs as solutions for women's life stresses and role conflicts. In contrast, alcohol and tobacco rather than psychotropic drugs seem to be the main chemical comforters used by men in many societies.

Case study: psychotropic drug advertisements in the UK

Stimson[36] in the 1970s studied advertisements for psychotropic drugs in British medical journals, and found that images of women in the adverts outnumbered men by 15 to 1. In the adverts, the women's place in society was predominantly shown 'as one which generated stress, anxiety, and emotional problems'. Images of the tired and tearful 'harassed housewife' in a cluttered kitchen, surrounded by crying children, were common. According to Stimson, these adverts reveal that

This medicalization of the stress and anxieties of some women's lives is part of a wider medicalization of social and personal problems such as bereavement, loneliness, divorce, political upheaval, poverty and unemployment. It is also part of the growing trend towards 'chemical coping', and the search for a stressless and painless utopia, as a modern way of life (see Chapter 8).

THE FEMALE PHYSIOLOGY AND LIFE CYCLE

In looking at the concept of 'medicalization' put forward by many critics of modern medicine, it should always be remembered that many women have not seen this process as necessarily a bad thing.[33] Instead they have welcomed the development of medical treatments for the premenstrual syndrome, dysmenorrhoea, menopausal symptoms and some of the pain and difficulties of childbirth.

Menstruation

Menstruation is a normal part of female physiology from the menarche until the menopause. Nevertheless, it is often a process surrounded by a variety of taboos and special behaviours designed to protect symbolically the menstruating woman from harm during this vulnerable period, and to protect men from the dangerous polluting power of her menstrual blood.

Women in Western industrial countries, especially in urban areas, have very different experiences of menstruation compared with women in many developing countries. In developing countries, especially in rural areas, menstrual periods are relatively uncommon for a number of reasons – just as they were a century ago in the Western world. This is because of a number of major changes in women's lives that have occurred in the industrialized countries over the past 100 years. These include a fall in the birth rate, a reduction in the average number of pregnancies per woman, a lowering of the age of menarche, a decline in infant and maternal mortality, and increased life expectancy and therefore a greater proportion of women who live to the menopausal age.[37] In the 1890s the average British working-class woman spent 15 years in a state of pregnancy and in nursing a child for its first year of life, while the time so spent today would only be 4 years,[37] so many more years of menstruation are likely. In the developing world, two other factors may also contribute to amenorrhoea or to infrequent periods; first, prolonged breast-feeding after birth, which is common in many of those countries, and second inadequate nutrition, which may have the same effect. Nutrition is particularly important, since women require about 17 per cent of their body weight as fat in order to have menarche, and about 22 per cent in order to have regular cycles.[38]

In recent years one aspect of menstruation, the *premenstrual syndrome* (PMS), has increasingly been seen not as a physiological phenomenon but as a problem of pathology and hormonal deficiency. Dalton,[39] for example, has described PMS as 'the commonest endocrine disorder', and one that is caised by a deficiency of progesterone. This contrasts with menopause, which has also been defined by some clinicians as a deficiency disease, though this time of oestrogen (see below).

Gottlieb[40] described the symbolic nature of the premenstrual syndrome in contemporary culture in the USA. She sees the negative moods (such as irritability and hostility) that define the PMS as the opposite of what is normally expected of women in the USA; this is a form of symbolic inversion of the idealized behaviour expected of them the rest of the month (to be always nice, quiet, kind, selfless and compassionate to others). Women are permitted, and even encouraged, to oscillate between these two extremes of personality within certain times of the month. According to Gottlieb, many American women have internalized this split model of feminine behaviour. However, their monthly 'ritual of reversal' of these values has a largely conservative effect, since it turns women's experience against themselves because they 'in effect choose, however unconsciously, to voice their complaints at a time when they know their complaints will be rejected as illegitimate'. Furthermore, Lupton[41] quotes studies noting how PMS is represented in the American media in a way that harks back to nineteenth century imagery of the woman being 'closer to Nature'. Descriptions of PMS in popular texts as the 'monthly monster' or the 'inner beast' all suggest that women are controlled by their menstrual cycles 'as if they were lower order animals on heat'.

Johnson,[42] too, sees the PMS (and the ways that it is described in American women's magazines) as a 'culture-bound syndrome' (see Chapter 10). He argues that in modern industrial society women's roles are changing, and they are increasingly placed in situations of role conflict: they are expected to be 'both productive and reproductive; to have both careers and families'. However, at the same time society criticizes them if they exclusively choose either of these options, or if they try to do both at the same time. Premenstrual syndrome thus symbolizes and encapsulates this role conflict between productivity and generativity by simultaneously denying the possibility of each: 'in menstruating, one is potentially fertile but obviously nonpregnant; in having incapacitating symptomatology one is exempted from normal work role expectations'. In this way, the cultural idiom of PMS is a symbolic cultural safety valve which recognizes the need for women to turn away simultaneously – at least temporarily – from both of these conflict-laden alternative role demands. In the process, however, it also solidifies stereotypes of women being delicate and frag-

ile, and thus incapable of assuming male roles in the public domain.

As well as the PMS, menstruation itself may be medicalized; in some cases this may act to disguise more traditional beliefs about the vulnerability of the menstruating woman to outside forces, and the polluting or poisonous properties of menstrual blood (see Chapter 3). For example, in their study of menstrual beliefs in Taiwan, Furth and Shu-Yueh[43] found that traditional images of the vulnerable menstruating woman's unclean or shameful menstrual blood were couched – especially among younger women – in the language of health or cleanliness. Most of them took 'health precautions' during their periods, to avoid invasion by infection and 'germs'. These precautions included herbal medicines, keeping warm, not washing one's hair, and avoiding baths, heavy exercise, iced or raw foods. Sexual intercourse during menstruation was thought to be dangerous to women ('It can cause a fever in the womb') and also to men.

Menopause

Like regular and frequent menstrual periods, the menopause is more a feature of modern, industrialized societies, where women have a longer life expectancy and most now live to the menopausal age and beyond.

Lock[44] has pointed out significant changes in the way menopause has been defined over the past century or so by Western medicine. In the nineteenth century, for example, menopause was thought to *cause* disease, but since the mid-twentieth century it has itself been redefined *as* a disease. Thus a normal feature of the female life cycle has increasingly become medicalized, though there are often important differences between lay and medical models of menopause.

Kaufert and Gilbert[45] noted that the biomedical definition of menopause as primarily an *endocrine* disorder (oestrogen deficiency) often leads to the defining as 'menopausal' of only those symptoms that can be attributed to an oestrogen deficiency (such as hot flushes, night sweats, osteoporosis and atrophic vaginitis), while ignoring those symptoms (especially social or psychological ones) that are not easily corrected by hormone replacement therapy (HRT). A further problem of seeing menopause as primarily a medical condition is that once it is defined as a hormonal deficiency disease, it can only be diagnosed by a physician and by laboratory tests, treatment can only be prescribed by a physician, and thus it often becomes 'a permanent condition to be permanently managed' by the medical system.

However, as Lock[44] points out, the medical model itself is not uniform, and there is much dispute within the medical literature on the defining symptoms and appropriate treatment of the menopause, as well as on the relation of oestrogen deficiency to both symptoms and other pathological changes (such as osteoporosis). There is also disagreement about other, more vague, menopausal symptoms, such as irritability, depression, tiredness, headaches, dizziness and loss of libido, and whether these are caused by a hormonal deficiency or not. There is of course a physiological change – the end of the menses and of fertility – that occurs at this time. However, this also coincides with a series of socio-cultural events in the woman's life (hence it is often called a 'change of life'); these are often associated with other social transitions, such as retirement, children leaving home (the 'empty nest syndrome') or ill health, and may also be responsible for some of the symptoms associated with menopause.

In her own study, carried out in Montreal, Canada, Lock[44] found that the medical management of menopausal symptoms was often very variable, and while some doctors always prescribed HRT, others hardly ever did. In some cases the decision to prescribe HRT seemed to be determined by the context in which consultation took place, as well as by the personality, training, age, sex and experience of the clinician and the social and cultural attributes of the patient herself. Similar findings, also from Canada, are illustrated in the following case history.

> ## Case study: medicalization of the menopause in Manitoba, Canada
>
> Kaufert and Gilbert[45] in 1986 studied 2500 women in Manitoba, Canada, aged between 40 and 59 years. Thirty-seven per cent were premenopausal, 14 per cent perimenopausal and 30 per cent postmenopausal; 19 per cent had previously had a hysterectomy. They found that in this sample of women, menopause was much less medicalized than anticipated. Overall, just under half the women said they had never discussed their menopausal status with a physician. Kaufert and Gilbert concluded that, within the sample, the experience of menopause was not a highly medicalized process, and was one in which some women involved their physicians not at all. This was unlike childbirth, which is highly medicalized in Canada; childbirth is a publicly visible process with little choice over whether to disclose it, unlike menopause. In Canada, the culture of pregnancy usually includes seeing a physician and, like the USA, nearly all births involve some form of medical intervention. However, North American society attaches a relatively light weight to menopause, compared with childbirth, and this may explain why it has only been partly medicalized.

In the case of both the premenstrual syndrome and menopause, it can be argued that two of the natural physiological events of women's lives have been redefined by some clinicians as 'endocrine deficiencies', or 'diseases'. This medicalization means that some women have become more dependent on the medical profession and its treatments than their mothers ever were. However, as mentioned earlier, many women have also welcomed the development of those medical treatments that have relieved the unpleasant symptoms of both menstruation and menopause.

GENDER CULTURES AND HEALTH

The gender roles prescribed by a particular gender

culture may, like other cultural beliefs and behaviours, be either protective of health or pathogenic, depending on the context. This section will briefly describe how being allocated at birth to the social category of either 'male' or 'female' may, under some circumstances, have a negative effect on an individual's health. Those conditions where the beliefs, expectations and behaviours inherent in a particular gender culture can be said to contribute towards ill health may be termed 'diseases of social gender'.

DISEASES OF MALE SOCIAL GENDER

Several aspects of male gender culture can be said to contribute to men's ill health, or to the risk of such ill health developing. For example, compared with women, men are encouraged to drink more alcohol, smoke more cigarettes, to be more competitive and take more risks in their daily lives. In almost all cultures, both warfare and hunting are exclusive male pursuits, and men's health – particularly that of younger men – is often put at risk by the dangerous and competitive sports, bodily mutilations, rituals of initiation and public trials of manhood and 'machismo' characteristic of so many cultures.

In the face of suffering and pain men are usually expected to have an unemotional language of distress; to be stoical and uncomplaining, and thus to have a high threshold for consultation with a doctor or other health professional (especially if they are also male). In many cases this stoicism may be counterproductive to health, since it may lead some men to ignore early symptoms of serious disease, or to the doctor underestimating the seriousness of that disease.

Another example of the relation of male gender cultures to ill health is the Type A behaviour pattern (TABP), which is described in more detail in Chapter 11. This is a type of competitive, ambitious and time-obsessed behaviour, which has been found to increase the risk of coronary heart disease (CHD) in some individuals. Waldron[46] has explained the fact that death rates in the USA from CHD are twice as high for men as for women as being due partly to cultural factors, especially to different American child rearing practices. Competitiveness, ambition and other features of the TABP are more likely to be encouraged and rewarded in men than in women. Men are expected to succeed in the occupational sphere while women are expected to succeed in the domestic sphere, and each sphere requires different behavioural adaptations if success is to be achieved. Later in life this type of socialization may be protective of women, but not of men, in contributing to the development of CHD.

DISEASES OF FEMALE SOCIAL GENDER

Some of these have already been discussed in Chapter 2 in the context of the many alterations of body image that occur world-wide, especially among women. In the Western world these include mammoplasty, rhinoplasty and other forms of plastic surgery, all of which carry with them the risks inherent in surgery and anaesthesia, as well as of postoperative infection. Other more exotic changes in the body surface and appearance, such as foot-binding, scarification, tattooing and lip-piercing, all carry with them clear risks to health. More recent fashions of clothing and body adornment can also be damaging to health; for example, orthopaedic problems may result from wearing platform heels and high-heeled shoes, and contact dermatitis or urticaria can follow the use of cosmetics, bath salts, deodorants and hair dyes. Furthermore, major changes in body shape to conform to current cultural images of female beauty may lead to 'food fads' and 'diet fads', which can be dangerous for nutrition and health. In some individuals, the cultural emphasis on female slimness may even contribute to the development of anorexia nervosa[47] (see Chapter 2) in Western countries and in those undergoing economic development. It may also lead to depression and a poor self-image among those women with obesity or those whose bodies do not conform to the current cultural images of female beauty.

Unlike males, women are socialized to have a low threshold for consultation with a doctor, and to display a more emotional language of distress, such as the various forms of 'nerves' described by anthropologists in different parts of the world (see Chapter 11).[48] This in turn may lead to a misdiagnosis of hysteria or hypochondria by male clinicians,[49] to the medicalization of their life events and physiological changes, and to the unnecessary use of drug therapy (especially psychotropic drugs). Conversely, frequent consultations with a doctor may sometimes aid in the early recognition of certain diseases.

Finally, in modern industrial societies many women are increasingly the focus of contradictory influences from their gender culture. On one hand their domestic role is emphasized and they are expected to remain at home with their families, but on the other hand they are expected at the same time to follow careers and to contribute towards the wider economy. These role conflicts have greatly increased the stresses in the lives of many modern women.

REPRODUCTION AND CHILDBIRTH

Anthropologists have reported widespread differences in the perceptions of conception, pregnancy and birth among different cultural groups. This inherited belief system, which Hahn and Muecke[50] call the *birth culture* of a particular society, 'informs members of a society about the nature of conception, the proper conditions of procreation and childbearing, the workings of pregnancy and labour, and the rules and rationales of pre- and postnatal behaviour'.

A key aspect of any birth culture are beliefs about the functioning of the body, and the nature of conception and pregnancy – especially when the woman is most likely to conceive. In a study in Sri Lanka, the Nichters[51] describe how the majority of women interviewed believed that they were most fertile from day 4 to day 14 after menstruation ceased. There was also a view among some that the uterus 'opened' and 'closed' each month, and that just after childbirth, especially in the first 14 days, a woman was at high risk of pregnancy as the uterus was still 'open'. This concept is similar to the Latin American group described in Chapter 2, who believed that the uterus was 'closed' for most of the month, and only opened at the period, so that pregnancy was most likely just before, during, or just after the period, and that contraception was unnecessary for the rest of the month.

Many different 'birth cultures', from both the industrial and non-industrialized worlds, have been described by anthropologists in recent years. In modern middle-class Europe and North America, for example, pregnancy and birth – like menopause and menstruation – have increasingly become seen as medical conditions, and thus the proper subjects for medical diagnosis and treatment.

WESTERN BIRTH CULTURE

In all cultures, women giving birth are assisted during the labour by one or more helpers. These people may be female relatives or friends, a traditional midwife or birth attendant or, in a hospital setting, a medically qualified obstetrician.

Stacey[52] has described how in the UK midwifery was an exclusive female profession until the seventeenth century, when a few male midwives (or *accoucheurs*) began to appear – though today it is still an overwhelmingly female profession.[24,26] Much of the knowledge of the traditional midwives came from their own experience of pregnancy and childbirth. Although many physicians were opposed to the idea, during the latter half of the nineteenth century midwives were gradually incorporated into the medical system, though they were only allowed to attend 'normal' births. Their position as practitioners in their own right was eventually formalized in the Midwives Act of 1902, though they still remained subordinate to the medically qualified obstetricians. According to Leavitt,[53] a similar process has taken place in the USA. Before 1880, women giving birth were aided mainly by female relatives and birth attendants. Only occasionally were doctors called in to help with difficult labours, but even then the power to make decisions about the birth remained with the woman, her family and friends. From 1880 to 1920, however, although most births still took place at home, the medical profession gradually increased its authority over the birth process and how it was to be managed. By the 1930s, for the first time, childbirth in the USA took place more often in hospital than at home. In this new hospital setting, control over the management of the birth process became almost exclusively a medical matter.

The growth of hospital obstetrics

In 1959 one in three of all births in the UK took place at home or in a nursing home, while by the 1980s, 99 per cent of births took place in a National Health Service hospital.[18] In the USA, too, approximately 98 per cent of births take place in a hospital setting.[53] The decline of home deliveries in the UK, and the gradual shifting of childbirth into a hospital environment, is shown by the changes in the numbers of hospital midwives and those still working in the community; between 1974 and 1980, hospital midwives increased from 15 002 to 17 163, while the number of community midwives declined from 4237 to 2773.[18] As noted above, by 2005 the total number of midwives practicing in the UK was over 30 000.[24,26]

In the past half-century or so, modern obstetrics has achieved notable successes in reducing both maternal and neonatal mortality and morbidity, preserving the lives of premature infants, diagnosing congenital abnormalities *in utero*, and successfully treating infertility with *in vitro* fertilization (IVF) and other techniques. However, for all its technical success, the birth culture of Western society, like other aspects of modern medicine, has been criticized by many women on a number of counts. These include:

- its overemphasis on the physiological, rather than the psychosocial, aspects of pregnancy and birth

- its tendency to medicalize a normal biological event, turning it into a medical problem, and thus converting the pregnant woman into a passive and dependent patient.

In particular, as in the distinction between disease and illness described in the previous chapter, medicine has been criticized for ignoring the meanings that women give to both their pregnancy and their childbirth experiences.

This overemphasis on birth as a technical problem often seems to imply a 'plumbing' model of the woman's body, as described in Chapter 2. In the minds of some obstetricians, birth seems to be seen as merely the technical problem of getting a living object (the baby) from one tube (the uterus) down another (the birth canal) and then out into the hands of the physician.

The origins of Western 'birth culture'

What are the origins of the birth culture of modern Western obstetrics? Davis-Floyd[54] traces it to the seventeenth century image, developed by Descartes, Bacon and Hobbes, of a mechanistic universe, following predictable laws, which could be discovered by science and controlled by technology. The Cartesian model of mind–body dualism led to the metaphor of the body as a machine, and the conceptual divorce of body from soul removed the body from the purview of religion and placed it firmly in the hands of science. Davis-Floyd argues further that Christian theology held that women were inferior to men and closer to nature. Consequently, the men who established the idea of body-as-a-machine also firmly established the male body as the prototype of this machine; in so far as the female body deviated from the male standard, so it was regarded as inherently abnormal, defective, dangerously unpredictable and under the influence of nature, and in need of constant manipulation by men. The demise of midwifery and the growth of the metaphor of the female body as a defective machine formed the philosophical basis for modern obstetrics. A further feature, especially in American obstetrics, is the hospital as a high-tech factory, dedicated to the production of perfect babies: 'the most desirable end product of the birth process is the new social member, the baby; the new mother is a secondary by-product'.

Furthermore, the conceptual separation of mother and infant is basic to this technological model of birth. The baby is removed from the mother and handed to a nurse, who inspects, tests, bathes, diapers and wraps the newborn, administers a vitamin K injection and antibiotic eye drops, then – having been 'properly encultured' or 'baptized' into the world of technology – the baby is handed back to its mother for a short time before being placed in a plastic bassinet for 4 hours of observation and again returned to its mother. To Davis-Floyd, therefore, 'the mother's womb is replaced, not by her arms but by the plastic womb of culture'. This separation is further intensified by assigning a separate doctor – the paediatrician or neonatologist – to the newborn infant.

Davis-Floyd describes how during the birth itself, the mother lies surrounded by medical technology: by external and internal foetal monitors, intravenous drips, charts and instruments (see Figure 6.1). To the woman, 'her entire visual field is conveying one overwhelming perceptual message about our culture's deepest values and beliefs: technology is supreme, and you are utterly dependent on it and on the institutions and individuals who control and dispense it'. This impression is strengthened by the frequent use of an episiotomy, which 'transforms even the most natural of childbirths into a surgical procedure'.

The medicalization of birth

As Davis-Floyd[54] describes, medicine (including obstetrics) has increasingly defined health and ill health mainly in terms of physiological dysfunction (see Chapter 5). As it has done so, the gap between lay and obstetrical birth cultures seems to have widened considerably and the possibility of a 'culture clash' between them seems more likely than before. This is especially true in many parts of the industrialized world, where some women have

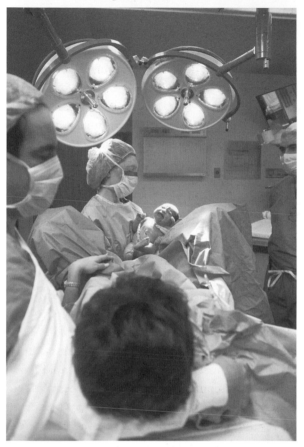

Figure 6.1 A hospital delivery room. Despite its success in reducing maternal and infant mortality, modern obstetrics has been criticized for 'medicalizing' birth, and transforming 'even the most natural of childbirths into a surgical procedure'. (Source: © Phototake Inc/Alamy. Reproduced with permission.)

expressed considerable dissatisfaction with certain aspects of the medical management of birth.

For example, Graham and Oakley[55] have described some of the fundamental differences between doctors' and mothers' perspectives on childbearing, particularly whether it is a natural or a medical process. This conflict is part of the wider differences in perspective inherent in all doctor–patient interactions. The medical view of pregnancy abstracts it from the rest of the woman's life experience, and treats it as an isolated medical event. The patient enters medical care at the onset of pregnancy, and leaves medical care after giving birth. However, for the mother it is integrated with *other* aspects of her life, for she acquires (with a first birth) a new social role, as well as profound changes in her financial situation, marital status, housing situation and personal relationships. There are also differences in how she and the obstetrician assess the quality of the childbearing experience, how they measure a successful outcome, and how they decide who should control the method and pace of the birth itself. Thus there is an inherent clash between the obstetricians – clinicians (usually male) who have a specialized knowledge of childbirth – and the mothers, whose expertise 'stems not primarily from medical science but rather from a woman's capacity to sense and respond to the sensations of her body'.

As well as having a technical purpose, many of the procedures of modern obstetrics can also be described as rituals of social transition or *rites de passage*, which will be described later in Chapter 9. For the purposes of this section, however, it is important to note that in all human societies pregnancy and childbirth are more than just biological events. They are also part of an important transition of the woman from the social status of 'woman' to that of 'mother'. As with all social transitions, during the dangerous journey from one status to another the individual must be protected from harm by the observance of certain ritual beliefs and behaviour. In many of these transitions the person concerned goes through a temporary period of withdrawal from ordinary life, before being 're-born' into their new social status; as Kitzinger[56] observes, the initiate often 'goes through an act of infantilization, in which he or she is reduced to the state of a small, dependent, submissive child' and 'it is as if only by going back to the beginning can re-birth take place'. The practice in some hospitals of shaving women's public hair and giving them an enema before they give birth can also be seen as part of this infantilization, or at least of returning the woman to a pre-pubertal state. However, as Davis-Floyd[54] has argued above, many of the rituals of obstetrics are also ways of transmitting some of society's most basic values to the woman undergoing childbirth. According

to her, these values include her powerlessness in the face of patriarchy, the 'defectiveness' of her female body, the need of medicine to control her natural processes, her dependence on science and technology, and the enduring importance of institutions and machines over individual beliefs and meanings. This type of cultural message is more likely to be transmitted to the new mother in the impersonal atmosphere of a hospital obstetric unit than when the birth takes place in the familiar atmosphere of the home. As Kitzinger[56] states 'in large centralized, hierarchical institutions existing outside and apart from the family there is a special likelihood of these rituals being used to reinforce the existing system and maintain the power structure'.

Despite this, Browner[57] notes that many pregnant women in the USA are deeply ambivalent about the value of medical technology, especially in prenatal care and diagnosis. Although they trust their own experience and 'embodied knowledge', few reject the findings of medical science. She predicts that as the role of clinical technology in childbirth grows, so will the consensus that biomedicine alone holds 'authoritative knowledge', especially in the domain of prenatal care. This ambivalence towards medical technology is confirmed in the national *Listening to Mothers* survey in the USA carried out in 2002.[58] A majority of the women interviewed had had 'technology-intensive' labours, with the following interventions during birth: electronic fetal monitoring (93 per cent), intravenous drip (86 per cent), epidural anaesthesia (63 per cent), artificially ruptured membranes (55 per cent), artificial oxytocin to strengthen contractions (53 per cent), bladder catheter (52 per cent), and stitching to repair an episiotomy or tear (52 per cent). Despite this, an overwhelming proportion of the women were pleased with the care that they received, and noted that they 'generally understood what was happening' (94 per cent), felt comfortable asking questions (93 per cent), got the attention they needed (91 per cent), and felt that 'were as involved as they wanted to be in making decisions' (89 per cent).[58]

In their study of antenatal ultrasound scans among primiparous women in Australia, Harris and colleagues[59] point out another aspect of these ambiguous effects of medical technology in the pre-natal period. Seeing the fetus on the scan transforms the woman's experience of her pregnancy. On one hand, it is a pleasurable experience, relieving her anxiety and confirming that the fetus is normal and the pregnancy is proceeding as expected. On the other hand, these scans also emphasize the growing power of medical technology over her body, for with its ability to 'see' right into her it now makes her, and her fetus, more closely subject to medical surveillance and control.

NON-WESTERN BIRTH CULTURES

Hahn and Muecke[50] described the discrepancies between the birth culture of middle-class USA and those of some of the social and ethnic groups in that country, such as working-class black people, Mexican-Americans, Chinese and the Hmong (from Laos). In each case, some of the basic assumptions of white middle-class obstetricians – for example, that the husband should be present at the birth – might *not* be shared by the members of those groups (or by men from other groups in society). Among some traditional Chinese groups, for example, women and their bodily products are regarded as dangerous and polluting for men, who therefore avoid the scene of birth and any contact with the woman in the month following the birth. As with other traditional groups, female obstetricians and birth attendants may be preferred to males.

In many cultures in the non-industrialized world, giving birth in the lithotomy or supine position favoured by Western obstetrics is not at all common. In her 1982 review of the literature on the subject, MacCormack[60] states that 'throughout the world, in Latin America, northern Thailand, India, Sri Lanka and West Africa, women either stand, squat or sit reclining against something or someone in the latter stages of labour'. In the second stage of labour, the midwife is often seated on the floor in front of the labouring woman. With breach or transverse presentations, traditional birth attendants are often skilled at manipulating the baby into the cephalic position by external massage.

Reviewing the literature covering Vietnam, Thailand, Burma, India, East and West Africa, Jamaica, Guatemala and Brazil, MacCormack[60] points out that, unlike in Western obstetrical practice, the umbilical cord is usually cut *after* the placenta is expelled, and not before. In some areas, dung is rubbed into the infant's umbilicus to stop bleeding, and this can increase the risk of neonatal tetanus.[60]

These traditional practices are changing rapidly, however, with social and economic development, and the gradual 'medicalization' of birth, even in poorer countries. In some cases, this medicalization may be welcomed because it fits in with certain traditional concepts. In Tamil Nadu, South India, for example, van Hollen[61] described how many women giving birth in government hospitals insisted on having their labour induced and accelerated by drugs such as oxytocin, even though this greatly increased the pain of their childbirth. This was because this pain, known as *vali* – a word which also means 'strength' or 'power' – was said to increase the woman's level of *sakti* or female regenerative power: 'the activating principal of life, the principle of endless change that is both celebrated and feared'. Enduring a greater pain resulted in greater *sakti*. Thus, according to van Hollen, 'as birth becomes increasingly biomedicalized throughout the globe, modern medical technologies may be used in different ways and be given different meanings in particular contexts'.

The postpartum period

After the birth, women in most cultures observe a special postpartum rest period, during which they have to follow certain dietary and other taboos and are cared for mainly by other women. This period of rest and seclusion usually lasts between 20 and 40 days. In some cases (see Chapter 9) the end of this post-partum rest period is marked by a special religious ritual for mother and body, signaling their re-entry into everyday life, such as the 'forty day blessing' (*sarantismos*) in the Greek Orthodox Church. Among Tamils in Sri Lanka, the period of 'childbirth pollution' is 31 days, followed by special rituals which purify the house, as well as a ritual bath for the mother and the shaving of the child's head.[62] Pillsbury[63] describes how in rural Chinese communities, in both the People's Republic of China and Taiwan (where it is called the *tso yueh*), 'doing the month' involves one full month of postpartum convalescence, during which time the woman is confined to her home, looked after by relatives, and has to eat a special diet and observe special taboos. She points out how, in contrast, the 'lying in' period of Western birth culture has given way to the puerperium, which does not have the same symbolic importance and 'no longer connotes the specificity of behaviour that continues to characterize "doing the month"'. A further important aspect of the postpartum period is that many cultures prohibit sexual relations between husband and wife for a period of time after the birth. In some cases this may last for several months; among many traditional Chinese in the USA, for example, sexual contact is sometimes proscribed for anything up to 100 days postpartum.[50] The implications of these customs for family planning are discussed in more detail, in Chapter 18.

Traditional birth attendants

In contrast to the modern, technological model of birth, most babies world-wide – especially in rural areas of the developing world – are delivered in a very different way, usually by female birth attendants such as the *parteras* of Mexico, the *comadronas* of Puerto Rico, the *nanas* of Jamaica, the *dais* of India, the *dayas* of Egypt and the *jiddas* of Yemen.

In Africa and in rural India, an estimated 80 per cent of women are assisted during birth by TBAs. World-wide, it has been estimated by the WHO that about 60–80 per cent of babies are delivered by TBAs.[64]

Traditional birth attendants are found in almost every village and in many urban neighbourhoods throughout Africa, Asia, Latin America and the Caribbean. As well as delivering babies, they also supervise antenatal and postnatal care, perform important rituals during pregnancy and birth and, in some parts of the world, carry out female circumcisions. In 1979 and 1990, WHO reports[65,66] supported the further training of TBAs. The aim of the WHO has been to increase their numbers and further training, and to increase consultation with them in order to eventually integrate them into the overall health programmes in developing countries while ensuring at the same time the continuation of the traditional art and respect for their roots in traditional cultures. After training, it was intended that they would take on other roles in the community, such as providing first aid, giving advice on family planning and distributing oral rehydration solution (ORS) in cases of infantile diarrhoea. As community health educators, they were to give advice on nutrition, the prevention of human immunodeficiency virus (HIV) infection, the importance of personal and environmental hygiene, and the need to bring babies and children to health clinics to monitor their development and get them vaccinated.[66] Various international aid agencies, such as the United Nations Children's Fund (UNICEF) have developed training programmes for TBAs, and after training supply with them with kits of basic equipment designed to reduce the risk of maternal infection during childbirth (Figure 6.2) . These kits usually include items such as booklets, soap, scrubbing brushes, disposable razor blades, a pair of scissors, a metal jug (for hot water), and sterile dressings, sutures and clamps.

In countries where TBAs are recognized by the authorities, considerable numbers have been trained and used in basic health services during the past 30 years, including in Ghana, Indonesia, Malaysia, Pakistan, the Philippines, Sudan and Thailand. In Egypt, for example,[67] where 80–90 per cent of babies are still delivered by *dayas*, the training programme has had four main objectives:

Figure 6.2 Traditional birth attendants or *dayas* in the Nile Delta, Egypt, holding equipment kits and pamphlets given to them by UNICEF. (Source: © Sean Sprague/Panos Pictures. Reproduced with permission.)

1 To expand the scope of their practice.
2 To increase the safety of their techniques.
3 To increase their referral to hospitals of babies and mothers who are at risk.
4 To increase cooperation between them and local health staff.

Despite their lack of formal training, and the shortcomings of some of their techniques, TBAs therefore offer the possibility of non-technological birth care, at little or no cost, in many parts of the non-industrialized world.

Case study: the nana in Jamaica

Kitzinger[56] in 1982 described an example of a traditional birth attendant, the *nana* or folk midwife of Jamaica. She estimated that about 25 per cent of Jamaican babies, especially in rural areas, are delivered by a *nana*. Because these women are not legally recognized by the state, most of these births are registered as 'born unattended' or 'delivered by mother' (or by a friend or relative). In the villages, the *nana* is a person of high standing and great authority, 'a key figure in the cohesion of women in Jamaican rural communities'. Together with the village schoolteacher and the post-mistress, she forms 'the political centre' or core of the social networks that tie the community together. *Nanas* are familiar figures, deeply rooted in their communities, and are often called upon for help in a variety of family crises. The midwifery skills of the *nana* are handed down within families, from mother to daughter. *Nanas* are always mothers themselves, for 'to be a *nana* is really an extension of the mothering role, so all *nanas* are mothers who are seen to be successful in their role'. They see their role as shepherding the women safely from conception to birth by facilitating their natural processes, and in doing so assisting in the drama of 'the re-birth of a woman as a mother'. Their care usually continues from pregnancy until the ninth day postpartum. The *nanas* supervise all the many rituals and taboos of pregnancy and birth (see Chapter 9) that mark the woman's transition from pregnancy to motherhood, and which help give meaning to her experience, by placing it in the context of the wider cultural values of her religion and community. Kitzinger contrasts this intimate, culturally familiar approach with the Western-style, technological birth procedures used in many Jamaican hospitals, where nurses and midwives value 'efficiency, speed of delivery of the patient, hospital routines concerning hygiene and order, and the suppression of emotional factors in childbirth so that they can get on with the work in an organized way, and treat the greatest number of patients in the shortest possible time'.

According to Kitzinger, the Jamaican *nanas*, who do things in 'the old time way', tend to be derided both by the medical profession and the educated middle-class as inefficient and harmful to health, and as echoes of a past of slavery and subjugation. However, she points out that the *nanas* are very experienced in the techniques of midwifery, are keen to learn more from modern obstetrics and are quick to call in a trained midwife or send the woman straight to hospital if anything goes wrong with the birth. Many rural women now use *nanas* during pregnancy and the first stage of labour, and then transfer to a qualified midwife for the birth itself.

Although they are still active in the countryside, a more recent study by Sargent and Bascope[68] suggests that the use of *nanas* is in overall decline in Jamaica, especially in urban areas. This is partly due to government policy and health education campaigns. Increasingly, pregnant women are placing their trust in hospital obstetrics, especially in the government nurse-midwives based in those hospitals.

FERTILITY AND INFERTILITY

Fertility is a universal human concern, as is anguish over infertility, whatever its cause. Most cultures include a series of rituals or prayers or special precautions to help a woman successfully conceive, and to carry her through to a safe delivery. Where a woman fails to conceive, a wide variety of cultural explanations usually come into play to explain her infertility and how to deal with it. As described in the previous chapter, such lay explanations for misfortune usually place the blame on the individual's behaviour, on the natural world, on the malevolence of other people, or on supernatural forces or gods. In addition, they often draw on deep cultural images of what constitutes 'a woman' and what 'a man'. Becker[69] described the poignant narratives of American women who have found that they are infertile. She shows how this knowledge strikes at the very sense of their own identity, unravelling their basic understanding of who they are. In the USA, as elsewhere, the ability to nurture others, and thus to be fertile, is the very basis of womanhood. The women compared themselves repeatedly with this cultural ideal of the 'natural mother': 'one who nourishes her child with the riches of her body'. While the pregnant body – 'a body that is nurturant, natural, and healthy' – stands as the very embodiment of the cultural values of womanhood, their own infertile bodies seemed somehow 'abnormal' by comparison.

Concepts of fertility and infertility are also partly dependent on how people conceptualize the inner workings of their bodies and the processes of conception and birth. For example, Cosminsky[70] described how in a Guatemalan village some of the traditional midwives believed that infertility was caused by a 'cold womb', which was not 'hot' enough to receive the semen. One form of treatment was to administer 'hot' herbal teas and to 'warm the womb' in a special sweatbath. If, however, the villagers believed that the sterility was caused by divine intervention, then the midwife was not expected to cure it.

In small-scale societies particularly, a 'barren woman' is often a marginalized figure, and seen as someone both personally unfulfilled and socially incomplete. In most traditional societies, blame for the infertility is usually placed on the woman. In many communities world-wide, producing a child – especially a son – is considered to be public proof of a man's virility, as well as of his adulthood. As a result, men are often reluctant to admit to any responsibility for infertility. According to McGilvray,[62] among Tamils in Sri Lanka and throughout most of South Asia, infertility is seen as primarily a problem with the woman and not the man. Sometimes a supernatural cause for the infertility is suggested, but rarely is the potency of the husband questioned, and most men would never acknowledge the possibility of their own sterility. In this type of setting, the very suggestion that they, and not their wives, are sterile may be very threatening to many men. For example, Palgi[71] describes the case of a Yemenite man from a traditional background who had emigrated to Israel. When his first wife failed to produce a child, he divorced her. When the second marriage was also childless, and doctors told him that he was the sterile one, he suffered a severe emotional collapse, with fearfulness, insomnia and a feeling of being tormented by evil spirits. Palgi links this reaction to cultural beliefs in his community that a man's dignity and respect are linked to the number of his progeny, especially sons. Furthermore, a common belief was that if there were no heirs to pray for a father's soul after death, then 'his peaceful life after death is endangered'. Similarly, Inhorn[72] described how in two other Middle Eastern settings – Cairo, Egypt, and Beirut, Lebanon – Arab men also saw their infertility as a stigmatized and problematic condition, and one that threatened their very sense of virility and manhood.

It should be noted, however, that these definitions of who is responsible for the infertility are not static. They are susceptible to significant changes during Westernization, migration, urbanization and other major social changes.

ASSISTED REPRODUCTION: THE NEW REPRODUCTIVE TECHNOLOGIES

In recent decades, in most industrialized countries, there have been major advances in the medical treatment of infertility, both male and female. Although they have helped many infertile couples to conceive, the new reproductive technologies (NRTs) remain controversial. This is largely because they have challenged the very notions of family, kinship and parenthood, especially the relationship between social and biological parenthood.

They have also altered perceptions of the physical functions and boundaries of the individual body, particularly the female body.

Despite this, their popularity continues to grow. By 2006 it was estimated that about 3 million children had been conceived from *in vitro* fertilization world-wide.[73] In some countries such as Japan, however, there has been both public and official opposition to the use of these procedures.[73]

Although a whole range of NRTs is now available, and in different combinations, the best known of them are:

- *in vitro fertilization* (IVF), involving ovum or sperm donation, either by the spouse of the infertile person or by an anonymous donor
- *surrogate motherhood*, whereby one woman carries a baby on behalf of another, and then gives it to her once it is born; the foetus may be either the surrogate mother's own child by the husband of the infertile woman, or the implanted, fertilized egg of another couple.

Other, more advanced techniques of assisted conception which may become freely available in the future (at least to the population of richer countries), include *intracytoplasmic sperm injection* (ICSI), *genetic cloning*, and the use of *embryonic stem cells*.

Before the development of the NRTs, ovulation, fertilization and pregnancy were events that all took place within the same woman's body. Now one or more may take place outside her body, or even in the bodies of three different women. In 1983, Snowden and colleagues[74] divided the maternal role into three parts: 'the genetic mother, the carrying mother, and the nurturing mother'. A woman who performs all three roles they described as a 'complete mother'. As a result of the development of IVF and surrogate motherhood, however, it is now possible for each of these roles to be carried out by a different woman: one providing the egg (also known as the 'commissioning mother'), another bearing the child (the 'carrying mother') and a third caring for the baby once it is born. Does the child therefore have one mother, or two, or even three? And which one, from its point of view, is the 'real' one?

A potential effect of the NRTs is thus to widen the split between biological and social parenthood. This does not apply only to motherhood; it has been estimated that up to 20 per cent of children born in the UK are not biologically related to their 'fathers',[75] and the use of IVF with sperm donation is likely to increase this percentage. Another result has been the creation of new and complex webs of kinship between, for example, 'carrying mothers' and 'commissioning mothers', children and their unknown genetic 'mothers' or 'fathers', couples and the anonymous donor of their child's ovum or sperm, and grandparents and grandchildren who are not genetically related to one another. Konrad,[76] for example, described the sense of 'relatedness' felt by both ova donors and recipients, even if they never meet one another in person.

The long-term effects of the NRTs on people's perceptions of parenthood and kinship, remain to be seen. Research indicates, however, that while they are welcomed by infertile couples, they are also provoking some unease in the general population. For example, in her study of women an English town, Edwards[77] found that they expressed anxiety about the possibility of incest, or other forbidden types of biological union, resulting from the NRTs. They feared that if two people, born of the same donated ova or sperm (in effect half-siblings) were to meet one day, marry, and produce a child, without knowledge of their genetic relationship, this would amount to incest (and interbreeding), and their child would be in danger of being born insane, disabled or otherwise damaged. The same anxiety was expressed about children born from the same surrogate mother, even if they were not biologically related, because they were both nourished by the same 'mother's blood'. In their view, 'a surrogate mother, though not genetically related to the fetus she carries, is inevitably and literally connected by the blood that flows between them.' There was also unease about a man donating sperm to his son's wife, if the son was infertile, as this would also be 'like incest'. Overall, the under-lying anxiety was about the breaching of 'natural' boundaries between people, and between generations, by these new technologies and the 'unnatural' consequences that might follow from this. This applied even if the 'incest' did not result from sexual intercourse, but only from a technological intervention. In other societies, too, there is unease about some of the NRTs, and even outright rejection of them. Inhorn[72] pointed out that some Middle Eastern societies reject surrogate pregnancies on religious grounds, as well as rejecting IVF if it involves a third-party donation of sperm, ova, or embryos; Gatrad and Sheikh[78] note that in Islam sperm donation is only acceptable if it originates from the woman's spouse.

In Western industrialized societies, where nuclear families are often the rule, social and biological parenthood usually coincide, except in the case of adoption, or where remarriage takes place following divorce or death of a spouse. Although the new forms of kinship created by the NRTs appear novel and unusual to Western culture, anthropologists have described many examples of what amounts to 'surrogate parenthood', with social and biological parenting being provided by different people. This is particularly common in traditional societies where large extended families are the rule and children may be cared for by a variety of adults – aunts, uncles, grandparents, older siblings and neighbours – as well as by their own biological parents. For example, Evans-Pritchard,[79] in the early 1950s, described unusual patterns of kinship and marriage among the Nuer people of the Sudan. Here, the failure to have any children, especially males to carry on the name, was regarded as a great tragedy by every Nuer family, and they adopted various strategies to overcome this problem. For example, in 'ghost marriage', which occurs when a man dies without legal male heirs, a kinsman of his (such as brother or nephew) marries the widow 'in the name of his dead kinsman'; as a result, the children of that union are regarded as belonging to the dead man, and the sons will carry his name. The woman is known as *ciekjooka*, the wife of a ghost, and her children are *gaatjooka*, children of a ghost. In another pattern, 'woman marriage', a barren woman 'marries' another woman and then arranges for a male kinsman or friend to make her pregnant. The children of this union become part of the 'husband's' family (who would not otherwise have any descendants); she is regarded as their legal father, they will carry her name, and sometimes they even refer to her as 'father'.

Both 'ghost marriage' and 'woman marriage' among the Nuer can be regarded as analogous to the sperm donation of IVF, although the donor, of course, is not anonymous. Ovum donation, however, was technically impossible until recent developments in reproductive technology. Overall, though, the growth of the NRTs in most Western countries is likely to result in a gradual weakening of the neat equation between biological and social parenthood, in new definitions of family and kinship, and in a growing anxiety about whether fertilization, pregnancy and parenthood are still the 'natural' processes that they once were.

CONTRACEPTION, ABORTION AND INFANTICIDE

Different attitudes to contraception, abortion and infanticide, all of which can be seen as forms of population control, seem to vary widely between cultures. Part of the reason for a society practising infanticide, for example, may be the size of the population, its food supply and the particular ecological niche that it occupies. In some cases the infants of one gender may be killed, but not the other, as in the case of the Tenetehara, a Brazilian Indian tribe, who believed that a woman should have three children, but not all of the same sex; if she had two daughters (or two sons) and gave birth to a third, then the baby would be killed (see Chapter 12). Overall, as Keesing[80] noted, in the past 'there is little doubt that peoples with finite space and resources in many parts of the world practised infanticide, of both sexes or of females, so as to restrict population numbers'. Infanticide of female babies still persists in different parts of

the world, especially in rural areas. The reasons for this are a complex mixture of cultural values, economic imperatives, government policy and sexist ideology. For example, Miller[81] described female infanticide, as well as the fatal neglect of some female children, in a society with a strongly patriarchal culture in the Punjab, northern India. A similar situation has been reported for many years from parts of rural China, even before the government's current 'one-child' policy.[82]

The particular 'population policy' of a culture may include a widespread tolerance of abortion, acceptance of abortion under certain limited circumstances, or strict taboos against it at any stage of pregnancy or for any reason. In the Western world, the debate on abortion centres both on whether the woman is entitled to control over her own body and fertility, and on whether the foetus is regarded as a 'person', with the same rights as other members of the society, or merely as an organ or collection of cells.

Abortion is a controversial issue in many societies, and there are many different cultural attitudes towards it. It is illegal in some societies, but accepted in others. Much of this definition depends on when – or whether – the fetus is regarded as a complete 'person', with all the rights that this implies. Different societies, with different religious and legal frameworks, place this point of 'becoming human' at different stages of the pregnancy: some at the very moment of fertilization, others several months later.[83] Societies also vary as to whether, and how, they help women who have had an abortion or miscarriage, deal with the emotional consequences of these events. An interesting example of this are the *Mizuko* shrines in Japan, dedicated to *Jizo*, a Buddhist *bottisatva* or enlightened being who is the guardian of all unborn, aborted, miscarried or stillborn babies. The shrine is a sacred place which allows women (and men) to grieve openly for the souls of their unborn babies. In the case of an abortion, the mother may carry out the *mizuko kuyo*, a ritual of apology and remembrance, and leave offerings at the shrine of toys, flowers, or food. In general, Western society, with its more secular and medicalized approach to bodily functions, lacks rituals such as these to help women grieve for an incomplete pregnancy, whatever the cause.

INDIGENOUS FORMS OF FERTILITY CONTROL

All human societies practice some form of population control, and many indigenous forms of controlling fertility are found world-wide.[84] Family planning and contraception have existed long before the arrival of modern methods such as 'the pill', the condom and the intrauterine contraceptive device (IUCD). In each case, these traditional approaches need to be understood in the context of people's beliefs about the functioning of their bodies, and about the nature of sexuality, fertility and pregnancy. They are also shaped by gender relationships, relationships of power, the role of children in their lives, and the social and economic *milieu* in which they live. Some of these methods of fertility control are the responsibility mainly of the woman, others of the man, while some involve both partners equally.

One should differentiate between the Western concept of *contraception* – used before, or during intercourse to prevent fertilization – from methods used *after* fertilization has taken place, and which may include induced abortions as well as 'menstrual regulation' (MR). Islam and colleagues[85] have defined MR as 'any chemical, mechanical or surgical process used to induce menstruation and thus to establish non-pregnancy'. It involves vacuum aspiration of the uterine lining by a syringe or other device, and is usually done within 8 weeks following a missed period, but without doing a pregnancy test. In Bangladesh, for example, where abortion is illegal or very restricted, they describe how MR is carried out ostensibly for 'removing menstrual irregularity' or 'bringing on the period', but the authors see it also as 'an unrecognized form of contraception'.[85]

Indigenous methods of fertility control that have been reported include:

- *prolonged breast-feeding*, which is perhaps the commonest way of reducing fertility in poorer parts of the world. In a process called *lactational amenorrhoea*, full breast-feeding (especially in the first few months) can stop menstruation and prevent conception.[86] It has been estimated that women who breastfeed fully in the first 6 months after delivery have a risk of pregnancy of less than 2 per cent,[87] though the risk rises somewhat after that time. If the period of breast-feeding is reduced by introducing bottle feeding, this obviously will greatly reduce its protective effect

- *post-partum sexual abstinence* is also one of the commonest forms of fertility control, and is often supported by strong religious taboos. In the Islamic tradition, for example – as in some other religious groups – intercourse must be avoided for about 40 days after delivery, until the postpartum bleeding (*nifas*) has ceased. Post-partum sexual abstinence is particularly common in sub-Saharan Africa, but it is also found in many other parts of the world.[84] The period of abstinence can vary from several weeks to several years. It can also vary by social class, region or ethnic group. In a study in Malawi, for example, Zulu[88] found that ethnic groups in the north of the country abstained for about 17 months, those in the south for 10 months, and those in the centre for only 6.6 months. Often the rationale people give for sexual abstinence is not so much fertility control, but rather for preserving the health of the child, or of its parents.[88,89] However, in a study in Ghana, Awusabo-Asare and Anarfi[89] point out the dangers of this prolonged abstinence (31 per cent of their sample abstained for 12–23 months, 21.6 per cent for 24 months or more) in a society threatened by AIDS, since abstinence is more strongly expected from women than from men. Given the decline in polygamy, this can increase the risk of the men contracting AIDS or other sexually transmitted diseases from other women during that period, and then infecting their wives when they resume conjugal relations

- *abstinence from sexual intercourse* – both pre-marital and post-marital – has been widely used in different societies, religions, and periods in history. As well as promoting pre-marital chastity and virginity, several groups have advocated chastity within marriage. In nineteenth century America, for example, abstinence for birth control in marriage was advocated by groups such as the Voluntary Motherhood Movement and the White Ribbon Campaign. Today, among the Airopai tribe of the Peruvian Amazon, Belaunde[90] describes how the men are encouraged to practice sexual restraint with their wives (a process called 'a man looking after his woman'), and how this is maintained by a number of cultural beliefs: such as avoiding intercourse before the frequent hunting and fishing expeditions 'lest he lose his shooting skills' as a result. The men also take part in lengthy shamanic rituals, and sexual relations are prohibited during these rituals 'because the divinities dislike the smell of sexual fluids'
- *coitus interrruptus* or withdrawal just before ejaculation is a commonly used, though often unreliable form of contraception. While it is forbidden by some religions and social groups, it is sanctioned by others. In Uzbekistan, for example, Krengel and Greifeld[91] report that it 'remains the most popular and widespread method of natural contraception and is in accordance with the Koran'. *Coitus reservatus* is withdrawal without ejaculation, and has been advocated by some groups in China and India (especially practitioners of Kundalini yoga), as a way of preserving the balance of vital energies within the man's body
- *rhythm or calendar methods*, favoured by many churches, advocate sexual abstinence during the days of the woman's fertile period, but they depend on an understanding of female physiology and the likely timing of ovulation (see above). They may also involve monitoring the quality of cervical mucus as a way of identifying the times when intercourse should be avoided
- '*outercourse*' refers to the various alternatives to penile–vaginal intercourse, especially among adolescents and young adults, and includes masturbation, oral sex, mutual petting, 'thigh intercourse', and practices such as 'bundling' in Colonial New England, where an unmarried young couple were allowed to share a bed, but only with a wooden partition between them.[92] Also included here should be anal intercourse, widely used in parts of Latin America among young people to preserve the girl's virginity, but also to prevent pregnancy, especially before marriage.[93] However, this practice may increase the risk of sexually transmitted diseases such as hepatitis B or AIDS
- *herbal oral contraceptives* used by women are usually taken in the form of potions, raw plants or fruits, and have been reported from many different cultures. They include women eating papaya daily in Sri Lanka,[92] and the use of *cada nuni* – an indigenous plant related to ginger – by the Airopai Indians of the Peruvian Amazon.[90] In the Philippines, Quijano[94] has described how drinking *Kamias* and other herbal concoctions has long been used by women as a traditional method of contraception, especially in rural areas
- *intravaginal spermicides and barrier methods* have included the use of various herbs, vegetable seedpods, crushed roots, plugs of grass, algae and seaweed, as well as the use of sponges, sometimes soaked vinegar or other liquids.[92] Herbal or other douches used after intercourse should also be included here
- *primitive condoms*, usually made from animal gut, have reportedly been used for centuries, mainly to avoid sexually transmitted diseases, but also to prevent pregnancy. The first known condom in England, made of animal gut, apparently dates from 1640, and mass-produced rubber condoms only appeared after 1843[92]

- *abortion* – either self-induced, or induced by others – has long been used for fertility control. In many societies it has involved the use of herbal or mineral abortifacients, as well as mechanical means, and both have sometimes resulted in high maternal morbidity and mortality. Molina[95] has described how *criollo* women in Argentina use up to 20 different plant infusions as contraceptives and abortifacients; they include querbracho (*Shipsis balancae*) whose bark is boiled, and the resultant fluid drunk over several days until expulsion of the fetus occurs. It can, however, cause both liver and kidney damage. Abortion as a form of fertility control was common in many countries of the Soviet Bloc. In Uzbekistan, abortion (together with the IUCD) was the commonest form of 'birth control' in Soviet times, though this situation is changing considerably.[91] In more developed societies, there is now the possibility that revealing the gender of a child before birth by amniocentesis or ultrasound scan may result in a request for abortion, if the parents are unhappy with that particular gender. The increased selective abortion of female fetuses has also been reported in several Asian countries, including India[96]
- *infanticide* of unwanted or deformed babies has been long practiced by many human groups, as noted earlier. The infanticide of female babies has been especially reported from societies at a subsistence level, where a male child may be preferred for hunting, fighting or hard manual labour
- *magical and ritual methods* include the use of prayers, amulets, or specific rituals to control fertility, and prevent pregnancy. Among the Amazonian Airopai,[90] for example, male shamans perform 'contraceptive rituals' on behalf of women who consult them. If necessary, they also perform rituals to re-establish a woman's fertility, or to cause abortions
- *birth spacing* refers to the cultural concepts that underlie many of these indigenous forms of preventing or delaying pregnancy, and

which defines the 'optimal' or preferred time between pregnancies for that cultural group. For example, Davids[97] described how Ethiopian immigrants to Israel believe that 3 years is the optimal interval between pregnancies, since it gives the woman's body time to recover from childbirth; having two or more pregnancies too close together may seriously damage her health, by giving her 'weak blood' (*dam manes*).

Whatever their degree of efficacy, their dangers and side-effects, many of these traditional forms of fertility control have been used for many centuries, and are deeply trusted by those who make use of them. As such they need to be taken seriously, and to be evaluated as to their usefulness in the modern world. In some countries, traditional forms of birth control, and traditional remedies, are being adapted to modern needs and to the modern problems of overpopulation. In India, for example, the National Research Development Corporation (NRDC)[98] has researched the use of *neem oil* as a contraceptive. It is indigenous, cheap and easily available, and in rural parts of India is already widely used as a traditional remedy for wounds, skin diseases, infections, arthritis and other ailments. Recently, it has also been found to have spermicidal activity, and is therefore now seen as a promising precoital and postcoital vaginal contraceptive, as well as an abortifacient. The NRDC suggest that because neem is already so well known, and so available, 'the rural population will accept it easily' as a form of contraception.

MALES AND PREGNANCY

Although pregnancy and childbirth are female events, both physically and socially, most men are deeply involved in the birth of their children. In many cultures this emotional involvement is recognized by a series of rituals that the men must carry out during their wives' pregnancy, birth and postpartum period.

Heggenhougen[99] has reviewed much of the literature on the role of fathers in the birth of their children. He points out that in most modern middle-class Western industrial cultures, the husband has only a minimal role to play – usually that of anxious spectator – in the birth of his child. Overall, the majority of human cultures exclude men from the scene of birth. However, this is not true of certain Native American, Eskimo, African and Maori groups.

Where the father is present at the birth, his presence is almost always functional, and the role and rituals that are prescribed for him are believed to be integral to the actual birth process. He has certain tasks to perform which are designed to protect mother and child and make the delivery easier, and which may be termed the *ritual couvade*. In many non-industrialized cultures he is expected to follow certain strict taboos; in Java the husband follows many of the same taboos as his wife, and supports her during labour, and this is also found in some Guatemalan communities, among the Catiguan villagers of the Philippines and in parts of northern Europe. In the Lan tsu Miao tribe of Kweichew, South China, the husband not only takes to his bed during his wife's labour, but also takes care of and 'mothers' the baby. In the Buka, Ashanti and Chickchee tribes, men perform rituals to fool evil spirits and attract their attention until the child is safely born. Among the Arapesh people of New Guinea, the verb 'to bear a child' is used indiscriminately for either man or woman, and childbearing is believed to be as heavy a drain on the man as on the woman. Among the Hopi Indians of the USA and the Chiriguano Indians of Paraguay, both husband and the last-born child go into couvade during the wife's pregnancy. In the modern Western world, largely under the influence of the women's movement and the trend towards 'natural childbirth', men tend to be more involved in their partner's pregnancy and are often present at the actual birth,

but they lack the protection of a ritually prescribed role (see Chapter 9) characteristic of more traditional societies.

In many cultures, especially those where the ritual couvade is not practised, men have often been reported as suffering from physical and/or psychological symptoms during their wife's pregnancy, birth and postpartum period. This is known as the *couvade syndrome* (from the Basque word *couver*, to brood or hatch), and has been reported from many parts of the world. According to Heggenhougen,[99] one can view this couvade syndrome as 'a subconscious form of participation or perhaps even competition, with the wife', while ritual couvade is 'a conscious participation, though it may have a subconscious base'.

A contemporary illustration of this syndrome, from the USA, is described in the following case history.

Case study: couvade syndrome in Rochester, New York, USA

Lipkin and Lamb[100] carried out a study in 1982 on the couvade syndrome, in Rochester, New York. They defined this syndrome as the occurrence of new physical or psychological symptoms in the mates of pregnant women, for which they sought medical care, and which were not otherwise objectively explained. In their study of 267 mates of postpartum women, 60 (22.5 per cent) of the men were found to have suffered from this syndrome. This translates to a prevalence rate of 225 of 1000 husbands at risk due to their wife's pregnancy. Many of their symptoms were vague and non-specific, such as 'feeling rundown', 'feeling lowdown' and 'weakness', as well as more 'pregnant' symptoms such as backache, genital burning, water retention (not confirmed on physical examinations), retrosternal burning, groin pain, dizziness and abdominal cramps. One patient complained of a chest pain that felt like 'something was pushing out'.

Whatever the cause, the evidence is that men are physically, as well as emotionally, deeply involved in the birth of their children. Clinicians should therefore be aware of the possibility of unexplained symptoms – both physical and psychological – in many expectant fathers.

KEY REFERENCES

5 Keesing, R.M.and Strathern, A.J. (1998) *Cultural Anthropology: A Contemporary Perspective,* 3rd edn. London: Harcourt Brace, pp. 270–281.

8 Shepherd, G. (1982). Rank, gender, and homosexuality: Mombasa as a key to understanding sexual options. In: *The Cultural Construction of Sexuality* (Caplan, P. ed.). London: Tavistock, pp. 240–70.

22 World Health Organization (2005). *World Health Statistics 2005.* Geneva:World Health Organization, pp.45–52.

28 van Dongen, E. and Elema, R. (2001) The art of touching: the culture of 'body work' in nursing. *Anthropol. Med.* 8, 150–62.

33 Gabe, I. and Calnan, M. (1989). The limits of medicine: women's perception of medical technology. *Soc. Sci. Med.* 28, 223–31.

50 Hahn, R.A. and Muecke, M.A. (1987). The anthropology of birth in five US ethnic populations: implications for obstetrical practice. *Curr. Probl. Obstet. Gynecol. Fertil.* 10, 133–71.

51 Nichter, M. and Nichter, M. (1996) Cultural notions of fertility in South Asia and their impact on Sri Lankan family planning services. In: *Anthropology and International Health: Asian Case Studies* (Nichter, M. and Nichter, M. eds). Reading: Gordon and Breach, pp. 3–33.

55 Graham, H. and Oakley, A. (1981). Competing ideologies of reproduction: medical and maternal perspectives on pregnancy. In: *Women, Health and Reproduction* (Roberts, H. ed.). London: Routledge and Kegan Paul, pp. 99–118.

60 MacCormack, C. P. (1982). Biological, cultural and social adaptation in human fertility and birth: a synthesis. In: *Ethnography of Fertility and Birth* (McCormack, C. P. ed.). London: Academic Press, pp. 1–23.

69 Becker, G. (1997). *Disrupted Lives.* Berkeley: University of California Press, pp. 80–98.

76 Konrad, M. (1998). Ova donation and symbols of substance: some variations on the theme of sex, gender and the partible body. *J. R. Anthropol. Inst. (NS)* 4, 643–67.

95 Molina, A.I. (1997) Ethnomedicine and world-view: a comparative analysis of the incorporation and rejection of contraceptive methods among Argentine women. *Anthropology and Medicine* 4(2), 145–58.

See http://www.culturehealthandillness.com for the full list of references for this chapter.

RECOMMENDED READING

Davis-Floyd, R.E. (1992). *Birth as an American Rite of Passage.* Berkeley: University of California Press.

Hahn, R. A. and Muecke, M. A. (1987). The anthropology of birth in five US ethnic populations: implications for obstetrical practice. *Curr. Probl. Obstet. Gynecol. Fertil.* 10, 133–71.

Heggenhougen, H. K. (1980). Fathers and childbirth: an anthropological perspective. *J. Nurse-Midwifery,* 25(6), 21–6.

Lock, M. (1998). Menopause: lessons from anthropology. *Psychosom. Med.,* 60, 410–19.

Lupton, D. (1994) *Medicine as Culture.* London: Sage, pp. 131–160.

Russell, A., Sobo, E.J. & Thompson, M.S. (eds) (2000) *Contraception across Cultures.* Berg.

van Teijlingen, E., Lowis, G. McCaffery, P. & Porter, M. (eds) (1999) *Midwifery and the Medicalization of Childbirth: Comparative perspectives.* Hauppage: Nova Science Publishers.

7 Pain and culture

Pain, in one form or another, is an inseparable part of everyday life. It is probably also the commonest symptom encountered in clinical practice,[1] and is a feature of many normal physiological changes such as pregnancy, childbirth, or menstruation as well as of injury and disease. Many forms of healing or diagnosis also involve some form of pain; for example, surgical operations, injections, biopsies or venesection. In all of these situations there is more to pain than merely a neurophysiological event; there are social, psychological and cultural factors associated with it that also need to be considered. In this chapter some of these factors will be examined in order to illustrate the following propositions:

1 Not all social or cultural groups may respond to pain in exactly the same way.
2 How people perceive and respond to pain, both in themselves and in others, can be influenced by their cultural and social background.
3 How, and whether, people communicate their pain to health professionals and to others can also be influenced by social and cultural factors.

PAIN BEHAVIOUR

From a physiological perspective, pain can be thought of as 'a type of signalling device for drawing attention to tissue damage or to physiological malfunction'.[2] Pain arises when a nerve or nerve ending is affected by a noxious stimulus, either from within the body or from outside it. It is therefore of crucial importance for the protection and survival of the body in an environment full of potential dangers. Because of this biological role it is sometimes assumed that pain is culture-free, in the sense of there being a universal biological reaction to a specific type of stimulus such as a sharp object or extremes of hot or cold. However, the two forms of reaction can be differentiated into:

1 An *involuntary,* instinctual reaction, such as pulling away from the sharp object
2 A *voluntary* reaction, such as
  a removing the source of pain, and taking action to treat the symptom (by taking an aspirin, for example)
  b asking another person for help in relieving the symptom.

Voluntary reactions to pain that involve other people are particularly influenced by social and cultural factors, and will be described below in more detail, with examples.

According to Engel,[3] pain thus has two components: 'the original sensation, and the reaction to the sensation'. This reaction, whether voluntary or not, has been called *pain behaviour* by Fabrega and Tyma,[4] and includes certain changes in facial expression, grimaces, changes in demeanour or activity, as well as certain sounds made by the victim, or words used to describe his or her condition or appeal for help. It is possible, though, to exhibit pain behaviour in the absence of a painful stimulus or, conversely, not to exhibit such behaviour despite the presence of the painful stimulus. To clarify this point, it is useful to identify two types of pain behaviour or reactions to pain: *private* pain and *public* pain.

PRIVATE PAIN Ⓐ

Pain, as Engel[3] points out, is 'private data'; that is, in order for us to know whether a person is in pain we are dependent on that person signalling that fact to us, either verbally or non-verbally. When that happens, the private experience and perception of pain become a social, public event; private pain becomes public pain. However, when pain originates within the body, rather than from any outside injury, it is often 'invisible' since there is no injury, lesion or wound visible to other people. In that case, it may be difficult for the sufferer to communicate the fact that they are suffering, or to get others to acknowledge, understand and 'share' their pain. In that case, as Scarry[5] notes, this can result in a sense of isolation for the victim, for the pain has caused an 'absolute split between one's sense of one's own reality and the reality of other persons'.

In some social groups and cultures, the pain may deliberately be kept private, and there may be no outward clue or sign that the person is experiencing pain, even when it is very severe. This type of behaviour is common among societies that value stoicism and fortitude, such as the Anglo-Saxon 'stiff upper lip' in the presence of hardship.[4] It is more likely to be expected of men, particularly younger men or warriors. In some cultures the ability to bear pain without flinching – that is, without displaying overt pain behaviour – may be one of the signs of manhood, and part of initiation rituals marking the transition from boyhood to manhood. For example, among the Cheyenne Indians of the Great Plains, young men who wanted to display their manhood and gain social prestige would undergo ritual self-torture

in the Sun Dance ceremony, suspending themselves from a pole by hooks passed through the skin of their chests, and accepting the pain without complaint.[6] Other less dramatic forms of a lack of pain behaviour occur in those who are semiconscious, paralysed or too young to articulate their distress, or in situations where such behaviour is unlikely to bring a sympathetic response from other people. Therefore, an absence of pain behaviour does not necessarily mean the absence of private pain.

PUBLIC PAIN Ⓑ

Pain behaviour, especially its voluntary aspects, is influenced by social, cultural and psychological factors. These determine *whether* private pain will be translated into pain behaviour, and the *form* that this behaviour takes, and the social settings in which it occurs.

Part of the decision about whether to translate private into public pain depends on the person's interpretation of the *significance* of the pain; whether, for example, it is seen as 'normal' or 'abnormal' pain, the latter being more likely to be brought to the attention of others. An example of normal pain is dysmenorrhoea. In two American studies quoted by Zola,[7] women from both lower and upper socio-economic groups were asked to keep a calendar in which they recorded all bodily states and dysfunctions. Only a small percentage even reported the dysmenorrhoea as a 'dysfunction', and among the lower income group only 18 per cent even mentioned the menses or its accompaniments. Definitions of what constitutes an 'abnormal' pain, and which therefore requires medical attention and treatment, tend to be culturally defined, and to vary over time. As Zola notes, 'the degree of recognition and treatment of certain gynaecological problems may be traced to the prevailing definition of what constitutes the necessary part of the business of being a woman'. This in turn may be influenced by the social and economic context in which the women's lives are embedded, such as the need to care for children or carry on working despite being in pain. Other definitions of abnormal pain depend on cultural definitions of body image, and the structure and function of the body.[8] Commonly held beliefs that 'the heart' occupies the entire chest, for example, may lead to an interpretation of all pains in this area as 'heart trouble' or a 'heart attack'. A case has been described of a man with psychosomatic chest pains who clung to the idea that he had 'trouble with the heart', despite numerous diagnostic tests that excluded cardiac disease, because he still had 'pain over my heart'.[9]

Zborowski[10] has pointed out that a cultural group's *expectations* and acceptance of pain as a normal part of life will determine whether it is seen as a clinical problem that requires a clinical solution. Cultures that emphasize military achievements, for example, both expect and accept battle wounds, while more peaceful cultures may expect them, but not accept them without complaint. Similarly, Zborowski noted[10] how in Poland and in some other countries labour pains were both expected and accepted by women giving birth, while in the USA they were not accepted and analgesia was frequently demanded. These attitudes towards pain are acquired early in life, as part of growing up in a particular family and community, and are an essential part of any culture's child-rearing practices. They also tend to change over time, as new technologies and fashions of pain relief become available, especially in societies undergoing social and economic development.

Pain as misfortune

Although physical pain is a particularly vivid and emotionally laden symptom, it can only be understood in a cultural context by seeing it as part of the wider spectrum of *misfortune*. Pain, like illness generally, is only a special type of human suffering. As such, it can provoke the same types of questions in the victim as do other forms of misfortune: 'Why has it happened to me?', 'Why now?' or 'What have I done to deserve this?'.

Where pain is seen as divine punishment for a behavioural lapse, the victims may be unwilling to seek relief for it. Experiencing the pain without complaint becomes, in itself, a form of expiation. Alternatively, they may demand more painful treatments from a physician, such as a surgical operation or an injection. If pain is seen as the result of moral transgressions, the response might also be self-imposed penitence, fasting or prayer, rather than consultation with a health professional. If interpersonal malevolence, such as sorcery, witchcraft or 'hexing' is thought to have caused a pain, the strategy for pain relief may be an indirect one – by a ritual of exorcism, for example.

In many cultures, because pain is seen as only one type of suffering within the wider spectrum of misfortune, it is *linked* with other forms of suffering in a number of ways. These include having a common cause (such as divine punishment or witchcraft), and therefore requiring a similar form of treatment (prayer, penitence or exorcism). This wider view of pain is common in non-Western societies, and members of these societies may find the secular Western treatment of pain – the prescribing of a pain-relieving drug – both incomplete and unsatisfying. Although Western medicine does acknowledge the existence of 'psychosomatic' or 'psychogenic pain', its attitude to organic pain does not take into account the social, moral and psychological elements that many people associate with pain. Nevertheless, the idiom of pain in modern English does still show linkages to other forms of suffering, including emotional distress, interpersonal conflicts and unexpected misfortune. These are often described using the metaphor of physical pain, for example 'I was sore at him', 'she hurt him deeply', 'a biting comment', 'a painful experience', 'a mere pinprick', 'it was a blow to me', 'tortured soul' and 'heartsore'. In more traditional societies, the link between physical pain and the social, moral and religious aspects of everyday life is likely to be much more direct, and to influence closely how people perceive their own ill health.

A

Lecture

Case study: The language of pain in North Indian culture

Pugh[11] in 1991 described the many meanings of pain in North Indian culture, and the metaphors used to express it. In the absence of Western mind-body dualism, neither traditional practitioners (*hakims*) nor their patients see pain (*dard*) solely in physical terms. When talking about pain, they draw on a shared reservoir of words, images and metaphors derived from local culture and everyday life. The metaphors they use (such as a 'burning', 'gripping', or 'stabbing' pain) blend together physical and emotional experiences into a single image. Thus, the same word, phrase or metaphor often conveys the meaning of physical and psychological suffering at the same time. For example, the metaphors used for physical pain can also be used to describe certain emotional states; sadness and grief, like 'hot' foods, can make the heart 'burn', and Urdu poets describe 'the burning ache of the heart', and the 'wonderful feelings of love-pain'. Such metaphors for pain as 'hot' or 'burning' reflect, as Pugh puts it, 'the integrated mind–body system of Indian culture'. Thus 'physical pain in Indian culture incorporates psychological malaise, while emotional distress manifests itself simultaneously in both mind and body'.

Furthermore, many of the words used to describe different types of pain suggest both its cause and its probable cure. On the basis of 'like causes like', the description of 'hot' or 'burning' pains implies their causation by 'hot' or 'burning' foods, or by hot weather, or by certain 'hot' emotional states (such as anxiety or anger). Their treatment is by remedies that cause 'cooling', such as cool packs, or cold musk medicine that 'provides psychophysical relief for pain, palpitations, and anxiety by "cooling" the body's heat and "calming" the heart'.

Finally, the metaphors 'which imbue pain with its sensory qualities draw on the familiar surroundings of house, field, and workshop', and the experiences of daily life. A 'burning pain' of the stomach, chest or throat is often said to be accompanied by a 'sour' (*khatta*) or 'bitter' (*katu*) taste. Both these tastes are also found in most people's diet: sourness in limes, pomegranates and tamarind; bitterness in mustard-seed oil, certain lemons and turmeric. Thus, the experience of pain and the meanings given to that experience are linked to many other aspects of local culture, cuisine, language and tradition. Because different types of pain, at different times, in different places, and in different parts of the body, all carry with them so many associations – physical, emotional, social, spiritual, dietary and climatic – the Western model of pain as mainly a physical event may be inappropriate. Pugh concluded that this is because north Indian cultural patterning depicts pain 'not as a single, fixed entity but rather as a fluid, context-sensitive constellation of meanings'.

The types and availability of potential healers or helpers also determine whether a person will display pain behaviour, and in what settings. For example, such behaviour is more likely to bring sympathetic help from a hospital doctor or nurse than from a punitive army sergeant. The personality and idiosyncrasies of the clinician, as well as whether they come from a similar culture and social class to the sufferer, may influence the decision to display it or not. Such behaviour may be displayed to one clinician but not to an unsympathetic colleague, leading to different evaluations of the patient's condition by the two clinicians.

A further factor determining whether private pain is made public is the perceived *intensity* of the pain sensation itself. There is some evidence that this perception (and pain tolerance) can be influenced by culture. In a review of the literature on culture and pain in 1977, Wolff and Langley[12] pointed out the paucity of adequately controlled experimental studies in this area. However, those studies that have been done confirm that 'cultural factors in terms of attitudinal variables, whether explicit or implicit, do indeed exert significant influences on pain perception'. Also, as Lewis[13] has noted, the intensity of a pain sensation does not follow automatically from the extent and nature of an injury. Beliefs about the meaning and significance of a pain, the context in which it occurs and the emotions associated with that context can all affect pain sensation: 'Fear of implications for the future may intensify awareness of pain in the surgical patient, or, by contrast, the hope and likely chance of escape from deadly risks of battle may diminish the injured soldier's sense of pain and his complaints, though the injury be similar in both cases'. A common example of this is soldiers who only notice that they have been wounded once the battle is over; the intensity of emotional involvement in the battle may divert attention, at least temporarily, from a painful wound. In certain states of religious trance, meditation or ecstasy, the intensity of pain perception can also be reduced, although the physiological reasons for this are not well understood. Examples of this phenomenon are the *yogis* and *fakirs* of India, or the fire-walkers of Sri Lanka, who all undergo self-inflicted pain or discomfort, apparently without experiencing the full intensity of the pain.

Attitudes and expectations of a particular healer or treatment can also influence the intensity of pain, as in placebo analgesia; here, a pharmacologically inactive drug in which the patient 'believes' causes subjective pain relief in the sufferer. Levine and colleagues[14] have suggested that the release of endorphins or endogenous opiates within the brain is the physiological mechanism underlying placebo analgesia, since it can be counteracted by the use of nalorphine. Whatever the underlying mechanism, the perception of the intensity of a pain, as well as the meanings associated with it, may influence whether a privately experienced pain is shared with other people.

The presentation of public pain

Each culture and social group – and sometimes even each individual or family – has their own unique 'language of distress'; its own complex idiom by which ill or unhappy individuals make other people aware of their suffering. There is a specific, often standardized way of signalling, both verbally and non-verbally, that they are in pain or discomfort. The *form* that this pain behaviour will take is largely culturally determined, as is the *response* to this behaviour. According to Landy,[15] this depends, among other factors on 'whether their culture values or disvalues the display of emotional expression and response to injury'. Some cultural groups (and families) expect an extravagant, often theatrical display of emotionality in the presence of pain; others value stoicism, restraint and the playing down of their symptoms. Zola[7], in his 1966 study of reactions to pain by a group of Italian-Americans and Irish-Americans, pointed out that the Italian-American response was marked by 'expressiveness and expansiveness', which he saw as a defence mechanism (dramatization) – a way of coping with anxiety 'by repeatedly over-expressing it and thereby dissipating it'. Conversely, the Irish-Americans tended to ignore and underplay their bodily complaints; for example, 'I ignore it like I do most things'. They tended to deny or play down the presence of pain – 'It was more a throbbing than a pain … not really pain, it feels more like sand in my eye'. Zola saw this denial as a defence mechanism against the 'oppressive sense of guilt' that he, and other researchers, see as a feature of rural Irish culture. These two different languages of distress may have negative effects on the types of medical treatment that these patients are given, especially by clinicians from different cultural backgrounds. The Italian-Americans, for example, might be dismissed as over-emotional or hypochondriacal by a clinician who values stoicism and restraint, and the Irish-Americans might have their suffering ('private pain') ignored because they continually underplay it. Zola warned that this might perpetuate their suffering by creating a 'self-fulfilling prophecy'.[7]

Pain behaviour may be *non-verbal*, and this too can be patterned by culture. It may include immobility, grimacing, restlessness, agitated movements, groaning, crying, screaming, or using certain gestures. In his study of bodily gestures, Le Barre[16] pointed out that while gestures differ cross-culturally they can only be interpreted by taking into account the context in which they appear. For example, in the Argentine, shaking one of the hands smartly so that the fingers make an audible clacking sound, can mean 'wonderful', but also signify pain when one says '*Ai yai*' following an injury. Therefore, non-verbal languages of distress include not only gestures but also the various facial expressions, bodily posture and exclamations, all of which take their meaning from the context in which they appear. They may also include other changes in behaviour, such as withdrawal, fasting, prayer or recourse to self-medication. Thus, as noted in Chapter 4, different types of pain behaviour can be an intrinsic part of a non-verbal narrative of suffering, and one that is displayed over time to family, friends or health professionals.

Because pain behaviour, whether verbal or not, is often standardized within a culture, it is open to imitation by those who wish to get sympathy or attract attention, by displaying public pain without any underlying private pain. Examples of this are the hypochondriac, the malingerer and the actor. People with Munchausen's syndrome, for example, may exactly mimic real pain behaviour and therefore undergo repeated surgical operations or investigations before the syndrome is discovered.[17] Pain behaviour may also mask an underlying psychological state, such as an extreme anxiety state, depression or emotional conflicts, as in *somatization* – whether personal or 'cultural' (see Chapter 10). In this case, the primary symptom complained of will not be anxiety or depression, but rather physical symptoms such as weakness, breathlessness, sweating, vague aches and pains, or pains in a particular area of the body. This type of somatization is said to be more common among low-income groups in the Western world; however, it is also a feature of many other higher socio-economic groups, as well as of other cultures world-wide. For example, in Taiwan the open display of emotional distress is not encouraged; instead this state

is usually expressed in a mainly somatic or physical language of distress. In 1980, Kleinman[18] noted that in Taiwan, Chinese culture 'defines the somatic complaint as *the* primary illness problem', even if psychological symptoms are also present. In one period, 70 per cent of the patients who visited the Psychiatry Clinic at the National Taiwan University Hospital initially complained of physical symptoms.[18] In this and other cultures, a depressed person may complain of vague fleeting pains, or 'pains everywhere', for which no physical cause can be found. This type of somatic presentation of depression is found in all societies, both rich and poor, whether or not it is also accompanied by psychological symptoms. Just as culture can influence somatization, so can the personality and background of the clinician. A doctor orientated towards purely physical explanations of ill health, for example, may only acknowledge somatic symptoms, in contrast to a colleague more interested in psychodynamic or social processes.

How pain is described is influenced by a number of factors, including language facility, familiarity with medical terms, individual experiences of pain and lay beliefs about the structure and function of the body (seen in the 'glove-and-stocking' distribution of hysterical pain or anaesthesia). The use of technical terms borrowed from medicine to describe a pain may also confuse the clinician; the person who says, 'I've had another migraine, doctor', may be using the term to describe a wide variety of head pains and not only migraine. The cues from clinicians that help shape a diffuse, especially psychosomatic, pain into a recognizable medical form, are questions such as 'Does it travel down your left arm?', 'Does it come on when you climb stairs?' or 'Does it feel like a tight band across your chest?'. Medical history-taking, examinations, diagnostic tests and health education campaigns may all unwittingly train patients to identify and describe the characteristic form of a particular type of pain, such as angina, colic or migraine.[9] Clinicians should therefore be aware of this process of 'clinical mimicry' and the difficulties it poses for reliable diagnosis.

Social aspects of pain

Public pain implies a *social relationship*, of whatever duration, between the sufferer and another person or persons. The nature of this relationship will determine whether the pain is revealed in the first place, how it is revealed, and the nature of the response to it. Lewis[13] notes how the *expectations* of sufferers are important here, particularly the likely response to their pain and the social costs and benefits of revealing it: 'Possibilities of care, of sympathy, the allocation of responsibility for sickness in others, affect how people show their illness'. People will receive maximum attention and sympathy if their pain behaviour matches the society's view of how people in pain should draw attention to their suffering, whether by an extravagant display of emotions or by a quiet change in behaviour. According to Zola,[7] 'It is the "fit" of certain signs with a society's major values which accounts for the degree of attention they receive'. There is thus a dynamic between the individual and society (Figure 7.1) whereby pain behaviour, and the reactions to it, influence each other over time.

The types of permissible pain behaviour within a society are learned in childhood and infancy. Engel[3] points out that pain plays an important role in the total psychological development of the individual: 'It is... intimately concerned with learning about the environment and its dangers... and about the body and its limitations'. It is integral to all early relationships: in infancy, pain leads to crying, which leads to a response from the mother or another person. In early childhood, pain and punishment become linked; the adult world inflicts pain for 'bad' behaviour. Pain may therefore signal

to the individual that he or she is 'bad', and therefore should feel guilty; it may also become an important medium for the expiation of guilt. Pain is also part of relationships of aggression and power, and of sexual relationships. Engel has described the 'pain-prone patient' who is particularly liable to 'psychogenic pain', and whose personality is characterized by strong feelings of guilt. In his view, this patient is more likely to complain of pains of one sort or another as a means of self-punishment and atonement; penitence, self-denial and self-deprecation may all be used as forms of self-inflicted punishments to ease the feelings of guilt. One could hypothesize that cultures characterized by a pervasive sense of guilt are also those that value 'painful' rituals of atonement and prayer, including fasting, abstinence, isolation, poverty and even self-flagellation.

Child-rearing practices

Child-rearing practices can help shape attitudes towards and expectations of pain later in life – particularly, as Zborowski[10] notes, the cultural values and attitudes of parents, parent-substitutes, siblings and peer groups. In his 1952 study in the USA, he described how parents from some religious or ethnic groups manifested 'over-protective and over-concerned attitudes towards the child's health, participation in sports, games, fights, etc.'. The child was often reminded to avoid colds, injuries, fights and other threatening situations. Crying in complaint was quickly responded to with sympathy and concern. In Zborowski's view, the parents thereby fostered an over-awareness of pain and other deviations from normal, as well as anxiety about their possible significance. In contrast, 'Old American' Protestant families tended to be less overprotective; the child was told 'not to run to mother with every little thing', to expect pain in sports and games, and not to react in too emotional a way to them.

Later in life, when these people actually suffered from severe physical pain, there was a variation in how that pain was displayed (or not displayed) compared with other people, ranging

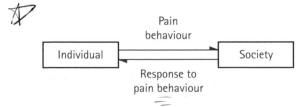

Figure 7.1 Pain behaviour relationship between the individual and society.

from a more emotional, exaggerated, theatrical display to a less emotional, more stoical or withdrawn one. All these culturally defined languages of distress will influence how private pain is signalled to others, and the types of reaction expected from them. Problems might arise, however, if the sufferer and those around them have different cultural origins, or come from different social classes, with different expectations of how a person in pain should behave and how they should be treated. In Zborowski's study,[10] patients with physical pain from the 'Old American' families, tended to be less emotional in reporting pain to health professionals, and to adopt a detached air in describing their pain, its character, duration and location. They saw no point in over-exaggerating their pain, because 'it won't help anybody'. Withdrawal from society was a common reaction to severe pain, and they often had a more idealized picture of how a person *should* react to pain, and what the appropriate response should be. As one patient put it, 'I react like a good American'. In hospital, they tended to avoid being a 'nuisance' and to cooperate closely with the ward staff, who also often had 'Old American' attitudes. These same staff might thus misinterpret the more emotional languages of distress of patients from other groups, leading them to conclude, quite wrongly, that these patients had a lower threshold of pain, were more neurotic or were more hypochondriacal.

As a result of social change and cultural assimilation, many of Zborowski's findings are no longer applicable to the groups that he described. However, his study did highlight how different cultural groups understand the meaning and significance of their pain, both for their present social and economic situation, and for the future, and how different groups, with similarly emotional languages of distress, may view the significance of the pain very differently. Thus, from the data collected in his study, he concluded that:

1 'Similar reactions to pain manifested by members of different ethnocultural groups do not necessarily reflect similar attitudes to pain'.

2 'Reactive patterns similar in terms of their manifestations may have different functions and serve different purposes in various cultures'.

Pain in childbirth

Expectations of pain in childbirth, and how it is displayed and understood, also vary widely. As described in Chapter 6, in some cultural groups the pain of childbirth may be welcomed by women, instead of feared. For example, Van Hollen[19] describes how in Tamil Nadu, South India, many of the women giving birth in government hospitals insisted on having their labour induced by the use of drugs such as oxytocin, though this greatly increased the level of their pain. This was because the pain of childbirth was said to increase the woman's level of *sakti*, the spiritual regenerative power of females and the 'active principle of life': the greater the pain endured, the greater the level of *sakti* that the woman could attain. This approach is very different from that of many women in Western countries, who have a less positive attitude towards labour pains, and who welcome analgesic drugs or anesthetics during childbirth.

Pain in religion and healing

In some cultural and religious groups, individual sufferers are encouraged to turn their private pain into public pain within a ritual context of healing. This is seen in some of the public rites of healing in Africa and Latin America, described in Chapter 4, but is also true of some religious groups in the West where, in a ritual setting, pain becomes a means of personal and spiritual transformation. Skultans,[20] for example, describes how women in a Welsh Spiritualist church are encouraged to share their painful symptoms with one another, and to each become 'possessed' by the pain of an ill member, thus helping to lessen her private pain by sharing it among themselves. Similarly, Csordas[21] describes how a healer in the Catholic Charismatic Renewal movement in the USA often 'embodies' the pain of a sufferer, as part of the ritual of diagnosis and healing. For example, an intense pain in the healer's heart means a 'heart healing' is taking place in the patient, while the healer may detect headache or backache in a supplicant 'through the experience of a similar pain during the healing process'. McGuire[22], in her study of ritual healing in suburban USA, describes how some Episcopalian communities see pain as a *positive* phenomenon, a type of lesson by which they can learn more about life and come closer to God. 'You ask the Lord what you're supposed to learn from this', one woman said, while another commented: 'Pain and illness aren't the end. You wouldn't know goodness and joy, if you hadn't experienced pain'. Members of some Eastern meditation groups also see pain as a potentially useful lesson or message to the individual. As one yoga adherent explained: 'Pain is your body's way of saying, "Hey, something's wrong, do something about it, don't block it out". It can be a way of turning your life around'. On a more individual level, the psychoanalyst McDougall[23] has described several cases of severe psychosomatic disorders where the experience of pain or other discomfort can play an important psychological role in reassuring certain patients, reminding them of their personal identity, the borders of their body, or even of their own existence. As she puts it: 'A body that suffers is also a body that is alive.'

Causing oneself intense pain – especially in the form of self-flagellation or 'mortifying the flesh'– has a long history in many religious groups. It has been used as a way of commemorating a particular event in the history of that religion, or of atoning for sins, placating the deity, attaining transcendence, or expressing the triumph of spirit over matter, soul over body. It was practiced during the Middle Ages by several Christian monastic orders as well as by some religious movements (known as 'flagellants'), and some Christian communities still do so today. In parts of the Philippines during Holy Week, some groups practice self-flagellation as a ritual re-enactment of the scourging of Jesus Christ, and sometimes on Good Friday the rituals of *penitencia* are accompanied by individuals hav-

ing themselves nailed to crosses to commemorate Christ's own crucifixion, even though this practice is disapproved of by the Catholic Church. In the Middle East and elsewhere, adherents of the Shi'ite branch of Islam also practice self-flagellation on certain religious occasions, flaying their upper backs with chains, often with small knives attached, especially in the public processions that take place on the 10th day of the month of *Moharram*, in commemoration of the martyrdom of Iman Husain at the Battle of Karbala in 680 AD. While in the annual *Kataragama Esala* festival in south-eastern Sri Lanka, some Hindu and Buddhist worshippers practice fire-walking over red-hot embers, or suspend their bodies from ropes attached to their skin by hooks, as part of expiatory rituals of penance, or of fulfilling a promise made to the god Si Skanda.

Pain in rites of passage

Hsu[24] points out that in many societies, the public infliction of acute pain is part of many of their *rites de passage* (see Chapter 9) – the rituals in which individuals acquire a new social identity – such as the circumcision of children or young people, or the painful initiation rituals of becoming a warrior. It is also part of many traditional forms of healing, such as cupping, cauterization, and acupuncture. She suggests that inflicting acute pain publicly in any of these situations can have a *social* function: making other people instantly aware of that person, and their suffering, and creating an emotional connection between them. Acute pain can break down the barriers between people, since it 'not only has a biological survival function for the individual, but... it also has an eminently social potential for enhancing a sense of togetherness between individuals and for making real social relatedness. In other words, the sensory experience of acute pain is essential for community building.' She suggests, too, that in traditional Chinese acupuncture, where inflicting acute pain by 'needling' is central to the therapeutic process, these pains also have another function: causing 'a bodily felt immediate social connectedness between patient and healer.

which, in unspecific ways, might be therapeutic'. This is very different to the approach of modern 'medicalized' society, where every effort is made to minimize pain at any cost, whether in medical treatment, surgery, childbirth or illness. But while visible displays of acute pain are increasingly uncommon in modern life, the more 'silent' chronic pain syndromes are continuing to increase (see below).

Thus as these examples indicate, pain, especially acute pain, is not always seen as an unwanted physiological experience. For some people it can also be a pathway to religious experience, a means of absolution, a way to a greater level of self-knowledge, a form of treatment or healing, or the means to a new social identity.

The politics of pain

The conscious infliction of physical pain on another person – in the form of *torture* – has been a feature of many political systems, religious organizations and repressive regimes throughout history. Historically, it has been used in times of war, as well as in times of peace. Today, despite various international agreements outlawing it, such as the United Nations *Convention against Torture* of 1985, it is still practiced by states in many parts of the world: sometimes openly, sometimes clandestinely. Physical torture is often accompanied by various forms of psychological abuse, such as social isolation or sexual humiliation, as well as by other forms of suffering. In repressive societies, torture is most commonly used on those accused of various crimes, as well as on prisoners of war, religious heretics, and political dissidents, in order to punish them, extract information, or both. However, as Scarry[25] points out, in these societies torture also plays an important *political* role, for it is also about making the experience of pain 'visible', of producing a 'wholly convincing spectacle of power' for the victim, the torturer, and the society at large. By causing 'private pain' to become 'public pain' as a result of torture, it demonstrates to all concerned the absolute power of the

state over its enemies, and over those who would challenge it or break its rules.

CHRONIC PAIN

One particular type of pain, chronic pain, poses unique problems for the sufferers and for those around them. As Brodwin[26] points out, chronic pain is truly a 'private disorder'. Unlike acute pain, which begins suddenly and lasts a short time only, the 'visibility' of chronic pain to other people tends to disappear over time, despite the individual's continued suffering. 'Even when it begins with a traumatic accident or major illness, it continues long after these events have faded from people's memory'. Often, few visual clues, such as a bruise, bandage, scar, or plaster cast, remain to remind family or friends of the pain and how it originally began. In short, chronic pain is often invisible. Brodwin[26] describes how in this situation chronic pain sufferers may evolve ways of displaying their private pain in a public performance to those around them, in order to get help and attention. Within families, particularly, their recurrent 'rhetoric of pain' may become an integral part of the family dynamics. It can also apply in relations with their employers and co-workers, since 'this rhetoric helps chronic pain sufferers communicate their wants and needs in crucial social relationships, especially when the use of other languages is not sanctioned'. However, as Hsu[24] notes, chronic pain, unlike acute pain whose effect is immediate, and visible to those around the sufferer, often 'alienates the person from the environment', rather than increasing their connection to other people. It does not necessarily reinforce social cohesion between individuals – sometimes just the reverse. Whatever its profound effect on the victim, it 'is unreal for the other, while it is so terribly present and all-encompassing for the sufferer, and this impossibility of the other to empathize with the sufferer enlarges the latter's pain experience'.

Chronic pain is often intimately linked with social and psychological problems. Interpersonal tensions, for example, may cause someone to develop chronic pain, and vice versa. In many families and cultural groups, a 'performance' of pain may be the only way of signalling personal distress, whatever its cause. This is an example of somatization and may take many forms, from 'pain everywhere' to recurrent pain in a particular organ or body part. As Kleinman and colleagues[27] put it, 'Depression and anxiety, serious family tensions, conflicted work relationships – all conduce to the onset of or exacerbation of chronic pain conditions and, in turn, may be worsened by chronic pain'. Thus, as described in Chapter 10, pain is one of the commonest manifestations of depression cross-culturally, and is often linked to a variety of other somatic symptoms.

In the decades to come, an increased life-expectancy in many parts of the world is likely to result in an increased prevalence of chronic diseases. Many of these, such as arthritis, and other degenerative conditions, will be characterized by a great deal of chronic pain, and dealing with this holistically will provide a new challenge for health professionals.

SUMMARY

In summary, in assessing the role of culture in pain behaviour, it is important to avoid using ethnic, social or religious stereotypes in understanding how, and why, different individuals respond to pain. While health professionals should be aware of cultural influences when evaluating people in pain, each case should always be assessed individually, avoiding generalizations or the use of stereotypes in predicting how a particular person from a particular background will respond to being in pain. Thus Kleinman and colleagues[27] emphasize the need to understand and to empathize with 'the peculiar qualities of the sting and throb of pain affecting a particular person – with a unique story, living in a certain community and historical period, and above all with fears, longings, aspirations'.

KEY REFERENCES

3 Engel, G. (1950). 'Psychogenic' pain and the pain-prone patient. *Am. J. Med.* 26, 899–909.

4 Fabrega, H. and Tyma, S. (1976). Language and cultural influences in the description of pain. *Br. Med. J. Psychol.* 49, 349–71.

7 Zola, I.K. (1966). Culture and symptoms: an analysis of patients' presenting complaints. *Am. Sociol. Rev.* 31, 615–30.

19 van Hollen, C. (2003) Invoking *vali*: Painful technologies of modern birth in South India. *Med. Anthropol. Q.* 17(1), 49–77.

23 McDougall, J. (1989). *Theatres of the Body*. London: Free Association Press, pp. 140–161.

See http://www.culturehealthandillness.com for the full list of references for this chapter.

RECOMMENDED READING

Good, M.D., Brodwin, P.E., Good, B.J. and Kleinman, A. (eds) (1992). *Pain and Human Experience: an Anthropological Perspective*. Berkeley: University of California Press.

Morris, D.B. (1993) *The Culture of Pain*. Berkeley: University of California Press.

Pugh, J.F. (1991). The semantics of pain in Indian culture and medicine. *Cult. Med. Psychiatry*, 15, 19–43.

Scarry, E. (1985) *The Body in Pain*. Oxford: Oxford University Press.

Wolff, B. B. and Langley, S. (1977). Cultural factors and the responses to pain. In: *Culture, Disease, and Healing: Studies in Medical Anthropology* (Landy, D. ed.). London: Macmillan, pp. 313–19.

8

Culture and pharmacology: drugs, alcohol and tobacco

In many cases, the effect of a medication or other chemical substance on human physiology and emotional state does not depend solely on its pharmacological properties. A number of *other* factors, such as personality, social or cultural backgrounds, can either enhance or reduce this effect, and are responsible for the wide variability in people's response to medication. This chapter examines some of these *non*-pharmacological influences, in relation to placebos, psychotropic and narcotic drugs, alcohol and tobacco.

THE 'TOTAL DRUG EFFECT'

Claridge[1] has pointed out that the effect of any medication on an individual (its 'total drug effect') depends on a number of factors *in addition* to its pharmacological properties. These are:

1 The attributes of the *drug* itself (such as taste, shape, colour, name).
2 The attributes of the *recipient* of the drug (such as their age, experience, education, personality, socio-cultural background).
3 The attributes of the *prescriber* or supplier of the drug (such as their personality, age, attitude, professional status, or sense of authority).
4 The physical *setting* in which the drug is prescribed or administered – the 'drug situation' (such as doctor's office, a hospital ward, a laboratory, or a social occasion).

To extend this model a step further, the physical setting of drug can be termed the *micro-context*, which can be differentiated from what can be called the *macro-context*. This is the whole social, cultural, political and economic milieu in which use of the drug takes place, and includes:

- the moral and cultural values attached to it, which either encourage or forbid its use
- the prevailing socio-economic climate, such as levels of poverty or unemployment
- the role of economic forces in producing, advertising and selling the drug
- the social grouping in which drug use actually takes place – such as a family, group of friends, members of a healing cult, or even a sub-culture of heroin addicts.

In each case of drug use (and irrespective of what the drug is), the cultural values and economic realities of the macro-context will always, to some extent, impinge on the micro-context. For example, they may help validate a particular type or appearance of drug, a particular way of using it, or the attributes of the individual who actually supplies it (such as a doctor or nurse).

Thus Claridge's model, which originally dealt mainly with medically prescribed drugs or placebos, can be extended to include all forms of drug use. It can be applied equally to the analysis of the placebo and nocebo effects, and to the use of psychotropic drugs or hard drugs, recreational drugs such as alcohol and tobacco, and the hallucinogenic drugs used by certain religious and cultural groups. Based partly on Claridge's model, Figure 8.1 summarizes all the *non*-pharmacological influences on the use of any particular drug, whether medically prescribed or not.

Because the 'total drug effect' is thus dependent on the mix of these many influences in any particular case, there can be wide variation in how different people respond to the same drug or medication. In the case of very powerful drugs, though, such as certain poisons, the effect is entirely due to its pharmacological actions.

THE PLACEBO EFFECT

The placebo effect can be understood as the 'total drug effect', but *without* the presence of a drug. Much research has been carried out in recent years into this phenomenon. This research, carried out mainly in medical settings, has also shed light on other phenomena such as drug addiction and habituation, alcoholism and the therapeutic effects of healing rituals in many cultures. In the medical literature, placebos are often viewed merely as pharmacologically inert substances administered

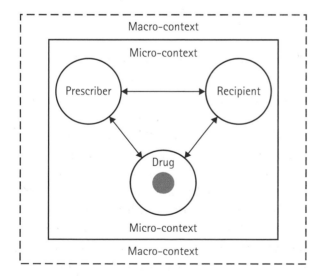

= Pharmacological effect of the drug

Figure 8.1 The 'total drug effect'.

as part of a double-blind trial of a new drug. Other writers have pointed out that the placebo effect is much wider than this. Wolf,[2] for example, defines it as 'any effect attributable to a pill, potion or procedure, but not its pharmacodynamic or specific properties'. For Shapiro[3] it is 'the psychological, physiological or psychophysiological effect of any medication or procedure given with therapeutic intent, which is independent of or minimally related to the pharmacologic effects of the medication or to the specific effects of the procedure, and which operates through a psychological mechanism'. It is therefore the *belief* of those receiving (and/or administering) a placebo substance or procedure in the *efficacy* of that placebo or procedure that can have both psychological and physiological effects.

In a review of the literature in 1975, Benson and Epstein[4] pointed out that placebos may affect practically any organ system in the body. Placebos had been reported to provide relief in a variety of conditions, including angina pectoris, rheumatoid and degenerative arthritis, pain, hay fever, headache, cough, peptic ulcer and essential hypertension. Their psychological effects included the relief of anxiety, depression and even schizophrenia.

Other studies indicate that, depending on people's expectations, placebos can even cause side-effects (such as drowsiness)[5] – about one-quarter of people taking placebos report such adverse effects[6] – or even psychological dependence on them.[5] Both these phenomena are examples of the *nocebo* effect; that is, the negative effects on health of belief and expectations (see Chapter 11). Hahn[7] points out that 'beliefs can make us sick as well as healthy'. In his comprehensive review of the subject, he cites numerous studies that show that a patient's negative expectations of a particular medical treatment or procedure can seriously affect many aspects of their mental and physical health. Barsky and colleagues',[6] too, point out that these 'non-specific side effects' of medical treatment can increase people's distress, add to the burden of their illness, and raise the costs of their medical care.

While the power of the placebo effect has been widely reported, its exact mechanism is still not clearly understood. Neither do we really understand how belief in a healer, and in their treatment, can in itself be healing. Some attempt, though, has been made to explain one particular phenomenon – placebo analgesia – from a scientific perspective. In a study by Levine and colleagues[8], postoperative dental pain was relieved by placebos, but this effect disappeared when the patients were given naloxone. It was hypothesized that placebo analgesia was mediated by endogenous opiates, or endorphins, whose effect was counteracted by the naloxone. Other physiological effects of placebos are still being investigated.

For the placebo effect to occur, a certain atmosphere or setting is required. Placebos, whether medications or procedures, are generally *culture-bound*, or rather *context-bound*; that is, they are administered within a specific social and cultural context that validates both the placebo and the person administering it. Placebos that work in one cultural group or context may not, therefore, have any effect in another.

According to Adler and Hammett,[9] the placebo effect is an essential component in *all* forms of healing and, from a wider perspective, it is an important component of everyday life. They see all forms of therapy, cross-culturally, as having two characteristics:

1 Participation by all those taking part (patient, healer, spectators) in a shared cognitive system.
2 Access to a relationship with a culturally sanctioned parental figure (the healer).

The shared cognitive system refers to the cultural world-view of the group – how they perceive, interpret and understand reality, especially the occurrence of ill health and other misfortunes.

In some societies this world-view is rationalistic, in others it is more religious or mystical. In either case, the perspective on ill health is part of their wider view of how the world operates or how things 'hang together'. This world-view 'enables man to locate himself spatially and historically', and 'provides a conceptual–perceptual structure beyond the limits of which few men transgress even in imagination'. This cognitive system, shared with other members of one's culture or society, makes the chaos of life (and of ill health) understandable, and gives a sense of security and *meaning* to people's lives.

The other component of the placebo effect is the emotional dependence of members of society on prominent people, especially their *healers*. Whatever their form, sacred or secular, these healers occupy a social niche of respect, reverence and influence comparable with the parental role. The therapeutic potency of this relationship probably results from 'a reactivation of the feelings of basic trust adherent to the original mother–infant dyad'. In Adler and Hammett's view,[9] both these aspects 'are the necessary and sufficient components of the placebo effect'; what people take from a placebo may be what they need from life – a sense of meaning and security derived from membership of a group with a shared world-view, and a relationship with a caring, parental-type authority figure. Both these aspects are also part of Western healing rituals, such as the doctor–patient consultation, and of most forms of symbolic healing (see Chapter 10).

All medications prescribed in this specialized setting are likely to have some placebo effect. In Joyce's[10] view, there is a placebo or symbolic element in *all* drugs prescribed by doctors, whether they are pharmacologically active or not. In 1969 he estimated that nearly one in five of all prescriptions written by general practitioners in the UK were for their placebo or symbolic functions, and that there were at least 500 000 people in the UK who each year were 'symbol-dependent' patients. In his view, any drug given for more than 2 years has a large symbolic component for the individual taking it. Any drug prescribed by a doctor can be seen as a 'multi-vocal' symbol, having a range of meanings for the individual patient. Some of these are discussed below, in the section on drug dependence.

THE DRUG

The placebo effect of the drug itself has been studied by several researchers. For example, Schapira and colleagues[11] studied the effect of the *colour* of drugs used for treating anxiety in 48 patients at a psychiatric outpatient department. It was found that anxiety symptoms and phobic symptoms seemed to respond best to green tablets, while depressive symptoms responded best to yellow. The yellow tablets were least preferred by patients for alleviating their anxiety. The authors conclude that one 'cannot ignore any ancillary factor which might enhance the response of patients to drug treatment'. In 1996 a review by de Craen and colleagues[12] of 12 published studies of the perceived influence of a drug's colour on its effectiveness, also found that green or blue tablets had a more sedative effect, and that red, orange or yellow tablets were best for stimulant drugs. One of the studies they quoted found that capsules seemed more effective in treating anxiety than tablets, though the reasons for this were not clear. Another study, by Branthwaite and Cooper,[13] focused on the influence of the tablet's *brand name*. They found that self-prescribed analgesic tablets used for headaches varied in their effectiveness, depending on whether the analgesic was labelled as a well-known, widely marketed proprietary analgesic. Patients found these branded or labelled analgesics much more effective in relieving headaches than unbranded forms of the same drug. The brand name can be seen as having a symbolic aspect for those that take it, and to stand for a drug with a general reputation for efficiency over many years. Yet another example of the potency of branded drugs in the eyes of their users was shown by Jefferys and colleagues[14] in their 1960 study of self-medication on an English working-class housing estate. Aspirins were found to be widely used for a range of complaints, including insomnia, anxiety and 'nerves'. In the author's study[15] in 1981 of a group of long-term users of psychotropic drugs in London, 36 per cent said they would take a proprietary analgesic (such as Aspro, Panadol or Veganin) for the relief of insomnia or anxiety if their psychotropic was withdrawn or unobtainable. Colour and name are not the only attributes of a drug that may influence its effect: size, taste, texture, shape and overall appearance should also be considered. This applies as much to coffee, tea, alcohol, cigarettes and 'hard drugs' as to conventional medications.

THE RECIPIENT

The attributes of the *patient* receiving the drug can also influence the placebo response. Among these are, as Claridge[16] states, the patient's 'attitude towards and knowledge of drugs, [and] what he has been told about the particular drug he is taking'. Also relevant is whether he is part of the same shared cognitive system as the prescriber, and certain traits of his personality. Various attempts have been made to define a 'placebo type' of personality that is more likely to show this response. Among the attributes mentioned are over-anxiety, emotional dependency, immaturity, poor personal relationships and low self-esteem. As Adler and Hammett[9] have noted above, the placebo may supply some of what is lacking in their lives; a sense of meaning, security, belonging and a caring relationship with a 'parental' prescriber. One should note, however, that all ill people display some of these characteristics to a lesser or greater extent, especially in the presence of severe illness. This sense of anxiety, vulnerability and dependence may enhance the placebo effect in a ritual of healing.

THE PRESCRIBER AND THE CONTEXT

The characteristics of the *prescriber* or healer are crucial to the placebo effect, especially if their healing role is validated by their society. This validation is likely to be displayed by the use of certain ritual symbols, such as a white coat, stethoscope or prescription pad. By manipulating these potent symbols in a healing *context*, the prescriber is both expressing and reaffirming certain basic values of the society, and enhancing a feeling of security and continuity on which the placebo effect depends (see Chapter 9). Their age, appearance, clothing, manner and air of authority are also relevant here, as are their own beliefs and expectations of the drug or procedure. As Claridge points out, the authority of the prescriber can also be used to manipulate *how* people respond to a particular drug: 'Deliberately manipulating the individual subject's motives or expectations is one way... in which drug effects can be enhanced, diminished or reversed'.[17]

Rapport, mutual confidence and understanding between prescriber and patient also contribute to the placebo effect. For this effect to be maximized there must be congruence between the doctor's approach to therapy and the patient's attitudes towards illness and expectations from treatment. This atmosphere of prescribing is complemented by the social environment (the 'micro-context') in which ingestion of the medication actually takes place. The patient's perception of other people's behaviour with whom they are interacting may affect their response to the drug. This type of response is more clearly seen in the public healing rituals of some small-scale non-Western societies, where the patient is surrounded by a crowd of friends and relatives who share expectations of the treatment's efficacy. However, even in a Western setting the experience and expectation of a patient's family and friends of a particular drug (or doctor or treatment) may influence the degree of the placebo response.

The placebo effect is also intrinsic to the effect of recreational drugs, such as tobacco, alcohol or hard drugs. In these settings, the attributes of the 'prescriber' – whether waiter, barmaid or drug dealer – are likely also to contribute some influence to the total drug effect, as is the atmosphere in which ingestion takes place, whether it is a restaurant, café, bar, pub or addicts' 'shooting gallery'.

SUMMARY

The placebo effect may be seen with either pharmacologically inactive *or* active preparations,

though its effects have been more vividly described with the former. It is also a feature of double-blind trials of new drugs, where about one-third of the sample usually respond to a placebo. It is fashionable for some doctors, trained to look only for physiological data and to explain the reasons for every physical change, to dismiss this phenomenon as only 'the placebo effect' (and therefore not *real* medicine). This is in marked contrast to most folk healers in non-industrialized countries (and to many alternative and complementary healers in the West), who see the placebo effect as an ally, not an enemy, in any successful treatment. Instead of focusing only on pathology, and seeing the patient only as a passive recipient of treatment, they strive to work within the patient's belief system, and to create a therapeutic alliance with them as an active agent in the treatment of their own condition. Kienle and Kienle[18] suggest, therefore, that the placebo effect may be due mainly to the patient's *own self-healing powers*, which have somehow been influenced (and stimulated) by a variety of non-specific factors, such as the 'situational context' and the 'internal attitude' of physician or healer. This may apply also to process of 'symbolic healing', described in Chapter 10.

Whatever the exact mechanism of the placebo effect, it should always be noted that the therapeutic effects of belief, expectations, and a good healer–patient relationship have been used by healers in every human culture, in all parts of the world, and throughout all of human history.

The placebo effect depends on the beliefs and expectations of physicians, as well as those of patients. This was illustrated in the following case study.

Case study: placebo effect in angina pectoris

Benson and McCallie[19] in 1979 reviewed the effectiveness of various types of therapy for angina pectoris. Many of these had been tried, only to be abandoned later on. They included heart muscle extract, various hormones, X-irradiation, anticoagulants, monoamine oxidase inhibitors, thyroidectomies, radioactive iodine, sympathectomies and many other treatments. When each of these had been introduced, their proponents (or 'enthusiasts') had reported remarkable successes in their initial trials of treatment. Most of these non-blind or single-blind trials failed to control the strong placebo effect evoked by the investigators' expectations of success. Later, when more controlled trials were done by 'sceptics' (more sceptical investigators who operate under circumstances that minimize the placebo effect), the therapy was found to be no better than inert, control placebos. Quantitatively, there was a consistent pattern of a 70–90 per cent success reported initially by the enthusiasts, which was reduced in the sceptics trial to 30–40 per cent baseline placebo effectiveness. This 30 per cent, as already mentioned, is the usual proportion of placebo types in a group, or the degree of placebo effect from any drug or procedure.

Benson and McCallie analysed the results of five erstwhile treatments for angina pectoris, all of which 'are now believed to have no specific physiologic efficacy, yet at one time all were found to be effective and were used extensively'. These were the xanthines, khellin, vitamin E, ligation of the internal mammary artery, and implantation of this artery. Vitamin E, for example, was introduced as a therapy for angina in 1946. Initial enthusiastic reports noted that 90 per cent of 84 patients benefited from several months' treatment with it. Over the years, several more trials were carried out which found a gradually reduced level of effectiveness. By the 1970s, controlled trials were showing it to be no better than placebo pills. That is, 'the discrepancy between the results of advocates and sceptics may be attributed, in part, to the greater degree of placebo effect evoked by the enthusiasts'. More than 80 per cent of patients initially reported subjective improvement in symptoms, from any of these five treatments. There were also objective improvements, such as increased exercise tolerance, reduced nitroglycerin usage and improved electrocardiograph results. In some cases these lasted up to 1 year.

The authors pointed out that 'the placebo effect will most likely persist as long as the psychologic context in which it was evoked remains unchanged. Patient and physician belief in the efficacy of the therapy and a continuously strong physician–patient relation should maintain the effects for long periods'. This can even occur in the presence of angiographically verified coronary artery disease. They also point out that the history of angina treatments demonstrates that the advent of a 'new' procedure may impair the effectiveness of an old one, and that the expectation of better results transfers the placebo effect to the new procedure. In conclusion, they quote Trousseau's remark that: 'You should treat as many patients as possible with the new drugs while they still have the power to heal'.

DRUG DEPENDENCE AND ADDICTION

DRUG DEPENDENCE

Psychological dependence on drugs has been defined by Lader[20] as: 'The need the patient experiences for the psychological effects of a drug. This need can be of two types. The patient may crave the drug-induced symptoms or changes in mood – a feeling of euphoria or a lessening of tension, for example. Or the patient may take the drug to stave off the symptoms of withdrawal'.

Both personality and socio-cultural factors are as important as the pharmacology of the drug used in both psychological dependence and physical addiction. In some cases the pharmacology can be irrelevant, as in psychological dependence on a placebo, or on a drug taken for years that no longer has a significant physical effect. In understanding these phenomena, the social and cultural contexts in which drugs are prescribed, administered or taken – all of which contribute to the total drug effect – need to be taken into account.

Some of these factors have been examined in the case of psychotropic drugs such as tranquillizers and sleeping tablets, especially the benzodiazepines. From the early 1960s onwards, these drugs formed the single largest group of drugs prescribed each year in the Western world. In the UK from 1965 to 1970, prescriptions for benzodiazepine tranquillizers increased by 59 per cent, and for non-barbiturate hypnotics by 145 per cent.[21] In 1972, 45.3 million prescriptions for psychotropics were issued by National Health Service (NHS) general practitioners in England alone (17.7 per cent of the total number of prescriptions).[22] In the USA in the 1970s, benzodiazepine psychotropics were the most commonly prescribed drugs,[23] and in 1973 it was estimated that prescriptions for one of these, diazepam (Valium), was increasing at a rate of 7 million annually.[24] In recent years, though, the numbers of these drugs prescribed has begun to decrease, prescriptions for the newer types of psychotropic drugs, such as antidepressants like Prozac (fluoxetine), have greatly increased. Ever since 1987, when it was first launched, the popularity of Prozac has risen throughout the industrialized world. By 1990 it was the drug most commonly prescribed by psychiatrists in the USA, and by 1994 it was the second most commonly prescribed drug in the world after Zantac (ranitidine).[25]

Many psychotropic drugs are given by regular repeat prescriptions or 'refills', and are taken for many years. In Parish's[26] study in Birmingham in 1971, 14.9 per cent of the patient sample had taken psychotropics (benzodiazepines) regularly for 1 year or more, and 4.9 per cent for 5 years or more. Yet in 1981 Williams,[27] of the Institute of Psychiatry in London, quoted studies showing that most hypnotics lost their 'sleep-promoting properties' within 3–14 days of continuous use by the patient, and that there was little convincing evidence that benzodiazepines were effective in the treatment of anxiety after 4 months' continuous treatment. It would therefore seem that many people are taking psychotropics for reasons other than their pharmacological effect. The symbolic *meaning* of the drug for the individual taking it, is an

important component of the phenomenon of psychological dependence.

Both the psychotropic drug and the prescription for it can be viewed as 'multi-vocal' ritual symbols (see Chapter 9), the power of which is conferred in the ritual of prescribing, and which signify many different things for the patient and for those around them. Ostensibly the drug is meant to have a particular physical effect (its 'manifest function'), but it may have other dimensions of meaning ('latent functions') for those ingesting it. It may symbolize (for example): that the person is ill; that all personal failures are caused by this illness (or by the drug's side-effects); that they deserve sympathy and attention from family and friends; that the doctor – a powerful, respected, healing figure – is still interested in them; and that modern science (which produced the drug) is powerful, reliable and efficient. Smith,[28] in reviewing the literature on this subject, lists 27 of these latent functions, as well as seven more manifest ones. Perhaps most importantly, the drug carries with it some of the healing attributes of the doctor who prescribed it.

Social values and expectations

Psychotropic drug use is embedded in a matrix of *social* values and expectations – a crucial part of the 'macro-context'. In this setting, the drug can be used to improve social relationships by bringing one's behaviour (and emotions) into conformity with an idealized model of 'normal' behaviour. In the author's study[15] of 50 long-term users of psychotropics in 1981, for example, the drugs were often taken for their believed effect on relationships with others. With the drug, the patient was 'normal', self-controlled, good to live with, nurturing, non-complaining, sociable and assertive. Without it the opposite would occur, with damaging effects on their relationships. Without the drug, 'I'd be nervy, impatient with other people', 'I'd be nasty, jumpy, not nice to live with', 'I wouldn't want to see people', 'I couldn't help those I love'.

At a study at the Addiction Research Foundation in Toronto carried out by

Cooperstock and Lennard[29] in 1979, the findings were similar. Tranquillizers were taken as an 'aid in the maintenance of a nurturing, caring role', especially by women in role conflicts between work and home. Men saw tranquillizers particularly 'as a means of controlling somatic symptoms in order to perform their occupational role'. In both these studies, psychotropic drugs were seen as a means (both pharmacological and symbolic) of meeting social expectations, whether at work or within the family. These expectations include the culture's view of what constitutes 'normal', acceptable behaviour, and how this is to be attained. Several authors have pointed out that in Western industrialized society there is widespread social support for what Pellegrino[30] terms 'chemical coping' – that is, the regular use of medications (including alcohol, tobacco and psychotropics) to improve one's emotional state and social relationships and help one to conform to societal norms. Warburton[31] has called this phenomenon 'the chemical road to success'.

Social acceptance of psychotropic drug-taking as a normal part of life can lessen the stigma of psychological dependence on them. In the author's study[15] in 1981, for example, 72 per cent of the sample knew of another person taking the same drug and 88 per cent were known by others to be taking a psychotropic. Only 18 per cent reported disapproval by others, 10 per cent reported approval and 29 per cent said that those who knew they took the drug did not care either way. In this sample, at least, psychotropic drug ingestion took place openly, and in the absence of any major moral disapproval. This climate of acceptance makes possible 'fashions' in drug taking, and facilitates the exchange of drugs between people. In Warburton's[31] study in Reading, UK, in 1978, 68 per cent of young adults interviewed admitted receiving psychotropics from friends or relatives.

This 'normalization' of drugs, as part of the macro-context of Western culture, is illustrated by lay beliefs about what is, and what is not, 'a drug'. In Jones's[32] study, for example, while 80 per cent of patients interviewed agreed that heroin was 'a drug', only 50 per cent classified morphine, sleeping tablets and tranquillizers as such, while only one-third saw aspirin as a drug. While 84 per cent of patients in the author's study[15] saw psychotropics as 'drugs', they were at pains to point out that they were *not* powerful or 'hard' drugs – that is, they were not something they had little control over, and which interfered with consciousness: 'It's just a calmer, a help. I can cut it off when I want to', and 'It's soft, sweet. It's different. It's softer' (than other drugs).

The social values that support this normalization may partly be *learned* from doctors, who in turn may be influenced by colleagues, and by the extensive advertising of the pharmaceutical industry, in newspapers, magazines and television programmes, as well as on the Internet. Parish[26] has suggested that in prescribing these drugs for personal problems, doctors are communicating a model on how to deal with these problems, not by confronting them but by taking a drug. The issuing of repeat prescriptions or 'refills' can also be interpreted by patients as tacit approval of psychological dependence. People's experiences of taking psychotropics with medical sanction can have cumulative effects. As Joyce pointed out, 'People who have had one favourable outcome from drug treatment will more probably experience such an outcome on subsequent occasions as well', and this can lay the foundations for future dependence. In Tyrer's[33] view, this dependence on psychotropics is more likely if the drug is prescribed in a fixed dosage regimen (where it becomes a fixed point around which the day is organized), and for a long period of time.

THE 'CHEMICAL ROAD TO SUCCESS'

Overall, the widespread acceptance in Western, industrialized society of the 'chemical road to success', and the growing use of 'chemical comforters' (whether legal or illegal), means that in Western society the cultural formula for 'success' has become:

where 'success' can be defined in mental, physical, social, sexual or economic terms. The 'chemical comforters' used range from vitamins, nutriceuticals, tea, coffee, tobacco and tranquillizers through to alcohol, marijuana, cocaine, heroin, lysergic acid diethylamide (LSD), and the newer 'designer drugs' such as Ecstasy. This formula, and the pursuit of the 'success', can increasingly be applied to many different aspects of modern life. These include personal life, relationships, marriage, work activities, leisure pursuits and even sport, where the use of anabolic steroids as 'performance-enhancing drugs' is becoming more common in international competitions.[34] Increasingly, the definition of 'success' now also seems to include the absence of any anxiety, worry, guilt, anger and grief – emotions that were considered to be a normal part of human life in all previous generations.

The role of the pharmaceutical industry

A part of this phenomenon is the growing power of the medical prescription, a key component of the 'medicalization of everyday life' (see Chapters 6, 9 and 10), and which, in turn, is making considerable profits for the pharmaceutical industry (often known as 'pharma'). Thus a report in 2004[35] estimated that over 44 per cent of all Americans were taking at least one prescription drug, and 16.5 per cent take at least three. These rates were up from 39 per cent and 12 per cent since the period 1988–1994. In the USA prescription drugs made up about one-tenth of the total medical bill in 2004, and were the fastest growing item of expenditure, and drug expenditure had risen at least 15 per cent *every year* since 1998. Many of these prescribed drugs are essential for health, of course, but the question remains: how many of them are prescribed unnecessarily, as part of the growing process of 'medicalization'?

This raises another question, with many ethical implications: what role does the pharmaceutical industry itself play in bringing about this process? Elliott,[36] for example, has criticized the industry's role in funding medical research and medical education programmes that present its products in a favourable light. Sometimes this may involve getting academics to put their names to 'ghost-written' articles which give a positive view of a particular drug, and which are then published in scientific journals. It can also involve giving doctors expensive gifts, generous grants, and lavish trips and conferences, as an incentive to prescribe their drugs. As Elliott puts it: 'when research is funded by pharma, it tends to favor pharma', and that 'when doctors take gifts and fees from pharma, they are much more likely to prescribe the drugs produced by the company that has given them the gift'.[36] This process may therefore play a role, even if indirectly, in the growing importance of medications – whether prescribed or non-prescribed – in modern life, and in promoting the 'chemical road to success'.

DRUG ADDICTION

In *physical dependence*, or *addiction*, social and cultural factors can also play an important role. Claridge[37] pointed out that the distinction between psychological and physical dependence may be more theoretical than real: 'Medically recognized addiction is only the pathological end-part of a continuum of drug-taking that involves us all. Even the most upright of citizens have their chemical comforters, most of which are psychologically harmless when taken in small quantities'. These 'chemical comforters' include tea, coffee, tobacco, psychotropic drugs and, of course, alcohol. Cultures differ on what particular comforter is most commonly used, and under what circumstances, and there are usually tacit rules controlling their use. Historically, too, there have been many shifts in the ways that different chemical comforters have been regarded; several of them regarded as dangerous, addictive or immoral in one century have been considered harmless in another. In Europe, for example, chocolate, tea, coffee and snuff have all been regarded with moral horror at one time or another.[38] 'Among the many disorders which the intemperance of mankind has introduced that shorten life, one of the greatest, I believe, is the use of chocolate', wrote G. B. Felici of Florence in 1728.[39] 'The Spanish, and every other nation which goes to the Indies, once they become accustomed to chocolate, its consumption becomes such a vice that they can only with difficulty leave off from drinking it every morning', wrote the explorer Franceso Carletti in 1701.[39] It has been argued that what has freed chocolate, coffee and tea from being defined as addictive substances in modern industrial societies is not that they are completely harmless, but that – unlike 'hard' drugs – they do not stop their users from working.[39]

Addict subcultures

In the case of the 'hard' drugs, such as heroin or morphine, the socio-cultural matrix in which drug taking occurs also has its tacit rules and sanctions. Addicts often form an *outcast subculture*, with their own particular view of the world.[40] These subcultures may play an important part in the spread of certain disease, such as infectious hepatitis. Recently, there has been increased research on the role of needle sharing among intravenous drug users in the spread of acquired immune deficiency syndrome (AIDS). In Edinburgh, UK, for example, it was estimated in 1988 that about 60 per cent of injecting drug users in the city were now human immunodeficiency virus (HIV)-positive,[41] while a study in Spain[42] in 1994 also related the spread of AIDS to the growing numbers of intravenous drug users in the country.

The extent to which individual addicts are integrated into this subculture may determine whether they are able to give up hard drugs or not. If for any reason the subculture is dismantled, then addicts may overcome their physical addiction with unexpected ease. For example, in 1971 Robins and colleagues[43] conducted a follow-up study of drug use by US servicemen returned from Vietnam. They studied 943 men who had returned to the USA from Vietnam, 8–12 months after their return. Four-hundred and ninety-five of these had tested positive in urine tests for opiates at the time

of departure from Vietnam, and three-quarters of these felt that they had been addicted to narcotics while there. In the 8–12 months after their return, one-third had had more experience with opiates, but only 7 per cent of the group showed signs of physical dependence. Almost none of the urine-positive group expressed a desire for treatment or addiction rehabilitation programmes. As Robins and his colleagues pointed out, this result is surprising 'in the light of common belief that dependence on narcotics is easily acquired and virtually impossible to rid oneself of, [yet] most of the men who used narcotics heavily in Vietnam stopped when they left Vietnam and had not begun again 8–12 months later'. Part of the explanation for this is probably that the *milieu* or macro-context in Vietnam – psychologically, socially and economically – was favourable towards the persistence of an addict subculture without, as the authors put it, 'the deterrents of high prices, impure drugs, or the presence of disapproving family'.

Physical addiction, therefore, is *not* just a physical phenomenon; it also requires certain social or cultural factors for its persistence. A further example of this is a case quoted by Jackson,[44] from St Louis, Missouri, USA, in the mid-1960s. Here the lifestyle and activities of heroin addicts remained unexpectedly unchanged when the supply of heroin in the city dried up. It was temporarily replaced by metamphetamine – the pharmacological effect of which is the polar opposite of heroin – but the addicts carried on behaving exactly as before: 'They went to the same shooting galleries to shoot up, scored from the same connections, and bought the magic white powder (metamphetamine instead of heroin) in the same little glassine envelopes they knew so well'. As Jackson concludes, 'The addicts maintained the heroin subculture on a metamphetamine metabolism; obviously the subculture had had powerful and spectacular magic working for it'.

The two following case studies, both from the USA, illustrate the power that addict subcultures can exert over the lives, and world-view, of their members.

Case study: addict subculture in Lexington, Kentucky, USA

The power and nature of an addict subculture was studied in 1974 by Freeland and Rosensteil[45] at the Clinical Research Center in Lexington, Kentucky. They found that self-defined groups, such as narcotic addicts, 'tend to justify their own way of life by stereotyping the behaviour of others in a negative fashion'. The power of culturally based stereotypes to influence a person's life and perceptions depends on how committed the person is to that way of life. In the case of the narcotic addicts, this commitment was intense and all-embracing. Their cultural (or rather subcultural) belief system embodied a strong we–they dichotomy. 'They' were the 'squares', whose lives were seen as being boring, passive, hypocritical, fear-ridden and subordinate. This negative picture contrasted with their own idealized self-image as 'hustlers' – a hustler being 'an active, dominant, capable, self-motivated person who is highly aware of his surroundings and in control of them'. They saw themselves as living 'the fast life'; a hustler first and an addict second. Hustlers were seen as having a specialized type of knowledge about the world that 'maximizes one's abilities as a predator'. In the researchers' view, the maintenance of this we–they dichotomy, and the stereotypes of 'square' and 'hustler', tend to minimize the impact of any therapeutic or rehabilitative programmes directed towards the addicts.

As a strategy to overcome this situation, they organized lengthy discussions on these stereotypes between the addict group and a group of 'squares'. The aim was to reduce the addicts' tendency to stereotype by reducing their ethnocentrism – that is, by providing them with alternative ways of seeing the world, derived from other groups. The 'squares' included medical staff and students, as well as others from churches and schools. Both groups were encouraged to discuss the stereotypes of the others, and to examine how these stereotypes affected their interactions. The addicts were also shown films of other societies, and it was pointed out that stereotyping was a universal human feature, although it could be dangerous and inhibit communication. The outcome of this process was to convince the addict group that they could modify their lifestyle 'without being doomed to a life of subservience, boredom, inactivity, and passivity'. This was a major step in their rehabilitation into everyday life. It was also helpful in enhancing rapport between addict patients and medical staff.

Case study: 'crack' cocaine subculture in Spanish Harlem, New York City, USA

Bourgois[46] in the late 1980s studied the violent street culture of 'crack' cocaine dealers and their clients in Spanish Harlem, New York City. He described the bleak lives of the residents of this poor, inner-city area, many of them Puerto Ricans, and the role played by the underground economy of drug dealing, distribution and consumption within the community. He pointed out that in order to understand the origins of this violent and crime-ridden drug subculture, larger social issues, such as the 'objective, structural desperation of a population without a viable economy, and facing systematic barriers of ethnic discrimination and ideological marginalization' cannot be ignored.

However self-destructive their lives, Bourgois did not see the drug dealers as propelled by an 'irrational cultural logic distinct from that of mainstream USA'. On the contrary, although completely excluded from the mainstream economy and society, many of their values are ultimately derived from it. The participants in the underground crack economy are frantically pursuing their own, distorted version of the American dream. As in conventional society, their ambitions include rapid upward economic mobility, the respect of their peers and the accumulation of flashy consumer objects.

Faced with the prospects of unemployment, low wages and discrimination in the outside world, some of the residents of Spanish Harlem have chosen to become aggressive, self-employed private entrepreneurs – like Papito, who owns a 'string of crack franchises' run by street sellers. People like him are, wrote Bourgois, 'the ultimate rugged individualists braving an unpredictable frontier where fortune, fame and destruction are all just around the corner'. Much of the crack economy is run on conventional business lines, with a recognizable hierarchy of bosses, wholesalers, messengers and street salesmen (who have to meet sales quotas set by their bosses). However, the entire crack economy is based on violence and a culture of terror and, ultimately, on self-destructiveness. Dealers have to be tough and violent enough to intimidate competitors, impress their clients and cement partnerships with other dealers. As a result, homicides, woundings, robberies and high rates of crack addiction are common in the community.

Despite their violent, and ultimately doomed lifestyle, Bourgois emphasized that for these marginalized inner-city young men, employment (or even better, self-employment) in the underground crack economy 'accords a sense of autonomy, self-dignity and an opportunity for extraordinary rapid short-term upward mobility'.

Treatment and prevention of drug addiction

These studies, like the others mentioned above, stress the importance of the *non*-pharmacological variables in producing and maintaining drug addiction, and the complexity of trying to deal with it. In any individual addict, these variables will always include a mix of socio-cultural, economic, geographical and personality factors. For this reason, drug addiction – and the culture of drug production and drug dealing that feeds upon it – is very difficult to change. This is especially so because the 'chemical road to success' has become so imbedded in modern daily life. Solutions to drug addiction cannot, therefore, be based solely on the treatment of individuals. In the long term, wider economic, social and cultural issues must

also be addressed in order to reduce demand for these drugs, as well as their supply.[47]

In the short term, however, a variety of approaches to reducing drug addiction have been tried, some of them making positive use of the cultural milieu in which the addict lives. In several cases, traditional healers or religious figures have been used to help people come off hard drugs and change their lifestyles. These include *curanderos* in Latin America, Buddhist monks in Thailand, acupuncturists in the Far East, and many religious and missionary groups in the Western world. In Malaysia, for example, the traditional Malay folk healer or *bomoh* has been found to be effective in treating some forms of mental illness.[48] However, since the 1970s, many of the 200 000 *bomohs* in the country have also been used to help prevent addiction and to treat and rehabilitate heroin addicts.[49] During their treatment, the addicts live in a controlled environment within the *bomoh's* compound. There they are treated with a mixture of herbal remedies, purificatory baths and religious rituals. *Bomohs* are said to have their own familiar 'spirits' (*hantu raya* or *pelisit*) to help them in their treatments, and some former patients have stated that the reasons for their continued abstinence after treatment was fear of this 'spirit', and the punishment it might bring if they were to relapse. In many cases, *bomoh* therapy has proved to be as effective, or even more effective, than orthodox medical treatments of addiction.[49]

ALCOHOL USE AND ABUSE

Alcohol is probably the most widely used 'chemical comforter' in the world. As well as being taken for its mood-altering properties, it is also used for many other purposes, including as a food, medicine, narcotic, energizer, aphrodisiac, payment, preservative, disinfectant, or sacramental drink. Its use in human communities is as old as agriculture, as a byproduct of the fermentation of fruits, grains and vegetables. Different regions of the world produce different forms of alcohol, depending on climate and local crops and vegetation. Whisky, vodka, gin and beer are all derived primarily from grains, Japanese *sake* is made from fermented rice, rum from sugar-cane, as is the Brazilian drink *cachaça*, and hundreds of types of wine are available from a variety of grape species. In general, Southern Europe can be regarded mostly as a 'grape' region, while Northern Europe is more of a 'grain' region.[50]

In addition to these better-known alcoholic drinks, many different local and traditional beverages are found worldwide, many of them home-brewed, and sometimes illegal. Some of them can have a relatively high alcohol content per volume. They include drinks such as *pito* in Ghana (2–3 per cent), *tonto* in Uganda (6–11 per cent), *talla* (2–4 per cent) and *dagim-araki* (46 per cent) in Ethiopia, *bouza* in Egypt (3.8–4.2 per cent), *arrack* in India (25–45 per cent), *ogogoro* or *kinkana* in Nigeria (40 per cent or more), *cachaça* or sugar cane spirit in Brazil (40 per cent or more) and *kachasu* in Zimbabwe (10–70 per cent).[51] Other home-brewed beverages, such as *pontikka* in Finland, can have even higher levels of alcohol content.

The excessive use of alcohol is a feature of many groups and individuals world-wide, especially those of lower social status and income. Alcohol abuse, and its many social, economic and psychological effects, is now one of the most serious public health problems world-wide, responsible for an estimated 1.8 million deaths each year.[52]

Various studies of the problem have indicated that the incidence of alcoholism, and the regular consumption of alcohol on ritual and other occasions, differs markedly between cultural and social groups, even within the same society. In the USA, in various studies from the 1960s to the 1980s, Italian-Americans and Jewish-Americans were found to have low rates of alcoholism, while Irish-Americans[53] and some Native Americans[54] had very high rates. In the UK, alcohol consumption in the 1990s was relatively low among some immigrant and ethnic minority groups (Afro-Caribbeans, Indians, Pakistanis and Bangladeshis) but was rising in some sections of the Sikh community.[55] Among the many reasons for these differences must be the ways that alcohol intake is embedded in the matrix of *cultural* values and expectations of different groups.

A number of anthropological and other social science theories, some of which are outlined below, have been advanced in order to explain how and why some cultural and social groups drink more than others. Although they are useful, their predictive value at the individual level is limited. They can never fully explain why one particular person from a particular group has an alcohol problem, while another from the same group does not. In each case, the reasons for alcohol use and abuse are always a complex mix of influences, not all of which can be explained by the social sciences.

At the level of the individual drinker, the effect of alcohol depends, as with all 'total drug effects', on a number of factors: physical, psychological and socio-economic. The physical factors include the body build of the drinker, the presence or absence of liver damage, whether drinking took place on an empty stomach or not and, possibly, an inherited intolerance of alcohol. They also include the pharmacological properties of the drink itself, especially its volume, type and concentration. These physical and pharmacological factors are not enough, however, to explain how and why people drink, and how it affects their behaviour. One should also consider the *socio-cultural* characteristics of drinkers, their family and friends, and the setting in which drinking takes place. In particular, the attitudes of their cultural group towards two different types of drinking – 'normal' and 'abnormal' – should be examined. Furthermore, the *economic* status of the drinker is an important factor, since the stress of poverty is often associated with alcohol abuse. Finally, the *psychological* influences on an individual drinker need always to be considered, including the drinker's personality, early experiences and current emotional state (especially depression).

MODELS OF ALCOHOLISM

Given the many factors that can influence the rates of alcoholism, it is not surprising that many different theoretical models have been put forward to understand this type of human behaviour, and how to deal with it. Each represents a different conceptual framework, and a different way of making sense of socially deviant behaviour. Each focuses on a different aspect of the 'Total Drug Effect'. Faced with this plethora of models, Miller and Hester[56] suggest that one needs to have an 'informed eclecticism', and to use aspects of *all* these various models, wherever they are useful, in order to truly understand alcohol abuse, and how to deal with it. Historically, the most influential of these models have been:

1 Moral Models
2 Disease models
3 Political and economic models
4 Socio-cultural models.

Moral models

Moral models – often with a religious basis – emphasize alcoholism as the consequences of personal choice, and usually define most drinking behaviour (especially excessive drinking) as 'wrong', 'bad' or 'immoral' and a sign of sinfulness, weak character, poor self-control, or social irresponsibility. Responses to this should therefore involve punishment, rather than treatment.[50] From the early nineteenth century, beginning with the American Temperance Society in 1826,[56,57] a number of other 'Temperance Movements' were founded in the USA, UK and Ireland, whose members 'took the pledge' to be 'teetotal' and never to drink alcohol. In the USA this movement was particularly strong among the dissenting Protestant churches: the Quakers, Congregationalists, Presbyterians, Baptists and Methodists.[57] Later that century, Temperance movements focused not only on moral disapproval of drinking, but also saw alcohol itself as a dangerous drug – a chemical that could seriously injure health and well-being.

Alcoholism could therefore only be prevented by avoiding this chemical: by temperance, abstinence, and eventually by social legislation to control its availability ('prohibition'). Moral models against alcohol use are still common in many parts of the world, especially in the Middle East, as described below.

Disease models

These models see alcoholism as a type of 'disease – whether physical, psychological or both – that requires treatment, but is not necessarily curable'. Their focus is mainly (though not exclusively) on the individual as the site of diagnosis and treatment rather than on their social, cultural or economic contexts. As alcoholics are in some way 'ill', they required treatment by a health professional, rather than punishment by a law enforcement agency.

Medical models of alcoholism have a long history. In the USA in 1784 Dr Benjamin Rush, a signer of the Declaration of Independence, published his famous tract '*An Enquiry Into the Effects of Ardent Spirits Upon the Human Body and Mind With An Account of Prevention and of the Remedies for Curing Them*', where alcoholism was described as a 'disease of the will'.[38] In Britain in 1804, Thomas Trotter published his *An Essay, Medical, Philosophical, and Chemical, on Drunkenness, and its Effects on the Human Body*, stating that 'In medical language, I consider drunkenness, strictly speaking to be a disease'.[38] This process of 'medicalization' – a shift from a moral to a medical model – still continues today. In 1957 the American Medical Association officially endorsed the concept of alcoholism as a 'disease',[58] and many other medical organizations in other countries have done likewise. From the 1970s onwards, various biological models have been put forward to explain this condition, focusing mainly on genetic and physical processes as a cause of alcohol dependence. They include theories of genetic vulnerability or predisposition to the increased effect of alcohol (the so-called 'alcohol gene' or ALDH2-2 allele),[59] or of some other innate biological inability to metabolize alcohol. Another aspect of the medical model has been an emphasis on pharmacological treatments such as diazepam, naltrexone and disulfiram – often combined with counseling – to help in withdrawal, or to discourage drinking in the future.[60]

Psychological models see alcoholism primarily as a 'mental illness', often in the form of a psychological or 'characteriological' predisposition (the so-called 'alcoholic personality').[61] A number of different psychological models exist, each with its own conceptual approach: whether psychodynamic, behavioural, cognitive, or other. They include: the various *psychodynamic* (Freudian) models, with their focus on unconscious needs, such as the idea of the 'oral personality', fixated at an early stage of emotional development, who is characterized by dependency, lack of self-control, and a search for oral gratification;[61] various *behavioural* models, such as Tension Reduction Theory, whereby individuals learn to drink in order to reduce unpleasant stress symptoms; and *social learning* models such as Classic Conditioning, Modelling, Instrumental Learning, and the Alcohol Expectancy Theory, where people choose behaviours based on their expected outcomes, and the values they ascribe to those outcomes, both of which they have learned, or been taught, in the past.[61,62]

Political and economic models

This approach, exemplified by that of Baer and colleagues,[63] focuses on the social and economic *inequalities* of the 'world system' – both within and between countries – and its role in producing alcoholism in poorer, disadvantaged communities. They emphasize how high rates of alcoholism can often be correlated with poverty, unemployment and social marginalization. They also focus on other aspects of the macro-context, such as the political economy of drinking and alcoholism, especially the role of global corporations in promoting alcohol use, particularly in poorer countries, as well as the role of government in promoting the 'legal addictions'[63] (see below).

These authors are critical both of socio-cultural theories which ignore these macro economic influences, and of the 'disease' perspectives (whether medical or psychological) which tends to see alcoholism mainly as an *individual* problem, while ignoring the impact of wider social forces (such as poverty, unemployment, poor housing, discrimination, or racism) on that individual, their family, and their community.

Socio-cultural models

These derive mostly from anthropology and other social sciences. They focus on aspects of the macro-context, rather than on the individual drinker; in particular, they look at cultural beliefs and behaviours related to alcohol, and how and when it should (or should not) be drunk. McDonald[50] points out that 'alcohol and its consumption are inherently cultural matters': wherever alcohol is used, it is always invested with special *cultural meanings*, and is subject to specific *rules* and norms of behaviour. These rules define what constitutes normal' and 'abnormal' forms of drinking: who can drink, how much they can drink, with whom they can drink, and where and when this drinking can take place. These cultural 'drinking norms' are also important for understanding the many *social* roles that alcohol can play: in creating and reinforcing identity, as well as relationships. Some of these socio-cultural models are described below:

Drinking norms: 'Normal' versus 'abnormal' drinking

Here the emphasis is on the drinking norms of a country or community, and how it differentiates between 'normal' (socially acceptable) and 'abnormal' (socially unacceptable) forms of drinking. 'Normal' drinking refers to the everyday use of alcohol at mealtimes, or on social and ritual occasions. In these cases, the moderate use of alcohol is an accepted part of daily life. However, even in these conditions, the type and amount of alcohol, and when and by whom it is consumed, are strongly controlled by cultural rules and sanctions. In 'abnormal' drinking, these mores are transgressed and there is frequent and excessive intake of alcohol, with resultant uncontrolled, drunken behaviour. Cultural groups vary in how and under what circumstances abnormal drinking takes place, and in how they define the behavioural characteristics of drunkenness. The boundary between normal and abnormal drinking is not clear-cut, however. In an Irish wake, for example, drunkenness is sometimes acceptable, but it is considered abnormal in other social contexts. O'Connor[64] has pointed out that, 'If one looks at the patterns and attitudes of drinking in a society, one may come to some understanding of drinking pathologies or alcoholism'. That is, one should look at the culturally defined 'normal' drinking behaviour of a group in order to understand the 'abnormal' forms of drinking that may be found within it.

On this basis, O'Connor classified cultures, in relation to drinking, into four main groups:

1 Abstinent cultures
2 Ambivalent cultures
3 Permissive cultures
4 Over-permissive cultures.

This classification refers to attitudes towards drinking as a normal part of everyday life, and also towards drunkenness. In *abstinent* cultures the use of alcohol is strictly prohibited under any circumstances, and there are strong negative feelings towards alcohol use. Examples of this are the Muslim cultures of North Africa and the Middle East, and certain Protestant ascetic churches in the Western world (such as Baptists, Methodists, Mormons and Seventh Day Adventists). While normal drinking is rare (and sometimes illegal) in these cultures, problem (abnormal) drinking is slightly higher here than in more permissive cultures, especially as a result of personal problems. O'Connor quotes studies that show that, in the American South, which has a strong abstinence tradition, 'a relationship was found between parental disapproval of drinking and an increase in the percentage of problem drinkers'. Similarly, another study showed a high incidence of heavy drinking and intoxication among a group of Mormon students; because drinking by members of abstinent groups is not controlled by any drinking norms, therefore alcoholism is more likely among such groups.

'Drinking norms' are tacit rules about who can drink, in whose company, in which settings, and how much can be consumed. 'Alcoholism', therefore, is the overuse of alcohol, and behaviour *uncontrolled* by social norms. The implication here is that in some cultures people are more familiar with how to drink as an ordinary part of everyday life. They know when to drink, the amounts to drink safely, and when to stop. In other groups, though, unfamiliarity with alcohol means that if they start drinking, they do so in a chaotic, uncontrolled and potentially dangerous way.

Ambivalent cultures have two, mutually contradictory attitudes towards alcohol. O'Connor applies this label to the Irish. On one hand, drinking is a normal part of Irish life: 'From the womb to the tomb the Irish were seen to use drink at christenings, weddings and funerals. All social and economic life was centred around the use of alcohol'. On the other hand, there has been strong disapproval of all drinking by various abstinent temperance movements in the past 150 years.[57] This has led to the absence of a consistent, generalized and coherent attitude in Ireland towards alcohol intake. In this situation, 'the culture does not have a well-integrated system of controls, the individual is left in a situation of ambivalence which may be conducive to alcoholism'.

In a *permissive* culture, however, there are norms, customs, values and sanctions relating to drinking which are widely shared by the group. Everyone is allowed to drink, but only in a controlled way and on certain occasions. In this type of culture, the moderate intake of alcohol at mealtimes, and on certain social or festive occasions, is encouraged as being normal, though there are strong sanctions against drunkenness or other forms of uncontrolled drinking behaviour. In these groups, such as Italians, Spaniards, Portuguese and orthodox Jews, the rate of alcoholism is low. For example, as Knupfer and Room[53] pointed out, Italian-Americans see wine as a type of food, to be consumed only as part of a meal, while among orthodox Jews wine is an integral part of many religious rituals, such as Passover and the Sabbath. Both groups tend to despise drunken behaviour. Among both, intoxication is regarded as a personal and family disgrace, and the use of wine between meals is frowned upon. France, too, is a permissive culture towards drink, though in O'Connor's view it is *over-permissive*. While less wine is taken in France than in Italy, alcoholism is much higher in France, and the pattern of drinking in the two countries is very different. Not only are French attitudes towards normal drinking favourable, but cultural attitudes 'are also favourable to other forms of deviant behaviour while drinking'. Drinking is also associated with virility, and 'there is widespread social acceptance of intoxication as fashionable, humorous or at least tolerable'.

In general, therefore, both 'permissive' and 'over-permissive' cultures, where drinking is allowed (but only in a controlled form), have lower rates of alcoholism – that is, abnormal, uncontrolled drinking behaviour – than either 'abstinent' or 'ambivalent' cultures. These socio-cultural patterns are passed on from generation to generation, and partly determine whether a particular member of the society is likely to seek solace in drink at times of crisis or unhappiness.

However, while O'Connor's model of different cultural macro-contexts is useful, it is limited in its applicability. As noted at the beginning of this book, cultures are never homogeneous, particularly in complex, modern industrial societies. Within the same society or community, or even within the same family, there may be very different attitudes among different groups of people, towards what constitutes normal or abnormal forms of drinking. These attitudes towards drink may be influenced by a variety of factors, including education, gender, age group, generation, religious faith, social class, or even region. Nevertheless, the model does highlight the value of looking at 'normal' drinking patterns before trying to understand the origins of 'abnormal' alcohol problems within a community.

Ethnic, religious and cultural variables

This perspective focuses more closely on the role of ethnic, religious and cultural variables within a community, in either increasing or decreasing rates of alcoholism. It pays particular attention to the role of upbringing and family environment, and in that way has some similarity to the 'social learning' models mentioned above. For example, Greeley and McCready[65] in the late 1970s examined the differences in alcohol use and abuse among ethnic and cultural groups in the USA in some detail, using data gathered by the National Opinion Research Center. Their study was based on almost 1000 families of Irish, Jewish, Italian and Swedish origin. They developed a model to examine how children learn drinking behaviour, and to explain much of the ethnic diversity in drinking patterns that has been found in the USA. In their view, five variables, from both the individual's upbringing and their present situation, can influence drinking behaviour, both 'normal' and uncontrolled.

1 *Family drinking* – that is, whether and how frequently both parents drank; a 'drinking problem' within the family; and parental approval of their children drinking.
2 *Family structure* – in particular, the decision-making style in the home, that is, whether decisions regarding the children are made by one parent or jointly by both; also the degree of explicit affection and mutual support within the family.
3 *Personality variables* – particularly orientations towards achievement, efficacy and authority. It has been suggested that an authoritarian family structure produces men with a particular type of personality, with an especially great need to be the only (and powerful) decision-maker, and

that this attitude may predispose to problem drinking.

4 *Spouse's drinking behaviour* – alcoholism is more likely if a spouse drinks heavily as well.

5 *Drinking environment* in which the person lives – that is, the prevalence of drinking and the availability of drink in their socio-cultural environment, including on social, ritual or festive occasions.

These five groups of variables, taken together, account for many of the differences in drinking patterns and rates of alcoholism among ethnic and cultural groups; they may also help in understanding why an individual in a particular group is at risk of becoming a problem drinker. However, the socio-economic environment of different groups should also be included, since poverty, unemployment and a sense of helplessness may also predispose to the overuse of alcohol.

O'Connor[64] has developed a similar model to show 'that for groups that use alcohol to a significant degree, the lowest incidence of alcoholism is associated with certain habits and attitudes'. Most of these factors apply, on a national level, to the 'permissive' societies described earlier, and which are generally associated with lower levels of problem drinking and drunken behaviour. These attitudes include:

1 Exposing the children to alcohol early in life, within a strong family or religious group.
2 Use of alcohol in a very diluted form (to give low blood-alcohol levels).
3 Alcohol being viewed mainly as a 'food', and usually consumed with meals.
4 Parents presenting an example of moderate drinking.
5 Drinking not being given any moral importance, as either a virtue or a sin.
6 Drinking not being considered proof of adulthood or virility.
7 Abstinence being socially acceptable.
8 Drunkenness being socially unacceptable and not considered 'stylish, comical or tolerable'.

9 Wide agreement among members of the group on 'the ground rules of drinking' – that is, the norms governing drinking behaviour.

Social functions of alcohol use: creating identity and relationships

Here the focus is on the roles of alcohol in creating – and maintaining – social *identity* and social *relationships*. Part of this process is the *setting* (micro-context) in which alcohol consumption takes place (such as a pub, club, bar, *taverna*, restaurant or home), and the social functions performed by that setting. Another aspect is whether drinking takes place in private or public, and whether it takes place in what is culturally defined as a 'male' or a 'female' space. Each type of setting has its own implicit rules governing the types of drinking behaviour that are permissible within it, including how and what and how much to drink, and who drinks with whom.

Drinking patterns in public settings such as bars or clubs, are often independent of the drinkers' social or cultural backgrounds (though there are more overtly ethnic settings, such as 'Irish pubs'). For example, Thomas[66] studied public drinking in bars and taverns in an urban working-class community of 50 000 people in New England, with the pseudonym 'Clyde Cove'. He found that these 'laboring-men's bars' functioned mainly as social clubs after work, where working-class men could meet together in an atmosphere of relative equality and mutual acceptance. In this setting, alcohol was merely a social lubricant and not the main reason why the men came together. According to Thomas, 'In the after-work hours of 4–6 p.m., nothing more is derived from bar life than a light form of *communitas* and a short period of time-out from the workaday world'. There were implicit rules governing their normal drinking behaviour; drunkenness or problem drinking was very infrequent and was considered to be deviant behaviour within the bar. The bar customers were drawn from many ethnic groups, but ethnicity did not affect the content of bar life and in many bars blacks and whites drank freely together.

In Mars's study[67] of longshoremen in Newfoundland, Canada, drinking played the role of a badge of *identity*; it defined and strengthened the boundaries of one group of men ('regular men'), while excluding the members of another ('outside men'). 'Regular men' – those with secure jobs unloading the boats – always drank beer together in taverns near the waterfront. Groups or 'gangs' of these men who worked together provided mutual help and 'insurance facilities' for their members, collecting funds for a sick member or donating blood for an injured one. They also formed a collective unit for bargaining with employers. Although ostensibly a leisure activity, drinking only took place with other members of one's work gang. Thus, drinking together and buying each other drinks acted to strengthen the relationships between fellow workers, while linking the world of work with that of leisure. Conversely, 'outside men' – those without regular employment, who were only hired to work erratically and on a temporary basis – never drank in the taverns. Marginal to the waterfront economy, and excluded from these mutually supportive groups of workmates, they tended to drink in the street or in parked cars, sharing the same bottle of cheap wine or rum with different men each time. Similarly, in a study of the small Irish fishing community of 'Clontarf', Peace[68] has shown how social drinking also plays a crucial role both in the creation of masculine identity and in relation to the world of work. Drinking heavily together in the village pubs every weekend gives men the opportunity to display their physical toughness to their mates, and to show that they can 'hold their beer well'. It helps to create and cement the bonds between men, many of whom will work together during the week, while at the same time clearly separating them from the world of women.

Thus, as Gefou-Madianou[69] has described, alcohol often plays an important part in creating gender identity in many different cultures, both in Europe and elsewhere. Reviewing studies from Greece, Spain, France, Hungary, Sweden and Ireland, she illustrates the very different ways that men and women consume alcohol. Whatever the cultural milieu, they generally obey different drinking norms, consume different types of alcohol, in different amounts, and drink in very different settings. Although in Mediterranean societies such as Greece alcohol is often consumed together by men and women, on religious occasions or at family gatherings, their behaviour differs markedly from when they drink in single-sex settings, such as the males-only *taverna* or local café. Contrasting north and south Europe, McDonald[50] suggests that in the south men drink together, but drunkenness is rare, since the men feel they 'have responsibility for social propriety', and it is they 'who suffer dishonour when priorities are breached'. In the north, drunkenness is much more common when men drink together, because responsibility for social propriety is not in the hands of men, but is given to women because of 'women's attributed sensitivity'.

As well as creating gender identity, alcohol can also be used as a way of reinforcing ethnic, religious, regional, or class identity. Often this depends not only on how one drinks, but also on the types of alcohol that are consumed. Ethnic or regional identity is often linked to the consumption of locally produced, or even home-brewed drinks. Class identity is often displayed by the types of drinks one can afford, such as expensive spirits or liqueurs, or rare vintage wines. Religious identity can be expressed in the ritual use of alcohol (especially wine) as a sacramental drink, such as the Christian Communion wine or *eucharist*, or the wine drunk on Jewish Sabbaths and festivals.

From an anthropological perspective, therefore, alcohol intake should always be viewed against its social, cultural and economic backgrounds. These include patterns of 'normal' and 'abnormal' drinking, the role of gender and social background, and the settings in which it occurs and the values associated with these factors. Other relevant factors are the economic interests involved in alcohol production and marketing (see below) and the meaning given to drinking by individuals or groups, such as proof of virility, manhood, adulthood or rebelliousness. All these elements, in addition to personality traits and socio-economic status, should be taken into account in understanding why and how a particular individual abuses alcohol.

The different uses of alcohol in creating new relationships, and in maintaining them, is illustrated in the following case study from the UK.

Case study: social uses of alcohol in two pubs in Cambridgeshire, UK

Hunt and Satterlee[70] in 1986 described the different social uses of alcohol in two pubs in a village in Cambridgeshire. One pub, 'The Griffin', was frequented mainly by newcomers to the village, who were predominantly upwardly mobile and middle-class, and about one-third of them were women. Here alcohol was a way of creating and sustaining new relationships, especially by the ritual of 'round buying', which involved taking turns to buy drinks for as many as 20 people in the group. Much of their bonhomie spilled over into social events in one another's homes, either before or after visiting the pub. In contrast, the clientele of 'The Three Barrels' were predominantly male, mainly working-class and middle-aged. Most of them had been born in the village, lived nearby, had known one another for many years and were often related to one another. In this ambience, 'round buying' was rare and unnecessary, since group cohesion was already maintained by a shared history, shared kinship and shared neighbourhood. In each pub, therefore, the same form of alcohol had a different meaning, and played a different social role in maintaining the cohesion of the group of drinkers.

TOBACCO USE

Tobacco, like tea, coffee, alcohol and psychotropic drugs, is a commonly used 'chemical comforter'. It is also very dangerous to health (over 60 carcinogenic chemicals have been identified in tobacco smoke).[71] Tobacco was first brought to Europe in the fifteenth century, after the discovery of the Americas. As with the other 'comforters', the widespread psychological dependence on smoking cannot be explained only by reference to the pharmacological properties of nicotine or tobacco. Socio-cultural factors also play an important role in determining who smokes, under what circumstances and for what reasons. As with alcohol use, it is important to understand the symbolic meanings of tobacco smoking – for the individual smoker and for those around him. In some cases, cultural background may *protect* against smoking and its effects. For example, studies in the UK in the early 1980s indicated that among immigrants from the Indian subcontinent, smoking was still rare among men and almost unknown among women,[72] at least in the first generation.

In the USA, cigarette smoking is believed to be the single greatest cause of disease and death,[73] and by 2005 was considered to be responsible each year for 438 000 deaths – about one in five of all American deaths.[74] The cost of tobacco-related illnesses is also high. In 1979 the annual cost of morbidity from smoking-related diseases was estimated at $27 billion,[75] but by 2002, the World Health Organization (WHO) estimated that smoking-related diseases cost the USA more than $150 billion every year.[76] Worldwide, the WHO estimated in 2002, that each year smoking-related diseases kill about one in 10 adults, and cause 4.9 million deaths.[77] They estimated that, if current trends continue, by 2030 smoking will kill one in six people on the planet.[76]

There are several studies that examine the demographic characteristics of these smokers, especially their age, sex, education, marital state and socio-economic position, and from these data some of the influences on smoking behaviour can be inferred. Reeder[78] in 1977 reviewed most of the literature then available on this subject. He pointed out that, in the USA and Europe, consumption of cigarettes had increased threefold since 1930, despite antismoking propaganda. While the proportion of adult smokers in the USA had dropped, that of teenagers has risen. The proportion of smokers had been declining among males, but increasing among females. Men and women who were 21 years old in the late 1970s now smoked at equal rates, but many men in their fifties had given up the habit. Smoking rates were lowest among better-educated groups, but this was less true for women. In general, there was a greater prevalence of smoking among women employed outside the home compared with housewives, and female white-collar workers were more likely to smoke than women in other occupations. Men in upper income categories were less likely to smoke, while women in the same bracket were more likely to be current smokers. Reeder related these contradictory statistics to the changing sex roles of females, a greater proportion of whom (in the USA) have a college education and paid employment. There is a general trend towards equality 'in virtually all domains of social and economic life' and smoking rates reflect this equality. However, 'In the case of socio-economic status the pattern is delayed, so that the smoking behaviour may be perceived as in some way an indicator of increased social power and/or independence – even before there is equality in economic status'. Many of Reeder's conclusions are still valid today.

Tobacco smoking is also an increasing problem among the young, and early onset of the habit can lead to longer-term problems. In a 1994 report, the US Surgeon General noted that nearly all first use of tobacco occurred before high school graduation, and that if adolescents could be kept tobacco-free until that time, most of them would never start smoking.[79] Despite this, in 2002 the WHO estimated that among young teens (13–15 years) about one in five smokes worldwide, and that *every day* between 80 000 and 100 000 children start smoking for the first time.[76]

The reasons why teenagers smoke are complex and varied. Quintero and Davis,[80] for example, in their study of Hispanic and Native American teens in New Mexico, USA, found that their reasons for smoking included:

1 To control their mood ('When I'm all stressed out or like I'm about to explode, I just like, I'll get a cigarette, and I'll be relaxing all good').
2 To fit in with their friends and peer group, who are also smoking.
3 To create or maintain a social image ('It would make you feel older, make you feel like you're grown up').
4 Because they had become dependant on the physical and psychological effects of smoking ('You just have to do it. It relieves you').

These factors, in addition to curiosity, personal choice and family influences, played a major part in maintaining their smoking habits. They therefore need to be taken into account when designing any antismoking campaigns aimed at teenagers.

Other studies[78] relate heavy smoking to a perception of powerlessness by the smokers, and a sense of 'anomie' and futility in the daily lives. Other correlations of high adult smoking rates were a drop in socio-economic status (in men) and experience of divorce or separation. Among teenagers, those less academically successful or from one-parent families were more likely to smoke. As with alcohol, teenagers were more likely to smoke if parents, siblings and friends already did so, the likely mechanisms in this case being imitation and role-modelling behaviour.

Considerable numbers of people continue to smoke, despite all the health warnings from government and other agencies about its dangers. Some studies indicate that many smokers still do not believe that smoking could damage their health. For example, Marsh and Matheson[81] studied beliefs about smoking among 2700 British smokers and 1200 non-smokers aged 16–66 years. Forty-five per cent of the smokers rejected outright the concept that they were more liable to heart disease due to their smoking, and 33 per cent that smoking made them more prone to lung cancer. Overall, only 14 per cent completely accepted the idea that smoking causes heart disease, and 11 per cent that it causes lung cancer.

Doherty and Whitehead[82] suggested that cigarette smoking may also persist because it can be a way of communicating a wide range of social messages, especially among family and friends. Among other messages, smoking may signal to other people 'let's talk', 'let's relax together', 'I need to be alone' or 'I'm not going to tell you how I'm feeling'. Smoking, like alcohol, may therefore play a variety of social roles, and may help define a sense of social cohesion or of social withdrawal.

ECONOMIC ASPECTS OF TOBACCO USE

Cigarette smoking does not, however, only persist because of smokers' anomie, ignorance or use of cigarettes as a social message. An overall picture of smoking must include the *economic* interests involved in tobacco production, advertising and use. In 1991 Nichter and Cartwright[83] estimated that world-wide, the tobacco industry spends about $12.5 billion annually on advertising and promotion ($2.5 billion of it in the USA). The WHO[76] estimated that in 1997 in the USA, the tobacco industry was spending about $15 million a day ($5.7 billion for the year) on advertising, while in Russia foreign tobacco companies were apparently the largest advertisers, accounting for 40 per cent of all TV and radio advertising (Figure 8.2). These figures contrast markedly with the amount spent by governments urging people to avoid smoking. In the UK in 1991, for example, the government's Health Education Authority (HEA) spent £5.5 million a year urging people not to smoke, while the tobacco industry spent about £130 million telling them that they should smoke.[84] The HEA estimated in 1991 that each year 284 159 people are admitted to NHS hospitals with smoking-related illnesses, that 110 703 premature deaths are caused in the UK annually by these diseases and that the cost to the NHS in inpatient bills alone is £437 million per year.[84] Overall, the WHO[76] has estimated that 12 times more British people have died from smoking than died in World War II.

In 1986, the *Bulletin of the Pan American Health Organization*[85] reviewed tobacco use world-wide, based on data from the World Health Organization. It pointed out that tobacco is produced in about 120 countries, and that the contribution of developing countries to world tobacco production increased from 50 per cent in 1963 to 63 per cent in 1983. The major tobacco producing and consuming countries are China, the USA, the CIS (formerly the USSR), India and Brazil. About 37 per cent of the world's cigarettes are produced by state-controlled industries in centrally planned countries, and a further 17 per cent are manufactured by state monopolies whose aim is to maximize government revenue. The remainder of the market is dominated by seven international con-

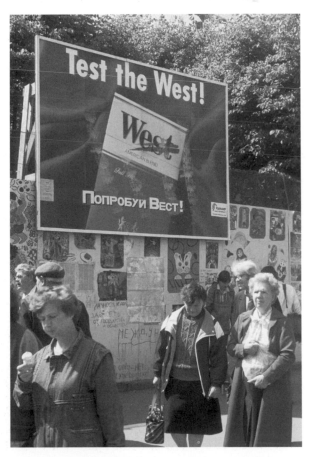

Figure 8.2 Advertisement for cigarettes in a street in St Petersburg, Russia. (Source: © Sean Sprague/Panos Pictures. Reproduced with permission.)

glomerates. By 2002, China had become the world's largest tobacco producer, accounting for about one-quarter of all the global tobacco leaf production.[76]

In many countries the tobacco industry provides thousands of jobs; it also provides income for the advertising industry, tax revenue for governments, and foreign currency for nations short on foreign exchange. Against this economic background, the *Bulletin* deplores 'the common government reluctance to act on tobacco, which is demonstrably a cause of avoidable disease and death on a scale unmatched by any other currently available product for human consumption'. By 2002, however, the overall situation of tobacco consumption had worsened, and the WHO[76] estimated that about a third of the male adult global population was a smoker, and that about 15 billion cigarettes were sold daily – or 10 million *every minute*.

THE 'LEGAL ADDICTIONS'

Both tobacco and alcohol have been termed 'legal addictions' by anthropologists Baer and colleagues.[86] They argued that, in the USA, both are sanctioned by society in ways that other 'chemical comforters' (such as heroin or marijuana) are not. The reason why they are the 'most commonly used non-medical legal drugs in US society' is partly because of pressure from the tobacco and alcohol industries. These firms, often multinational corporations, have not only tried to prevent these substances being classified as drugs, but have also often denied that they are addictive or harmful (although in the case of tobacco, recent court cases in the USA have ruled otherwise). Over the years their advertising campaigns and sponsorship activities have had a major impact on sales of their products, especially on the young. Stebbins,[87] for example, describes how in South America tobacco promotion by large transnational tobacco companies is ubiquitous, and especially targets women and the young; this is done by television adverts and billboards, but also by sponsoring many sporting and cultural events. Increasingly, both alcohol and tobacco products are being exported from Western countries into the developing world (like the pharmaceuticals described below). For example, studies quoted in the *World Mental Health* report in 1995[88] indicate that the expansion of mainly Western alcohol conglomerates into low-income countries, and their dominance of the markets there, is advancing swiftly. The countries of Africa, Asia and Latin America are now one of the fastest-growing import regions for both hard liquor and beer, with 15 per cent and 25 per cent respectively of the global import totals. An estimated 15–20 per cent of adults in Latin America are said to be alcoholics or excessive drinkers, and there is increasing alcohol consumption in parts of China.[45]

Thus on both a local and an international level, any fuller understanding of these legal chemical comforters must always take this macro-context of economic issues and profit motives into account.

WESTERN PHARMACEUTICALS IN DEVELOPING COUNTRIES

In recent decades, a significant development has been the huge influx of pharmaceutical products, mainly manufactured by Western multinational firms, into the developing world. There is now a growing dependence on these imported drugs in many Third World countries, and this has important implications.[89]

Ferguson[90] describes how these drugs are produced by a relatively small number of firms (50 per cent of the world's pharmaceuticals are supplied by only 25 firms), based in a small number of countries – mainly in the USA, Europe and Japan. Furthermore, these firms 'tend to manufacture medications designed to meet the health needs of populations in the developed countries', rather than those of the poorer countries. Despite this, enormous quantities of expensive pre-packaged medications are being exported to the Third

World, backed by advertising campaigns that stress their advantages over both traditional remedies and locally produced pharmaceuticals. Imported drugs are now a major drain on the finances of the less developed countries, where 75 per cent of the world's population live. In 1992 the Director General of the WHO pointed out that these poor countries accounted for only 20 per cent of the world consumption of pharmaceuticals, but it cost them annually about $170 000 million, and still about 'half the world's population lacked regular access to the most-needed 57 medicines'.[91]

These imported drugs significantly influence how people regard and treat their own ill health. Anthropologists have shown how, in different cultures, and in different groups within those cultures, the same drugs may be conceptualized and used in very different ways.[92] Embedded in local cultural and social contexts, their use is often based more on inherited folklore and traditional beliefs than on medical criteria.[92] They have described the large 'informal sector' of pharmaceutical use in many Third World societies, parallel to their more 'formal' use by the medical profession, although there is often overlap between the two. In many developing countries, drugs that are only available on prescription in the Western world can be bought over-the-counter (often at relatively high cost) from local pharmacies, shopkeepers or street vendors, or administered by traditional practitioners or untrained folk healers (such as the 'injectionist').

Many Western pharmaceuticals *do* have a very useful role to play in developing countries, especially in the hands of health professionals or trained primary care workers. Even in the informal sector, when bought from vendors or over-the-counter, they are often useful in alleviating various symptoms and treating many common disorders.[92] Also, the informal sector helps distribute the pharmaceuticals widely, even to areas where there are no available doctors or nurses or other sources of health care[93]. In some cases people with stigmatized conditions such as sexually transmitted diseases may even prefer the anonymity of treatment by some itinerant injectionist to a consultation with a local health professional; sometimes it may also be cheaper.

However, as well as their high cost, these imported drugs carry with them many dangers, especially when used as self-medication. These include: severe side-effects, drug allergies, self-poisoning, accidental overdoses, inappropriate use (treating viral infections with antibiotics, for example) and the development of drug-resistant strains of microbes or parasites, such as tuberculosis and malaria. Some of the drugs used are also out of date and therefore ineffective or perhaps even toxic. Furthermore, in many parts of the world they have stimulated a growth in the number of injectionists, with all the dangers associated with this (see Chapter 4). Overall, anthropologists have argued that the massive inflow of pharmaceuticals into Third World countries contributes towards a gradual 'medicalization' of ill health and suffering[90] and a moving away from more social, holistic or indigenous approaches to illness towards an emphasis on only one form of therapy, drug treatment. That is, towards the 'chemical road to success' outlined above.

In many developing countries, the main retail outlet for imported pharmaceuticals is local pharmacies. For example, in her study of the town of Asuncion, El Salvador, Ferguson[90] found that these pharmacies were also the main source of health care for poorer people, providing them with advice and information as well as over-the-counter medicines. However, most of the time the pharmacies in Asuncion were actually run by unqualified, sometimes illiterate, pharmacy clerks. Often the advice given by them was inappropriate, or a blend of folk and biomedical modes of treatment: for example, advising clients with a mild viral infection to avoid certain behaviours or 'cold' foods or drinks, but at the same time selling them tetracycline or another strong antibiotic. Furthermore, many of the drugs sold may also be counterfeit drugs, whether locally made or imported, and with little or no pharmacological effect.

THE ESSENTIAL DRUGS PROGRAMME

To deal with this chaotic situation, and to ensure a more rational and fairly distributed use of drugs world-wide, the WHO has, since 1977, developed a 'Model List of Essential Drugs' (now numbering about 250), which is regularly updated.[94] These are the basic drugs that should be available to any population, and the list excludes many of the more expensive or exotic patented drugs available in the West. A further step, in 1981, was the establishment of the WHO's Action Programme on Essential Drugs to help member countries develop national drugs policies for 'selecting, procuring, storing and distributing essential drugs, and through training and monitoring to see that drugs are used properly'.[95] Above all, the policy aimed to ensure 'regular supplies of affordable drugs of good quality'.[94] Many of these would be locally produced, or else bought cheaply in bulk from pharmaceutical firms in their generic forms (that is, without brand names and expensive packaging). As well as improving the quality of available drugs and reducing their price, the aim was to achieve a more rational use of drugs and greater coverage of the world's population.

Opposition to this programme has come not only from sections of the pharmaceutical industry, but also from local populations. In many Third World communities, these beautifully packaged imported drugs, adorned with internationally renowned brand names, seem to offer greater healing power to consumers than the cheaper, poorly packaged, locally produced alternatives on a government's Essential Drugs list (Figure 8.3). In El Salvador, for example, Ferguson[90] describes how, as a result of the penetration of these expensive imported drugs into local markets, there has been a marked shift towards them and away from the use of equally effective but much cheaper pharmaceuticals produced by Salvadorean firms, as well as from self-treatment with home remedies (which are sometimes also very effective).

As with the psychotropic drugs and other chemical comforters described earlier, belief in the 'quick fix' of a tablet (or of an injectionist's needle) may not provide an adequate solution to the social and psychological stresses faced by many in Third World countries. Although these drugs do have a role in treating or preventing, ill health, many of the health problems of these poor communities cannot be solved solely by expensive antibiotics or other drugs. Overall, there is the danger that an overemphasis on drug treatment – especially on treating the symptoms of disease rather than their cause – 'fosters the notion that the solution to illness resides in the consumption of medicines rather than improvements in living conditions'.[90] In other words, the cultural formula of 'drug + individual = success', mentioned earlier, may in its medical forms spread to include much of the non-Western world.

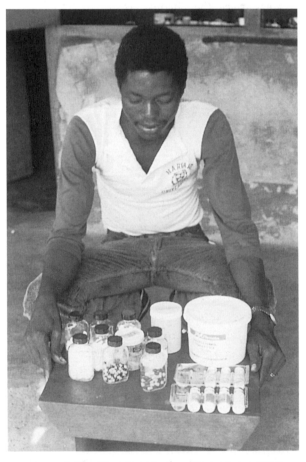

Figure 8.3 Selling Western pharmaceuticals to the public: a street vendor in Ghana. (Source: World Health Organization/Goldschmidt, *World Health*, No. 3, May–June 1998, page 26. Reproduced with permission.)

SACRAMENTAL DRUGS

In many cultures, drugs are used as sacramental substances, intrinsic to the rituals of religion, divination and healing, and to certain social interactions. Like the 'social foods' described in Chapter 3, their ingestion may contribute to the continuity and cohesion of a particular group of people. World wide, the most common ritual drug is obvi-

221

ously *alcohol*, and some of its social and religious uses have been described above. Other common substances important to the rituals of social encounters are the chemical comforters of tobacco, tea, coffee and chocolate.

In some cultural groups hallucinogenic drugs are used to obtain states of transcendence and fervour, and in their trance state those who take them are 'possessed' by the power inherent in the drug. Such rituals may take many hours or even days to perform. Sometimes the drug is used only by a shaman or ritual healer, whose visions will reveal the source of individual or collective misfortune. Dobkin de Rios[96], for example, described the use of the hallucinogen *ayahuasca* by folk healers (*ayahuasqueros* or *vegatalistas*) in an urban slum in Iquitos, Peru. As part of the ritual of healing the healer or *vegatalista* imbibes the *ayahuasca*, and the visionary content of his drug experience helps to identify the cause of the individual's illness (such as witchcraft, evil eye, or *susto*), and how it should then be dealt with.

In Medieval Europe, certain hallucinogens were used as part of 'witches' brew' or as unguents rubbed into the skin. They included belladona (*Atropa belladona*), henbane (*Hyoscyamus niger*), mandrake (*Mandragora officinarum*) and the fly agaric mushroom (*Amanita muscaria*).

Although most hallucinogenic drugs have powerful pharmacological effects on individuals, the cultural context of their use also influences the drug experience. In a ritual of divination, for example, it will influence the structure and timing of the ritual itself and the expectations and behaviour of its participants, as well as shaping the content of the shaman's visions and how they are communicated to those around him.

Among the more well-known hallucinogenic drugs used in a ritual context today are:

- marijuana (*Cannabis sativa* and *Cannabis indica*), known as *hashish* or *kif* in the Middle East and North Africa, as *dagga* in Southern Africa and as *ganja* among Rastafarians in the Caribbean[97]

- psilocybin (*Psilocybe mexicana Heim*), used by some Mexican Indian groups
- peyote cactus (*Lophophora williamsii*), used by Native Americans in the south-western USA and members of the Native American Church (which claims about 250 000 members)[98]
- *ayahuasca* or *yagé* vine (*Banisteriopsis caapsis* and *Banisteriopsis inebrians*), a hallucinatory drink used by South America Indians (especially in Brazil, Ecuador, Peru and Colombia)[99]
- morning glory seeds (*Rivea corymbosa* and *Ipomoea violacea*), used by Mexican Indians in healing and divinatory rituals
- iboga (*Tabernanthe iboga*), used as a hallucinogen in parts of Zaire and Gabon
- jimson weed (*Datura stramonium*), used among the Algonquin Indians in the north-eastern USA, and other species of *Datura* used in parts of South America, Africa and Asia.[100]

In Yemen, leaves of *qat* (or khat) (*Catha edulis Forssk.* and *Catha spinosa Forssk.*) are chewed for their stimulant or hallucinogenic properties. *Qat* is also used in parts of Ethiopia, Somalia and Kenya (where it is known as *miraa* or *marongi*).[101] Cola nuts (*Cola nitada* or *Cola acuminata*) are also widely chewed for their stimulant and hunger-relieving effects in parts of West Africa, especially in Senegal, Sierra Leone, Ivory Coast, Ghana and Nigeria.[102] Sometimes they are seasoned before use with pepper, salt, ginger or tobacco flowers. Coca (*Ethroxylum coca*) is grown in highland areas of Peru, Ecuador and Bolivia.[102] Mixed with lime paste, the leaves are commonly chewed to alleviate the symptoms of hunger, thirst and fatigue, as well as for their stimulant effect. Its use in rituals dates back to the time of the Incas. Among its producers, it is rarely used in either the form or dosage preferred by those addicted to its derivative, cocaine. In Melanesia, including parts of New Guinea, the Solomon Islands, Fiji and Vanuatu, kava (from the shrub *Piper methysticum*) is either chewed or drunk as an infusion. It induces feelings of tranquillity and wellbeing.[102] Pituri (from the shrub *Duboisia hopwoodii*) is chewed by Australian

222

Aborigines as a hallucinogen, or to alleviate the symptoms of pain, fatigue and hunger; it also plays an important role in certain male initiation rituals.[102,103]

In recent years, use of many of these hallucinogenic plants has spread beyond their groups of origin and their original ritual context. Instead of being taken as part of a public and highly controlled religious ritual, they are being increasingly being used – or rather misused – by individuals in other cultures, who take them in an uncontrolled way.[104] In the industrialized world, many have been used as recreational drugs, in either their original or synthetic forms. In some susceptible individuals they are known to have caused addiction, habituation, acute psychosis, suicidal behaviour and various other disorders. Even in those groups that have traditionally used sacramental drugs in a controlled way, their overuse and abuse is now becoming more common. This is now true of drugs such as cannabis, *qat*, coca and, of course, alcohol.

KEY REFERENCES

1 Claridge, G. (1970). *Drugs and Human Behaviour*. London: Allen Lane.

7 Hahn, R.A. (1997). The nocebo phenomenon: concept, evidence, and implications for public health. *Prev. Med.* 26, 607–11.

15 Helman, C.G. (1981). 'Tonic', 'fuel' and 'food': social and symbolic aspects of the long-term use of psychotropic drugs. *Soc. Sci. Med.* 15B, 521–33.

35 National Center for Health Statistics (2004) *Health, United States, 2004*, pp. 4, 17–18. Atlanta: Centers for Disease Control.

43 Robins, L.N., Davis, D.H. and Goodwin, D.W. (1974). Drug use by US army enlisted men in Vietnam: a follow-up on their return home. *Am. J. Epidemiol.* 99, 235–49.

46 Bourgois, P. (1989). Crack in Spanish Harlem. *Anthropol. Today*, 5(4), 6–11.

51 World Health Organization (2004) *Global Status Report on Alcohol 2004*, pp. 18–21. Geneva:

WHO, Department of Mental Health and Substance Abuse.

64 O'Connor, I. (1975). Social and cultural factors influencing drinking behaviour. *Irish J. Med. Sci.* (Suppl.), June, 65–71.

76 World Health Organization (2002) *Fact Sheets: Smoking Statistics*. Manilla: WHO Regional Office for the Western Pacific: http://www/wpro.who.int/media_centre/fact_sheets/fs_20020528.htm (Accessed on 7 July 2005)

80 Quintero, G. and Davis, S. (2002) Why do teens smoke? American Indian and Hispanic adolescents perspectives on functional values and addiction. *Med. Anthropol. Q.* 16(4), 439–57.

94 World Health Organization (1992). *The Use of Essential Drugs*, WHO Technical Report Series 825. Geneva: WHO.

104 Grob, C. and Dobkin de Rios, M. (1992) Adolescent drug use in cross-cultural perspective. *J. Drug Iss.* 22 (1), 121–138.

See http://www.culturehealthandillness.com for the full list of references for this chapter.

RECOMMENDED READING

Douglas, M. (ed.) (1987). *Constructive Drinking*. Cambridge University Press.

Gefou-Madianou, D. (ed.) (1992). *Alcohol, Gender and Culture*. Abingdon: Routledge.

McDonald, M. (ed.) (1994) *Gender, Drink and Drugs*. Berg.

Rudgley, R. (1993). *The Alchemy of Culture: Intoxicants in Society*. British Museum Press.

Van Der Geest, S. and S.R. Whyte (eds.) (1988) *The Context of Medicines in Developing Countries*. Kluwer.

RECOMMENDED WEBSITES

Centre for International Ethnomedicinal Education and Research: *http://www.cieer.org/directory.html*

International Society for Ethnopharmacology: *http://www.ethnopharmacology.org*

9 Ritual and the management of misfortune

Rituals are a feature of all human societies, large and small. They are an important part of the way that any social group celebrates, maintains and renews the world in which it lives, and the way it deals with the dangers and uncertainties that threaten that world. Rituals occur in many settings, take on many forms and perform many functions, both sacred and secular. This chapter will describe the type of rituals that relate to health and illness and the management of misfortune.

WHAT IS RITUAL?

Anthropologists have defined the various attributes of ritual in a number of ways, and they have pointed out that, for those that take part in it, ritual has important social, psychological and symbolic dimensions. A key characteristic of any ritual is that it is a form of repetitive behaviour that does not have a direct overt technical effect. For example, brushing the teeth at the same time each night is a repetitive form of behaviour, but it is not a ritual; it is designed to have a specific physical effect – the removal of food and bacteria from the teeth. If, however, this action is accompanied by others that do not directly contribute towards the effect, such as always using a toothbrush of a particular colour or saying certain words or prayers before, during or after brushing the teeth, then these extraneous actions can be thought of as having a private ritual significance for the person. In some cases, *all*

actions in a repetitive pattern of behaviour have no technical effect – as in private prayers or religious observance, or in some of the actions of the person with obsessive–compulsive disorder. In general, though, this form of private ritual behaviour is of less interest to anthropologists than the public rituals that take place in the presence of one or more other people.

Loudon[1] defined these public rituals as 'those aspects of prescribed and repetitive formal behaviour, that is those aspects of certain customs, which have no direct technological consequences and which are symbolic'. That is, 'the behaviour or actions say something about the state of affairs, particularly about the social conditions of those taking part in the ritual'. In a social setting, rituals both express and renew certain basic values of that society, especially regarding the relationships between people, between people and nature, and between people and the supernatural world – relationships that are integral to the functioning of any human group. According to Turner,[2] 'ritual is a periodic restatement of the terms in which men of a particular culture must interact if there is to be any kind of coherent social life'. He sees two functions of ritual: an expressive function and a creative function. In its *expressive* aspect, ritual 'portrays in a symbolic form certain key values and cultural orientations'. That is, it expresses these basic values in a dramatic form, and *communicates* them to both participants and spectators. Leach[3] and other anthropologists see this aspect of ritual as being the most important. For them ritual has some of the properties of a language, which can only be understood within a specific cultural context and by those who can decode its meaning. Leach[3] states that 'we must know a lot about the cultural context, the setting of the stage, before we can even begin to decode the message'. In its *creative* aspect, ritual, according to Turner,[4] 'actually creates, or recreates, the categories through which men perceive reality – the axioms underlying the structure of society and the laws of the natural and moral orders'. It therefore restates, on a regular basis, certain values and principles of a society and how its members should act *vis-à-vis* other people, gods and the natural world, and it helps to *recreate* in the minds of the participants their collective view of the world. In some cases rituals may act to reinforce ideas of social inequality, based on class, caste, occupation or gender.

THE SYMBOLS OF RITUAL

These two functions of ritual – expressive and creative – are achieved by the use of *symbols*. These include certain standardized objects, as well as the special clothing, movements, gestures, words, sounds, songs, music and scents used in rituals, which are mentioned below, as well as the fixed order in which they appear. Turner[4] has examined the forms and meanings of ritual symbols, particularly those used in healing rituals. He points out that, especially in pre-literate societies, rituals have the important function of storing and transmitting information about the society; each ritual is an aggregation of symbols, and acts as a 'storehouse of traditional knowledge'. He sees each symbol as a 'storage unit' into which is packed the maximum amount of information. This is because ritual symbols are 'multivocal', that is, they represent many things at the same time. Each symbol can be regarded as a multifaceted mnemonic, with each facet 'corresponding to a specific cluster of values, norms, beliefs, sentiments, social roles and relationships within the cultural system of the commu-

nity performing the ritual'. Therefore, to the outsider observing a ritual, there is always more to the symbols than meets the eye. Each symbol has a whole range of associations for those taking part in the ritual. It tells them something about the values of their society, how it is organized and how it views the natural and supernatural worlds. This restatement of basic values is particularly important at times of danger or uncertainty – when people feel that their world is threatened by misfortunes such as accident, famine, war, death, severe interpersonal conflicts or ill health.

THE RANGE OF RITUAL SYMBOLS

Although Turner's concept of ritual symbols concentrated mostly on physical *objects*, there are many other components of ritual that can also be regarded as having a strong symbolic value. When included in a ritual, they can signal important information to both participants and observers. They include

- *clothing* (such as a priest's vestments, a doctor's white coat, or a Jewish prayer shawl)
- *colours* (such as purple worn by higher clergy, black worn for mourning, white worn by health professionals)
- *body decorations* (such as special face paints, cosmetics, jewellery, or talismans)
- *smells* (such as incense in a church or temple)
- *tastes* (such as the 'bitter herbs' eaten at the Passover meal or *seder*)
- *foods* (such as the Communion wafer, or Thanksgiving turkey)
- *sounds* (such as organ music, chants, bells, drums, cymbals, or the sounds of a Tibetan prayer wheel)
- *words* (such as special words, phrases or statements used in prayer or supplication, either spoken or sung)
- *silences* (such as moments of silence observed at special points in a religious service, meditation, or service of remembrance)
- *rhythms* (such as choral performances, songs, clapping, or rhythmic dances)

- *movements* (such as dancing, swaying, or kneeling during prayer); and
- *gestures* (such as crossing oneself on entering a church).

In addition, important rituals usually take place at a specific and designated *time* (such as a particular time of the day or the week, or on a particular date every year), and in a particular *place* set aside for them (such as a house of worship, a hospital, a doctor's clinic, a shrine, a cemetery, or the house of a traditional healer). These components of ritual, whether they are physical objects or not, usually occur in a standardized order and at specific parts of the ritual, and in a specified way. They are important parts of the *choreography* of a ritual, and help determine whether it will be successful or not.

The doctor's white coat

As mentioned above, ritual symbols can be 'decoded' only by looking at the context in which they appear. For example, a white coat worn in a hospital setting has a different range of associations from one worn by a supermarket attendant. Although both may be worn as a hygienic measure, the context in which they are worn adds many other associations to them. The white coat worn by a doctor in a healing context (hospital or doctor's office) may be regarded as a ritual *symbol*. While it does have a technical aspect (maintaining hygiene and avoiding dirt and contamination) it also carries a number of associations with it. For those taking part in medical healing (doctors, nurses, patients) it symbolizes or represents a number of attributes associated with doctors in general. Some of these associations are shown in Table 9.1. The potency of this multivocal symbol is shown by its widespread use in television or newspaper advertisements for patent medicines, which feature an 'expert' whose white coat symbolizes 'science' and 'reliability'.

Table 9.1 Some associations of the physician's white coat as ritual symbol

A training in medicine
A licence to practise medicine
Membership of the medical profession
Being answerable to a professional organization
A repository of specialized and inaccessible knowledge
Power to:
    take a medical history
    obtain intimate details of patients' lives and examine patients' bodies
    order a wide range of tests
    prescribe medication or other treatments and make life or death decisions
    hospitalize patients, some against their will
    control those lower in the professional hierarchy, e.g. junior doctors, nurses, medical students
Orientation towards caring, and the relief of suffering
A scientific orientation in concepts and techniques
Confidentiality
Reliability and efficiency
Emotional and sexual detachment
Cleanliness
Respectability and high social status
High income
Familiarity with situations of illness, suffering and death

Similarly, these coats are often worn by medical secretaries and receptionists, though this is often not crucial for hygienic reasons. Here the coat symbolizes membership (however peripheral) of the healing profession, and carries with it some of the attributes of doctors. Because of the proliferation of white coats among hospital nurses, paramedical staff and technicians, however, other subsidiary symbols, such as a stethoscope, bleeper, or specially coloured nametag, are required to complete the message to others involved in the healing context.

The sum of these symbols communicates information about the wearer of the coat, and reinforces ideas of how 'a doctor' should dress and behave. These symbols refer less to the individual doctors than to the attributes of their role as representatives of that special category of persons who constitute the official healing profession – a group that is empowered to use the forces of science or technology for the benefit of their patients. Thus, individual doctors employ the potent symbols of medical science (such as a white coat, stethoscope, or computer) in their rituals of healing in the same way that non-Western healers employ certain religious symbols or artefacts (such as certain plants, talismans, divination stones, holy texts or statuettes) that also symbolize powerful healing forces (such as gods, spirits or ancestors). In this way, the use of these symbols brings the wider values of the society directly into the doctor–patient interaction.

Despite recent trends towards a more informal, less hierarchical relationship between doctor and patient, several studies suggest that many patients prefer this relationship to remain more formal, and that the physician's white coat still retains its symbolic power. A study of 200 hospital patients in Boston and San Francisco found that 65 per cent believed that their doctors should wear a white coat, (and 52 per cent that they should not wear blue jeans), while only 10 per cent wanted to address their physician by their first name.[5] A similar study of psychiatric inpatients in London found that 71 per cent preferred their doctors to wear white coats or formal attire, as well as a name-badge,[6] because these 'may facilitate role recognition and the establishment of boundaries' – an important element in psychiatric treatment. In the UK, unlike in the USA and some European countries, most general practitioners (GPs) and many hospital doctors do not wear white coats, but even here *other* aspects of their dress still play an important ritual role. One study[7] found that for 64 per cent of patients the way that their GP dressed was important in inspiring confidence in their professional skills. They preferred their family doctors not to dress too informally, but to wear more traditional, formal dress; a suit and tie in men, but a white coat in women. Another British study[8] found that while children saw formally dressed paediatricians as competent but not friendly, they saw casually dressed paediatricians as friendly but not as competent.

Turner[4] has pointed out another attribute of ritual symbols; 'polarization of meaning'. This refers to the clustering of the associations of a particular multivocal symbol around two opposite poles. At one pole the symbol is associated with 'social and

Figure 9.1 The physician's white coat: a potent ritual symbol of the healing powers of medical science. (Source: © Corbis MED 2016. Reproduced with permission.)

moral facts'; at the other with 'physiological facts'. This is seen in both healing rituals and rites of social transition. For example, in some societies a girl's first menstruation, the menarche, is marked by a special ritual. Some of the symbols used in this ritual are associated, in the minds of the participants, both with the *physiological* event (the menarche) and the *social* event of her new membership of the community of adult, fertile women. The ritual symbol acts as a 'bridge' linking the physiological and social stages of human life. These stages include birth, puberty, marriage and death. The symbols are a way of integrating physiological changes (especially at puberty), which might potentially be socially disruptive if left unchecked, with the laws and values that help keep society together. According to Turner, 'powerful drives and emotions associated with human physiology, especially with the physiology of reproduction, are divested in the ritual process of their antisocial quality and attached to components of the normative order'.[4] In the Western world, many of the rituals that used to mark life stages such as birth, puberty and death have disappeared. This means that these major life changes are not surrounded by ritual symbolism that gives meaning to the event far beyond its physiological significance. In contrast, in many non-Western societies, the symbols associated with physiological changes link these changes to wider social or cosmological events. Pregnancy, for example, is not only a physical event, but is also the social transition of 'woman' to 'mother'. Death is a physical event, but is sometimes seen as a simultaneous 'birth' into the society of ancestors. Some of these rituals will be described further in this chapter.

Case study: colour symbolism of Zulu medicines, South Africa

Ngubane's description[9] in 1977 of the symbols used in healing rituals by the Zulu people of South Africa illustrates the multivocal and bipolar aspects of ritual symbols. In this community, it is the *colour* of the medicines rather than their pharmacological properties that is considered the most important attribute. This colour symbolism is particularly important in medicines used for prophylactic purposes, or in dealing with illnesses thought to have a supernatural origin. The medicines are divided into three groups – black (*mnyama*), red (*bomvu*) and white (*mhlope*) – and each colour is associated with a cluster of meanings, physiological, social and cosmological. Black represents night-time, darkness, dirt, pollution, faeces, death and danger. Defecation, dirt and death can be seen as antisocial elements, all of which should be absent from normal social encounters. Also, night is the time when people cannot see, when they withdraw from their usual social activities; at night, sick people become sicker and sorcerers are said to work. Ancestral spirits visit their descendants in dreams, so that sleep is a point of contact with the dead. Ngubane states that sleep 'may be regarded as a miniature death that takes a person away from the conscious life of the day'.[9] In contrast, white symbolizes the good things of life, good health and good fortune. It represents daylight and the events that take place during it, such as eating or social interactions. During the day, people participate in social activities and live their lives. They see clearly, and there is no sense of danger. White represents the social values of life, eating and seeing. The third colour, red, symbolizes the states of transition between black and white, much as sunset and sunrise are between day and night. It represents an in-between position, slightly more dangerous than white but less so than black. It also stands for other states of transition or transformation, such as growth, regeneration or rebirth. The association of blood with states of transition (such as birth, or a fatal wound) is also relevant here. In treating an ill person the Zulu traditional healer aims to restore health, which is seen as a *balance* between the person and the environment. This is achieved by expelling from the body what is bad by the use of black and red remedies, and then strengthening the body by the use of white medicines. The medicines are always used in a fixed order: black, red, white. This is meant to achieve a transformation from illness to health, 'from the darkness of night to the goodness of daylight', from death to life, from danger to safety, from antisocial to social behaviour. As Ngubane states: 'the daylight represents life and good health. To be (mystically) ill is likened to moving away from the daylight into the dimness of the sunset and on into the night ... The practitioner endeavours to drive a patient out of the mystical darkness by black medicines, through the reddish twilight of the sunrise by red medicines, and back into daylight and life by white medicines'.[9]

TYPES OF RITUAL

While there are many different types of private ritual, anthropologists have described three main types of public ritual:

1 Cosmic cycle or calendrical rituals.
2 Rituals of social transitions (*rites de passage*).
3 Rituals of misfortune.

CALENDRICAL RITUALS

Calendrical rituals celebrate changes in the cosmic cycle, such as the changing of seasons and the division of the year into segments such as months, weeks or days, as well as certain festivals and holy days. The identity and world-view of the group is linked symbolically to events in the cosmic cycle, or to certain specified points within that cycle. Examples of this are harvest festivals, midsummer festivals, holy days such as Christmas and Easter, or commemorative days such as Thanksgiving or Remembrance Sunday. These social occasions are usually based on the cycle of the seasons, or the position of the moon, sun or planetary bodies. In many of these rituals, the symbols used link the social and cosmological dimensions and help rein-

force and recreate the social organization and values of the society.

RITUALS OF SOCIAL TRANSITION

The rituals of social transition are present in one form or another in every society. They relate changes in the human life cycle to changes in social position within the society by linking the physiological to the social aspects of an individual's life. Examples of this are rituals associated with pregnancy, childbirth, puberty, menarche, weddings, funerals and severe ill health. In each of these stages the ritual signals the *transition* of the individual from one status to another, such as from 'wife' to 'mother' in pregnancy. As Standing[10] points out, the ritual taboos and prescriptions surrounding pregnancy in many societies help prepare the woman, in terms of her behaviour, for her future role as a mother, as well as dramatizing this change in status to the society at large. In Western society, puberty rituals (such as confirmation or *barmitzvah*) still exist, and signal the transition between child and young adult. Birth rituals such as baptism, christening or circumcision signal 'social birth' (new membership of society), shortly after biological birth.

Leach[11] sees the origin of these transition rituals in the human tendency to divide things or actions into *categories*, each with its own boundary and name (see Chapter 1). According to Leach, 'When we use symbols (either verbal or non-verbal) to distinguish one class of things or actions from another we are creating artificial boundaries in a field which is "naturally" continuous'. These 'boundaries in the continuous field of perception' are characterized by a sense of ambiguity and danger. When things lie in the no man's land between definitions or categories, when they are 'neither fish nor fowl', they provoke a sense of uneasiness, especially in those who prefer things to be more clearly defined. This process, according to Leach, applies also to the progress of the individual through various social identities during the course of their life – such as 'child', 'adult', 'mother' and 'widow'. In the period of transition between these identities, the individual is considered to be in an interval of 'social timelessness', in a vulnerable, 'abnormal' position, dangerous both to themselves and to others; for this reason, special rituals of social transition are invoked that mark the event and protect both individual and society by various ritual taboos and observances. For example, many Western wedding customs still specify that in order to avoid bad luck the bride should not be seen by her groom the night before the wedding, and she is kept protectively veiled until well into the wedding ceremony, after which she is no longer considered vulnerable. In many non-Western societies the vulnerable period of transition may last for months or even years.

In Leach's view, most ritual occasions in any society are concerned with this 'movement across social boundaries from one social status to another'.[11] In these circumstances, ritual has two functions: 'proclaiming the change in status' and 'magically bringing it about' (though the two are closely related). To the participants, the belief is that without the ritual the change would somehow not take place.

Stages of social transition

Van Gennep[12] described three stages in these *rites de passage*. They are:

- separation
- transition
- incorporation.

In the first stage, the person is removed from his or her normal social life and set apart by various customs and taboos for a variable period of time. After this stage of transition, other rituals celebrate the third stage of incorporation, whereby the person is returned to normal society, and into their new social role. Often this last stage is marked by ritual bathing or other rites of symbolic purification. Based on Van Gennep's and Leach's work, the three stages of these rituals of social transition are illustrated in Figure 9.2.

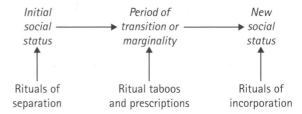

Figure 9.2 Rituals of social transition.

Rituals of pregnancy and childbirth

In all societies, pregnancy and childbirth are more than just biological events. As described more fully in Chapter 6, they are also social events marking the transition of the woman (especially with a first birth) from the social status of 'woman' to that of 'mother'. During pregnancy, the woman is in a state of transition between these two social statuses. In this state of limbo she is often considered to be in an ambiguous and socially abnormal situation, vulnerable to outside dangers and sometimes dangerous to other people. In many traditional societies pregnant women withdraw from social activities and live somewhat apart from other people, subject to certain taboos about diet, dress and behaviour. These taboos are designed to protect the pregnancy, but they are also ways of marking the transition between social statuses. In some cases these taboos may extend well into the postpartum period. Among the Zulu people of South Africa, for example, a woman is considered to still be vulnerable to outside dangers until all her postpartum bleeding ceases.[13] Furthermore, this blood is considered to be dangerous to her husband's virility, as well as to plants in the field and even to livestock.

Many of the practices and beliefs associated with modern Western obstetrics can also be seen as having an important ritual component,[14] and the ritual symbols used here are those of medical science and technology. Some of the culturally specific messages transmitted to pregnant women and their families by these symbols have been described earlier in this book. Overall, pregnancy and childbirth in the Western world are as ritualized, in their own way, as they are elsewhere. According to Kitzinger[15]: 'Baptism, circumcision, naming ceremonies, segregation of the new mother and baby, churching of women, taboos on sexual intercourse following birth, even the postnatal checkup, are all often complicated steps in a kind of dance which continues until mother and child are safely established in their correct social places and are considered no longer at risk'.

The three main stages of social transition in pregnancy and childbirth are illustrated in Figure 9.3.

Rituals of death and mourning

Hertz[16] examined one form of rituals of social transition; those associated with death and mourning. He examined the funerary customs of many societies, and saw common themes among them. In most human societies people have, in effect, *two* types of death: one biological and the other social. Between these two there is a variable period of time, which may be days, months or even years. While biological death is the end of the human organism, social death is the end of the person's social identity. This takes place at a series of ceremonies, including the funeral, where the society bids farewell to one of its members and reasserts its continuity without him or her. Hertz points out that, in most non-Western societies, death is seen not as a single event in time but as a *process* whereby the deceased is slowly transferred from the land of the living into the land of the dead; simultaneously, there is a transition between social identities from living

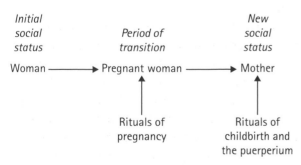

Figure 9.3 Rituals of pregnancy and childbirth.

person to dead ancestor. During the period between biological death and final social death, the deceased's soul is often considered to be in a state of limbo, still a partial member of society and potentially dangerous to other people as it roams free and unburied. In this transitional phase the soul still has some residual social rights, especially over its bereaved relatives. They have to perform certain ceremonies, act or dress in a special way, and generally withdraw from ordinary life. Like the deceased's soul, they, too, are in a socially ambiguous state between identities, dangerous both to themselves and to others. In many cultures a widowed woman is prohibited from remarrying for a specified period (sometimes forever) after her husband's death. In Hertz's model she is considered to be in a transitional state, still married to the soul of her husband, until his final moment of social death and even beyond it.

Many different ways exist for disposal of the dead.[17] These range from burial and cremation to the 'sky funerals' of Tibet, where the body is dismembered and then exposed to vultures and other carrion. In Parsee funerals, too, the dead are exposed to the elements on structures known as 'Towers of Silence'. In the Malay Archipelago, the corpse is given a first, temporary burial while it decomposes, before being reburied months or even years later at a final ceremony. During the period between the two funerals, 'the deceased continues to belong more or less exclusively to the world he has just left. To the living falls the duty of providing for him; twice a day till the final ceremony ... [they] bring him his usual meal'. During this period 'the deceased is looked upon as having not yet completely ended his earthly existence'. The final funeral ends this existence, and the ritual is one of incorporation, whereby the deceased is initiated or reborn into the society of dead ancestors, and the mourners reincorporated into normal society and liberated from the special taboos and restrictions of their transitional state. The final ceremony also removes the danger from the soul, which is no longer in limbo.[16]

Eisenbruch[18] described some of the culturally patterned ways of taking leave of the deceased among different social and cultural groups in the USA, including urban African-Americans, Chinese, Italians, Greeks, Haitians, Latinos and South East Asian refugees, and showed the wide variations in their bereavement beliefs and customs. In the UK, Skultans[19] also described some of the range of bereavement practices among different cultural and religious groups. The Irish *wake*, for example, involves watching of the corpse by relatives for several days and nights, and sometimes involves feasting and drinking. Among Greek Cypriots there is 'socially patterned weeping and wailing', followed by a defined period of mourning and wearing black. Among orthodox Jews, the *shiv'ah* has a precise structure of mourning, lasting 7 days after the funeral, during which time the bereaved remain at home and are visited by consolers, who bring them food. Mourning dress is worn until the thirtieth day, and recreation and amusement are forbidden for 1 year. In this case the transitional period lasts from the funeral (shortly after biological death) until the tombstone is dedicated a year later and mourning officially ends. The dedication of the tombstone can be seen as the last of a series of 'funerals', during which the deceased gradually leaves the world of the living. In this group, as in many others, 'social death' takes place slowly, in a series of culturally defined stages.

To some extent, all funerary practices are influenced by a culture's view of the existence, or nature, of an afterlife. In ancient Egypt, for example, prominent people were buried together with texts from the *Book of the Dead* – a guidebook for the deceased, telling them about the world to come and how they should behave within it. Cultures that believe in reincarnation, who see time as circular or spiral, and expect the souls of the dead eventually to be 'recycled' back onto Earth are likely to have very different attitudes to mourning from those without such a belief, who see death as a final, permanent event, rather than as part of a more cyclical process.

Traditional death attendants

In some societies, the care and preparation of the corpse is carried out only by close family members. In others, however, it is done by certain specialized individuals within the community – individuals whom I would term *traditional death attendants* (TDAs). These individuals are also familiar with all the rituals necessary for the funeral itself and subsequent mourning. Among orthodox Jews, for example, the *chevra kadisha* or Burial Society of each community, made up of volunteers, carries out this ritual role of caring for the corpse and preparing it for burial. In many cases, therefore, people who have emigrated from societies where either family members or TDAs usually take care of the corpse, may find the rather impersonal approach of professional undertakers rather difficult to accept, especially where they are unfamiliar with the cultural background of the grieving family. In recent years there has been a growing shift away from TDAs towards to use of these undertakers, as described below.[20,21]

The 'medicalization' of death and dying

In Western industrialized society, death, like birth, is increasingly 'medicalized', and is more likely now to take place in hospital than at home. The natural stages of biological dying are now often seen as being, in some way, unnatural or even pathological. In many such societies, the concept of death by 'natural causes' has almost disappeared. In the USA, according to Kaufman and Morgan,[22] a death in hospital is now considered to be a 'socio-medical failure'. Sometimes this may lead to the bereaved family blaming the death on the supposed incompetence of the physicians, rather than on old age or severe disease. Furthermore, Konner[23] has criticized the growing emphasis on the quantity of life expectancy rather than the quality, especially where resuscitation involves heroic, aggressive, uncomfortable and painful forms of treatment. He contrasts two poignant examples: an elderly American man, semi-comatose and subject to a variety of intense, painful treatments in Sun City,

Arizona, 'his body poked full of needles and tubes surrounded by busy strangers'; and the slow, dignified, natural death of an elderly Indian woman, dying among her close family in Benares (Varanasi) on the Ganges. In the USA, as in other Western societies, there is now a considerable conflict between the notion of a 'natural death', which takes place without medical intervention, and the pressure on the family, and physicians, to delay death and extend life, whatever the financial and emotional cost. For example, Kaufman and Morgan[22] describes how in many American hospitals, with their advanced high-tech environments, the process of dying is now 'open to endless negotiation' between the medical personnel, the family and the even the dying person about whether, or for how long, the dying process should be postponed, with the aid of feeding tubes, mechanical respirators, and powerful drugs. In a culture that values autonomy and individual choice, responsibility for these key decisions is often handed over to the family, sometimes putting them in a difficult, if not impossible situation. At a time of extreme emotional stress, they are expected to decide whether or not to carry on 'treating' the dying person, whether or not to resuscitate them, and whether, and when, to withdraw treatment and allow death to take place 'naturally'.

This Western 'medicalization' – and 'psychologization' – of death and dying can also extend to the mental state of the mourners who are often expected to do their 'grief work' in a standardized period of time, and in a standardized way. However, if they have 'unresolved grief' or 'pathological grief' (as defined by the intensity or duration of their mourning) then they may require 'grief therapy', or even antidepressant medication. In the UK and elsewhere, there has been a proliferation in recent years of 'bereavement counsellors' who offer this 'grief therapy' to those who have been bereaved.[24]

'The dead never die'

In most traditional societies the dead do not really die – at least, not in a social (or emotional) sense.

In much of sub-Saharan Africa and Asia, and in parts of Latin America, they remain as an omnipresent part of the lives of their relatives and an invisible member of the family (see Chapter 10). Their death as a member of society is followed by their birth into the community of ancestors. Here they remain forever, observing, protecting and sometimes punishing those who survive them. Thus, as invisible members of society, they still have a major influence on their descendants. In the words of Kaufman and Morgan, 'the dead make the living'.[22] In societies such as these, *ancestor worship* is common, and frequent and regular offerings are made at special shrines to appease them. The ancestors may communicate with their families in dreams or visions, or as part of certain rituals, or with the aid of traditional healers. In much of sub-Saharan Africa, they remain as permanent guardians of the social order, causing ill health or misfortune to those of their descendants who break the moral code. In Mexico, their continuing membership of the family is celebrated at the beginning of each November, when a meal is 'shared' between the living and their dead relatives at the graveside as part of the annual 'Day of the Dead' (*El Día de los Muertos*).[25] This ritual is believed by anthropologists to combine aspects of Catholicism (All Souls Day) with elements of the religion and ancestor-worship of the ancient Aztecs. In Europe and North America, the care of cemeteries and gravestones, the planting of memorial gardens, and the erection of memorials, are all ways of not only memorializing the dead, but also of keeping in some continuing contact with them.

Summary

As these examples illustrate, there is a wide variation in the care of the dying, bereavement practices and beliefs about death in different social and cultural groups. Because of these differences, Eisenbruch[18] has emphasized that although there are certain constancies in how human beings grieve; it cannot be assumed that the states of grieving in different cultures all occur at the same rate, or even in exactly the same sequence.

The three main stages of social death are illustrated in Figure 9.4.

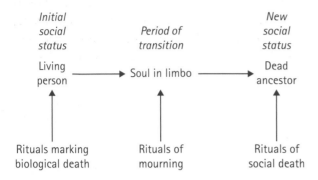

Figure 9.4 Stages of social death.

Birth and death: social and biological

The relationships described above, between biological and social birth and death, are summarized in Figure 9.5.

Figure 9.5 Social and biological birth and death.

In most societies, *social birth* follows biological birth and can be said to extend over many years. Growing up involves a whole series of social births. At each stage individuals are 'born' into a new social identity, until finally they acquire the status of a full adult member of their community. In Western societies these stages usually begin with acquiring a name, and being christened, baptized or circumcised. Thereafter, each stage – beginning at school, going through puberty, leaving school, being allowed to drive, drink alcohol, have sexual intercourse, vote, inherit property, enter work or college, get married and have children – is a form of social birth. However, in some cases social birth can be regarded as preceding the moment of biological birth. As mentioned earlier, much of the debate around the abortion issue centres on whether the foetus is a person, with social and legal rights, or not, either from conception

onwards, or from some other point during the pregnancy. For some women, viewing the ultrasound image of their growing foetus as part of an antenatal check-up may help increase the social identity of the foetus long before the actual delivery takes place, and this may have major emotional and social implications for the mother.[26] At the same time, in those countries where male children are more valued than female children, discovering the gender of the fetus may well lead to selective abortion of female fetuses. In India, for example, the increasing availability of ultrasound scans over the past 20 years has led to an increased abortion of female fetuses (estimated at about 10 million, over this period) resulting in a fewer girls than boys being born in India, especially in urban areas.[27]

As with social birth, *social death* usually takes place after biological death, in a series of stages, including the funeral, mourning and annual rituals of remembrance (outlined above). However, in some circumstances a form of social death can be said to *precede* biological death, often by many years. Here individuals are still alive physically, but in a subtle way less 'alive' socially, both in the eyes of the wider society and sometimes their own families. For example, those who have been confined to institutions for the rest of their lives (prisons, old age homes, geriatric wards, hospices for the terminally ill, or homes for the mentally handicapped), or those who have developed dementia or major mental or physical disabilities, may sometimes be said to have undergone a form of social death, long before the date of their biological death. In many societies, retirement or unemployment may also have the same effect, as may childlessness, widowhood or divorce, or the diagnosis of a serious disease such as acquired immune deficiency syndrome (AIDS), cancer or leprosy. Some religious or ethnic groups who emphasize endogamy (marrying within the group) may regard those who have 'married out' as socially 'dead', or at least as no longer full members of that group. In each of these cases, these social deaths may contribute to the *nocebo* effect, since the changed and negative attitudes of other people towards the individuals concerned may seriously affect both their mental and physical health. The most extreme example of social death followed shortly afterwards by biological death is 'voodoo death' or 'hex death', described in more detail in Chapter 11.

Modern medical technology has had an important impact on the nature of death. In some cases of severe illness or extreme old age, it now enables doctors for the first time to more-or-less control the exact timing of death. Modern life-support systems make it possible to widen the duration of biological death and postpone social death almost indefinitely (see Chapter 14). They can now convert death from a single point in time to a period of time. In the case of brain death, technology can now maintain the patient in a comatose state for months or even years, thus increasing the period of transition or liminality for them as well as for their family. This in turn may have profound emotional implications for all concerned. Technology also enables doctors to end this period, whenever they decide to do so, by switching off the machine. The effects of these changes on our perceptions of death are likely to be profound.

Changes in death rituals

Rituals of death and bereavement are not static in an age of globalization and rapid social change, especially after immigration. Laungani,[20] for example, described how the bereavement practices of Hindu immigrants to the UK have changed over the years, compared with those practiced in India. This is particularly so in relation to the open display of the dead, cremation and the subsequent scattering of the ashes in a holy river (such as the Ganges). Where once family members handled and prepared the corpse, this is now done by professional undertakers. Where once the timing of funerals was more flexible (and sometimes only carried out at an auspicious time determined by a Hindu priest), cremations in the UK tend to be carried out on a fixed, and strict schedule. Nevertheless, compared with Christian burials in the UK, these Hindu funerals are still characterized

by a more communal approach and by a more public and volatile display of emotions. Similar changes in funerary practices are happening worldwide, with the increased mobility of populations, shrinking size of the family, rushed time schedules and the decline of tradition. Some of these changes are described in the case study from Japan.

Case study: changes in Japanese funerary practices since World War II

Suzuki[21,28] in 2003 described the major changes in Japanese funerary practices since World War II, especially the shift from 'funeral rituals' (*sôshiki*) before the War to 'funeral ceremonies' (*o-sôshiki* or *osôgi*) today – a shift not only in funerary practices but also in the values surrounding death itself. In pre-War 'funeral rituals', the funeral was a highly elaborate ritual, predominately Buddhist in character, and took place gradually in a series of clearly-defined stages. Death took place mainly at home, and the funeral itself was a very public event involving much of the community. It reflected the participants' fear of death, which they believed caused the release of malevolent spirits (*koku-fujô*) that could be dangerous to them, as well as to their deities. The purpose of the ritual was to usher the deceased's spirit safely to the next world – converting it from a malevolent (*ara-mitama*) to a peaceful (*nigi-matama*) state – and to strengthen the relationships between surviving family members, and between them and their community. The actual funeral was carried out by a Buddhist priest, and by members of the local mutual-aid group (*kôgumi*), drawn from five to seven nearby households. In contrast, in contemporary Japan, death has been transferred from home to hospital. For most people it now takes place among strangers, and in an unfamiliar environment. Responsibility for the funeral, too, has been increasingly transferred to professional undertakers, and cremation has become more common. Whereas traditional rites were dedicated to protecting both bereaved and deceased from evil spirits, the modern commercialized funeral ceremony is less concerned with this, and instead 'centers on beautification of the deceased life and memories', as if the deceased remained 'alive' until the moment of cremation. Japanese undertakers have adopted an industrialized, standardized, mass-produced model of funeral practices (she call these 'McFunerals'), which are often rushed, and follow rigid time schedules. Unlike traditional funerals, 'McFunerals' are characterized by efficiency, predictability, standardization, and a precise price range for different types of funeral.

In contrast to this Japanese example, many changes in funerary rituals are becoming more individualized, and more adapted to the personality or attributes of the deceased person. These 'consumer-invented' funerals often include a variety of new rituals such as reading poetry, or playing the favorite music of the deceased, but they may also include innovations such as the elaborately carved wooden coffins – in the shape of automobiles, airplanes, birds, animals, fish or vegetables – sometimes used in Ghana, and often based on the previous occupation or interests of the deceased.[29] Mourning for dead has also reached cyberspace, with the growth of 'virtual donor cemeteries' – memorial sites on the Web for the donors of transplanted organs, which include their names, dates of birth and death, and details of their previous lives.[30] One other major development, particularly in the industrialized world, has been the gradual 'medicalization' of mourning, with the proliferation of paid or voluntary 'bereavement counselors' and 'grief therapists', whose aim is to help the mourners in their 'grief work', and 'work through' the pain of their loss.[24]

Mourning for non-humans

People not only grieve for their deceased relatives or friends. They may also grieve for many other parts of their life which are permanently lost, such as the loss of a body part (after amputation, hysterectomy or mastectomy), the loss of physical attractiveness (after burns or major scarring of the face), the loss of normal bodily functioning (after accidents, severe heart attacks or colostomies), the loss of mental functioning (after strokes, head injuries or the development of dementia), the loss of favourite pets (or livestock), the loss of social position (after redundancy, retirement or demotion), the loss of a house or other dwelling place (after war or natural disasters) or the loss of one's familiar home environment and cultural background – the phenomenon of 'cultural bereavement' (see Chapter 12) most marked among immigrants and refugees, especially those from rural, agrarian societies. For these people, whose sense of self often includes a particular patch of land, ancestral graves or religious shrines, migration may feel like a form of 'amputation' of their identity, and they would mourn for that loss, as well as for the loss of their homes and livelihood.

In each of these cases, the grieving process may be very intense, and the way that people mourn these various losses is patterned not only by their individual personalities, but also by their religious, social and cultural backgrounds.

Rituals of hospitalization

Many healing rituals are also rituals of social transition whereby an 'ill person' is transformed into a 'healthy person'. This often involves the patient's withdrawal from everyday life while certain treatments are followed and taboos observed. If the patient recovers he or she is ritually reincorporated into normal society, but in the phase of transition the sufferer is considered especially vulnerable, as well as dangerous to other people. To some extent, the hospital can be seen as a setting for these rites of social transition. Patients admitted to hospital leave their normal life behind and enter a state of limbo characterized by a sense of vulnerability and danger. As with other institutions, such as the army or prison, they undergo a standardized ritual of entry in which they are divested of many of the props of their social identity. Their clothing is removed and replaced by a uniform of pyjamas or nightdress. In the ward they are allocated a number, and transformed into a 'case' for diagnosis and treatment. Later, when they have recovered, they regain their own clothes and rejoin their community in the new social identity of either a 'cured' or a 'healthier' person. While hospital treatment is designed to provide intensive medical care and observation, and to remove patients with infectious disease from the community, it also follows Van Gennep's three stages of separation, transition and incorporation, as illustrated in Figure 9.6.[12]

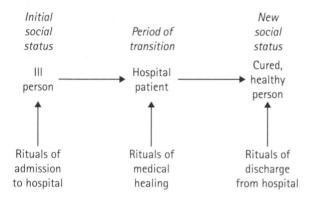

Figure 9.6 Hospitalization as a ritual of social transition.

Clinicians should be aware of these social dimensions of hospitalization, especially patients' feelings of unease and anxiety about their ambiguous or abnormal social status.

THE SYMBOLIC POWER OF 40

One interesting and recurrent feature of many rituals of transition, especially after birth and death, is the symbolic power of the number 40. Schimmel[31] points out that the number 40 is particularly important in the religious traditions and folklore of Judaism, Christianity and Islam: from the 40 days and 40 nights of Noah's Flood, to the 40 days of Lent, and the 40 disciples of Ali, the first Imam of Shi'ite Islam. She notes that in many cultures the number 40 represents the time of waiting, preparation, purification and transition, such as the 40 weeks of pregnancy, and the 40 days of quarantine.

In many human groups, rituals after childbirth which end the liminal state of the puerperium –

where the mother is still ritually 'unclean' – also take place 40 days or 6 weeks after the birth, after which time she is allowed to resume her everyday activities. In the Christian tradition the feast of Candlemas on the 2nd of February marks the end of Mary's 40-day confinement after the birth of Jesus. In the UK a ritual of religious re-incorporation known as the 'churching of women' used to take place at this time, but this has largely given way to the more secular ritual of the 6-week postnatal check-up. In the Greek Orthodox church the '40-day blessing' (*sarantismos)* for new baby and mother still continues, while among Mexicans and Mexican-Americans, *la cuarentena* is a 40-day postpartum period during which the mother is expected to rest and to adjust to her new baby, while family members take responsibility for her household chores, a process that has some similarities to 'doing the month' in Chinese communities (see Chapter 6). In Islam, sexual intercourse is discouraged for the first 40 days after childbirth, until the postpartum bleeding (*nifas)* has stopped. In several religions, including Islam, the main mourning period after bereavement is also about 40 days long.

RITUALS OF MISFORTUNE

These usually come into play at times of unexpected crisis or misfortune, such as accidents or severe ill health. Loudon[1] sees two functions of this type of ritual; a manifest function (the solution of specific problems) and a latent function ('the re-establishment of disturbed relationships between human beings'). In many small-scale non-industrialized societies they also function to repair disturbed relationships with the social and supernatural worlds. As Foster and Anderson[32] pointed out, in these societies 'illnesses are often interpreted as reflecting stress or tears in the social fabric. The purpose of curing therefore goes well beyond the limited goal of restoring the sick person to health; it constitutes social therapy for the entire group, reassuring all onlookers that the interpersonal stresses that have led to illness are being healed.

237

Illness is therefore seen as a *social* event. The illness of one member, especially if blamed on witchcraft or sorcery resulting from interpersonal conflicts, threatens the cohesion and continuity of the group. The group has an interest in finding and resolving the cause of the illness, and restoring both the victim and themselves to health. As a result, such healing rituals usually take place in *public*, in marked contrast to the privacy and confidentiality that characterize doctor–patient consultations in the Western world. The aim of these public rituals is visibly to restore the harmonious relationships between Man and Man, Man and his deities, and Man and the natural world.

Rituals of misfortune usually have two consecutive phases: the phase of *diagnosis* or divination of the cause of the misfortune and the *treatment* of the effects of the misfortune, and removal of the cause. In the case of ill health, the first phase includes giving the condition a label or identity within the cultural frame of reference. This implies a concept of how misfortune is caused, its probable natural history and its prognosis, which is shared by healer, patient and spectators. There are many techniques used by different cultures to diagnose ill health, ranging from divinatory séances to the use of sophisticated diagnostic technology. Several of them have been mentioned in Chapter 4. As an example, Beattie[33] described a divinatory séance among the Nyoro people in Uganda, where the diviner goes into a trance, speaking in a small falsetto voice and using a special vocabulary 'so people knew that the spirit had come into his head, and they began to ask him questions'. These questions related to the diagnosis of a variety of misfortunes, such as marital conflicts, theft and ill health. It was the 'spirit' who diagnosed their cause and prescribed treatment, speaking publicly through the mouth of the diviner. In contrast, the private diagnosis of Western medicine refers mainly to disorders of the patient's body or emotions; in general, neither mystico-religious beliefs nor social relationships are considered major factors in diagnosis and treatment. In both cases, there is an overlap between these rituals and rites of social transition. Many involve the transition of the sufferer from the social identity of 'ill person' towards that of 'cured person', via the three stages described by Van Gennep.[12]

TECHNICAL ASPECTS OF RITUAL

In looking at all forms of healing ritual, it is important to distinguish the ritual aspect from the practical or *technical* aspect that often coexists with it. In practice, the division between the two is not absolute; a purely sacred ritual can have the practical, technical effect of permanently altering people's behaviour or emotional state, for example. The technical aspect is often interwoven with the ritual, and includes such practical techniques as the use of medicines, surgical operations,[34] inhalations, massages, cupping, injections and bone-setting, as well as techniques of psychotherapy and midwifery. Even in the most primitive society, where the purely ritual aspect of healing is strongest, there is likely to be a component of shrewd observations and experience on the part of the healer as to why and how people get ill, some knowledge of human nature, and a mastery of certain theatrical and practical techniques.

In Western society, medical diagnosis and treatment also take place in ritual time and ritual space – that is, at certain times and in certain settings carefully marked off from the rest of everyday life (such as a hospital clinic or a doctor's office). In this setting even the most technical treatments are influenced by the ritual atmosphere, and this is clearly illustrated in the case of the placebo effect. Also, as Balint[35] has pointed out, the most important 'drug' that can be administered in this setting is the personality of the doctor.

FUNCTIONS OF RITUAL

Rituals fulfil many functions, both for the individual and for society. Depending on the perspective from which they are viewed, these functions can be classified into three overlapping groups; *psychological*, *social* and *protective*.

PSYCHOLOGICAL FUNCTIONS

In situations of unexpected misfortune or ill health, rituals provide a standardized way of explaining and controlling the unknown. The sudden onset of illness causes feelings of uncertainty and anxiety in the victims and their family. They ask: 'What has happened?', 'Why has it happened?', 'Why to me?', 'Is it dangerous?'. As Balint[36] describes it, in the consultation 'the patient is still frightened and lost, desperately in need of health. His chief problem, which he cannot solve without help, is: What is his illness, the thing that has caused his pains and frightens him?'. Part of the function of a healing ritual (as well as treating the condition) is to provide explanations for the illness in terms of the patient's cultural outlook – that is, to convert the chaos of symptoms and signs into a recognizable, culturally validated condition, whether it is pneumonia or *susto*, with a name and a known cause, treatment and prognosis. In a psychological sense, therefore, diagnosis itself *is* a form of treatment, converting the unknown into the known, and reducing the uncertainty and anxiety of patient and family. In the words of Phineas Parkhurst Quimby, a famous folk healer born in New England in 1802:[37] 'I tell the patient his troubles, and what he thinks is his disease, and my explanation is the cure. If I succeed in correcting his errors I change the fluids in the system, and establish the patient in health. The truth is the cure'.

Ritual also lessens anxiety at times of physiological change, such as pregnancy. These rituals, many of them public, help to control the sense of anxiety or unease associated with this vulnerable transitional state. Standing[10] has noted how it is impossible to eradicate *all* risk in pregnancy, but following prescribed rituals and taboos at least provides some kind of assurance that everything possible is being done to minimize that risk. Some diagnostic rituals can also be used to explain misfortune or failure *post hoc*, and thus lessen feelings of guilt or responsibility. For example, in some communities a woman who has given birth to a deformed child might be told that she had been bewitched by an unknown person during pregnancy, and that therefore the deformity was not her fault. However, in some cases the modern rituals of childbirth that are heavily dependent on technology may have a much more negative effect, causing the woman to feel more anxious, more helpless, and less in control of her own body at a crucial time for her.[38]

At times of extreme crisis, such as bereavement, rituals usually provide a standardized mode of behaviour that helps to relieve the sense of uncertainty or loss. Everyone knows what to do and how to act under those circumstances, and this restores a sense of order and continuity to their lives. It also enables the bereaved slowly to adjust to the fact of death, and to see it not as the end of one cycle but as the beginning of another. This gradual acceptance occurs in well-defined ritual stages, which vary between cultures.[18,39] The normal phases of grieving in most Western communities (though not necessarily elsewhere), from 'numbness' to 'reorganization', described by Murray Parkes,[40] can therefore be placed in a ritual context, and at each stage the mourners can be given much-needed social support and understanding. For example, in previous generations in the UK and other European countries, the status of mourner was signalled by wearing black clothes or a black armband. This marked mourners out from other people, and for a period of time ensured a special, protective attitude towards them. Skultans[19] has speculated that the increased risk of death among the recently bereaved (see Chapter 11) may be partly due to the disappearance of this type of protective ritual. She points out that in modern, middle-class Britain, while 'some rituals are maintained at the actual time of death and funeral in that the family gathers and mourning dress is worn ... the absence of ritual is most marked during the subsequent period of mourning. Most noticeably, the bereaved are given no guidance on how to behave in their precarious position: they are not, as in non-industrialized societies, set apart from the rest of society for a prescribed period of time, nor are they given ritual protection in this severe crisis'.

Today there is thus little outward change in behaviour and dress, and often grieving is seen as a 'pathological state', to be treated by antidepressants or other medication. Mourning rituals that encourage emotional displays of grief and define precisely when the mourning period ends probably limit the possibility of excessive or pathological mourning.

Rituals also provide a way of expressing and relieving unpleasant emotions; that is, they have a *cathartic* effect. This is especially true of the public rituals of small-scale, non-Western societies. As Beattie[33] puts it, 'they provide a way of expressing, and so of relieving, some of the inter-personal stresses and strains which are inseparable from life in a small-scale society'. In this setting, this 'safety valve' function benefits both the individual and society. Both diagnosis and treatment take place in the presence of all the family, friends and neighbours of the patient, and their part in the causation of the illness is openly discussed, as well as what they can do to help the patient. In Western clinical practice, as Turner[41] remarked, 'relief might be given to many sufferers from neurotic illness if all those involved in their social networks could meet together and publicly confess their ill will towards the patient and endure in turn the recital of his grudges against them'. In most cases, however, this type of emotional catharsis only takes place in private, in the presence of only one other person, whether psychotherapist, counsellor, psychiatrist or priest.

In some cases, the psychological catharsis in a ritual is followed by initiation of the victim into a new social group: a 'community of suffering', made up of others who have also suffered from the same affliction. Al-Adawi and his colleagues,[42] for example, describe how in Oman people 'possessed' by a *zar* spirit, which has caused them either mental or physical illness, are exorcised at a *ramsa*, a public ritual that can last from 1–7 days. The client or *mobtala'a* undergoes a lengthy ritual of exorcism by the traditional healer, with songs, exhortations, rhythmic drumbeats, and fasting. Because it is believed that the effect of an exorcism, even if successful, will only be temporary, the *ramsa* itself also functions as an initiation ritual, whereby the healed person now joins the community of fellow victims of the same *zar* spirit. This group in turn will officiate at other exorcisms in the future; it will act both as a collective healer, and as a sort of 'self-help' or support group for its members. Some of them may even become exorcists in their own right. Thus, the victim of the *zar* has not only been healed – they have also acquired a new, and supportive, social identity.

Finally, rituals of healing can also function to reduce anxiety and uncertainty in the healers themselves. Bosk[43] has suggested that many of the occupational rituals of American physicians, such as case conferences, grand rounds and mortality and morbidity conferences, may help the physicians to cope with their *own* sense of anxiety and uncertainty, and to make the necessary treatment decisions. Katz's detailed study[34] of surgical rituals in the USA has come to the same conclusion.

SOCIAL FUNCTIONS

These overlap with the psychological functions. Particularly in small-scale societies, the cohesion of the group is threatened by interpersonal conflicts. By ascribing ill health to these conflicts, the group can use this misfortune to bring conflicts into the open and publicly resolve them; this is a feature of societies where ill health and other misfortune is ascribed to interpersonal malevolence, such as witchcraft or sorcery. Illness also creates a temporary caring community around the victim, and old antagonisms are forgotten, at least for the moment. Because ill health reminds the community of its own vulnerability to death and decay, both rituals of misfortune and those of social transition (such as mourning rites) help reassert the continuity and survival of the group after the illness or death of one of its members.

Another social function of rituals is to create or recreate the basic axioms on which the society is based. By the use of multivocal symbols, the rituals dramatize these basic values and remind people of them. According to Turner[2], the way a society lives can be seen as an attempted imitation of models portrayed and animated by ritual. As such, rituals can modify behaviour towards a more sociable form, and resolve the tensions between self-interest and the interests of the group. In the colour symbolism of Zulu healing, for example, the colours are always used in the sequence black, red, white; that is, from 'anti-social' symbols, through a transitional phase towards more positive social symbols – from defecation, death and dirt towards life, eating and cleanliness. In other societies, rituals of social transition help control or tame potentially antisocial sexual impulses at puberty by restrictive taboos during the period of 'becoming an adult'.

PROTECTIVE FUNCTIONS

Rituals dealing with ill health can protect the participants in two ways; psychologically or physically. The role of rituals in protecting against the anxiety and uncertainty associated with illness, death and other misfortune has already been described. In other ways, ritual observances can protect the ill or weak person from physical dangers such as infection. Some of the rituals surrounding pregnancy, birth or the postpartum period, for example, may protect the woman and her newborn child from sources of infection or injury, especially if they involve withdrawal from normal social life. Secluding an ill person, as part of a ritual of social transition, may also limit the spread of infectious diseases to the community, while a healing ritual held in public may have exactly the opposite effect. Other protective functions arise from cleansing and purification rites, which, although carried out for ritual purposes, may also remove dirt and bacteria and promote physical cleanliness.

SUMMARY

This section has listed some of the main functions of ritual, psychological, social and protective, especially in rituals of illness and misfortune. If Douglas[44] is correct, and the industrialized world is moving away from ritual and 'there is a lack of commitment to common symbols', then the individual's management of misfortune, disease, death and the stages of the human life cycle might all become more difficult.

In the following case studies, three types of ritual of misfortune are contrasted: a public healing ceremony in a non-Western community; the more private diagnostic ritual in a Western society; and the ritual setting of a new type of syncretic, traditional healer (one increasingly common in many countries, whose rituals and practices use a mixture of Western and traditional elements).

Case study: curative rites among the Ndembu of Zambia

Turner[41] in the 1960s described curative rites among the Ndembu people of Zambia. The Ndembu ascribe all persistent or severe ill health to social causes, such as the secret malevolence of sorcerers or witches, or punishment by the spirits of ancestors. These spirits cause sickness in an individual if his or her family and kin are 'not living well together', and are involved in grudges or quarrelling. Because death, disease and other misfortunes are usually ascribed 'to exacerbated tensions in social relations', diagnosis (divination) takes place publicly, and becomes 'a form of social analysis', while therapies are directed to 'sealing up the breaches in social relationships simultaneously with ridding the patient ... of his pathological symptoms'. The Ndembu ritual specialist or traditional healer, the *chimbuki*, conducts a divinatory séance attended by the victim, his kin and neighbours. The diviner is already familiar with the social position of the patient, who his relatives are, the conflicts that surround him, and other information gained from the gossip and opinions of the patient's neighbours and relatives. By questioning these people, and by shrewd observation, he builds up a picture of the patient's 'social field' and its various tensions. Actual divination takes place by peering into medicated water in an old meal mortar, in which he claims to see the 'shadow soul' of the afflicting ancestral spirit. He may also detect witches or sorcerers, who have caused the illness, among the spectators. The diviner calls all the relatives of the patient before a sacred shrine to the ancestors, and induces them 'to confess any grudges ... and hard feelings they may nourish against the patient'. The patient, too, must publicly acknowledge his own grudges against his fellow villagers if he is to be free of his affliction. By this process, all the hidden social tensions of the group are publicly aired and gradually resolved. Treatment involves rituals of exorcism to withdraw evil influences from the patient's body. It also includes the use of certain herbal and other medicines, manipulation and cupping, and certain substances applied to the skin. These remedies are accompanied by dances and songs, the aim of which is the purification of both the victim and the group. Turner doubted whether the medicines he saw used in these rituals had much pharmacological effect, but he pointed out the psychotherapeutic benefits, to both the victim and the community, of the public expression and resolution of interpersonal conflicts, and the degree of attention paid to the victim during the ceremony.

Case study: consultation with a general practitioner in the UK

In Britain, the consultation between the average general practitioner (GP) or family physician and his or her patients is markedly different from the Ndembu example, but it too is a form of healing ritual. General practitioners are part of the National Health Service, and access to a GP is free and unrestricted, though most prescriptions have to be paid for. Consultations take place at defined times and places (the office or *surgery*), and are governed by implicit and explicit rules of behaviour, deference, dress and subject matter to be discussed. Events take place in a fixed order: entering the surgery; giving one's name to a receptionist; sitting in a waiting room; being called in turn to see the doctor; entering the doctor's room; exchanging formal greetings; and then beginning the consultation. From this point onwards, Byrne[45] described six stages in the procedure:

1 The establishment of rapport between GP and patient.
2 The doctor discovering why the patient has come.
3 The doctor's verbal and/or physical examination.
4 Both parties' 'consideration of the patient's condition'.
5 The doctor detailing treatment or further tests.
6 The termination of the consultation, usually by the doctor.

The patient's symptoms and signs are recorded, during the consultation, on the medical card, and the present condition is seen against the background of previous illnesses recorded there. Particular attention is paid to questions such as 'when did the pain begin?' and 'when did you first notice the swelling?' as part of the verbal diagnosis. As Foster and Anderson[46] point out, this historical approach is characteristic of Western diagnosis; in other cultures, the healer is expected to know all about the patient's condition without asking so many probing questions. As well as gathering clinical information by taking a history, physical examination or tests, GPs – like the Ndembu *chimbuki* – use informal knowledge gathered over the years in the community. As a result, assessment of a patient is based not only on the consultation but also on the GP's knowledge of the patient's environment, family, work, past medical history, pattern of behaviour and the culture of the neighbourhood.

The consultation is characterized by privacy and confidentiality, and usually involves only one patient and one doctor at a time. Its form is the ritual exchange of information between the two; symptoms and complaints flow in one direction, diagnoses and advice in the other. The patient receives practical advice (e.g. 'Spend a day or two in bed') or a prescription for medication. The prescription form itself resembles a contract, with the name of the doctor, the name of the patient and the prescribed medication linking the two written on it. It is assumed that the authority of the doctor extends beyond the consultation, because the drug must be taken as prescribed once the patient gets home (e.g. 'Take one tablet three times a day, after meals, for 7 days'). As with other healing rituals, the consultation takes place at specified times and in a setting set aside for this purpose. The GP's room, although designed for a technical purpose, includes many objects that will not be used in a particular consultation, and can therefore take on the significance of ritual symbols. These may include: a framed diploma on the wall; a stethoscope, otoscope and ophthalmoscope; a sphygmomanometer; tongue depressors; scalpels, forceps, needles and syringes; a glass cabinet full of instruments; bottles of antiseptic and other medicines; one or more telephones; a bookshelf filled with impressive-looking textbooks or journals; a large desk; family photographs; sheaves of special forms or notepaper; an ink pad and rubber stamps; and a pile of previous patients' medical cards. Most GPs now have a computer on their desks – an object that plays an increasingly important role in the consultation, and which can now be regarded as ritual symbol in its own right (see Chapter 13).

In this formalized setting of ritual time and place, the patient's diffuse symptoms and signs are given a diagnostic label and organized into the named diseases of the medical model. As well as prescribed medication, the most powerful drug administered in this setting is faith in the healing powers of the doctor.[23]

Case study: 'Doctor John' – an innovative traditional healer in Transkei, South Africa

Simon[47] in 1991 described the setting and healing rituals of 'Doctor John', a Xhosa traditional healer in rural Transkei, eastern South Africa. 'Doctor John' used many of the ritual symbols and practices of Western medicine, but blended them with certain aspects of traditional African healing. Situated in a village back street, his consulting room was in a small, dilapidated shack. Although without formal qualifications, a lavishly painted sign hung outside proclaiming: '*Dr John: Homeopath, Naturopath, Herbalist. Welcome*'. At any one time, 20–30 people were waiting for him, some standing in the courtyard outside, others sitting in his tiny waiting room in which an assortment of herbs, bulbs, roots, dried skins, and calabashes were crammed onto makeshift shelves. Many of the bottles of herbs had labels with popular brand names; others had illegible instructions scrawled on them. Within the actual consultation room (its door labelled '*Dr John's Office*'), the healer sat behind a desk, dressed in a white coat, a suit and tie, and wearing a pair of green-tinted spectacles. On the table, illuminated by two candles, lay a number of significant ritual objects: burning incense, small calabashes, beads, a stethoscope, a syringe and a stack of medical publications, ranging from scientific journals to home doctor books. His assistant was an elderly woman, who also wore a white coat. All the patients who entered the room were asked how they were feeling, and then each one was examined with the stethoscope. Then 'Dr John' announced that he would implore his *amakhosi*, or spirits, to aid in the diagnosis and discover the cause of the patient's illness. Afterwards, he told the patient that he would use a 'doctor's book' to find the most appropriate treatment for them. He then read out a passage from one of his books, translating its meaning to the patient. To strengthen the effect, he often repeated sentences aloud from it in English. He then scribbled instructions on a piece of paper (the 'prescription'), and asked the patient to hand this to his assistant, who then dispensed the appropriate herbs. Like other traditional healers in that area, he always also included one or two pharmaceutical products in the prescription, such as cough mixtures, aspirins, laxatives or milk of magnesia, which he kept in a small closet nearby. Simon noted that his syncretic mix of Western and African healing practices, his 'commitment to the parallel utilization of medical traditions, and not a singular devotion to either form of practice', had made him a popular and effective healer locally.

Whatever the success or otherwise of his treatments, the case of Dr John and his ritual setting shows that in the modern age traditional medicine is not static. 'Like any form of therapy, local (traditional) healing is a dynamic, changeable profession, with shifting ideas and practices tailored to suit the times'.

KEY REFERENCES

1 Loudon, J. B. (1966). Private stress and public ritual. *J. Psychosom. Res.* 10, 101–8.

2 Turner, V. W. (1968). *The Drums of Affliction.* Oxford: Clarendon Press and IAI, pp. 1–8.

9 Ngubane, H. (1977). *Body and Mind in Zulu Medicine*. London: Academic Press, pp. 111–39.

11 Leach, E. (1976). *Culture and Communication.* Cambridge: Cambridge University Press, pp. 33–6, 77–9.

15 Kitzinger, S. (1982). The social context of birth: some comparisons between childbirth in Jamaica and Britain. In: *Ethnography of Fertility and Birth* (MacCormack, C.P. ed.). London: Academic Press, pp. 181–203.

16 Hertz, R. (1960). *Death and the Right Hand.* London: Cohen and West, pp. 27–86.

20 Laungani, P. (1996). Death and bereavement in India and England: a comparative analysis. *Mortality* 1(2), 191–212.

21 Suzuki, H. (2003) McFunerals: the transition of Japanese funerary services. *Asian Anthropol.* 2, 49–78.

22 Kaufman, S.R. and Morgan, L.M. (2005) The anthropology of the beginnings and ends of life. *Annu. Rev. Anthropol.* 34, 317–14.

41 Turner, V. W. (1964). An Ndembu doctor in practice. In: *Magic, Faith and Healing* (A. Kiev, ed.). New York: Free Press, pp. 230–63.

See http://www.culturehealthandillness.com for the full list of references for this chapter.

RECOMMENDED READING

Bryant, C.D. (ed.) (2003) *Handbook of Death and Dying* (2 volumes). Sage.

Katz, P. (1981). Ritual in the operating room. *Ethnology* 20, 335–50.

Kaufman, S.R. & Morgan, L.M. (2005) The anthropology of the beginnings and ends of life. *Annual Review of Anthropology* 34, 317–14.

Kaufman, S. (2005) *And a Time to Die: How American Hospitals Shape the End of Life.* Scribner

Robben, A.C.G.M. (ed.) (2004) *Death, Mourning and Burial: A Cross-cultural Reader.* Oxford: Blackwell.

Turner, V. W. (1974). *The Ritual Process.* London: Penguin.

10 Cross-cultural psychiatry

Cross-cultural psychiatry – also known as *cultural psychiatry* – is the study and comparison of mental illness, and its treatment, in different cultures and social groups. It is one of the major branches of medical anthropology, and has been a valuable source of insight into the nature of health and ill-health in different parts of the world. Historically, research into the subject has been carried out by two different types of investigator:

1 Western-trained psychiatrists who have encountered unfamiliar, and what seemed to them bizarre, syndromes of psychological disturbance in parts of the non-Western world, and who have tried to understand these syndromes in terms of their own Western categories of mental illness, such as 'schizophrenia' or 'manic depressive psychosis'.

2 Social and cultural anthropologists, whose main interests have been the definitions of normality and abnormality in different cultures, the role of culture in shaping personality structure, and cultural influences on the cause, presentation and treatment of mental illness.

Although these two approaches have led to different perspectives on the subject, they share a concern with two types of clinical problem:

1 The diagnosis and treatment of mental illness where health professional and patient come from different cultural backgrounds.

2 The effect on mental health of migration, urbanization and other forms of social change, as well as of poverty and deprivation.

The focus of cross-cultural psychiatry is mainly on mental *illness* rather than on mental disease. That is, it is concerned less with the organic aspects of psychological disorders than with the psychological, behavioural and socio-cultural dimensions associated with them. Even when the condition clearly has an organic basis, as in neurosyphilis, delirium tremens, cerebral malaria or dementia, anthropologists are more interested in how *cultural* factors affect the patient's perceptions and behaviour, the content of their hallucinations or delusions, and the attitudes of others towards them.

In general, the relationship of culture to mental illness can be summarized as:

- it defines 'normality' and 'abnormality' in a particular society
- it defines the difference between 'abnormality' and 'mental illness'
- it may be part of the aetiology or cause of certain illnesses
- it influences the clinical presentation and distribution of mental illness
- it determines the ways that mental illness is recognized, labelled, explained and treated by other members of that society – including by health professionals.

NORMALITY *VERSUS* ABNORMALITY

DIMENSIONS OF SOCIAL BEHAVIOUR

Some of the many dimensions of social behaviour are illustrated in Figure 10.1. This represents the range of possible *perceptions* – by members of a particular society or culture – of a particular form of social behaviour: whether they see it as 'normal' or abnormal for their society, and whether it is controlled, or not, by the norms or rules of that society. It also reflects the fact that all human groups recognize that there are certain times and places when people can be allowed to behave in an 'abnormal' way, provided that they are seen to conform to the strict guidelines (explicit or implicit) laid down by their culture for this type of situation. In this case, even if their behaviour is bizarre or unconventional, it is still to some extent controlled by social norms. In contrast, most cultures disapprove of forms of public behaviour that are obviously *not* being controlled by the rules of their society: and which they usually label as either 'mad' or 'bad'. Thus in Figure 10.1 there are four possible zones of social behaviour (A, B, C, D) according to the perceptions of that society, or of groups or individuals within that society.

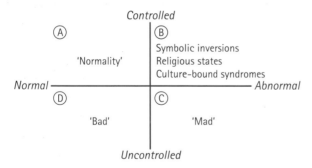

Figure 10.1 Perceptions of social behaviour.

It should always be emphasized, however, that these zones, and the definitions of behaviour they encompass, are *not* static. Rather, they are a series of fluid categories, a spectrum of possibilities, that are likely to change with time and circumstance and the particular perspective of the onlooker. Thus, behaviour seen as 'bad' in one generation may be seen as 'mad' in the next, and 'normal' behaviour in one group of people may be regarded as 'abnormal' in another. Alcohol consumption, for example, has, at various times and places (sometimes within the same society), been seen as normal, as morally bad, as a symptom of psychological disorder, and as an accepted part of certain ritual or religious occasions. Furthermore, these broad social categories do not necessarily take into account *individual* factors such as personality, motivation, experiences, emotional state or physiology. Their focus is not primarily on an individual's perspective, but rather on that of society as a whole – or, at least, of a section of that society. However, in the case of 'controlled normality' (A), 'uncontrolled normality' (D) and 'controlled abnormality' (B) it is assumed that the individual is at least *aware* (consciously or not) of what the social norms are, whether they conform to them or not. That is, that they have some degree of self-awareness, or insight, into their own behaviour.

'Normality'

Definitions of 'normality', like definitions of 'health', vary widely throughout the world, and in many cultures these two concepts overlap. Mention has already been made in Chapter 4 of some of the medical definitions of health that are based upon the measurement of certain physiological and other variables that lie within the normal range of the human organism. At its most reductionist, this approach concentrates mainly on the physical signs of brain dysfunction before diagnosing mental illness. In this chapter, some other ways of looking at the problem will be examined, especially the *social* definitions of normality and abnormality. These definitions are based on shared beliefs within a group of people as to what constitutes the ideal, 'proper' way for individuals to conduct their lives in relation to others. These beliefs provide a series of guidelines on how to be culturally 'normal' and, as will be described below, how also to be temporarily 'abnormal'. Normality is usually a *multidimensional* concept. Not only is the individuals' behaviour relevant, but also, for example, their dress, hairstyle, body adornments, smell, personal hygiene, posture, gestures, movements, emotional state, facial expression, tone of voice and use of language – all of which are taken into account – as well as their *appropriateness* to certain contexts and social relationships. That is, 'normality' is a series of clusters of attributes, with each cluster being appropriate for a particular type of context: such as work, leisure, personal relationships, or social occasions. 'Normal' behaviour on a beach or a holiday, is very different from that at a workplace or religious festival.

The social definition of normality (Figure 10.1, A) is never uniform within a population. Most cultures have a wide range of social norms that are considered appropriate for different age groups, genders, occupations, social ranks and cultural minorities within the society. Attitudes towards foreigners or minorities often include stereotyped views of their normal behaviour, which may be seen as bizarre, comical or even threatening.

'Controlled abnormality'

Most societies, especially those with rigid codes of normal behaviour, often make provision for certain specified occasions where these codes are deliberately flouted or *inverted*, and 'abnormal' behaviour, whether of the individual, or of the group, becomes the temporary norm (Figure 10.1, B). Despite this, their behaviour is actually tightly controlled in terms of when it happens, how it happens, and for how long it lasts, although to the outsider it may appear wholly 'abnormal'. One example of this, has been called by anthropologists 'rites of reversal' or 'symbolic inversions', which Babcock[1] defines as 'any act of expressive behaviour that inverts, contradicts, abrogates or in some fashion presents an alternative to commonly held cultural codes, values and norms be they linguistic, literary or artistic, religious, or social and political'. Often they are ways of 'letting off steam', of allowing people to express themselves, and feel free of social constraints, but only under controlled conditions.

Group behaviour

These special occasions, such as certain festivals, bacchanalia, parades, *mardi gras* and carnivals (like those in Brazil, the Caribbean, southern Europe and London's Notting Hill Gate), sometimes involve a collective inversion of normal behaviour and roles. For example, in their study of the carnival in St Vincent, West Indies, and 'belsnickling' (a form of Christmas mumming) on La Have Islands, Nova Scotia, Abrahams and Bauman[2] described how they both involve 'a high degree of symbolic inversion, transvestism, men dressed as animals or supernatural beings, sexual licence and other behaviours that are the opposite of what is supposed to characterize everyday life'. In a Western setting, such temporarily 'abnormal' social behaviour is often found at New Year's Eve parties, April Fool's Day, fancy dress balls, university 'Rags', Christmas office parties, Halloween, as well as at major sporting events, and on vacations far from home. Many tourists, especially those on trips to distant, poorer countries, dress and act in ways that are opposite to their normal life back home, especially in terms of sexual and drinking behaviour. Similar alterations or inversions of normal role behaviour are found in some of the spirit possession cults of African women, described by Lewis,[3] where women who seek power and aspire to roles otherwise monopolized by men 'act out thrusting male parts with impunity and with the full approval of the audience'. To some extent, *war* can also be described as a form of 'controlled abnormality', whereby soldiers are permitted to break one of the major taboos of social life – killing another person – but only under 'controlled' conditions. All these forms of 'abnormal' behaviour in public by large crowds of people are, however, strictly *controlled* by norms, since their timing and location are clearly defined and structured in advance, and after they end the participants are expected to return, as soon as possible, to their 'normal' everyday behaviour.

Individual behaviour

On a more individual level, displays of behaviour that are 'abnormal' by the standards of everyday life must also be seen against the background of the culture in which they appear. Like the crowd behaviour at a carnival or 'rite of reversal', they are also controlled (to a variable extent) by implicit cultural norms that determine how and when they may appear. In many cultures, especially in the non-industrialized world, individuals involved in interpersonal conflicts, or who are experiencing feelings of unhappiness, guilt, anger or helplessness, are able to express these feelings in a standardized language of distress (see Chapter 5). This may be purely verbal, or coded in a language of physical symptoms or involve extreme changes in dress, behaviour or posture. To the Western-trained observer, some of these languages of distress may closely resemble the diagnostic entities of the Western psychiatric model. For example, they may involve statements such as 'I've been bewitched', 'I've been possessed by a spirit (or by God)' or 'I can hear the voices of my ancestors speaking to me'. In a Western setting, people making this type of statement are likely to be diagnosed as 'psychotic, probably schizophrenic'.

However, it should be remembered that in many parts of the world people freely admit to being 'possessed' by supernatural forces, to having 'spirits' speak and act through them, and to having had dreams or visions that conveyed an important message to them. In most cases this is not considered by their communities to be evidence of mental illness. One example is the widespread belief, especially in parts of Africa, of *spirit possession* as a cause of mental or physical ill health. Women especially are the victims of possession by malign, pathogenic spirits that reveal their identity by the specific symptoms or behavioural changes that they cause. In these societies, Lewis[3] notes that possession is a normative experience and, whether or not people are actually in a trance, they are only possessed when they consider they are, and when other members of their society endorse this claim. That is not to say that spirit possession is 'normal',

in the sense that most people expect to be possessed during their life. Rather, it is a culture-specific way of presenting and explaining a range of physical and psychological disorders in certain circumstances. In these societies: 'belief in spirits and in possession by them is normal and accepted. The reality of possession by spirits, or for that matter of witchcraft, constitutes an integral part of the total system of religious ideas and assumptions. Where people thus believe generally that the affliction can be caused through possession by a malevolent spirit (or by witchcraft), disbelief in the power of spirits (or of witches) would be a striking abnormality, a bizarre and eccentric rejection of normal values. The cultural and mental alienation of such dissenters would in fact be roughly equivalent to that of those who in our secular society today believe themselves to be possessed or bewitched'.[3]

Possession, then, is an 'abnormal' form of individual behaviour, but one that conforms with cultural values, and whose expression is closely controlled by cultural norms. These norms provide guidelines as to who is allowed to be possessed, in what circumstances and in what way, as well as how this possession is to be signalled to other people.

Another form of controlled abnormal behaviour by individuals is *glossolalia*, or speaking in unknown tongues. To those who believe in it, it is thought to result from a supernatural power entering into the individual, with 'control of the organs of speech by the Holy Spirit, who prays through the speaker in a heavenly language'.[4] It is a dissociative, trance-like state in which the participants 'tend to have their eyes closed, they may make twitching movements and fall; they flush, sweat and may tear at their clothes'. It is a feature of religious practices in parts of India, the Caribbean, Africa, Southern Europe, North America and among many Pentecostal churches in the UK (including those with West Indian congregations). There are believed to be about two million practitioners of glossolalia in the USA in various denominations, including some Lutheran,

Episcopalian and Presbyterian churches. Glossolalia usually takes place in a specified context (the church) and at specified times during the service. It can be seen as a form of 'controlled abnormality' that, to a Western-trained psychiatrist, might seem evidence of a mental illness. However, there is no evidence that this is the case. On the contrary, there is some evidence from various cultures that 'in any particular denomination, those members of it who speak in tongues are better adjusted than those who do not'.[4] In one study, a comparison between a group of schizophrenic patients from the Caribbean and West Indian Pentecostals suggested that the Pentecostals believed that the patients 'were unable to control their dissociative behaviour sufficiently to conform with the highly stylized rituals of glossolalia in church'.[4] Although both groups might appear to practise similar glossolalia, it was the culturally *uncontrolled* form that was regarded as mental illness by members of that community.

As described above, the 'abnormal' behaviours at the controlled end of the spectrum (Figure 10.1, B) frequently overlap with religious and cosmological practices, as in glossolalia, spirit possession and the use of hallucinogens in religious rituals, and also the healing rites of the *shaman* (see Chapter 8). The latter is a form of sacred folk healer who is found in many cultures. The shaman, often known as a 'master of spirits', becomes voluntarily possessed by them in controlled circumstances and, in a divinatory séance, both diagnoses and treats the misfortune (and illness) of the community. In some cases, such as the *vegatalistas* of the Andes region, they may go into a trance with the aid of a hallucinogenic drug (such as *ayahuasca*). To a Western psychiatrist, the behaviour of the shaman during his trance may closely resemble that of the schizophrenic. However, shamans in their ritual performances act in conformity with cultural beliefs and practices, and in the selection of shamans, frankly psychotic or schizophrenic individuals are screened out as being too idiosyncratic and unreliable for the rigours of the shamanic role.[3]

Another example of long-term 'controlled abnormality' is the Hindu *sadhu*, the holy man or wandering ascetic who renounces all material possessions and, relying on charity for their daily needs, devotes themselves exclusively to religious practices. Often they walk about naked, their bodies smeared with ashes, their hair, beards and nails long and uncut. To some Western observers, this may appear evidence of 'self-neglect' or even of mental illness, but to the communities in which they live and wander the *sadhus*' ascetic behaviour makes cultural sense, and is greatly revered.

At various points along the spectrum of 'controlled abnormal' behaviours (Figure 10.1, B), the different *culture-bound* or *context-bound* mental illnesses can also be located. These conditions, described below, are all under the control of social norms to a variable extent. For example, their timing and setting may be unpredictable, but the clinical presentation of their symptoms and behaviour changes are not chaotic but patterned by the culture in which they appear. Also, unlike the severe uncontrolled psychosis in the East African example (Figure 10.1, C), a culturally explicable cause for them can usually be found – such as *susto* following an unexpected accident or fright, or *evil eye* resulting from, for example, an extravagant lifestyle that was bound to attract envy. These conditions do not occur in the formalized setting of temple or ritual, but cultural factors influence their presentation, recognition and treatment.

'Uncontrolled abnormality'

In every society, there is a spectrum between what people regard as 'normal' and 'abnormal' social behaviour. However, as the examples of glossolalia, spirit possession and carnivals illustrate, there is also a spectrum of 'abnormal' behaviour – from controlled to uncontrolled forms of abnormality. As with the abnormal, uncontrolled drinking behaviour (drunkenness) described in Chapter 8, it is behaviour at the *uncontrolled* end of the spectrum that cultures regard as a major social problem, and that they label as either 'mad' (Figure 10.1, C) or 'bad' (Figure 10.1, D). According to Foster and Anderson[5] 'there is no culture in which men and women remain oblivious to erratic, disturbed, threatening or bizarre behaviour in their midst, whatever the culturally defined context of that behaviour'. According to Kiev[6], the symptoms that would suggest mental disorder include uncontrollable anxiety, depression and agitation, delirium and other gross breaks of contact with reality, and violence both to the community and to self. In one study by Edgerton,[7] lay beliefs about what behaviour constitutes madness or psychosis was examined in four East African tribes; two in Kenya, one in Uganda and one in Tanzania (Tanganyika). It was found that all four societies shared a broad area of agreement as to what behaviours suggested a diagnosis of 'madness'. These included such actions as violent conduct, wandering around naked, 'talking nonsense' or 'sleeps and hides in the bush'. In each case, the respondents qualified their description of psychotic behaviour by saying that it occurred 'without reason'. That is, violence, wandering around naked, and so on, occurred without an apparent purpose, and in the absence of any identifiable and acceptable external cause (such as witchcraft, drunkenness or simply malicious intent). Edgerton notes how this catalogue of abnormal behaviours is not markedly at variance with Western definitions of psychosis, particularly schizophrenia. In these cultures, as elsewhere in the world, behaviour is labelled as 'mad' (Figure 10.1, C) if it is abnormal, not controlled by social norms, and has no discernible cause or purpose. Cross-culturally then, the extremes of 'uncontrolled abnormality' largely overlap with psychiatry's classification of the major psychoses, such as schizophrenia and bipolar disorder.

On rare occasions, the label of 'temporary madness' may be also applied to certain types of behaviour – usually to cases of mass hysteria, intoxication by alcohol or drugs, or 'crimes of passion' (the *crime passionnel* in France).

'Uncontrolled normality'

Certain other behaviours, also uncontrolled by social norms, are still regarded by society as being 'normal', even though they are classified as socially undesirable and often illegal. These are the behaviours classified as 'bad' or 'criminal' (Figure 10.1, D); in these cases, persons convicted of a crime would be regarded as guilty but 'normal'. Society recognizes that wherever there are rules, there are some individuals that will break those rules. If brought to trial, the issue debated by their lawyers and by forensic psychiatrists would be the accused's awareness (or lack of awareness) of what the social norms or laws of their society are and whether they had 'insight', were responsible for their actions and 'knew right from wrong'. If they did know, then they would be guilty and deserve punishment, as opposed to being mentally ill, and deserving treatment. Historically, in some Western countries, a number of behaviour patterns that were once considered 'crimes' were later reclassified as a 'disease' or 'disorder': they have included illegitimacy, truancy, substance abuse, masturbation and homosexuality – which was included as a 'sociopathic personality disturbance' in the 1952 *Diagnostic and Statistical Manual of Mental Disorders* (DSM-I), then as a 'sexual deviation' in the 1968 version (DSM-II), and only completely declassified as a mental disorder by the American Psychiatric Association in 1973 (see below).[8]

Advantages of 'abnormality'

Under certain circumstances, 'abnormal' behaviour – whether 'controlled' or 'uncontrolled' – can be of definite advantage to some individuals: emotionally, socially, or even economically. Examples of this may include adopting the 'sick role' (see Chapter 5), suffering 'spirit possession', being the victim of witchcraft or entering a shamanic trance, as well as some forms of malingering or hypochondria. In each case, a certain type of behavioural 'performance' may well bring the individual a great deal more care and attention, more sympathy, more social support, or even financial benefits.

On a group level, taking part in a carnival or festival may also be very satisfying, bringing with it a joyful catharsis and a strong sense of community. In economic terms, behaviour at the less extreme end of 'uncontrolled abnormality' may also be advantageous, at least in the short-term. An example of this is the 'Type-A Behaviour Pattern' (TABP), described by cardiologists: the type of individual who is aggressive, ambitious, competitive, chronically impatient, and obsessed with deadlines (see Chapter 11). Although they are apparently more prone to coronary heart disease than more relaxed people, 'Type A's' are often very successful (at least in their early years) in business, politics or the professions, and often become top managers, executives, politicians or academics. Is the TABP therefore as 'pathological' as the medical textbooks suggest? Similarly, Martin[9] has suggested that in contemporary USA, changes in economic and social patterns have increased the focus on a new type of individual: one who is entrepreneurial, competitive, flexible, creative, hyperaware of their environment, and the 'proprietor or his or her self as a portfolio'. This type of person is highly valued in the new economic milieu, as well as in the artistic and creative professions, and for that reason 'manic-depression' (bipolar disorder) and 'attention deficit hyperactivity disorder' (ADHD) are increasingly being redefined as an *asset*, not as a liability. As Martin states: 'the qualities of the "manic style" fit well with the kind of person frequently described as highly desirable in corporate America: always adapting by scanning the environment for signs of change, flying from one thing to another, while pushing the limits of everything, and doing it all with an intense level of energy focused totally on the future'.[9]

THE COMPARISON OF PSYCHOLOGICAL DISORDERS

Given the marked variation in cultural definitions of 'normal' and 'abnormal' throughout the world, can meaningful comparisons be made between mental illness in different groups and societies? Landy[10] has summarized two of the questions faced by medical anthropologists and cross-cultural psychiatrists who have examined this problem:

1 Can we speak of some aspects of behaviour as normal or abnormal in a pan-human sense (that is, specific to the human species)?
2 Are the psychoses of Western psychiatric experience and nosology universal and transcultural, or are they strongly shaped by cultural pressures and conditioning?

The answers to both these questions are important, since they determine whether mental illness can be adequately diagnosed and treated cross-culturally, and whether the prevalence rates of mental illness in different cultures can be compared. They would also shed light on why some forms of mental illness seem to be more common in some parts of the world than in others.

In examining notions of 'abnormality' in the section above, most of the emphasis has been on abnormal *social behaviour* rather than on organic disorders or on emotional state. For most medical anthropologists the social and cultural dimensions of mental illness are the main areas of study. This is because cultural factors influence the clinical presentation and recognition of many of these disorders, even those with an organic basis. In addition, in many parts of the Third World (and elsewhere) mental illness is perceived as 'abnormal action' rather than 'mistaken belief'.[11] Diagnosing mental illness by psychological state, such as the presence of a delusion, may be difficult where the content of the delusion is shared by other members of the society. For example, in some cultures a person who accuses a neighbour of having bewitched him may initially be perceived as acting in an acceptable, rational way for that society. He will only be viewed as 'mad' or psychotic if his accusations are then followed by 'mal-adaptive personal violence rather than the employment of the accepted communal technique for dealing with sorcery'.[11] In this case, the diagnosis of mental illness by a Western-trained doctor would depend not only on his or her own clinical observations, based on assessment of the affected person's behaviour, biological changes (such as anorexia, insomnia and loss of libido) and response to certain psychological tests, but also on how the affected person's behaviour is perceived by his own community. The problem, therefore, in comparing mental illness in different societies, is whether to compare Western clinical evaluations of patients in different cultures, or the perceptions by various cultures of those that they regard as mentally ill.

Those who have examined this problem in more detail have tended to take one of three approaches; the *biological* approach, the *social labelling* approach or the *combined* approach.

THE BIOLOGICAL APPROACH

This approach sees the diagnostic categories of the Western psychiatric model as being universally applicable to mankind, despite local variations caused by cultural factors, since they have a *biological* basis. In Kiev's[12] view, the forms of psychiatric disorders remain essentially constant throughout the world irrespective of the cultural context in which they appear. According to Kiev,[12] for example, 'the schizophrenic and manic-depressive psychotic disorders are fixed in form by the biological nature of man, while the secondary features of mental illness, such as the *content* of delusions and hallucinations are, in contrast, influenced by cultural factors'. On this basis, Kiev[13] proceeds to classify the various culture-bound disorders within the diagnostic categories of the Western model. For example, *koro*, *susto* and bewitchment are forms of anxiety; the Japanese *shinkeishitsu* is an obsessional compulsive neurosis; evil eye and voodoo death are examples of phobic states; and spirit possession, *amok* in Malaya and *Hsieh ping* in China are all examples of dissociative states. In Kiev's opinion, these conditions 'are not new diagnostic entities; they are in fact similar to those already known in the West'.[13]

This approach, which is similar to the view of diseases as universal entities (see Chapter 5), has been criticized for the primacy it gives to the Western diagnostic and labelling system[14,15]. In addition, Western categories of mental illness are also 'culture-bound', as well as being the product of specific social and historical circumstances, and are therefore not necessarily pan-human in their applicability. For example, Kleinman[16] has criticized the World Health Organization (WHO) International Pilot Study of Schizophrenia, which compared schizophrenia in a number of Western and non-Western societies. He points out that the study enforced a definition of schizophrenic symptomatology, and that this definition may have distorted the findings by 'patterning the behaviour observed by the investigators and systematically filtering out local cultural influences in order to preserve a homogeneous cross-cultural sample'. Applying the Western model of, say, schizophrenia to other parts of the world may therefore be an example of what Kleinman[16] terms a *category fallacy* – that is, 'the reification of a nosological category developed for a particular cultural group that is then applied to members of another culture for whom it lacks coherence and its validity has not been established'. The danger of category fallacies is therefore implicit in much of the biological approach, and in its attempt to fit exotic illnesses into a universal, diagnostic framework[17]. Kirmayer and Minas[18] point out that the increasing 'biologization' of psychiatry in recent years – with its growing emphasis on brain dysfunction, and the physical or genetic basis of mental illness – increases this possibility, even if modern psychiatry does pay some lip-service to the role of culture.

A further critique of the biological approach is that the *same* mental illness may play *different* social roles in different societies. For a fuller understanding of an episode of that mental illness in another culture, one must always know something of the *context* – social, cultural, political and economic – in which it has taken place. For example, in some small-scale societies a psychotic episode may be viewed as evidence of an underlying social conflict, which must be resolved by a public ritual, while the same psychosis is unlikely to play such a central role in the life of a Western, urban community.

THE SOCIAL LABELLING APPROACH

This perspective, developed by sociologists, sees mental illness as a 'myth', essentially a *social* rather than a biological fact, and one that can appear with or without biological components. Society decides what symptoms or behaviour patterns are to be defined as deviant, or as that special type of deviance called 'mental illness'. This mental illness does not appear until it is so labelled, and had no prior existence. Once the diagnostic label is applied, it is difficult to discard. According to Waxler,[19] mental illness is only defined relative to the society in which it is found and cannot be said to have a universal existence. She notes how, in Western societies, social withdrawal, lack of energy and feelings of sadness are commonly labelled 'depression', while in Sri Lanka the same phenomena receive less attention and very little treatment. The definition of mental illness is thus culture-specific. The process of labelling involves a first stage, where an individual's minor deviant behaviour is labelled as 'mental illness'. There are, however, certain culture-specific contingencies under which potential deviants are immune from this labelling, and these include the individual's power relative to the labeller (based on his or her age, sex, race, economic position, etc.). Once individuals are labelled as 'mentally ill', they are subject to a number of cultural cues that tell them *how* to play their role; that is, 'the mentally ill person learns how to be sick in a way his particular society understands'. Once labelled, individuals are dependent on the society at large for 'de-labelling' them and releasing them from the sick role, and in some cases they may never be able to free themselves from this role. The value of the social labelling perspective is that it sheds light on the *social* construction and maintenance of the symptomatology of mental illness. Since this mental illness only exists by virtue of the society that

defines it, 'mental illness' is a relative concept and cannot easily be compared between different societies. This perspective has been criticized for its neglect of the biological aspect of mental illness, especially in those conditions where this is a definite feature (such as brain tumours, delirium tremens, dementia or cerebral malaria). It also ignores the more extreme psychoses, which do seem to be universal in distribution.

THE COMBINED APPROACH

This uses elements of both the biological and the social labelling perspectives, and is the one most medical anthropologists would agree with. In this view, there *are* certain universals in abnormal behaviour, particularly extreme disturbances in conduct, thought or affect. While there is wide variation in their form and distribution, the Western categories of major psychoses, such as 'schizophrenia' and 'manic depressive psychosis', are found throughout the world, though of course they may be given different labels in different cultures. An example of this, the similarity to Western definitions of psychosis of folk categories of 'mad' behaviour in four East African tribes, has already been described above.[7] The major psychoses, therefore, as well as disorders arising from organic brain disease, seem to be recognized in all societies, though their clinical presentations are usually influenced by the local culture. For example, psychotics in a tribal society may say that their behaviour is being controlled by powerful witches or sorcerers, while Western psychotics may feel controlled by spacemen, Martians or flying saucers. Those who suffer these extreme psychological disorders are usually perceived by their own cultures as exhibiting 'uncontrolled abnormal' (Figure 10.1, C) forms of social behaviour. To a variable extent their clinical pictures can be compared between societies. Foster and Anderson[5] have suggested that this comparison should be between their *symptom patterns* rather than between diagnostic categories (such as schizophrenia); on this basis, the problem of trying to fit other cultures'

mental illnesses into Western diagnostic categories can be overcome.

The comparison of symptom patterns can also be carried out for the culture-bound disorders described below, many of which could be classified as 'neuroses' or 'functional psychoses' in the Western psychiatric model. These conditions, especially those with a preponderance of neurotic or somatic symptoms, are probably more difficult to compare than are the major psychoses. Many of them do seem to be unique clusters of symptoms and behaviour changes, which only make sense within a particular context and within a particular culture, and have no equivalent in other societies. The specific symptom patterns of *susto*, for example, are unlikely to be found in the UK, at least not among the native-born population. Not only does culture closely pattern their clinical presentations, but the *meanings* of these conditions for the victim, their family and community are difficult for a Western observer to evaluate or quantify. Nevertheless, anthropologists such as Rubel[20] believe that these folk illnesses have a fairly constant clinical presentation within a culture, and can therefore be quantified and investigated using standard epidemiological techniques (see Chapter 15).

CULTURAL AND SOCIAL INFLUENCES ON PSYCHIATRIC DIAGNOSIS

Before psychological disorders can be compared, they have to be diagnosed. In recent years a number of studies have indicated some of the difficulties in standardizing psychiatric diagnoses, particularly among psychiatrists working in different countries. Variations in the clinical criteria used to diagnose schizophrenia, for example, have been found between British and American psychiatrists and British and French psychiatrists, and among psychiatrists working within these countries. Some of the diagnostic categories in French psychiatry, such as 'chronic delusional states' (*délires chroniques*) and 'transitory delusional states' (*bouffées delirantes*), are significantly differ-

ent from the diagnostic categories of Anglo-American psychiatry.[21] A further example was the diagnostic category 'sluggish schizophrenia' in Soviet psychiatry, which was virtually limited to the former USSR.[22] All of these discrepancies in diagnostic behaviour among psychiatrists are important, since they affect both the treatment and prognosis of mental illness as well as the reliability of comparing morbidity statistics for these conditions between different countries.

Part of the reason for these differences lies in the nature of psychiatric diagnosis, and the categories into which it places psychological disorders. Unlike the diagnosis of medical 'diseases', there is often little evidence of typical biological malfunctioning, as revealed by diagnostic technology. Where biological evidence does exist, it is often difficult to relate this to specific clinical symptoms. Most psychiatric diagnoses are based on the doctor's subjective evaluation of the patient's appearance, speech and behaviour, as well as performance in certain standardized psychometric tests. The aim is to fit the symptoms and signs into a known category of mental illness by their similarity to the 'typical' textbook description of the condition. However, according to Kendell,[23] the way that psychiatrists learn how to do this may actually make diagnostic differences among them more likely. He points out how the majority of patients encountered by trainee psychiatrists do not possess the 'typical' cluster of symptoms of a particular condition. They may have some of the symptoms but not others, or have symptoms typical of another condition. As a result, trainee psychiatrists learn how to assign diagnoses largely by the example of their clinical teachers: 'He sees what sorts of patient his teachers regard as schizophrenics, and copies them'. So while young psychiatrists see many 'typical' cases of various disorders during their studies, their diagnostic behaviour tends to be modelled on that of their teachers, rather than using the stricter criteria of their textbooks. As a result, 'diagnostic concepts are not securely anchored. They are at the mercy of the personal views and idiosyncrasies of influential teachers, of therapeutic fashions and innovations, of changing assumptions about aetiology, and many other less tangible influences to boot'.[23]

Among these influences, Kendell[24] cites the personality and experience of the psychiatrist, the length of his diagnostic interview, and his styles of information-gathering and decision-making. To this list can be added the psychiatrist's social class, ethnic or cultural background (especially its definition of 'normality' and 'abnormality'), as well as prejudices, religious or political affiliations, and the context in which diagnosis takes place.

An example of how these influences work in practice was provided by Temerlin's[25] classic experiment in 1968. Three groups of psychiatrists and clinical psychologists were each shown a videotaped interview with an actor who had been trained to give a convincing account of normal behaviour. Before the viewing, one of the audiences was allowed to overhear a high-prestige figure comment that the patient was 'a very interesting man because he looked neurotic but actually was quite psychotic'. The second group were allowed to overhear the remark, 'I think this is a very rare person, a perfectly healthy man', while the third group was given no suggestions at all. All three audiences were asked to diagnose the 'patient's' condition. In the first group of 95 people, 60 diagnosed a neurosis or personality disorder, 27 diagnosed psychosis (usually schizophrenia), and only eight stated that he was mentally normal. In the second group, all 20 people diagnosed the 'patient' as normal, while only 12 of the 21 members of the third group also diagnosed normality; the other nine diagnosed neurosis or personality disorders.

Another factor enhancing the subjective element in psychiatric diagnosis is the diffuse and changeable nature of the diagnostic categories themselves. Kendell[26] points out that many of these categories tend to overlap, and ill people may fit into different categories at different times as their illnesses evolve. Each category or syndrome is made up of the 'typical' clinical features, but as he notes: 'Many of these clinical features, like depression and anxiety, are graded traits present to vary-

ing extents in different people and at different times. Furthermore, few of them are pathognomonic of individual illnesses. In general, it is the overall pattern of symptomatology and its evolution over time that distinguishes one category of illness from another, rather than the presence of key individual symptoms'.[26]

However, psychiatrists differ on whether to adopt this historical approach or whether to focus mainly on the individual's current mental state, as indicated by the degree of 'insight' displayed, or behaviour at the clinical interview. There is also a difference of opinion as to what explanatory model should be used to shape this diffuse clinical picture into a recognizable diagnostic entity. Eisenberg[27] notes that Western psychiatry is not an internally consistent body of knowledge, and that it includes within it many different ways of viewing mental illness. For example, its perspective on the psychoses includes 'multiple and manifestly contradictory models', such as the medical (biological) model, the psychodynamic model, the behavioural model and the social labelling model. Each of these approaches emphasizes a different aspect of the clinical picture, and proposes a different line of treatment. The choice of explanatory model, and of diagnostic label, may sometimes be as much a matter of temperament as of training.

THE POLITICAL ROLE OF PSYCHIATRY

Political and *moral* considerations can play a part in the choice of psychiatric diagnosis. In some cases, psychiatrists may be called upon to decide whether a particular form of socially deviant behaviour is 'mad' or 'bad'. In the Western world this is common as part of the judiciary system, but has also been applied to such conditions as homosexuality, alcoholism, truancy or obesity. Critics of psychiatry such as Szasz[28] have also argued that confining lawbreakers to psychiatric hospitals, ostensibly for treatment (that is, labelling them as 'mad' rather than 'bad'), is just another form of punishment, but without the benefits of a proper defence and trial. Psychiatrists making these decisions are likely to be under the influence of social and political forces, the opinions of their colleagues, and their own moral viewpoints and prejudices. In some societies, many forms of political dissent are labelled as mental illness. The state and its supporters are assumed to have a monopoly of truth, and disagreement with them is considered to be clear evidence of psychosis. Wing[29] has described a number of these cases in different countries where state psychiatrists have labelled dissent as 'madness', especially in the former USSR, where, according to Merskey and Shafran[22], political dissidents who opposed the Soviet system were often diagnosed as having 'sluggish schizophrenia' and then confined to mental hospitals against their will.

The mislabelling of dissenting behaviour as 'madness' has a long history. In 1851, for example, before the American Civil War, a certain Dr Samuel A. Cartwright writing in the *New Orleans Medical and Surgical Journal* argued that black slaves were suffering from two types of mental illness. One was *drapetomania*, whose main symptom was 'absconding from service' – the uncontrollable urge to escape from slavery. He described it as 'as much a disease of the mind as any other species of mental alienation, and much more curable'.[30] The treatment recommended included whipping the slave, or even amputating their toes. Another syndrome he described was *dysathesia aethiopica*, where the slaves' 'abnormal' behaviour included being disobedient, destroying the plantation, and refusing to work – a disorder their overseers called 'Rascality'. In this way, slave owners in the South were reassured by Dr Cartwright that it was mental illness, not the harsh conditions of slavery, that made their slaves seek freedom.

In their study of mental illness among immigrants to the UK, Littlewood and Lipsedge[11] suggest that psychiatry can still sometimes be used as a form of social control, by misinterpreting the religious and other behaviour of some Afro-Caribbean patients (as well as their response to

discrimination) as evidence of schizophrenia. Although there is a high rate of schizophrenia among Afro-Caribbeans, depression is rarely diagnosed, and the authors suggest that 'whatever the empirical justification, the frequent diagnosis in black patients of schizophrenia (bizarre, irrational, outside) and the infrequent diagnosis of depression (acceptable, understandable, inside) validates our stereo-types'.[31] In dealing with immigrants and the poor, they warn against psychiatry's role in 'disguising disadvantage as disease'. Other researchers, however, while agreeing that ethnic and racial prejudices do exist among UK psychiatrists, dispute that this alone leads to an overdiagnosis of schizophrenia among Afro-Caribbeans. Lewis and colleagues,[32] for example, in their 1990 study of 139 British psychiatrists, did find evidence of stereotyping and 'race-thinking' towards Afro-Caribbean patients – judging them as potentially more violent, less suitable for medication, but more suitable for criminal proceedings than white patients. Presented with identical vignettes of black and white patients, they were more likely to diagnose cannabis psychosis and acute reactive psychosis among the black patients, but less likely to diagnose schizophrenia. Thus, while confirming the role of prejudice in psychiatric diagnosis, they found no evidence of a 'greater readiness to detain patients compulsorily or to manage them on a locked ward merely on the grounds of "race"'. Thomas and colleagues,[33] in a study of compulsory psychiatric admissions in Manchester in 1993, found that second-generation (UK-born) Afro-Caribbeans had nine times the rate of schizophrenia of whites. However, this could largely be explained by their greater socio-economic disadvantage, with poor inner-city housing and higher rates of unemployment – all of which have been correlated with high rates of schizophrenia – rather than by psychiatric misdiagnosis. They therefore suggest that 'efforts aimed at improving social disadvantage and the provision of employment for ethnic minority groups may improve the mental health of such groups'. Wesseley and colleagues[34] in 1991 also found higher rates of schizophrenia among Afro-Caribbeans in south London, irrespective of their place of birth, compared with other groups, but these differences could also mostly be explained by the greater social adversity they suffered rather than by their ethnicity. However, many of these studies have not yet been replicated in ethnic minorities throughout the UK, and some aspects of their methodology can be seen as problematic. It is difficult, for example, to define the precise inter-relationships of 'race', 'culture', 'ethnicity' and 'social class' within a society. Furthermore, the classification of people by ethnic group – such as 'Afro-Caribbean', 'Asian' or 'white' – is in itself problematic, since each of these groups is not homogeneous and contains within it people from very different backgrounds. Rates of a particular psychiatric diagnosis in a particular community are also not the whole story; the political and socio-economic *context* in which this diagnosis takes place, and the *meanings* attached to it, are equally important. A final, relevant issue is the degree to which different communities have been offered equal access to treatments such as psychotherapy, and whether this psychotherapy was culturally appropriate or not.

Eisenberg[27] mentioned another example of how deviant behaviour can be given a moral (bad) or medical (mad) diagnosis. The same constellation of symptoms and signs (including weakness, sweating, palpitations and chest pain on effort) can, in the absence of physical findings, be diagnosed either as 'neurocirculatory aesthenia' or 'Da Costa's syndrome' (and thus as a medical problem), or as the symptoms of cowardice (and thus a moral problem) if they appear in a soldier during battle. This is illustrated also by the gradual shift, since the turn of the century, from moral definitions of 'cowardice' or 'weakness' among military personnel to more recent medicalized definitions such as 'shell shock', 'battle fatigue' or 'post-traumatic stress disorder' (PTSD). More recently, Blackburn[35] has also suggested that the psychiatric definition of the 'psychopathic personality' is 'little more than a moral judgement masquerading as a clinical diagnosis'.

SUMMARY

In summary, this section suggests that, to some extent, both psychiatric knowledge and practice are themselves cultural constructions.[15] It also suggests that there are a number of factors that can affect the standardization of psychiatric diagnostic concepts between different societies. These include the lack of hard physiological data, the vagueness of diagnostic categories, the range of explanatory models available, the subjective aspect in diagnosis, and the influence of social, cultural and political forces on the process of diagnosis. Some of the differences in diagnosis between psychiatrists in different Western countries, and within a single country, are illustrated in the following case studies carried out between 1969 and 1993.

Case study: differences in psychiatric diagnosis in the UK and the USA – 1

Cooper and colleagues[36] in 1969 examined some of the reasons for the marked variations in the frequency of various diagnoses made by British and American hospital psychiatrists. Hospitals in the two countries differ in their admission rates (as noted on the hospital records) for the condition 'manic-depressive psychosis'. In the UK, for some age groups, admission for this condition is over 10 times more frequent than in US state mental hospitals. The authors posed the problem: 'Are the differences in official statistics due to differences between the doctors and the recording systems, or do both play a part?' That is, was the actual prevalence of manic-depressive psychosis different in the two cities (London and New York), or were the differences in admission rates caused by the diagnostic terms and concepts used by the two groups of hospital psychiatrists? At a mental hospital in each city, 145 consecutive admissions in the age range of 35–59 years were studied. These were assessed by the project psychiatrists, and diagnosed according to objective, standardized criteria. These diagnoses were then compared with those given by the hospital psychiatrists. Hospital staff in both cities were found to diagnose 'schizophrenia' more frequently and 'affective disorders' (including manic-depressive psychosis and depressive neurosis) less frequently than did the project psychiatrists. Both these trends were more marked in the New York sample. While differences in the incidence of the various disorders were found by the project staff between the cities, these differences were less significant than the hospital diagnoses suggest. The hospital psychiatrists appeared to exaggerate these differences by diagnosing schizophrenia more readily in New York, and affective illness more readily in London. The study does not reveal, however, how the cultural differences between the two groups of psychiatrists affected their diagnostic behaviour.

Case study: differences in psychiatric diagnosis in the UK and the USA – 2

Katz and colleagues[37] in 1969 examined the process of psychiatric diagnosis among both British and American psychiatrists in more detail. The study aimed to discover whether disagreements among these diagnoses were 'a function of differences in their actual perception of the patient or patients on whose symptoms and behaviour they are in agreement'. Groups of British and American psychiatrists were shown films of interviews with patients, and asked to note down all pathological symptoms and make a diagnosis. Marked disagreements in diagnosis between the two groups were found, as well as different patterns of symptomatology perceived. The British psychiatrists saw less pathology generally, less evidence of the key diagnostic symptoms 'retardation' and 'apathy', and little or no 'paranoid projection' or 'perceptual distortion'. Conversely, they saw more 'anxious intropunitiveness' than did the American psychiatrists. Perceiving less of these key symptoms led the British psychiatrists to diagnose schizophrenia less frequently. For example, one patient was diagnosed as 'schizophrenic' by one-

third of the American psychiatrists, but by none of the British psychiatrists. The authors conclude that 'ethnic background apparently influences choice of diagnosis and perception of symptomatology'.

Case study: differences in psychiatric diagnosis within the UK

Copeland and colleagues[38] in 1971 studied differences in diagnostic behaviour among 200 British psychiatrists, all of whom had at least four years in full-time practice and possessed similar qualifications. They were shown videotapes of interviews with three patients, and asked to rate their abnormal traits on a standardized scale and to assign the patients to diagnostic categories. There was fairly good agreement on diagnoses among the sample, except that psychiatrists trained in Glasgow had a significant tendency to make a diagnosis of 'affective illness' in one of the tapes, where the choice of diagnosis was between affective illness and schizophrenia. In addition, psychiatrists trained at the Maudsley Hospital, London, gave lower ratings of abnormal behaviour on the patients than the rest, while older psychiatrists and those with psychotherapeutic training rated a higher level of abnormalities than did younger psychiatrists. The authors point out that rating behaviour as 'abnormal' is 'likely to be affected by the rater's attitude towards illness and health and what is normal and abnormal'. The survey illustrates, therefore, that differences in these attitudes are associated with differences in postgraduate psychiatric training, as well as with age.

Case study: differences in psychiatric diagnosis in England and France

Van Os and colleagues[39] in 1993 studied the concepts of schizophrenia held by a sample of 92 British and 60 French psychiatrists. They found major differences in how each group conceptualized the aetiology, diagnosis and management of the disorder. Overall, they seemed 'to have been particularly affected by the traditional divide between Anglo-Saxon empiricism and continental rationalism – between trying to reach the truth through experiment and trying to reach it through ideas'. In France, psychoanalytic theories, which emphasize the aetiological role of family dynamics and parental factors, have been more influential, while in the UK psychiatry has been more linked to physical medicine and has focused more on neurodevelopmental and genetic causes. Similarly, in treatment the British psychiatrists preferred more biological and behavioural approaches compared with the French psychiatrists. The study also found major differences in the incidence of schizophrenia in the two countries. In France, the number of first admissions to psychiatric hospitals for this condition under the age of 45 years was much higher than in the UK, but much lower after 45 years. Also, rates of first admission for the period 1973–1982 were rising in France but falling in the UK. These apparent differences in the incidence of schizophrenia could largely be explained by the cultural and conceptual differences between the two groups of psychiatrists, and differences in the diagnostic criteria used. French psychiatrists were reluctant to diagnose schizophrenia after 45 years, and before that age the French concept of schizophrenia encompassed a number of other chronic psychological states (such as *heboidophrenic* or 'pseudopsychopathic' schizophrenia), which in the UK would not be included under the diagnosis of 'schizophrenia'.

CULTURAL PATTERNING OF PSYCHOLOGICAL DISORDERS

Each culture provides its members with ways of becoming 'ill', of shaping their suffering into a recognizable illness entity, of explaining its cause, and of getting some treatment for it. Some of the issues raised by this process, in the case of physical illness, have already been discussed in Chapter 5, and they apply equally to cases of psychological disorder. Lay explanations of these conditions fall into the same aetiological categories: personal behaviour and influences in the natural, social and supernatural worlds. Mental illness can therefore be explained by, for example, spirit possession, witchcraft, the breaking of religious taboos, divine retribution, and the 'capture' of the soul by a malevolent spirit. Foster and Anderson point out how these types of 'personalistic' explanations for mental illness are much more common in the non-Western world; in contrast, the Western perspective on mental illness emphasizes psychological factors, life experiences and the effects of stress as major aetiological factors. In recent years, it also increasingly emphasizes genetic and other biological causes of mental illness.

As with physical illness, cultures influence the 'language of distress' in which personal distress is *communicated* to other people. This 'language' includes the many culturally-specific definitions of 'abnormality', such as major changes in behaviour, speech, posture, facial expression, dress or personal hygiene. When it includes the verbal expression of emotional distress, including the description of hallucinations and delusions, it usually draws heavily on the symbols, imagery and motifs of the patient's own cultural milieu. For example, in Littlewood and Lipsedge's[40] study, 40 per cent of their patients with severe psychoses who had been born in the Caribbean and in Africa structured their illness in terms of a religious experience, compared with only 20 per cent of the white patients born in the UK. Similarly, Scheper-Hughes[41] points out that in rural Kerry in western Ireland, psychiatric patients showed a greater tendency to delusions of a religious nature, including the motifs of the Virgin and the Saviour, than would occur among American schizophrenics, who would be more likely to have 'secular or electromagnetic persecution delusions'. While possession by a malign spirit may be reported in parts of Africa, possession by 'Martians' or 'extra-terrestrials' is more likely among Western psychotics. Each culture thus provides a repertoire of symbols and imagery in which mental illness can be articulated, even at the 'uncontrolled abnormality' end of the spectrum. As with the ritual symbols described in Chapter 9, the symbols in which mental illness is expressed show polarization of meaning. On one hand they stand for personal psychological or emotional concerns and on the other they stand for the social and cultural values of the wider society. Where mentally ill people come from a cultural or ethnic minority, they often have to use the symbols of the dominant majority culture in order to articulate their psychological distress and obtain help.[42] That is, they have to internalize (or appear to internalize) the value system of the dominant culture, and to use the vocabulary that goes with these values. In some cases this may lead to an over-identification with the very people who are persecuting them, and with their prejudiced or racist beliefs. For example, Littlewood[4] described the case of 'Beatrice Jackson', a 34-year-old Jamaican widow in London, from a very religious background: as part of a psychotic breakdown, she strongly rejected her own 'blackness' as something within her that was evil, ugly and unacceptable, and believed that her breakdown had been caused by the machinations of the (black) devil. Littlewood describes how she had thus internalized the dominant racialist symbolism of both colonial Jamaica and of the England she had encountered, where 'black' represented badness, 'sin, sexual indulgence and dirt'. In her religion, too, 'black' represented hatred, evil (evil people were 'blackhearted'), devils, darkness and mourning, while 'white' was associated with 'religion, purity and renunciation', and both brides and angels were always dressed in white. She was therefore not only the victim of racism, but the content of her delusions was also expressed in a racist idiom, in terms of a white/black moral dichotomy.

SOMATIZATION

A problem frequently encountered in making psychiatric diagnoses cross-culturally is that of somatization (see Chapters 5 and 7), i.e. the cultural patterning of psychological and social disorders into a language of distress of mainly physical symptoms and signs. According to Swartz,[44] somatization is 'a way of speaking with the body'. This phenomenon has been reported from numerous cultures world-wide, and from a variety of socio-economic groups within those societies. It is particularly a feature of the clinical presentation of depression,[15] and of personal suffering and unhappiness. In these cases, depressed people often complain of a variety of diffuse and frequently changeable physical symptoms, such as 'tired all the time', headaches, palpitations, weight loss, dizziness, 'pains everywhere', and so on. They frequently deny feeling depressed, sad, or having any personal problems. Hussain and Gomersall[45], for example, described how depression among Asian immigrants in the UK often manifests primarily as somatic symptoms, especially generalized weakness, 'bowel consciousness', exaggerated fear of a heart attack, and concern about the health of genital organs, nocturnal emissions, and the loss of semen in urine (known as *dhat* or *jiryan*),[46] though the presence of these specific symptoms does not, of course, always mean depression.

Kleinman[47,48] points out how different cultures and social classes sometimes pattern unpleasant effects, such as depression, in different ways. For some, somatization represents a culturally specific way of coping with these effects, and functions to 'reduce or entirely block introspection as well as direct expression'. Unpleasant effects are expressed in a non-psychological idiom: 'I've got a pain' instead of 'I feel depressed'. He points out that in the USA this tends to be more common among poorer social classes – blue-collar workers with a high school education or less, and who have more traditional life styles – while *psychologization* (seeing depression as a psychological problem) is more common among upper middle-class professionals and executives with a college or graduate school education. Overall, however, the pattern of 'speaking with the body' is probably much more common world-wide, across a wide variety of social and cultural groups, than expressing distress and anxiety in purely abstract, psychological terms.[44]

In many cases, however, the distinction between somatization and psychologization is more theoretical than real. As illustrated in the case history by Ots (see below), ostensibly somatic symptoms may actually carry a powerful *emotional* message, clearly understood by both healer and patient. In a study in the UK in 1989, Krause[49] found that although Punjabi immigrants tended to somatize, they *were* able to articulate their distress in psychological terms, and even where somatic symptoms were present these were considered to express psychological as well as physical distress. Furthermore, even though psychologization – the use of abstract psychological terms or concepts to describe subjective mental states – is the notional opposite of somatization, it is also often couched in a somatic or non-psychological idiom. In everyday English, for example, emotional distress is often expressed in a somatic idiom: examples of this include 'broken hearted', 'a pain in the neck', 'full of joy', 'can't stomach something', 'a painful experience' and 'hungry for attention'. In the author's study in Massachusetts, USA in 1985,[50] patients with psychosomatic disorders often described their emotions and feelings as if they were tangible 'things' that somehow entered them and caused damage to their bodies: 'I tend to hold lots of things inside … Anger, tension, hostility, any kind of fear – I think of them as being crammed into my colon', 'I put negative feelings inside myself … Doctors often say anger gets stored in the colon'. This Western view of certain emotions (especially antisocial ones such as anger, fear or envy) as 'pathogens' or 'forces' that cause ill health or unhappiness, and which originate either within the self or in the outside world, has become increasingly common. In many cases they are believed to somehow accumulate within the individual, causing distress or illness in a particular part of the body, unless they 'can get it all out'.

In its modern form this echoes the remark by Henry Maudsley, the famous nineteenth century anatomist, that 'The sorrow that has no vent in tears makes other organs weep'.[51]

In Taiwan, Kleinman[47] describes how somatization is extremely common. In both Hokkien and Chinese, the two languages spoken on the island, there is an impoverishment of words referring to psychological states, and often words meaning 'troubled' or 'anxious' express these emotions in terms of bodily organs. Self-scrutiny is not encouraged, and as an American psychiatrist working there he found it 'extremely difficult to elicit personal ideas and feelings' from his Taiwanese patients.

Kirmayer and Young[52] have summarized the different ways that clinicians, psychiatrists and anthropologists have interpreted the phenomenon of somatization. Depending on their interpretive stance, they have seen such somatic symptoms as indicating one or more of the following:

- an index of disease or disorder
- a symbolic expression of intrapsychic conflict
- an indication of a specific psychopathology
- an idiomatic expression of distress
- a metaphor for experience
- an 'act of positioning' within a local world
- a form of social commentary or protest.

They point out both the complexity and widespread occurrence of somatization, and how our understanding of it may be a reflection of Western cultural ways of thinking – especially of our mind-body dualism.

Depression cross-culturally

Reviewing the cross-cultural literature on depression, Patel[15] points out the Western psychiatry focuses primarily on *mood change* as the core feature of depression: these usually include feelings of sadness, hopelessness and despair. However, he points out that in fact the commonest clinical presentation of depression is actually multiple *somatic* symptoms, of long duration, and that this applies to both Western and non-Western societies. These symptoms can include feelings of tiredness, weakness, multiple aches and pains, dizziness, palpitations, and sleep disturbances. However, the clinical presentation of depression is not only somatic: psychological symptoms can also be elicited relatively easily on enquiry – even in 'non-Western' communities. These may include a loss of interest in daily or social activities, suicidal thoughts, poor concentration, and excessive anxiety. Overall, whatever its presentation, the prevalence of depressive illness seems to be high across *all* cultures, whether in the industrialized world or not.

One problem in assessing depression cross-culturally, is that the Western diagnostic category of 'depression' – a condition closely linked to mood changes – often has no clear equivalent in some non-European languages. As Patel[15] notes, this often leads to 'the mistaken belief that the experience of sadness is an essential presenting feature of the disorder'. Furthermore, no clear differentiation is made in many of these languages between 'depression' and 'anxiety'. He suggests, therefore, that in trying to diagnose depression in a such a community, psychiatrists should strive to identify local concepts, such as *kufungisisa* in Zimbabwe, 'neurasthenia' in China, or *susto* in Latin America, which are similar (though not identical) to the psychiatric construct of depression, rather than imposing that construct upon them (the 'category fallacy').[16]

Overall, the use of somatization as a main language of distress (and expressing both psychological or social stresses), and across so many cultures, illustrates how important it is to understand it from a holistic point of view. This is particularly true in the case of depression. In any interpretation of somatization, then, the complex interweaving of psychological, physical and social states, in different contexts, must be taken into account in order to understand why some people somatize while others do not.

Two examples of somatization from China, one from Hong Kong, the other from Nanjing, are illustrated in the following case studies.

Case study: depression in Hong Kong

Lau and colleagues[53] in 1983 studied 213 cases of depression (142 females and 71 males) presenting to a private general practice in Hong Kong over a period of 6 months. The chief complaints that had prompted patients to consult their doctor were: epigastric discomfort (18.7 per cent); dizziness (12.2 per cent); headache (9.8 per cent); insomnia (8.4 per cent); general malaise (7.5 per cent); feverishness (4.7 per cent); cough (4.7 per cent); menstrual disturbances (3.3 per cent); and low back pain (3.3 per cent). Somatic symptoms were complained of initially by 96 per cent of the sample. Practically no depressed patient mentioned emotional distress initially as the chief complaint. Many of the sample had pain as the sole or coexisting complaint; 85 per cent in all had pains or aches of some description. Headaches, for example, were present in 85.4 per cent of the sample. The authors thus warn of the dangers of missing the diagnosis of depression because of the possible facade of somatic symptoms.

Case study: psychosomatic symptoms in Nanjing, Peoples Republic of China

Ots[54] in 1990 studied 243 patients, many of whom had 'psychosomatic disorders', attending a traditional Chinese medicine (TCM) clinic in Nanjing. He points out that in China, as in Taiwan and Hong Kong, the open expression of emotion is not encouraged. Instead, the main 'medical care-seeking behaviour' of people suffering from severe unhappiness or psychosocial stress is the presentation of physical complaints, mostly of the 'liver' and 'heart'.

Unlike Western medicine, TCM is not dualistic and does not strictly separate emotions and physical functions; both are seen as part of the same phenomenon. That is, 'specific emotional changes and specific somatic dysfunctions are viewed as corresponding with each other and often as identical'. Although TCM ostensibly focuses on the abnormalities of a particular organ, such as those of the 'liver', 'heart' or 'kidney', these diagnoses must be understood as not referring (in most cases) to an actual physical disease, but to *metaphors* for certain emotional states. Each diagnosis (such as 'liver disease') is really 'a metaphor whose primary referent is not a particular organ but an emotion diagnosed via the patterns of somatic symptoms'. Thus, although TCM emphasizes *physical* symptoms (and treatments) rather than psychological ones, the practitioners are able to 'read' these somatic symptoms as essentially an emotional message, and thus identify the underlying psychological problem. In the nosology of traditional Chinese medicine, 'liver' is a metaphor for anger, 'heart' for anxiety, 'spleen' for depression and 'kidney' for a decline in reproductive powers. In the clinic, about 80 per cent of the liver-related diagnoses given did *not* relate to actual physical diseases of the liver (such as hepatitis), but rather to aspects of *anger*. For example, a diagnosis of 'liver-*yang* flaring up' meant that the individuals were suppressing their anger, and this had affected their body, particularly their liver. If not treated, it might even lead to 'liver attacking spleen' – a disorder of the spleen. In other words, anger turned inwards might eventually cause depression.

Therefore, Ots points out that although traditional Chinese practitioners focus mainly on somatic symptoms, they do *not* ignore emotional states, whatever their cause; to them 'emotions are merely understood as pathogenic factors which cause disturbances of the organs and their functions'. Treatment here would consist not of psychotherapy or catharsis (which cultural norms would not permit), but would aim instead 'to harmonize the emotions by harmonizing bodily functions'. In the case of 'liver-anger', it is the liver itself that is treated, usually by a combination of 10–15 herbal medicines.

Ots suggested, therefore, that Western models of psychosomatic disorders may not be easily applied to China, since the culture there gives both patients and practitioners a different body awareness, and the Chinese 'are culturally trained to "listen" with their body' in a way unfamiliar to Western medicine.

CULTURAL SOMATIZATION

Somatization often takes the form of vague, generalized symptoms, such as tiredness, weakness, fever or 'pains everywhere'. However, in some cultural or social groups a special form of somatization takes place: the selection of one particular organ as the main focus of all symptoms and anxiety. I would term this phenomenon *cultural somatization*, and the organ chosen often has a symbolic or metaphoric significance for the group concerned, such as the liver, spleen, kidney or heart. Examples of this are the heart in Ots's study in China,[54] in Iran (*narahatiye qalb* or 'heart distress') and in the Punjab (*dil ghirda hai* or 'sinking heart'), the liver in France (*crise de foie*), the bowels in the UK[55] (and other countries) and the penis in some Chinese groups (*koro*). In each case, not only do individuals suffer from a particular symptom but they also become the 'embodiment'[56] of core cultural themes of the society in which they live.

This shared focus on a particular organ or body part must be differentiated from the more personal, idiosyncratic forms of somatization described by Western psychoanalysts. For example, Freud and Breuer's[57] model of hysteria suggests that certain localized physical symptoms (such as pain or paralysis in a limb or body part) could be the expression of a particular intrapsychic conflict, unique to that individual. In this case, the selected body part had a special, symbolic significance for the person concerned. Researchers of psychosomatic disorders have adopted a similar approach in trying to understand the reasons for 'organ choice' – that is, why one organ in an individual is selected as a target organ while another is not. In many individual cases, though, and irrespective of the cultural context, the choice of target organ is likely to be based on both cultural *and* individual criteria.

263

Mumford[58] proposed a useful model for understanding how somatization relates to cultural background. He suggested that there are three levels at which culture may shape the evolution of somatic symptoms, from first awareness to actual clinical presentation. They are:

1 *Language and idiom*, without which the sensation cannot be expressed.
2 *Concepts of health and disease*, without which the symptom cannot be interpreted.
3 *Culturally sanctioned illness behaviour*, without which the symptom cannot be presented to other people in order to obtain treatment of relief.

In most communities, all three of these levels are necessary in order for cultural somatization to take place and to be recognized as such by all concerned.

THE CONCEPT OF 'PSYCHOSOMATIC'

Although first used in 1818,[59] the term psychosomatic has been most widely applied since World War Two. It refers to conditions that have both a psychological *and* a physical component, often with some causal connection between the two. Generally, it is used to describe conditions whose origin is entirely psychological and where no physical abnormality can be found (such as tension headaches or irritable bowel syndrome), or those where there *is* a physical disorder, but it is precipitated or worsened by psychological factors (such as asthma attacks precipitated by family conflict). However, both anthropologists and medical researchers have criticized this term for the mind–body dualism that it implies. As Lipowski[60] states, 'psychosomatic connotes an assumption that there exist two classes of phenomena, i.e. psychic (mental) and somatic, which require separate methods of observation and distinct languages for their description'. That is, the term imposes a 'methodological and semantic dualism' onto the nature of human suffering. Despite its attempts to combine the 'disease' and 'illness' perspectives, the essential dualism of the concept still remains. Furthermore, psychosomatic disorders are an anomalous category within biomedicine. Unlike many 'real' diseases in the medical textbooks, they often include conditions that are difficult to diagnose, explain, predict, treat or prevent, and there is often no definite physical abnormality to be found. In some cases, therefore, this may lead to 'victim-blaming' (putting the responsibility for therapeutic failure on patients and supposed defects in their psyche).

A further problem is the linear, *causal* relationship that the term implies between certain psychological factors (such as personality, character, traits, conflicts or emotions) and specific symptoms or physical changes. Earlier last century, this 'psychogenicity' hypothesis suggested that certain personality types or people with certain character traits suffered from certain types of physical diseases – for example, asthmatics were often said to be 'passive and dependent people'.[61] Each psychosomatic disorder, therefore, was said to be associated with its own specific form of psychopathology. Some of the psychoanalytic literature has further implied a spatial model of body and mind, whereby an inner (psychic) reality somehow acts upon an outer (physical) one to cause psychosomatic symptoms. According to McDougall,[62] a psychoanalyst, 'such somatic phenomena arise in response to messages from the psyche'. This image of active psyche and passive body ('the mind is making use of the body in order to communicate something, to tell a story') [62] is now common in much of the psychosomatic literature, including discussions of somatization. It sometimes includes the notion of an inherited or acquired 'weakness' of the part of the body where these mental forces have their greatest effect.

Other authors have tried to widen the definition of psychosomatic to include social and contextual factors, and to develop more *multicausal* models. Engel,[63] for example, proposed a 'biopsychosocial model', which would be less dualistic and would integrate mental and physical factors with social ones – especially the events surrounding the origin of the disorder. Other multicausal models included that of Alexander and colleagues,[64] who proposed that these disorders were due to three factors:

1 The individual's 'characteristic psycho-dynamic conflict pattern', present from childhood.
2 A specific 'onset situation', which involved activation of this conflict pattern.
3 'Factor X', defined as a specific organ vulnerability or weakness.

From a family therapy perspective, Minuchin and colleagues[65] developed the 'family systems theory', whereby the family is seen as a system of inter-relationships that strives to maintain equilibrium – even at the cost of causing a psychosomatic disorder (such as anorexia nervosa) in one of its members (see below).

More recently, psychosomatic research has concentrated on sophisticated *physiological* models, which seek to connect certain psychological states with specific physiological changes in the body, especially in the immune, endocrine and neural systems. The relatively new field of psychoneuroimmunology (PNI),[66] for example, has shown how sensitive the immune system is to changes in psychological state, such as depression. Other work has focused on how physical factors – such as chromosomal, metabolic or endocrine abnormalities – can in turn influence the emotional and intellectual state, as well as behaviour. Like earlier models of psychosomatic disorders, many of these contemporary physiological models are also dualistic, since they often ignore the role of social and cultural factors in the origin, interpretation and management of the condition.

In recent years, the term 'psychosomatic' has increasingly become a part of Western folk culture, just as it is in the discourse of biomedicine. Anthropology can help in understanding how this concept has diffused into the population, and how it is now understood. In English-speaking countries particularly, the word often suggests that the condition is somehow not as 'real' as physical illness, and that its origin and chronic course is somehow the patient's 'fault'. In some cases, prolonged contact with health professionals may contribute to this process. People may learn from them, and from other sources, the moral implications of these disorders, and of their failure to recover from them despite medical treatment. As one woman with ulcerative colitis in the Massachusetts study[50] stated, 'What I heard from all the doctors was that it was my fault, and if only you did what they said, everything would be OK', while a medical student, also with ulcerative colitis, remarked: 'I searched very hard and for a reason – why me? Everyone told me it *must* be psychological, there must be a large psychological component – it's in the medical textbooks'.

Psychosociosomatic disorders: the role of context

From an anthropological perspective, therefore, many of the current psychosomatic theories – whether dualistic, multicausal, systemic or physiological – are useful but often insufficient. For a fuller picture, they also need to include the role of context, whether cultural, social, political or economic, in the origin, presentation and understanding of the disorder. In this respect, some of the anthropological theories outlined in this book are particularly useful. They include concepts of the cultural constructions of body and self (Chapter 2), 'illness' (Chapter 5), pain (Chapter 7), placebos and nocebos (Chapter 8), ritual (Chapter 9) and stress (Chapter 11), as well as of cultural and symbolic healing (see below). The role of poverty and deprivation, and the sense of helplessness that can result from them, are also relevant here. Only in this way can a fuller, more holistic understanding of the subtle ways in which certain phenomena – physical, psychological, social and cultural – all blend together in certain situations of human suffering, and in certain individuals, be obtained. In this sense, it is proposed here that this field of study should be more accurately called the study of *psychosociosomatic* disorders.

This approach is best described in the case of what are known as the 'culture-bound disorders'.

CULTURE–BOUND PSYCHOLOGICAL DISORDERS

'CULTURE-BOUND' OR 'CONTEXT-BOUND'?

The 'culture-bound disorders' (CBDs) are a group of folk illnesses, each of which is unique to a particular group of people, culture or geographical area. Because 'cultures' are never homogeneous, and because these conditions tend to occur in certain types of contexts (time, place, and social circumstances) perhaps they should also be termed *context-bound disorders*.

Each is a specific cluster of symptoms, signs or behavioural changes recognized by members of those cultural groups and responded to in a standardized way (see Chapter 5). They usually have a range of symbolic meanings, moral, social or psychological, for both the victims and those around them. They often link an individual case of illness with wider concerns, including the sufferers' relationship with their community, with supernatural forces and with the natural environment. In many cases they play an important role in expressing and resolving both anti-social emotions and social conflicts in a culturally patterned way. The conditions in this group range from purely behavioural or emotional disorders to those with a large somatic component. Among the dozens that have been described[67] are:

- *spirit possession* in many parts of Africa and elsewhere[3]
- possession by *jinns* or the *zar* spirit in many Muslim countries[68]
- *amok* – a spree of sudden violent attacks on people, animals and inanimate objects, which afflicts males in Malaysia
- *Hsiehping* – a trance state among Chinese, where patients believe themselves possessed by dead relatives or friends whom they had offended
- *koro* – a delusion among Chinese males that the penis will retract into the abdomen and ultimately cause death
- *Dhāt* syndrome – a state of extreme anxiety about loss of semen in the urine, among men in India and elsewhere
- *mal de ojo* or evil eye among Latin Americans (and other groups), where illness is blamed on the 'strong glance' of an envious person
- *latah* – a syndrome of hyper-suggestibility and imitative behaviour found in South East Asia
- *voodoo death* in the Caribbean and elsewhere, where death follows a curse from a powerful sorcerer;
- *Shinkeishitsu* – a form of anxiety and obsessional neurosis among young Japanese
- *windigo* – a compulsive desire to eat human flesh among the Algonkian-speaking Indians of central and north-eastern Canada
- *susto* (or 'fright') in most of Latin America – a belief in 'loss of soul'
- *narahtiye qalb* –'heart distress' (described in Chapter 5)
- *dil ghirda hai* –'sinking heart' (described in Chapter 5).

Culture-bound syndromes are by no means all as 'exotic' as this list suggests. Elsewhere in this book it has been suggested that a number of common behaviours, idioms of distress, perceptions of bodily states and certain diagnostic categories can all, in certain contexts, be regarded as Western culture-bound disorders. These include obesity, anorexia nervosa, premenstrual syndrome and the Type A coronary-prone behaviour pattern. In a review of this subject, Littlewood and Lipsedge[69] added to this list a number of other conditions common in the contemporary UK, including:

- *parasuicide*, an overdose with medically prescribed drugs
- *agoraphobia*, 'The Housewives' Disease'
- *shoplifting* by well-off, middle-aged women
- *exhibitionism* (or 'flashing')
- *domestic sieges*, where a divorced man denied access to his children, for example, holds the family hostage in their home.

In each of these the authors saw certain recurrent patterns of public behaviour, each of which encapsulates some of today's core cultural themes and values. Like the conditions mentioned earlier, they can therefore be regarded as *culture-bound*. Housewives' agoraphobia, for example, can be seen as both a ritual display of (and a protest against) the cultural pressures and injunctions on women, especially those that state that 'a woman's place is in the home'. By 'over-conforming' to this stereotype, the woman is able to dramatize the situation, mobilize a caring family around herself, and at the same time also restrict her husband's movements by forcing him to stay at home and look after her.

NEW CULTURE-BOUND SYNDROMES

In addition to these, a number of new syndromes have recently appeared in the industrialized world. Although many are created mostly by the media and are not yet fully-fledged culture-bound syndromes, they have begun to penetrate widely into popular culture and discourse. Some have a more medical origin, and have even found their way into psychiatric textbooks. In an increasingly secular age, many of them represent medicalized images of antisocial or nonconformist behaviour (see Chapter 5) and often lie on the border between 'mad' and 'bad' behaviour. In the UK, these emerging culture-bound syndromes include:

- aggressive behaviour or 'rage' syndromes, such as *road rage* (conflict between motorists), *air rage* (violent behaviour on an air flight) and *trolley rage* (conflict between customers in a supermarket)
- violent, repetitive behaviour syndromes, such as *serial killing, child abuse, 'granny bashing'* (abuse of the elderly), *bullying* (among schoolchildren) or the *battered wife syndrome*
- addiction or dependency syndromes, such as *workaholism* (addiction to overworking), *shopaholism* (addiction to shopping), *chocoholism* (addiction to chocolate), *lottomania* (addiction to buying lottery tickets), *sex addiction*, and even *internet addiction* (see Chapter 13)

- energy-loss syndromes, such as *burnout* (especially among those in the caring professions), *stress* (see Chapter 11) and *yuppie 'flu* (myalgic encephalopathy, or ME)
- miscellaneous syndromes, such as *school refusal syndrome, ADHD* and *false memory syndrome*.

Even when there is some proven physical or psychiatric basis for them (as there is, for some on this list), these syndromes often condense wider social and cultural concerns into a single diagnostic image or metaphor, and often this is seen as the perverse product of modern life. Over the years, several of these syndromes have become more popular, while for various reasons others have gradually declined. As an example, Acocella[70] has detailed the rise and fall of the *multiple personality disorder* (MPD) in the USA over the past 20 years, and relates it clearly to certain social trends and intellectual fashions that have also ebbed and flowed within that same period.

In addition to the more specific and standardized culture-bound syndromes, both non-Western and Western, a more diffuse cultural patterning determines the language of distress in which certain types of psychological or social disorder are expressed in each society. Here, the mode of presentation is culture-bound, though not the exact pattern of symptomatology. Examples of this, quoted above, are the largely somatic presentation of depression among Chinese in Taiwan, Hong Kong and the People's Republic of China, Asian immigrants in the UK and working-class Americans. However, in other cases a particular pattern of symptoms and how people interpret them can be described as 'culture-bound', even though they do not form as standardized a syndrome as those listed above. Bose,[71] for example, has described a culture-specific idiom of distress among some British Bangladeshis in London. Here, a wide range of expressions of extreme personal distress are interpreted by the patients, their families and religious healers as evidence of *upridosh*, or possession by malign spirits (*jinns*).

These displays of distress, both emotional and behavioural, may include refusing to eat, muteness, crying, shouting, swearing, 'disrespectful behaviour' and visual hallucinations or visionary experiences. Bose points out how this idiom of distress has no exact equivalent in psychiatric nosology, and can only be fully understood from within the specific cultural frame of reference, and the life circumstances, of the individual patient concerned.

It could be argued, as Hahn does below,[72] that *all* syndromes, whether physical, psychological or social, are to some extent 'culture-bound'. That is, there is always some unique, local cultural perspective on the condition, even if it is a standard biomedical disease. However, with their dramatic changes in behaviour and mental state, the absence of clear physical changes, and the many symbolic meanings attached to them, the conditions mentioned above do constitute a specific class of phenomena of great interest to medical anthropologists.

The following three case studies describe an example of a well-known and widely spread culture-bound disorder from Latin America, another syndrome afflicting some Latino immigrants to the USA, and two inter-related syndromes found in South Africa.

Among Indians, it is believed to be caused by the soul being 'captured' because, wittingly or not, the patient disturbed the spirit guardians of the earth, rivers, ponds, forests or animals. The soul is believed to be held captive 'until the affront has been expiated'. Among non-Indians, this 'soul loss' is usually blamed on a sudden fright or unnerving experience. Its clinical picture consists of:

- becoming restless during sleep
- during waking hours, complaining of depression, listlessness, loss of appetite and lack of interest in dress and personal hygiene.

The healing rites, carried out usually by a folk healer or *curandero*, consist of an initial diagnostic session where the cause of the specific episode is identified and agreed, and then a healing session whereby the soul is 'coaxed and entreated to rejoin the patient's body'. The patient is massaged, rubbed and sweated to remove the illness from the body and to encourage the soul to return. Rubel relates the incidence of the condition to a number of epidemiological factors (see Chapter 15), including stressful social situations, especially where the individual cannot meet the social expectations of his own family and cultural milieu.

Case study: *susto* in Latin America

Rubel[20] in 1977 described the characteristics of *susto* (or 'magical fright'), which is also known as *pasmo, jani, espanto* and *pédida de la sombra*. It is found throughout Latin America in both rural and urban areas, among both men and women, and among both Indians and non-Indians. It is also found among Hispanic Americans, especially those in California, Colorado, New Mexico and Texas. It is based on the belief that an individual is composed of a physical body and of one or more immaterial souls or spirits which, under some circumstances, may become detached from the body and wander freely. This may occur during sleep or dreaming, or as the consequence of an unsettling experience.

Case study: *ataques de nervios* among Latinos in the USA

De La Cancela and colleagues[73] in 1986 described *ataques de nervios* (attacks of nerves) among Puerto Ricans and other Latino immigrants in the USA. These attacks are a specific and 'culturally meaningful way to express powerful emotion'. They usually have an acute onset, with a variety of physical symptoms including shaking, feelings of heat or pressure in the chest, difficulty in moving limbs, numbness or tingling of hands or face, a feeling of the mind 'going blank', and sometimes a loss of consciousness or abusive behaviour. These acute episodes usually follow the gradual buildup of *nervios* (nerves) from the general problems of life, especially with family relationships, housing or money. An 'attack' is then usually precipitated by some specific stressful event. The authors point out that for most Latinos it is not seen as an 'illness' needing medical attention, but rather as an expression of upset, anger, frustration or sadness at the stressful event, as well as a temporary escape from it and a way of getting sympathy and help from other people. However, they suggested that this disorder cannot only be understood at the micro-level; the social, political and economic status of Latinos in the USA, and 'the sense of hopelessness, helpless, and lack of control' many of them experience, need to be examined. Stressful experiences in the countries of origin (especially in Central America), coupled with the effects of migration – such as the disruption of family life, unemployment, discrimination, overcrowded housing and changes in gender roles – are all part of this wider context. Added to the sense of social and political helplessness are the constant 'demands to submerge cultural identity and assimilate to the United States culture', and the lack of respect accorded to their cultures of origin. The authors suggested, therefore, that as well as treating individuals with this condition, and their families, attention must also be paid to wider socio-economic realities, because 'in the long run *ataques* may be more effectively dealt with in the sociopolitical arena'. Therefore, health providers 'need to engage in social action and advocacy focusing on the social problems and material conditions that give rise to *ataques de nervios*'.

Case study: *amafufunyana* and *ukuthwasa* in South Africa

Swartz[74] in 1998 described two common culture-bound disorders among Xhosa- and Zulu-speaking African people in South Africa. Both are forms of spirit possession, though one is considered negative, the other positive. *Amafufunyana* is a form of hysteria, with agitated and uncontrolled behaviour and sometimes suicide attempts. It is believed to be caused by possession by malign spirits, sometimes sent by sorcery. Among the Zulu, according to Ngubane,[75] possession is sometimes by 'a horde of spirits' from different ethnic groups. It can occur in individuals, or in larger outbreaks, such as in a girls' school. Like *nervios* or 'nerves' (see Chapter 11), it afflicts mainly people (especially women) who are in a relatively powerless social and economic position, especially at times of major social change and disruption. As such, it helps to draw attention to their suffering and to mobilize a caring network around them. Treatment is usually a ritual of exorcism by a traditional healer. In contrast, *ukuthwasa* – a similar form of spirit possession – has a more positive outcome. It is 'the state of emotional turmoil a person goes through on the path to becoming an indigenous healer'. Here possession is a necessary sign of the victim's 'calling' to be a healer. It signals a positive relationship to the ancestors, who will one day help them in their healing task. However, as Swartz points out, neither of these conditions forms a discrete or standardized entity. While the labels *amafufunyana* and *ukuthwasa* do have meaning, 'these meanings shift in different circumstances', and in different contexts. Like 'nerves', they can cover a variety of conditions and human situations. *Amafufunyana*, in particular, offers victims a way of explaining *post hoc* what has happened to them, as well as placing blame for it elsewhere. Similarly, the definition of *ukuthwasa* 'lies partly in the experience of the person undergoing it, and partly in the way these are handled by existing healers'. However, where somebody with this condition fails to become a healer, they may be rediagnosed by the community as having *ukuphambana*, or madness.

THE POROUS SELF

Many of these conditions, such as *susto*, *amafufunyana*, various forms of 'spirit possession' and even shamanism only make sense when one understands that in many cultural groups both body and 'self' are regarded as *porous*. That is, under certain circumstances invisible (or sometimes visible) entities, such as souls, spirits, or even malevolent or envious thoughts, can either enter the body, or leave it. This is very different from the Western view, which usually regards the skin as the impenetrable boundary of the body and self – a bulwark against both human and natural environments. In some cultures, however, the skin is regarded as much more 'open' to outside influences, and in some circumstances, forces or objects can 'enter' the body via the skin. Examples of this are: spirit possession in many African communities; possession by a *jinn* or the *zar* spirit in many Arab countries;[68] and in Jewish folklore, possession by a *dybbuk* – the restless soul of a dead person. Sometimes this possession can have positive effects. A shaman may 'incarnate' the spirits of his or her ancestors, and while in this special state of possession now has the power to diagnose, and heal members of their community.[76] This type of positive possession can occur in private, or *en masse* such as during one of the *sessões*, or public trance rituals of the Umbanda religion in Brazil.[77] In other circumstances, some vital but invisible essence of an individual (soul or spirit) is believed to temporarily 'leave' their body through the skin, as in the case of *susto*, or in some forms of witchcraft. In some traditional societies, such as the indigenous San people of southern Africa,[78] this process could happen voluntarily to the shaman – usually in a trance state achieved after careful preparation, and induced by rhythmic dances, drumming, fasts, or hallucinogenic plants. In this altered state of consciousness, the shaman's spirit was believed to somehow 'leave' their body and travel afar, in order to discover the cause of an illness, to heal a suffering person, to fight off evil spirits, or even to transform themselves temporarily into an animal or a bird. Within these societies, these 'out-of-the-body' experiences are usually regarded as abnormal behaviour, but as a form of the 'controlled abnormality' described above.

This view of the porous self is much less common in Western, industrialized countries, where 'body' and 'self' are seen as essentially the same thing, and the 'individual' is thought of as an entity bounded, and contained, by its impenetrable boundary of skin, even though it can sometimes be penetrated by 'germs', the natural environment, or invisible radiation. In modern psychology traces of the idea of a porous self still persist, and may well underlie some of the spatial metaphors commonly used by psychologists, such as 'projection', 'introjection', 'ego boundaries' or 'containment'. Some echoes of the earlier way of thinking can also be found in modern English phrases such as 'He's too sensitive – he takes too much in', 'He jumped out of his skin', 'He was besides himself', 'What's got into you today?' or 'He drove like a man possessed'.

As the examples above illustrate, culture-bound disorders can only be fully understood by looking at the wider *context* in which they appear. In some cases, this context may include many of the political, economic, social and gender issues of the wider society.

CRITIQUES OF CULTURE–BOUND DISORDERS

Several critiques of the CBDs have been put forward, particularly their overemphasis on *culture*. As noted earlier in this book, culture is only one determinant among many of human behaviour, and is always part of a wider context of time, place, demography, and socio-economic conditions. Also, while CBDs may be relevant to very small-scale, homogeneous societies, applying them to complex and heterogenous societies is more problematic, since these may contain many different 'cultures' (of region, class, gender, occupation, or religion) within their own borders. As noted already, the label of *context-bound disorders* may therefore be more appropriate.

Hahn[72] has criticized the concept of 'culture-bound disorders' from a different perspective. He points out that all syndromes are, to some extent, 'culture-bound'. Confining the term therefore only to psychological or behavioural disorders (such as *susto* or spirit possession) implies that more physical conditions (such as measles, cancer or heart attack) are somehow 'culture-free', and thus more 'real'. In fact, this dichotomy duplicates the disease/illness (or body/mind) split already described in Chapter 5, and is another example of biomedicine's view of biological facts as being more objective, more real, and more universal. Hahn also points out that it is only conditions outside the DSM classification (see below) that are classified as 'culture-bound', and as almost all of these come from non-Western societies, it reinforces the idea that these societies are somehow 'exotic', 'strange' and 'primitive' compared with our own. It also reinforces the primacy and universality of the Western, psychiatric approach. According to Hahn, Western psychiatry is in danger of claiming 'too much of culture at the margins of our nosological scheme and too little of culture at medicine's core.'

Hahn[72] proposes instead a more inclusionist approach, similar to Engel's 'biopsychosocial' model, which could integrate psychological, social, and physical dimensions. He suggests that all episodes of human suffering have cultural, biological and psychodynamic aspects, and can be placed on a 'nature–culture continuum'. Some conditions (such as *susto*) tend to be more 'cultural', while others (such as cancer) are more 'biological', but each one of them shares all three dimensions – and the same is true of biomedicine itself. He contrasts this wider approach with the 'exclusionist' view of the CBDs as a unique group of disorders that are very different from 'real' diseases.

'MEDICALIZATION': THE GROWTH OF 'UNCONTROLLED ABNORMALITY'

One of the most important cultural developments in industrialized societies is the way that human behaviour, and emotional state, are increasingly 'medicalized' (see Chapter 6) – and this is particularly true of psychiatry. In terms of Figure 10.1, this means a gradual expansion of (C), with more previously 'normal' or 'bad' behaviours being reconceptualized as psychiatric problems.

There are two basic classificatory systems in Western psychiatry that are widely used to diagnose and treat mental disorders. They are the *ICD-10 Classification of Mental and Behavioural Disorders*,[79] produced by the World Health Organization and the *Diagnostic and Statistical Manual of Mental Disorders* (DSM),[80] produced by the American Psychiatric Association. Over more than a century, the number of recognized mental disorders – that is, of types of behaviour classified as 'abnormal', and situated in the 'uncontrolled abnormality' zone – has increased exponentially in both classificatory systems. In the USA, for example, the census of 1840 included only one category of mental illness ('idiocy/insanity'), but by 1880 it had risen to seven (mania, melancholia, paresis, dementia, dipsomania and epilepsy).[81] In 1918 the *Statistical Manual for the Use of Institutions for the Insane* included 22 principal categories of mental disorder. By 1952 when the first edition of DSM (DSM-1) was published, 106 diagnostic categories of mental illness were now listed, and the book itself was 129 pages long, while the DSM-IV of 1994 listed a total of 357 diagnostic categories, and was now 900 pages long.[81]

CRITIQUES OF THE DSM

While many of the new diagnostic categories in DSM-IV represent advances in the diagnostic techniques and understandings of psychiatry, some critics have suggested that this proliferation is further evidence of the increasing 'medicalization' of ordinary human behavior. That is, of a tendency to put more and more types of behaviour – previously seen as either 'normal' or 'bad' – within the zone of 'controlled abnormality'. This is despite the fact that DSM-IV admits that 'no definition adequately specifies precise boundaries for the concept of "mental disorder"'.[80] In the legal field, this has often meant a shift from defining deviant behaviour as 'bad' to 'mad', and therefore as requiring treatment, rather than punishment. A similar shift from a moral to a medical model, has occurred in attitudes to alcoholism, as described in Chapter 8.

Kutchins and Kirk[82] have criticized the DSM for 'pathologizing everyday behavior'. They have pointed out that many of these new 'syndromes' had once been forms of behaviour, or emotional state, that were regarded as either 'normal' (even if they were considered undesirable). DSM-IV, for example, includes 'Age-related Cognitive Decline', 'Caffeine-Induced Sleep Disorder', 'Hypoactive Sexual Desire Disorder', 'Male Erectile Disorder', 'Disruptive Behavior Disorder', and 'Separation Anxiety Disorder' (which in children may be associated with school refusal). Some diagnoses in DSM have come and gone. As mentioned earlier, in the USA homosexuality was once regarded as a criminal offence, then was classified as a mental 'illness' by DSM in 1952, and only finally de-classified as such in 1973.[8] 'Self-Defeating Personality Disorder' appeared in the Appendix of the revised DSM-III in 1987, but had been removed by 1994 in DSM-IV.[82] Other forms of behaviour have also become 'de-medicalized': masturbation was once considered an immoral act, was later was classified as a mental disorder, but is no longer seen as such.

This growth in this 'medicalization' of everyday behaviour is echoed in the growth of lay categories – the 'new culture-bound disorders' – mentioned above. The overall effect of this process, in both psychiatric and lay discourse, can be seen as a lessening of personal responsibility, and an increased tendency to blame outside influences (upbringing, early experiences, economic background, or even genetics or brain dysfunction) for one's personal or social suffering. This shift away from a punitive towards a treatment approach, from the involvement of law enforcement officials to that of health professionals, also means a greater role for the pharmaceutical industry in supplying drugs to treat these new 'disorders'. Also, as Kutchins and Kirk[81] note, once a form of behaviour appears in the DSM, this has legal, medical and economic implications. It may mean, for example, that insurance companies will now reimburse the cost of psychotherapy, hospitalization, or medication for people diagnosed as suffering from this condition.

The DSM has also been criticized for its failure to fully include cultural issues in psychiatric classification and treatment. Although DSM-IV-TR (2000)[80] does include an Appendix with some discussion of 25 'culture-bound syndromes', Kirmayer and Minas[18] suggest that these form 'a sort of museum of exotica at the back of the book', and that in the main text cultural considerations are included 'as just minor qualifications to what are presumed to be culture-free diagnostic categories'.

Overall, Kleinman[83] suggests that the DSM is, in itself, a culture-bound classificatory system, and that in some circumstances applying it could lead to the 'category fallacy' mentioned above. Criticising DSM-III, he noted also that it 'is so organized that every conceivable psychiatric condition is listed as a disease to legitimate remuneration to practitioners from private medical insurance and government programs.'. The same, it can be argued, is true of DSM-IV.

CULTURAL AND SYMBOLIC HEALING OF PSYCHOLOGICAL DISORDERS

In many non-Western societies, particularly in rural or small-scale communities, mental illness is often considered to be more of a *social* event, one that intimately involves the patient's family, friends and community. In many cases, both mental and physical ill health are interpreted as indicating conflicts or tensions in the social fabric. Kleinman[83] uses the term *cultural healing* for when healing rituals attempt to repair these social tears and 'reassert threatened values and arbitrate social tensions'. Healing takes place at many levels; not only is the patient restored to health, but so is the community in which he or she lives. The aim of the healer, like the Ndembu *chimbuki* described in Chapter 9, is to resolve the conflicts causing the patient's illness, restore group cohesion and integrate the patient back into normal society. Unlike in the Western world, emotional disorders are often seen as *useful* to the community. For example, Waxler[19] notes how in many small-scale societies mental illness can be useful, even necessary; it incurs obligations between people (such as the obligations of family, friends and neighbours to attend and pay for a public healing ritual), and this has an *integrating* function, strengthening the ties within and between groups. In these societies, few other specialized institutions (such as a centralized legal, political and bureaucratic organization) exist to promote integration, and deviance (such as mental illness) can play this role. This usually occurs within a shared cognitive system, where everyone shares similar views of the aetiology of misfortune and ill health. If mental illness in one individual is ascribed to sorcery or witchcraft from someone in another group (family, clan or tribe), the offender's group has incurred obligations to the victim's group, which must be repaid in a public ceremony. This helps recreate the ties between groups and also reasserts the boundaries between them, and in the process the mentally ill person is reintegrated into society. According to Waxler, this process, and the key role of the family in caring for the patient, means that in traditional non-Western societies mental illness seems to be more easily cured and much more short-lived. She contrasts this with the West, where psychiatric treatment does not have this integrating function (which is fulfilled by the political, bureaucratic system and so on), and mental illness serves to *alienate* the sick individual even further from society. It establishes boundaries around the patient, and does not create or re-establish social ties between kin and other groups (except perhaps within the nuclear family) or make clear the boundaries between groups. The Western schizophrenic is assumed to have a chronic, relapsing disease process that may always recur, and is 'a schizophrenic in remission' rather than 'a person who had schizophrenia'. She therefore relates this lack of an integrating function with the long illness careers and poor prognosis of Western psychotics.

However, Kleinman[84] points out that 'cultural healing' may heal social stresses 'independently of the effects they have on the sick person who provides the occasion for their use'. In some cultures,

the resolution of social conflicts may not be as beneficial to mentally ill patients as Waxler suggests; it may involve imprisoning, killing or driving them from the community. For example, in the past those 'possessed' by evil spirits in the New Hebrides and Fiji were routinely buried alive. However, in many non-industrialized societies the mentally ill are usually well cared for within their families or communities.

In more traditional societies, mental illness is usually dealt with by folk healers such as the Taiwanese *tâng-ki*, the Ndembu *chimbuki*, the Latin American *curandero*, the Moroccan *fqih*, the Malaysian *bomoh* or the Zulu *isangoma*. Some of the practices and psychotherapeutic functions of these ritual healers have already been described. Perhaps the most famous is the *shaman*, who appears in many different cultures,[76] from Alaska to Africa, and whose Western equivalents are mediums, clairvoyants and 'channellers'. Like the mentally ill person who is 'possessed' by spirits, the shaman also allows himself to become temporarily possessed by certain spirits. Lewis[85] points out that, unlike the patient, his possession is 'controlled' during the healing seance and thus occurs when and where he chooses. In this condition of controlled abnormality, the fact that he is able to master or neutralize the spirits is of great reassurance to the community. He is also able to identify and exorcise malign spirits possessing the ill person, and in the process alleviate anxiety, fears, guilt and conflicts. Murphy[86] has described some of the psychotherapeutic aspects of shamanism as part of his ritual of cultural healing. These include:

- working within the shared beliefs of the group, and thus reinforcing them
- involving the individual as well as the community in the ritual, during which time the patient remains surrounded by familiar friends and relatives
- by becoming 'possessed', illustrating his mastery over the other spirits causing ill health.

In his séance, the shaman identifies the cause of mental illness (such as breach of a taboo) and pre-

Mental illness short lived in Eastern Societies

scribes the appropriate expiatory acts, which are believed to effect the cure, and then demonstrates that the patient has indeed recovered. That is, 'through suggestion and the patient's personal involvement in the cure, these visible acts further promote in the patient a psychological realization that he is returning to a state of health'. According to Lewis, by the wide role that he plays in the religious and social life of his community, 'the shaman is not less than a psychiatrist, he is more'.[85]

SYMBOLIC HEALING

'Cultural healing', with its focus mainly on the social dimensions of healing, is really only a special form of what anthropologists have called *symbolic healing* – that is, healing that does not rely on any physical or pharmacological treatments for its efficacy, but rather on language, ritual and the manipulation of powerful cultural symbols. As well as the more traditional folk or religious healing described above, it also includes the various types of 'talk therapy' common in the West, such as psychoanalysis, psychotherapy and counselling.

This section examines a number of key questions raised by symbolic healing. How does it work? What are its effects on mental illness? Does it have common features in whatever society it occurs?

In understanding this phenomenon, the previous discussions of the placebo effect (Chapter 8), ritual healing (Chapter 9), folk healers (Chapter 4), illness narratives (Chapter 5) and even the 'total drug effect' (Chapter 8) are all relevant. In addition, the innovative work of Dow,[87] Kleinman,[88] Csordas,[89] Moerman[90] and others are particularly useful in helping to identify certain basic themes that seem to underlie virtually *all* forms of symbolic healing, whether sacred or secular, and wherever they occur.

Before this type of healing can take place – involving a particular healer, client and community – a number of conditions must be fulfilled. These conditions apply both to secular healing such as the Western 'talk therapies' and to the more religious forms of healing, and include the following.

1 The healer must have a coherent system of explanation, or frame of reference, for the origin and nature of the problem, and how it can be dealt with. Dow[87] called this the *mythic world* – 'a model of experiential reality', whose elements 'represent solutions to personal human problems', and which is composed of culturally specific beliefs, metaphors and idioms. It may consist, for example, of a belief that malign 'spirits' (or 'intrapsychic conflicts') are responsible for all mental illness and extreme emotional states. In many cases, especially in small-scale societies, the mythic world is common to most members of the group; however, it may also be created *de novo* by some charismatic healer or cult leader, or be shared by only a tiny group of adherents, as in the new cults, religions, lifestyles, talk therapies and healing systems that are now proliferating in Europe and the USA.[91] The mythic world may exist only in an oral form or be standardized in certain texts (or textbooks). It may take many forms, sacred or secular, for example, as a religious cosmology (Ayurveda), a folk tradition (spirit possession), a theory of personality (Freudian psychoanalysis) or a scientific model of the body (biomedicine).

2 The mythic world must include what Kleinman[88] describes as a *symbolic bridge* between personal experience, social relations, and cultural meanings. That is, suffering individuals in that society must be able to understand their own situation and its resolution in terms of its imagery and symbols (such as spirit possession, or intrapsychic conflict). In many cases these symbols are already familiar to these individuals since, as Finkler[92] puts it, they 'emerge from the depths of their cultural experience and... reach the bearers of that culture at the most profound levels of their existence'. They represent 'the deep cultural grammar governing how the person orients himself to the

world around him and to his inner world',[92] and serve to link the individual to the social world and often to the supernatural world as well.

3 When a suffering individual consults a healer, the healer aims to activate this 'symbolic bridge' by *convincing* the clients (if they require convincing) that their own particular problem *is* explicable in terms of the symbols of the mythic world. That is, the patients have to be persuaded that their suffering can be redefined or 'reframed' as, for example, evidence of spirit possession, neurosis or evil eye affliction. Thus the healer's aim at this stage is to get 'the patient to accept a particularization of the general mythic world as a valid model of the patient's experiences',[87] and to achieve this they may use many different theatrical or rhetorical techniques.

4 Once patient and healer have reached this consensus, the healer needs to get the patient *emotionally* (as well as intellectually) 'attached' to the symbols of their mythic world. That is, before therapeutic change can take place, patients must first become more self-aware, feel emotionally involved in the healing process, and see these symbols (whether they are spirits or intrapsychic conflicts) as relating to them personally and to their situation. This is done, for example, by interpreting a patient's excess rage as evidence of 'possession' by an angry evil spirit, or of severe inner 'conflicts' dating from childhood, or by interpreting feelings of depression as being caused by 'soul loss' (as in *susto*). In each case, the aim is not only to relate the patients' emotions (including their hopes and fears) to the symbols of the healer's mythic world, but also to link the individual patients thereby to wider social, cultural and cosmological concerns.

5 The healer now begins to guide *therapeutic change* by manipulating the symbols of their mythic world. For example, having identified the spirit possessing the patient, he goes through a complex ritual of exorcism, at the end of which the anxious patients are reassured that the spirit has left them and that they can now resume their normal life. Or, they may be reassured by a psychotherapist that they have at last 'worked through' certain archaic, inner conflicts. Or, as in the case of *susto*, they may be told after a ritual that their soul has, at last, been safely returned to their body. In each case, Kleinman[88] points out that the 'healing, as a sacred or secular ritual, achieves its efficacy through the transformation of experience'. The patients learn to re-evaluate and 'reframe' their past and present experiences. Furthermore, Kleinman[88] saw this process, and the symbols used within it, as a way of linking the patient's 'self' (both psychological and physical) to the social relations and cultural concerns of the wider society. Thus a successful transformation will affect not only their emotional state, but also their physiology, their relationships with other people and their relationship to the culture at large. In many cases the symbols that achieve this are not only the conceptual symbols of the mythic world, but also the more tangible ritual symbols described in Chapter 9.

6 The 'healed' patients have acquired a new way of conceptualizing their experiences in symbolic terms, and a new way of functioning – both of them confirmed by the healer. In the process, they have also acquired a newly fashioned *narrative* of their past and present, and of their likely future. Whether this narrative is short (as in spirit exorcisms) or lengthy (as in psychoanalysis), it summarizes *post hoc* what happened to them and why and how the healer was able to restore them to happiness or health.

Symbolic healing thus often takes place at *many* levels simultaneously: psychological, physical, social, cultural and spiritual. As with the placebo effect, the exact mechanisms of its effects on physiology (for example, relieving muscular tension, reducing pain sensation or lowering blood pressure) are not clearly understood, nor whether they are mediated by the autonomic nervous system, the endocrine system, the immune system or the neuropeptide (endorphin) system.

Secular symbolic healing: the 'talk therapies'

In the Western world most forms of 'talk therapy', with the exception of family therapy, focus mainly on the individual patient, as do many of the alternative/complementary therapies described in Chapter 4. Whatever their ideology, the majority of talk therapists will see their individual clients as the main 'problem', and their emotional state, behaviour, insights and delusions as the main areas of concern. Most of the clients' treatments will take place in specialized settings, such as a psychotherapist's office or a clinic, far removed from their social milieu, and characterized by both privacy and confidentiality. Where patient and therapist come from similar backgrounds, they may share many assumptions about the likely origin, nature and treatment of psychological disorders. However, the proliferation of talk therapies has meant that, in many cases, the patients may have to *learn* this world view gradually, acquiring with each session a further understanding of the concepts, symbols and vocabulary that comprise it. This can be seen as a form of 'acculturation' whereby they acquire a new mythic world couched, for example, in terms of the Freudian, Jungian, Kleinian, Laingian or other psychological models. This mythic world, shared eventually by patient and therapist, is often inaccessible to the patient's family or community who, in any case, are excluded from the consultation.

Karasu[93] examined some of the mechanisms by which psychotherapy seems to work, and his model is similar to the one above. Whatever the specific type of therapy (and reportedly there are 400 different types of psychotherapy now available), he identified three underlying 'therapeutic change agents' common to them all, and which are necessary for success, and usually used in sequence. They are:

1 *Affective experiencing* – a process of inducing emotional arousal, which is often followed by an increased responsiveness to suggestion, and an 'unfreezing' of previous attitudes, and this in turn prepares the client for new cognitive inputs.

2 *Cognitive mastery* – the therapist now provides the client with rational explanations, interpretations, information and clarifications, in order to ensure 'the acquisition and integration of new perceptions, thinking patterns, and/or self-awareness'

3 *Behavioural regulation* – the therapist undertakes a process of educating, and constantly encouraging the client to change or modify their habitual behaviour patterns, and to control certain negative actions and habits.

Different types of psychotherapy appear to focus mainly on just one of these change agents, for example EST, primal scream, and drama therapy focus on 'affective experiencing', cognitive therapy, sex therapy and supportive therapy focus on 'cognitive mastery' and biofeedback, aversion therapy and assertiveness training focus on 'behaviour regulation'. Despite this, Karasu argues that *all* of the three 'therapeutic change agents' are found, though in different proportions, in every form of successful psychotherapy.

Psychoanalysis

Psychoanalysis is a special and influential form of symbolic healing, found almost exclusively in the Western world and providing the basis for many of the other 'talk therapies'. To Dow,[87] it is 'probably the most significant psychotherapy in Western culture'. Stein[94] argued further that its concepts provide a useful way of understanding the universal characteristics of the human condition, whatever the cultural or social context. As a form of therapy, though, it has specific features that are very different from most forms of cultural healing. Its focus is only on the individual, irrespective of home environment and socio-cultural background, and healing sessions involve only a solitary analyst and a solitary client. The sessions take place in a specified place (the ana-

Change Agents

lyst's office) and at a specified time, and in most cases they last exactly 50 minutes. Lying on a couch in this office, with the analyst out of sight and sitting silently behind them, the clients are encouraged to 'free associate', to 'say anything that comes into your head'. As a form of healing, its emphasis is on phenomena believed to originate *within* the individual psyche as they emerge during the analytic session, especially the meanings given by the client to their past experiences. In the session, as Dow[87] describes, 'transactional symbols are developed by the analyst from the content of the mythic world constructed by the patient', and these will form the basis of the therapeutic stages outlined above. Above all, the emphasis of psychoanalysis is on the treatment of the individual rather than of the social domain. As one analyst[95] states, 'the wish for further insight in order to discover the unconscious meaning of unsatisfactory life situations or incomprehensible symptoms implies acceptance of the fact that ultimately the causes of psychological symptoms *lie within oneself*'.

Anthropologists have argued that, whatever the reasons for its efficacy, the practice of psychoanalysis can also be understood as the expression of certain core Western cultural values,[96] especially those of the educated middle-classes. Included here could be: the emphasis on self-awareness, insight, 'personal growth', individualism, privacy and confidentiality; the high value placed on language and the ability to verbalize one's distress; and the location of conflicts (especially sexual ones) deep within the psyche, rather than in the social world outside. Its metaphors of the psyche are often spatial (as well as dualistic); an 'inner' psyche hidden within an 'outer' body and the consequent need for 'insight'. Its view of time is, to some extent, paradoxical; on one hand, a rigid adherence to Western monochronic 'clock time', strictly enforcing the 50-minute consultation, and on the other hand, an open-ended period of therapy, sometimes lasting for many years. As in some other forms of symbolic healing, analyst and

client share in the creation of a personalized *narrative* of misfortune, and one embellished and refashioned over many years.

In contrast, more traditional forms of symbolic healing tend to be less structured, last a shorter time, take place in the presence of other people and be linked more to the social or supernatural aspects of daily life. They do not seek insight from the patient, or aim at their individuation or 'personal growth'. These differences, as Kleinman[97] points out, 'illumine the radical differences between egocentric Western culture and sociocentric non-Western cultures, and disclose that culture exerts a powerful effect on care'.

Case study: Religious healing among a Hasidic Jewish community in London, UK

Dein[98] describes attitudes to health and healing among orthodox Hasidic Jews of the Lubavitch movement in Stamford Hill, London. In dealing with illness (as well as conditions such as infertility), the community combine pragmatic with symbolic healing. They consult medical doctors and complementary practitioners, but also use religious healing if the condition is severe, long-lasting or unresponsive to treatment. This can include prayer, reciting the Psalms (*tehillim*), carrying out good deeds (*mitzvot*), giving to charity (*tzedakah*), consulting a rabbi for advice or checking religious artifacts in the house, such as the phylacteries (*tefillin*) for flaws, which would make them invalid, and therefore less protective of the individual. Before his death in 1994, seriously ill or troubled people – or their families – would write or fax to the *Rebbe*, the head of the movement in New York, for his advice or blessing. After his death, some continue to write to his tomb, asking for a blessing. This study illustrates, therefore, how medical pluralism can exist even in a relatively small community, and how people can freely combine biomedical and symbolic healing in dealing with illness and other misfortune.

The setting of symbolic healing

Symbolic healing usually takes place at specified times and in specified places. As described in Chapter 9, the *setting* itself plays a crucial role in the healing process, setting the stage, creating a mood of expectation and giving information to the clients about the healers – especially their interests, background, the source of their power and what they believe in. For example, patients entering Sigmund Freud's consulting rooms in Vienna or London would find the desk and shelves filled with artefacts from ancient Greece, Rome and Egypt, reflecting his interest in his clients' early, hidden childhood experiences, and his remark that the analyst's work 'resembles to a great extent an archaeologist's excavation of some dwelling-place that has been destroyed and buried'.[99]

In religious healing, the setting may be a church, a temple, a shrine, a tomb, the home of a religious leader or a sacred place of pilgrimage (Figure 10.2). For example, El-Islam[100] describes how, in many Arab countries, the families of people with severe mental problems (frequently blamed on the evil eye, sorcery or possession by *jinns*) often turn first to forms of ritual healing. These may include visits to the tombs of famous *sheikhs*, consultations with a respected *sheikh* or master (*Al-Asyaad*), the use of amulets containing holy verses, and purification rituals (*Mahuw* or *Mahaya*) that involve drinking or washing in water that has been washed off Koranic verses written on a plate. In *Umbanda*,[77] a popular Brazilian religion that has incorporated elements of Catholicism, Afro-Brazilian beliefs and European Spiritism, consultations and healing take place during public religious rituals (*sessões*). They are usually held in special centres (*terreiros*) decorated with brightly-painted images and murals of the various deities. During the service, Umbanda initiates can become possessed by these deities – such as the *orixas* (African deities or their Catholic equivalents), *caboclos* (spirits of indigenous Indians) or *Pretos Velhos* (spirits of old African slaves). In this altered state of consciousness they are able to act as 'spirit consultants' to other members of the congregation, divining the causes of their illness or misfortune with the aid of their spirits and then healing it, often by exorcism. Similarly, in the Venezuelan cult of María Lionza, the mediums or *materias* 'receive' a particular spirit, and in this state of possession give specific advice to those who consult them: how to remain healthy, how to deal with family or

Figure 10.2 A *jhārphuke vaidya*, or Hindu Tantric healer, and his clients in the Kathmandu Valley, Nepal. He offers healing for a variety of ailments, including physical disease, social problems, and mental illness, especially when caused by witchcraft or other supernatural causes. (Source: © David Gellner. Reproduced with permission.)

work problems, how to improve their economic situation, or how to answer certain questions that are troubling them.[101] The mediums main aim, therefore, is to make people feel better about themselves, and about their daily lives. If they are ill, however, they would refer them to a doctor or to a local traditional healer (*curandero*).

Whether symbolic healing is sacred or secular, the setting in which it occurs and the ritual symbols used within it are crucial parts of the healing process. Both play an essential, though non-verbal, role in the creation of the mythic world, in terms of which healing will take place.

The efficacy of symbolic healing

It is difficult to evaluate the efficacy of different forms of symbolic healing, since definitions of therapeutic success vary among them. Some seem to relieve one type of psychological distress, but not another. For example, in a detailed study of healing in a spiritualist temple in rural Mexico, Finkler[102] found that it was ineffective for the psychoses but useful for 'neurotic disorders, psychophysiological problems and somatized syndromes'. It enabled patients to abandon their sick roles, return to normal behaviour, and eliminate the feeling of 'being sick'. Similarly, in a study of therapeutic outcomes from a Taiwanese healer or *tâng-ki*, Kleinman[103] found that symbolic healing was mainly effective for episodes of neurosis and somatization, and its value more in healing the 'illness' than in curing the 'disease'. It was effective in fitting the illness episode into a wider context – explaining it in familiar terms, mobilizing social support about the victim and reaffirming basic values and group cohesion – and thus reducing anxiety in both the victims and their families. In a study in Tamil Nadu, southern India, in 1997 Campion and Bhugra[104] found that of 198 psychiatric patients attending hospital, 45 per cent had earlier sought help from a Hindu, Muslim or Christian religious healer. Of these, 30 per cent felt that they had got some benefit from the consultation, although the majority (90 per cent) had discontinued this treatment by the time of hospitalization.

Overall, most anthropologists would agree therefore that – for whatever reason – many people *are* helped by symbolic healing, whether religious or secular.

'Healing', however, is not identical to 'curing', especially in the case of severe psychosis or physical disability. Individuals and their families may feel that they have been 'healed', even though they have not yet been 'cured' in conventional psychiatric or medical terms. This distinction is clearer in some forms of religious healing, such as faith healing. As Csordas[105] points out, there are crucial differences between secular healing (with its mind–body dualism), such as medicine or psychotherapy, and religious healing (with its tripartite division of mind–body–spirit). In his study of Catholic Charismatic healing in the USA,[106] he described their four distinct types of healing: *physical healing* of bodily illness; *inner healing* of emotional scars or mental illness; *deliverance* from the adverse effects of demons or evil spirits; and *spiritual healing* of the soul injured by sin, primarily by means of the Sacrament of Reconciliation (confession). Even if the first three fail in a particular case, and the person remains mentally or physically ill, spiritual healing is still possible as what Csordas calls 'a hedge against the failure of healing prayer'.

It should be pointed out that, as described in previous chapters, *all* forms of healing, including medical and surgical treatments,[107] have some symbolic component to them. Both Western medicine and psychiatry are symbolic systems as well as technical ones. With the gradual diffusion of their concepts and techniques world-wide, there is an increasing likelihood of complex interactions or conflicts between the different mythic worlds of traditional and psychiatric approaches to mental illness, as illustrated in the following case studies.

Case study: a case of 'fox possession' in Sapporo, Japan

Etsuko[108] described the case of Michiko, a 43-year-old single woman complaining of possession by a fox spirit (*kitsune-tsuki*), a common idiom of mental disorder in Japan. Her illness began after her parents died, when she became distressed and 'strange voices and noises came to my ears. I felt very uneasy'. She was seen by psychiatrists but 'the medicine was no help, but it's natural that spirits can't be cured by medicine. And doctors would never understand spirit possession'. To get relief, and an explanation for her symptoms, she consulted in turn seven different shamans. With the seventh one, a shaman of the Shugendo sect of Buddhism, a series of séances confirmed that she was possessed by an evil fox spirit because – among other reasons – she and her ancestors had killed many foxes in their previous lives. After several rituals, Michiko claimed that the fox spirit had told her important facts; in particular, that she was really of noble birth, and that her misfortune was not her fault but the result of her being born under an unlucky star. Gradually the fox evolved from a possessing spirit to be her personal deity; at the same time, she became transformed from being a client into being a shaman in her own right. Her psychological state improved markedly, as 'the illness of possession was replaced by a shamanistic ability brought about by her steady effort in religious practice'. At the same time as this improvement was taking place, the psychiatrists judged her condition to have deteriorated, to have gone from auditory hallucinations and possession state to delusional perceptions, grandiose beliefs and signs of chronic schizophrenia. This case illustrates, therefore, the discrepancy between being 'healed' and being 'cured' – at least from a psychiatric perspective.

Case study: psychiatric and religious healing in Jerusalem, Israel

Bilu and colleagues[109] described how secular (psychotherapy) and sacred (Jewish mysticism) forms of healing can intersect in a medical milieu in Jerusalem, Israel. By using hypnosis, guided imagery and conventional psychotherapy, the therapists were able to treat Avraham, a religious psychotic patient, by working within his own mythic world, and its complex metaphors and symbolism drawn largely from Jewish mysticism. By encouraging him, under hypnosis, to confront the black 'demon' that was persecuting him, and chase it away ('Go, go, go away because you do not belong to our world!'), they were able to greatly improve his emotional state and social functioning. During the therapy sessions Avraham was symbolically led through a desert until finally he found peace in a quiet green oasis – a manifestation of Paradise and the Garden of Eden – filled with 'pure springs, sweet odors, beautiful gardens, and particularly pious inhabitants'. His personal cure was thus linked to the wider cultural themes of Exodus and redemption in Jewish tradition and theology, already familiar to the patient.

Case study: spiritist healing in Porto Alegre, Brazil

Greenfield[110] examined the healing practices of a new syncretic religion, a Spiritist group known as *Casa do Jardim,* in Porto Alegre, southern Brazil. Its imagery is an unusual fusion of Afro-Brazilian folk religion and ideas drawn from medical science; several of its healers are themselves physicians. They believe in two parallel worlds, one material and the other spiritual, with communication possible between the two. Each human being has a spirit as well as a body, and under some circumstances that spirit can also get ill. In that case, the healers will 'uncouple' it from the body and send if off to the spirit or astral world, where teams of 'spirit doctors' will diagnose and treat it in a 'spirit hospital' called the *Amor e Caridade* before returning it, healed, to its body. Mental illness is believed to be caused by disincarnate evil spirits from the astral plane imposing themselves on the living. Its treatment is by 'disobsession' – the healer 'incarnating' the offending spirit, lecturing it on the error of its ways and then sending it back to the astral plane. Like other healing groups, the *Casa do Jardim* provides social support, practical help and psychotherapy, especially for 'unaffiliated individuals who face the increasing uncertainty and insecurity of life in disorganized, anomic, urban Brazil'.

ANTHROPOLOGY AND FAMILY THERAPY

Anthropology is essentially the study of groups rather than of individuals, though sometimes individuals are studied within the context of certain groups. In all human societies, the primary social group is always the *family*. The composition of the family varies greatly between cultures, as does the role that it plays in the lives of its members.

Outside the urban areas of the industrialized world, where the nuclear family (a couple and their children) is often the norm, the extended multigenerational family (usually a couple, together with one or more married children and their children and spouses) is one of the commonest kinship patterns found world-wide. In poorer parts of the world, this larger family unit, though linked to the wider society, often acts as a miniature and self-contained community or self-help group, whose members share many of their resources and many of the tasks and responsibilities of everyday life. In whatever form it takes, and in whatever culture it appears, the family is always a *social* as well as a biological unit, and it always includes members who are not biologically related to it. As well as marriage partners and their families of origin, it may also include honorary relatives or 'fictive kin', such as close friends or neighbours, or even health professionals.

In recent years there has been an increasing overlap in interest between medical anthropologists, family therapists and some psychiatrists. All three are interested in widening the definition of 'patient' beyond the individual, to include their family and, where relevant, their community as

well. For many clinicians, like some of the folk healers described in Chapter 4, the family and not the individual has become the main focus for both diagnosis and treatment.

DEFINITIONS OF 'FAMILY'

One obvious problem is that the definition of 'family' is not universal. There is wide cross-cultural variation in patterns of kinship, and anthropologists have described many different types of family structure. Children in different parts of the world may be the result of different forms of marriage: *monogamy* (one wife, one husband), *polygyny* (one husband, several wives) or – more rarely – *polyandry* (one wife, several husbands).[111] As well as extended families and nuclear families, there are joint families (a household composed of married siblings, spouses and children) and one-parent families (usually mother and child). In some Islamic societies, the phenomenon of 'milk kinship' (see Chapter 3) means that children breast-fed by the same women are regarded as symbolic siblings' and forbidden to marry one another when grown up, even though they may not be biologically related at all.

In recent years, especially in Western countries, a number of new types of family structure have appeared. These include adoptive or fostering families, childless marriages by choice, lesbian and gay couples, and the complex combinations of step-children, step-parents, grandparents and in-laws that have resulted from high rates of divorce and remarriage[112] – sometimes called *blended families*. A growing number of *mixed marriages* have also arisen from the new population diversity (Chapter 12), and this may involve marriage between people from different cultural, racial or religious backgrounds. While many of these families find this an enriching experience, others may encounter problems with their families of origin, or when dealing with children, or with other issues, later in life. Medicine and science have also aided in the growth of new types of family structure, Advances in transplant surgery (Chapter 2) and in the 'New

Reproductive Technologies' (Chapter 6), for example, can mean that previously unrelated strangers now have a new sense of 'kinship' with one another. More recently, too, the growth of the global communications network means that families scattered by migration to many different countries can still keep up frequent and affective contact with each other, in a way impossible to previous generations of migrants. These *virtual families* can maintain a sense of family closeness, even though they are many thousands of miles apart and may never, in fact, see each other again. Thanks to the internet, emails, web-cams and telephones, they are now able to exchange news and family gossip, share feelings and ideas, as well as photographs and films. However, they cannot provide the practical assistance, emotional support, and tactile relationships that their members may need from a family on a daily basis.

Certain other social groupings can also function as quasi-families for some of their member, even though most of their members are not biologically related to one another. These groupings can provide their members with many of the benefits of family life – continuity, emotional closeness, social support, one or more parental or authority figures, a sense of belonging and identity, economic assistance, protection from outside dangers, as well as the sharing of responsibility for the young, the old and the unwell. Many different forms of these 'non-biological families' now exist, and in the future they are likely to increase in number and importance (especially in urban areas), as a byproduct of our age of mobility, individualism, secularism, family break-ups, the reduction in family size and the growth of the scattered 'virtual family'. These new 'families' include groups of close friends, the church or other religious organization, communes (often organized like large extended families), clubs, women's' groups, self-help or therapy groups, fraternities or sororities, youth gangs, military regiments, cults (often dominated by a single, powerful, polygynous male), business firms and corporations, voluntary organizations, addict subcultures (see Chapter 8), and even the personnel of a hospital

ward. To some extent the relationship between health professionals and their patients, especially if it is long-lasting, resembles that between close family members, even though emotional care usually flows only in one direction.

In many parts of the world, the concept of 'family' also includes the dead. In an emotional sense, therefore, as mentioned in Chapter 9, the dead never die. In much of Asia and Africa and in parts of Latin America the ancestors are still regarded as part of the family, and even though invisible they continue to play important roles in daily life. They are often consulted or worshipped, or shrines are erected to them. In many parts of Africa they are also the guardians of the social order, and punish transgressions among their descendants by causing them to suffer misfortune or fall ill. Contact with the ancestors is usually maintained by regular rituals, attended by most of the family. In the annual Mexican 'Day of the Dead' (*El Día de los Muertos*), for example, the family gathers at the graveside of their relative, decorates it with photos and mementos, and then 'shares' a communal meal with them.[113] This ritual also serves to remind the living that the dead are still very much part of their lives. In some cultures, the links between living and dead are more pervasive and constraining. Widows, for example, may be forbidden ever to remarry, since they are considered permanently married to their dead husbands.

THE FAMILY AS A SMALL-SCALE SOCIETY

However it is constituted, it is useful to view the family as a small-scale society, or even as a small 'tribe', with its own distinctive organization and culture. In many ways, what may be termed this *family culture*[114] is very similar to that of the wider society, but it also has certain unique and distinctive features of its own. As described at the beginning of this book, a culture includes a set of implicit and explicit guidelines telling people how to view the world, how to experience it emotionally and how to behave in it, especially in relation to other people, the natural world and supernatural entities or gods. Families, like larger cultural groups, also have their own particular view of the world, their own codes of behaviour, gender roles, concepts of time and space, private slang and language, history and myths and rituals. They also have ways of communicating psychological distress to one another and to the outside world.

This family culture can be either protective or pathogenic to health, depending on the context. For example, certain types of family structure may contribute to the development of alcohol abuse among the children later in life (see Chapter 8), while others may protect against this. The family can also be seen as a 'system', in which the pattern of inter-relationships can have important influences on both health and disease.[115] This *systems theory* or cybernetic model suggests that family dynamics are often aimed at maintaining a state of equilibrium between these various relationships, even at the cost of psychologically 'scapegoating' one of its members. For example, Minuchin and colleagues[65] have shown how certain types of family structure are more likely to cause psychosomatic disorders such as anorexia nervosa in some of its members. These 'psychosomatic families' maintain their cohesion, continuity and sense of equilibrium, not only by producing this disorder in one of its members, but also by helping to maintain it. The recovery of the 'identified patient' (in this case, the anorexic young girl) may well cause the breakup of such a pathological family. In this case, as in others, focusing only on the individual and not on their family makes a fuller understanding of the problem difficult to achieve.

Byng-Hall[116] described the concept of *family script*, which is transmitted from generation to generation. These scripts are ways of behaving, of viewing the world and of reacting emotionally to it. As with culture in general, most of these scripts are outside of conscious awareness. Their role is to provide a sense of stability and continuity, and a set of guidelines for performing the daily drama of a family's life. They often function to avoid potentially dangerous conflicts within the family. Each generation of the family knows its allocated role within this continuing drama, and sometimes this role may determine when and how they get ill, or even die. The script may also influence the clustering of certain symptoms within a particular family, and how these symptoms are passed on from parents to children.[117] Family scripts can be maintained by the family's own myths and folklore, which are passed on from generation to generation; in some cases, these myths may have originated centuries before the birth of its present members.[116] Many years later, these *family myths* may still be exerting a negative effect on both the mental and physical health of its members.

Like other societies, the family does not exist in a vacuum. It is always part of a *context*, which can be geographic, economic, social, cultural or historical. This context can influence family dynamics and act to either increase or decrease family coherence. Some of the impacts on the family of migration, for example, are described in Chapter 12.

CULTURE AND FAMILY DYNAMICS

The relation of *culture* to family dynamics is complex, and to some extent controversial. McGoldrick and colleagues[118] have provided a comprehensive selection of mini-ethnographies of the family cultures of different ethnic groups in the USA – such as the 'Irish family', 'the Italian family' and the 'British-American family' – and the problems that family therapists face when dealing with each of them. Although it is certainly possible, and useful, to make some generalizations about, say, Italian families, and the cultural themes they have in common, the danger of stereotyping *all* Italian families still applies. Furthermore, listing the supposed cultural traits of families from different ethnic groups often ignores major differences between families (based on region, economic position, social class, education etc.), even if they come from the same ethnic group. Maranhao,[119] in his critique of McGoldrick's book, has also argued that 'family oriented ethnic groups' are sometimes described in it as if their differences from the Anglo-Saxon family type (with its emphasis on

A family Members illness may be hold by the family system

individual rather than family goals) were 'pathological' by definition. Overall, in his view, knowledge of the cultural background of a family is useful but not essential for therapy to take place – 'the interviewer does not have to know anthropology, but just be a sensitive family therapist'.

DiNicola[120] has suggested two alternative ways of describing the relationship between a family's mental health and its culture of origin. *Cultural costume* is 'the particular set of recipes the individuals or families of a community have to give meaning and shape to their experiences and to communicate these experiences through shared ceremonies, rituals and symbols'. It is therefore the repertoire of cultural beliefs and behaviours of which each family culture is a particular (and sometimes unique) expression. The cultural costume becomes *cultural camouflage* 'when culture is invoked as a smokescreen to obscure individual states of mind or patterns of interaction in the family'. That is, the family claims that pathological behaviour patterns within it are only normal expressions of its cultural background. DiNicola quotes, as examples of this: 'My husband drinks very hard, he's Irish,' or 'My son had a breakdown because he stopped going to the Orthodox church and lost the Greek way'.

Lau,[121] like Maranhao, points out how west European or North American family therapists may misdiagnose family patterns from other cultures as pathological or deviant. This is especially likely where the family structure is less familiar to them, as in one-parent families (among some West Indians) or in multigenerational extended families (among Asians, Chinese and Greek Cypriots) who are living in the same household. She points out that in many cultures outside the Western world, 'breaks are not expected between the generations and continuity in the group depends on the presence of three generations'. Notions of individual autonomy and differentiation therefore have a different meaning in these groups from the Western nuclear family model. In dealing with families from ethnic minorities, Barot[122] has further suggested that a focus on their culture may be insuffi-

cient because a wider analysis of the institutional and structural factors (such as unemployment, racial discrimination, poor housing, inadequate social and health-care facilities and the effects of migration) that may also adversely affect their lives is required as well. Furthermore, these external factors may act to weaken the traditional culture and cohesion of those families, so that 'culture' is no longer a viable explanation for many of the pathological breakdowns in family life.

From an international perspective, several detailed studies have shown fundamental variations in family culture between different parts of the world, though, as noted above, these broad generalizations do not take into account variations within each country or community. Tamura and Lau,[123] for example, have contrasted Japanese and Western (particularly British) family structures. In Japan, the culture stresses the *interconnectedness* of relationships, especially within the family. A high value is placed on the unity and wellbeing of the group, and the 'family self' – the 'basic, inner psychological organization' of the Japanese – 'involves intensely emotional intimacy relationships, high levels of receptivity to others, strong identification with the reputation and honour of the family and others'. The individual is thus seen as part of a 'web of interconnectedness', rather than as merely a 'skin-encapsulated ego'. The core of a Japanese family is the mother–child dyad, rather than the husband–wife dyad in the West; because children are firmly in the woman's domain, many Japanese men may be reluctant to accompany their wives to a therapist if their children have problems.

In contrast, family structure in North America and north-western Europe stresses the *separateness* of individuals – their degree of autonomy and individuation from one another – rather than their interconnectedness. Westerners are expected to see themselves as autonomous, independent, individual units, with sharp boundaries between themselves and others. Human growth and emotional development in the family life cycle is seen as a process of individuation, while in Japan it involves the transition from one form of integration to another. Tamura and Lau thus warn against imposing the Western notion of 'hyper-individualism' on Japanese families, or misinterpreting connectedness as 'enmeshment' or inadequate individuation. Japanese therapists tend to see family problems as resulting from *too little* connectedness rather than too much, and therefore aim to strengthen integration of the family unit rather than fragment it. In carrying this out, their clients expect them to be authoritative, directive and also 'connected', almost as if they were senior family members. Finally, Japanese families may avoid seeing a therapist because of feelings of shame and guilt for their inability to deal with the problem within the privacy of the family.

In India, Shankar and Menon[124] stress that the traditional extended or joint family is a key resource in the care of people with serious mental illness, such as schizophrenia. Given the widespread poverty and unemployment – as well as the paucity of psychiatric hospitals, trained mental health professionals and social welfare benefits – therapists planning interventions with families of schizophrenics therefore 'need to take into account the complex matrix of social, economic, cultural, and infrastructural factors that exist in the country'. Thus the majority of the seriously mentally ill are managed by their families, who represent 'the cornerstone of client care in the community'. Because these families (unlike many of their Western equivalents) 'have at no time received the label of being aetiological agents of the illness', they do not feel any sense of guilt if asked to participate in their relative's therapeutic programme. In dealing with Indian schizophrenics, Shankar and Menon therefore suggest that no attempt should be made to blame the family either for causing the illness or for any relapses. Instead, they should be treated as an ally in treatment and not as a potential enemy. The therapist should be sensitive to their needs, as well as those of their ill relative, and should aim to strengthen their positive role in the care of the patient. They should be given ample information on schizophrenia, and encouraged to supervise the patient's medication and to identify any early signs of relapse.

El-Islam[100] has listed 'certain widely shared features of general relevance to psychiatry' in the Arab world, while also emphasizing the enormous cultural diversity within those communities. He describes the strong extended family structure, which favours 'affiliative behaviour' at the expense of 'differentiating behaviour'; that is, 'traditional child rearing instils behaviour oriented towards accommodation, conformity, cooperation, affection, and interdependence rather than behaviour oriented towards individuation, intellectualisation, independence and compartmentalisation'. Also, in more traditional communities, women 'are at a socio-cultural disadvantage in relation to men'; polygyny is still practised, arranged marriages are common, and divorce is more easily obtained by men than by women. In this setting, conflicts may arise between older family members and a more Westernized younger generation, especially over attitudes to sexual behaviour, education and the choice of marriage partner. However, El-Islam notes that, for those of its members who have a mental illness (such as schizophrenia), the extended family provides a more therapeutic setting, and with a better prognosis, than would institutionalization. In Oman, Al-Adawi and colleagues[68] described how individuals (mostly women) who have been 'possessed' by the malevolent *zar* spirit are exorcised by a shaman, and then join the community of those who have also been afflicted by that same spirit. This new group becomes a sort of quasi-family for them, 'a form of fictive kinship which enables these individuals to join supportive, cooperative groups of other afflicted people', and which can help create long-term relationships that last for many years.

Therefore, as this section illustrates, family therapy provides one of the most fruitful areas of co-operation between psychology, psychiatry and medical anthropology – especially in understanding the family's role in both the cause and cure of mental illness – and research in this area is likely to increase in the future.

CROSS-CULTURAL PSYCHIATRIC DIAGNOSIS

This chapter has illustrated some of the complexities in making cross-cultural psychiatric diagnoses, and especially the problems of defining 'normality' and 'abnormality' in the members of other cultures. A further problem is that clinicians may *over*emphasize culture as an explanation for patients' behaviour, and thus ignore any underlying psychopathology.[125] In making cross-cultural diagnoses, therefore, the clinician should always be aware of:

- the extent to which cultural factors affect some of the diagnostic categories and techniques of Western psychiatry
- the role of the patients' culture in helping them understand and communicate their psychological distress
- how the patients' beliefs and behaviour are viewed by other members of their cultural group, and whether their abnormality is viewed as beneficial to the group or not
- whether the specific cluster of symptoms, signs and behavioural changes shown by the patients are interpreted by them, and by their community, as evidence of a 'culture-bound' psychological disorder
- whether the patient's condition is indicative not of mental illness, but rather of the social, political and economic pressures upon them.

KEY REFERENCES

3 Lewis, I. M (1971). *Ecstatic Religion*, pp. 178–205. London: Penguin.

16 Kleinman, A. (1987). Anthropology and psychiatry. *Br. J. Psychiatry* 151, 447–54.

18 Kirmayer, L.J. and Minas, H. (2000) The future of cultural psychiatry: an international perspective. *Can. J. Psychiatry* 45, 438–446.

19 Waxler, N. (1977). Is mental illness cured in traditional societies? A theoretical analysis. *Cult. Med. Psychiatry* 1, 233–53.

58 Mumford, D. B. (1993). Somatization: a transcultural perspective. *Int. Rev. Psychiatry* 5, 231–42.

67 Tseng, W-S. (2003) *Clinician's Guide to Cultural Psychiatry*. London: Academic Press, pp. 89–142.

72 Hahn, R.A. (1995) *Sickness and Healing: an Anthropological Perspective*. New Haven: Yale University Press, pp. 40–56.

79 Cooper, J.E. (1994) *ICD-10: Classification of Mental and Behavioural Disorders*. Edinburgh: Churchill Livingstone/World Health Organization.

80 American Psychiatric Association (2000) *DSM-IV-TR: Diagnostic and Statistical Manual of Mental Disorders*, 4th edn. Arlington: American Psychiatric Association.

100 El-Islam, M.F. (1982). Arabic cultural psychiatry. *Transcult. Psychiatry Res. Rev.* 19, 5–24.

104 Campion, J. and Bhugra, D. (1997). Experiences of religious healing in psychiatric patients in south India. *Soc. Psychiatry Psychiatric Epidemiol.* 32(4), 215–21.

118 McGoldrick, M., Pearce, J. K. and Giordano, J. (eds) (1982). *Ethnicity and Family Therapy*. New York: Guildford Press.

119 Maranhao, T. (1984). Family therapy and anthropology. *Cult. Med. Psychiatry* 8, 255–79.

See http://www.culturehealthandillness for the full list of references for this chapter.

RECOMMENDED READING

Bhui, K. and Bhugra, D. (eds) (2007) *Culture and Mental Health*. London: Hodder Arnold.

Desjarlais, R., Eisenberg, L., Good, B. and Kleinman, A. (eds) (1995) *World Mental Health*. Oxford: Oxford University Press.

Kleinman, A. (1988). *Rethinking Psychiatry*. New York: Free Press.

Kutchins, H. and Kirk, S.A. (1997) *Making Us Crazy: DSM – The Psychiatric Bible and the Creation of Mental Disorders*. New York: Free Press.

Littlewood, R. and Lipsedge, M. (1997). *Aliens and Alienists*, 3rd edn. Abingdon: Routledge.

Swartz, L. (1998). *Culture and Mental Health: A Southern African View*. Oxford: Oxford University Press.

Tseng, W-S. (2003) *Clinician's Guide to Cultural Psychiatry*. London: Academic Press.

RECOMMENDED WEBSITES

Annotated Bibliography of Cultural Psychiatry: http://www.admsep.org/culture.html

Society for the Study of Psychiatry and Culture (USA): http://www.psychiatryandculture.org

World Psychiatric Association: http://www.wpanet.org/home.html

World Association of Cultural Psychiatry: http://www.waculturalpsychiatry.org

11

Cultural aspects of stress and suffering

Reflective essay

THE NATURE OF STRESS

'Stress' is one of the most commonly used words of the modern world. An internet search for the word 'stress' in 2005 revealed 185 million entries on Yahoo[1] and 126 million on Google,[2] though not all of them referred to psychological stress. At the level of popular culture, 'stress' has become one of the most pervasive metaphors for personal and collective *suffering,* and for all the difficulties that people encounter in everyday life. In more developed countries, it is a word that pervades everyday conversations, and which appears with increasing frequency on newspaper and magazine pages, and on the radio and television.

The concept of 'stress' was first described by Hans Selye in 1936,[3] and soon attracted much attention; by 1976 more than 110 000 papers had been published on it in the academic literature,[4] and it had become a widely-used concept in popular culture.

In Selye's original model (based on an engineering concept) 'stress' represents the generalized response of the organism to environmental demands. It is an inherent physiological mechanism which prepares the organism for action, and which comes into play when demands are placed on it. Not all stress is harmful to the organism: at a moderate level ('eustress') it has a protective and adaptive function. However, at a higher level ('dystress') the stress response can cause pathological changes and even death. The actual environmental influence – whether physical, psychological or socio-cultural – that produces stress is termed a *stressor*. Selye has described the sequence of events whereby an organism responds to a stressor as the General Adaptation Syndrome (GAS). This usually has three stages:

1 The *alarm* reaction, whereby the organism becomes aware of a specific noxious stimulus.
2 The stage of resistance or *adaptation*, in which the organism recovers to a functional level superior to that which existed before it was stressed.
3 The stage of *exhaustion,* where the recovery processes, under the continuing assault of stressors, are no longer able to cope and to restore homeostasis.

In this final stage, the physiological changes that have taken place in the organism now become pathological to it, and disease or death results. From a physiological point of view, the GAS is said to be mediated via the adrenal medulla and the hypothalamic–pituitary–adrenocortical axis, and involves a wide range of physical changes.[5]

CRITIQUES OF SELYE'S MODEL

Selye's early model, although widely accepted as basic for much stress research, has been criticized on several counts – in particular, for its rather mechanistic approach and its overemphasis on the physiological dimensions of the stress response. Psychologists such as Weinman[6] have pointed out the importance of the *psychological* responses or coping strategies of the individual confronted by a stressor. These range from an initial 'alarm and shock state', with feelings of anxiety or of being threatened, through attempts to cope with the subjectively unpleasant situation, to a range of more extreme psychological reactions such as depression, withdrawal, suicide or resorting to 'chemical comforters'. These responses, as well as the *meanings* people give to their stressful experiences, are all influenced by the individual's personality, education, social environment, economic situation and cultural background. As such, they are of more interest to the social scientist than the purely physiological stress responses.

A further salient critique of Selye's model, and of much of the subsequent literature on stress, comes from the anthropologist Allan Young[7]. He argues that 'stressors' are often described in the stress literature as if they were abstract 'things', separated from a particular social and political context, and a particular time and place. Sometimes they are described almost as if they were invisible pathogens or forces that cause illness or unhappiness to certain individuals. Furthermore, the focus on these decontextualized stressors and their physiological effects may lead to ignoring the larger economic and social forces acting upon the individual, which may also have an adverse effect on health.

Pollock,[8] too, has criticized Selye's approach, pointing out that his original model of how stress acts physiologically was a mechanical one, taken from physics and engineering. However, since then stress theory has become heavily 'psychologized', with an increasing emphasis on the pathogenic role of emotions and perceptions, but 'it still relies for its validation on the physiological models with which it is fundamentally non-compatible'. In addition, the key link in stress theory – the postulated process by which stress is actually transformed into illness – 'remains unclear and unproven', and many of the studies carried out on this link have produced 'inconsistent, contradictory or inconclusive results'.

Another critique of the model is that it overemphasizes the *external* origin of stress, so that the individual often appears in the stress literature as a passive victim of circumstances. However, from a psychological point of view, many sources of stress may originate *within* the individual. Whatever their origin in early development, these intrapsychic factors, such as exaggerated fears, chronic anxiety, aggressiveness, insecurity, oversensitivity or false expectations of life, may all contribute towards one individual having a much more stressful life than another.

Finally, the assumption that stress is always *negative* in its effect on the individual can also be challenged. McElroy and Townsend[9], for example, point out that in many cultures certain rituals can actually induce physical and emotional stress as part of a healing process. These rituals may include painful stimuli (such as fire-walking), physical exhaustion, sleep deprivation, extreme heat or cold, hyperventilation or altered states of consciousness – sometimes with the aid of hallucinogenic drugs (see Chapter 8). To members of these cultural groups, these stressful processes are an essential prerequisite to being healed. Furthermore, on a physical level, some of these culturally induced stressors may cause the release of endorphins, or endogenous opiates, which induce feelings of wellbeing, reduce pain perception and have a variety of other positive physiological effects.[9]

Despite these and many other criticisms, Selye's model of stressors and stress responses is useful as a starting point in understanding how human beings cope with the adversities of life. It can be used as an analytical tool, provided that there is an awareness of its limitations and that the role of *context* – psychological, social, cultural and economic – is always included when trying to understand why one individual or group finds some situations stressful, while others do not.

RELATION OF STRESSORS TO STRESS RESPONSE

By definition, a 'stressor', according to Selye, is an environmental influence or agent that produces a stress response in the organism. The range of possible stressors is therefore extremely wide, and a list could include such events as severe illness or trauma, natural disasters, bereavement, divorce, marital conflict, unemployment, retirement, interpersonal tensions at work, religious or other persecution, financial difficulties, changes in occupation, migration, wartime combat and excessive exposure to heat, cold, damp or noise. However, the relationship between stressors and their response is more complex than this list suggests. For example, the same event might cause stress in one individual but not in another. Also, as Parkes[10] points out, stress can arise from usually positive experiences such as promotion, engagement, the birth of a child or winning a great deal of money, all of which involve a change in lifestyle. Individuals vary in how they cope with and adapt to these life changes, and to more adverse circumstances such as bereavement. In both cases, as the World Health Organization (WHO)[11] point out, stress (and the diseases that result from it) represent an unsuccessful attempt on the part of the body to deal with adverse factors in the environment. Thus, 'disease is the body's failure to become adapted to these adverse factors rather than the effect of the factors themselves'. There are many reasons for this failure of adaptation, including the physical, psychological and socio-cultural characteristics of the individual. For example, elderly frail people are more likely to experience cold or very humid weather as 'stressful' than younger, more robust people. Also, some situations (such as retirement) may cause a stress response in one person but not in another. Weinman notes that 'specific situations or objects are threatening to the individual because they are perceived as such rather than because of some inherent characteristic'.[6] Some of the social or cultural factors that apparently predispose to, or protect against, the stress response will be described later in this chapter.

According to Selye,[4] the relationship between particular stressors and the response they elicit is marked by *non-specificity*. That is, it cannot be predicted what specific stress-related disease (such as peptic ulceration, psychiatric disorders, hypertension or coronary thrombosis) will result from a specific stressor (such as marital conflict, frustration at work, combat fatigue or burns). A stressor such as marital conflict may result in peptic ulceration in one individual and bronchial asthma in another. In psychosomatic research (see Chapter 10) this is known as the problem of *organ choice,* and many theories have been put forward to explain why one organ is 'chosen' and not another.[12] In practical terms, therefore, a stressor and its effect can only be linked circumstantially, and to some extent only *post hoc*, though more experimental evidence is accumulating on the nature and prevalence of this link.

Stress can also be viewed either as a causal factor in disease – or as a contributory one – by reducing the individual's 'resistance' to disease processes such as viral infections[13] or rheumatoid arthritis.[14] The relatively new field of *psychoneuroimmunology (PNI)* has tried to examine the relationships between psychological state, the endocrine system and the body's defences or immune system.[15] Although still characterized by non-specificity, there is evidence that depression and anxiety may adversely affect the immune system and thus increase susceptibility to infections and other illnesses.[15] In other cases, an individual with a pre-existing organic disease might have a relapse in response to stress, as described by Trimble and Wilson-Barnet[16] in the case of epileptic seizures. Finally, the physical disease itself may be a stressful experience which can delay recovery or cause other forms of ill health, especially if it involves loss of income or of job security or a change in personal relationships.

STRESS AND LIFE CHANGES

Many of the stressors mentioned above, such as bereavement, migration or the birth of a child, involve prolonged, major *changes* in the patterns of people's lives. In recent years, more attention has been paid to the possible negative effects of these changes on both mental and physical health. From this point of view, stress represents an inadequate adaptation to change, an unsuccessful attempt on the part of the individual to cope with and adapt to the changed circumstances of their lives – whether this is promotion at work or the loneliness of widowhood. Parkes[10] provides a useful way of viewing these changes or *psychosocial transitions*. He points out that the change is likely to take place in that part of the world which impinges upon the self – the *life space*. This consists of 'those parts of the environment with which the self interacts and in relation to which behaviour is organized; other persons, material possessions, the familiar world of home and place of work, and the individual's body and mind in so far as he can view these as separate from his self'. They also involve changes in the basic assumptions that people have made about their worlds, for these can no longer be taken for granted. In Parkes's view, the psychosocial transitions most likely to cause stress are those that are lasting in their effects, take place over a relatively short period of time, and affect many of the assumptions that people make about their worlds. In that sense, the sudden unexpected loss of a spouse or job is likely to be more stressful than other slower transitions, such as those involved in growth and maturation. Changes such as bereavement, losing a job, or migration will involve many aspects of an individual's life space, such as social relationships, occupational status, financial security and living arrangements, and are more likely to provoke a stress response.

The effects of these changes on both mental and physical health have been studied by several investigators. For example, in their classic study of bereavement in the late 1960s, Parkes and his colleagues[17] examined the death rates of 4486 widowers aged 55 years or older for 9 years following the death of their wives. Of these, 213 died in the first 6 months of bereavement – 40 per cent above the expected death rate for married men of the same ages. The death rate from degenerative heart disease was 67 per cent higher than expected. The mortality rate dropped to that of married men after the first year. The authors ascribed the increased death rate to 'the emotional effects of bereavement with the concomitant changes in psychoendocrine function'. Since then other studies have reached similar conclusions; in a significant number of cases, ill health is preceded by a high level of psychosocial transitions or 'life events', especially if these events are perceived as negative.

The precise causal link between these life changes and the occurrence of ill health remains unclear, though various hypotheses have been advanced. In 1980, Murphy and Brown,[18] in examining the question 'whether stressful situations bring about episodes of illness associated with pathological structural changes occurring in a tissue, system or area of the body', pointed out that in most cases illness will *not* follow from an experience of stress, but where it does the link is likely to be a psychiatric disturbance. They cited evidence that individuals with psychiatric disorders had a significantly higher rate of organic illness, and hypothesized that 'stressful circumstances lead to organic illness by first producing a psychiatric disturbance'. In their study of 111 women in London, 81 had developed a new organic disease (from which they had previously not suffered) in the previous 6 months. Of this latter group, 30 per cent (24) had had at least one severe life event before the onset of ill health, compared with 17 per cent of a matched comparison group. However, this association applied only to women aged between 18 and 50 years, where 38 per cent had had at least one severe event compared with 15 per cent of a control group. In this age group, 30 per cent had experienced the onset of psychiatric disturbance in an average period of 7 weeks before the start of their illness, compared with an expected 2 per cent in the control group. The authors concluded that 'it is the onset of psychiatric disturbance rather than a severe event that is the immediate cause of organic disorder for those [women] under 50'.

The events most likely to cause psychiatric disorders are those involving long-term threat to the 'life space', such as an unplanned pregnancy, or terminal illness in a relative. However, the exact physiological mechanism whereby life events, psychiatric disorder and organic illness are all interlinked remains unclear. Engel[19] has also pointed out how sometimes illness and even death can be preceded by a period of psychological disturbance, during which the person feels 'unable to cope'. He termed this the *giving-up–given-up complex*, and suggests that this state 'plays some significant role in modifying the capacity of the organism to cope with concurrent pathogenic factors'. It is characterized by a feeling of: psychological impotence or helplessness ('giving-up'); a lowered self-image as one who is no longer competent, in control or functioning in the usual manner; a loss of gratification from human relationships and social roles; a disruption of the sense of continuity between past, present and future; and reactivation of earlier memories of helplessness and giving-up. In this state, the person is less likely to deal with pathological processes, though the complex itself does not 'cause disease directly but rather contributes towards its emergence'. Once again, the precise physiological mechanism by which this occurs remains unclear. However, the three perspectives mentioned above – 'psychosocial transitions', 'life events' and the 'giving-up–given-up' complex – all provide useful ways of viewing the effects on health and illness of such dramatic changes in life space as migration, urbanization, conquest, refugee status, rapid social or technological change or 'voodoo death'.

FACTORS INFLUENCING THE STRESS RESPONSE

In Selye's original model, stress represented a pathological physical response to environmental demands. However, as noted earlier, this response is mediated by a number of other factors, including:

1 The characteristics of the individuals concerned.
2 Their physical environment.
3 The social support available to them.
4 Their economic status.
5 Their cultural background.

INDIVIDUAL CHARACTERISTICS

The individual's characteristics that influence response to stress are partly physical (such as age, weight, build, genetic make-up, state of nutrition and previous health) and partly psychological. Weinman[6] points out how differences in personality affect response to stress, from phlegmatic types to those whose response is primarily somatic – such as the 'gastric responders' or 'cardiovascular responders'. Infantile and childhood experiences also play some part, as do the individuals' perception of whether they have control over their lives or not. In the work situation, for example, Karasek and colleagues[20] have related a low sense of personal control to high levels of stress response. To a variable degree, the individual's outlook on life – including his or her hopes, fears and ambitions – is conditioned by socio-cultural background as well as by their early upbringing.

PHYSICAL ENVIRONMENT

Physical sources of stress include extreme heat, cold, dryness, damp and wind, as well as pollution and overcrowding, and sources of tissue damage such as pathogenic organisms, burns or trauma. In all these cases, the nature and extent of the environmental stressor will influence the severity of the stress response.

SOCIAL SUPPORT

Social and cultural factors tend to overlap in practice, but will be considered separately. Several authors have noted the importance of social support, at all stages of life, in protecting against stress. Weinman[6] notes how 'insufficient early support can give rise to physical and behavioural abnormalities, including a reduced ability to withstand stress' later in life. Brown and Harris[21] have demonstrated that women who lost their mothers before the age of 11 years are more vulnerable to depression in adulthood, and a close and confiding relationship with another person helps protect against stress and psychiatric disorder. Kiritz and Moos[22] also pointed out the relationships of social environment to stress. In their view, social support and a sense of group cohesion *protect* against stress, while a sense of personal responsibility for others increases the physiological stress response. It is also increased by work pressure (to complete a large number of transactions per unit time), uncertainty (about the possibility of physical or psychological harm) and change in their psychosocial environments (such as job relocation, unemployment or redundancy). Some social factors, such as violence – whether domestic, crime-related or political – can be important stressors, with a major impact on the mental and physical health of the individual.

ECONOMIC STATUS

Economic factors are especially relevant to the stress response. Unemployment, deprivation and poverty (and the associated poor housing, diet, sanitation, clothing, and exposure to crime and violence) are potent stressors in any community, as is loss of income and financial insecurity resulting from either physical or mental ill health. The competitiveness, high expectations, long hours and lack of job security associated with so many careers in the industrialized world today also leads to a heightening of the stress response.

CULTURAL BACKGROUND

Cultural factors play a complex role in the response to stress. In general, this role might considered to be either *protective* or *pathogenic* ('culturogenic stress'). Culture also helps to shape the *form* of the stress response into a recognizable language of dis-

tress. That is, different cultural groups exposed to similar stressors may display different types of stress response, as may men and women within the same cultural group. In their study of French, American, Filipino and Haitian college students in 1975, Guthrie and colleagues[23] found clustering of the different symptoms of stress in the four groups. The Americans, for example, reported more gastrointestinal symptoms, while the French reported more changes in mood or thought content. The Filipinos, especially the women, tended to emphasize cardiovascular symptoms, such as a rapid heartbeat and shortness of breath. Symptoms such as dizziness, headaches, nightmares and muscle twitches were more often mentioned by women in all four groups, and the authors suggest that 'in certain societies it may be less socially acceptable for males to admit and experience this constellation of symptoms'. The cultural values of a group may also *protect* against stress, for example, by strengthening social and family cohesion and mutual support, which enable the individual to cope better with the vicissitudes of life. A culture's world-view can also have this effect, by placing individual suffering in the wider context of misfortune in general. This is characteristic of religious world-views, especially those with a fatalistic view of misfortune as being an expression of divine will or fate. Membership of a group with such a shared conceptual system also helps give meaning and coherence to daily life, and reduces the stress of uncertainty. Cultures that value meditation and contemplation rather than competitiveness and material achievement are probably less stressful overall to their members. A further factor is that in many societies the rearing of children (and the stress that goes with it) is shared among several adults of an extended family as well as the parents, and this may also have a protective function. In looking at non-Western or pre-industrial societies, however, care should be taken to avoid what has been termed 'the myth of the stress-free "primitive" existence'.[24] Contrary to the WHO's contention[11] that stress as 'a traditional method of adaptation has become inadequate in the psychological, social and economic circumstances of modem society', the evi-

Figure 11.1 A *favela* or shanty town in Porto Alegre, Brazil. Poverty, unemployment, poor housing, and inadequate sanitation are all major sources of stress in many parts of the world.

dence is that traditional societies, too, have their full share of damaging stressors.

'CULTUROGENIC' STRESS: THE NOCEBO EFFECT "I Hurt" reverse placebo

While culture can protect against stress, it can also make it more likely. That is, certain cultural beliefs, values, expectations and practices are likely to *increase* the number of stressors that the individual is exposed to. For example, each culture defines what constitutes 'success' (as opposed to 'failure'), prestige (as opposed to loss of face), 'good' behaviour (as opposed to 'bad') and 'good news' (as opposed to bad tidings), and there is considerable variation between these in different societies. In part of New Guinea, for example, failure to have enough pigs or yams to exchange with other tribal members on certain occasions may lead to a stressful loss of face; in the Western world, failure to 'keep up with the Joneses' in terms of lifestyle or consumer objects may also result in subjective stress. In each society, individuals try to reach the defined goals, levels of prestige and standards of behaviour that the cultural group expects of its members. Failure to reach these goals, even if the goals seem absurd to mem-

bers of another society, may result in frustration, anxiety, depression and even the 'giving-up–given-up' complex described above. Some beliefs can be directly stressful, such as the belief that one has been 'cursed' or 'hexed' by a powerful person against whom there is little defence. In some cases, as in 'voodoo death', this may result in the victim's death after a short period of time. Other cultural values that may induce stress are an emphasis on warlike activities, or intense competition for marriage partners, money, goods or prestige. The unequal distribution of wealth in a society, based on its economic culture, is usually stressful to its poorer members, whose lives are a daily struggle for survival; however, economic privileges also sometimes involve high levels of stress owing to competitiveness and fear of the poor. Also, as Marmot[25] has described, *relative* social inequality, accompanied by a sense of not having control over one's life and work, is associated with higher levels of both morbidity and mortality – and this applies in both rich countries and poor countries.

In its effect upon the health of the individual, therefore, there are both negative and positive sides to belief. According to Hahn and Kleinman,[26] 'belief kills; belief heals'. Those beliefs and behaviours that contribute to stress, and are acquired by growing up within a particular society, can therefore be regarded as a form of culturally induced or 'culturogenic' stress.

This type of stress is also an example of the nocebo phenomenon (from the Latin root *noceo*, I hurt), which is the negative effect on health of beliefs and expectations, and therefore the exact reverse of the placebo phenomenon (see Chapter 8).

CULTUROGENIC STRESS: SOME EXAMPLES

Socio–cultural death

The most extreme form of culturogenic stress and the nocebo effect described by anthropologists is known as 'voodoo death', 'hex death' or 'magical death', which Landy[27] prefers to term *socio-cultural death*. This phenomenon has been reported from various parts of the world, including Latin America, Africa, the Caribbean and Australia, and is usually found in traditional, preindustrial societies. In magical death, people who believe they have been marked out for death by sorcery sicken and die within a short period, apparently of natural causes. Once victims and those around them believe that a fatal curse has been placed upon them, then all concerned regard them as doomed. As Landy states, a 'process is set in motion, usually by a supposed religious or social transgression that results in the transgressor being marked out for death by a sorcerer acting on behalf of society through a ritual of accusation and condemnation; then death occurs within a brief span, usually 24 to 48 hours'. The anthropologist Claude Levi-Strauss[28] provided a graphic account of this process, beginning with the individual's awareness that he is doomed, according to the traditions of his culture. His family and friends share this belief, and gradually the community withdraws from him. Often they remind the unfortunate victim that he is doomed, and virtually dead. Then: 'Shortly thereafter, sacred rites are held to dispatch him to the realm of shadows. First brutally torn from all of his family and social ties and excluded from all functions and activities through which he experienced self-awareness, then banished by the same forces from the world of the living, the victim yields to the combined terror, the sudden total withdrawal of the multiple reference systems provided by the support of the group, and, finally, to the group's decisive reversal in proclaiming him – once a living man, with rights and obligations – dead and an object of fear, ritual, and taboo'.

This situation is a classic example of Engel's 'giving-up–given-up' complex, which he sees as a life setting conducive both to illness and to sudden death. In 1971 he analysed the reports of 170 cases of sudden death,[29] and found certain common themes in most of them:

- they involved events that were impossible for the victim to ignore
- the individual experienced or was threatened with overwhelming emotional excitation
- the person believed he or she no longer had control over the situation.

Ten of the cases involved sudden death during loss of status or self-esteem; for example, two men who were confidently expecting promotion to important positions dropped dead when their expectations were unexpectedly dashed. Various hypotheses have been advanced to explain the mechanism of culturogenic sudden death. Cannon[30] believed it was caused by overactivity of the sympathetic nervous system – the 'fight or flight' response – in a situation where the victim is (culturally) immobilized and can do neither. According to Engel,[31] it is caused by vasovagal syncope and cardiac arrhythmias in a patient with pre-existing cardiovascular disease. This occurs in cases of emotional arousal and psychological uncertainty, where both the sympathetic ('fight-flight') and parasympathetic ('conservation-withdrawal') systems are simultaneously activated. In Lex's[32] view this simultaneous activation takes place in the settings characteristic of magical death. In this state the nervous system is 'tuned' or oversensitized, and the individual is more vulnerable to suggestions that he will die by magical means; he is also vulnerable to acute parasympathetic hyper-reactivity, or vagal death.

'Magical death' is an extreme and dramatic form of the culturogenic stress response. It represents the reverse of Hertz's[33] model of bereavement (see Chapter 9), for here social death *precedes* biological death by a variable period of time. In a Western setting, long-term admission to a psychiatric institution, old-age home, geriatric ward or prison can also be seen (in some circumstances) as a form of socio-cultural death, as can retirement, unemployment, or bankruptcy, or even – in some societies and cultural groups – childlessness, widowhood or divorce. Each of these involves a major change in the circumstances of daily life. In the case of people who have been institutionalized, they encounter a whole new set of stressors, of the sort well described by Erving Goffman[34] in the case of mental hospitals, but his findings apply also to other similar 'total environments'.

A modern form of social death was seen among the first to suffer from the acquired immunodeficiency syndrome (AIDS), in the early years of the epidemic – and this is still the case in some developing countries. Cassens[35] described the many stressful social consequences that occurred for homosexual men who had been diagnosed as having this condition at that time. As well as the physical illness itself, they had to cope with guilt, anxiety and the fear of certain death, and the strong prejudices of other people (see Chapter 16). There was also a loss of privacy about their sexuality, possible loss of employment, rejection by family and friends, and constant exposure to lurid stories in the media with their 'tones of sin and retribution', which could only increase their sense of social isolation and rejection. Since then the level of stigma attached to people with human immunodeficiency virus (HIV)/AIDS has reduced considerably, at least in the developed world.

The effect of diagnostic labels

Another, though much less extreme, example of culturogenic stress is the damaging effect on health and behaviour of certain diagnostic labels – for example, patients told by their doctor 'you've got cancer', 'you've got a weak heart' or 'you've got hypertension'. In Waxler's[36] view, certain diagnostic labels can affect patients' symptoms, behaviour, social relationships, prognosis and self-perception, as well as the attitudes of others towards them. This may even occur in the absence of physical disease. In this case, the nocebo phenomenon results from lay beliefs about the origin, significance, severity and prognosis of 'a weak heart' or 'hypertension', and about the behaviour appropriate to sufferers from that condition. Patients may see themselves as ill or disabled, while family and friends may begin treating them in a particular way, such as encouraging them to change their diet

or behaviour, or to take special precautions. Like the patient, the relatives' attitudes are shaped by cultural beliefs about the significance of certain diseases. In the case of children, this might have lifelong effects; parents of a child labelled 'asthmatic' may, based on their own childhood memories of what asthma entailed, prohibit the child from a wide range of social or sporting activities. A diagnostic label can thus become a form of self-fulfilling prophecy. Some individuals who are labelled as 'ill' may become enmeshed within certain institutions that sustain the label rather than encourage its disappearance. Waxler notes how organizations such as Alcoholics Anonymous (AA), for example, may inadvertently prolong an individual's label of 'illness' because 'a large percentage of AA members' social lives centres on the organization and other members, thus isolating them from normal relationships and further strengthening their role as "alcoholics"'. She quotes another study of a group of American farmers who had no evidence of cardiac disease, but who labelled themselves as having 'heart disease' because they misunderstood their doctors' diagnosis. As a result they took more heart-related precautions, and generally acted like cardiac invalids. As Waxler points out, the label itself – what the farmer or his family *believed* to be the case – had an important effect upon his behaviour, even when he had no symptoms and no disease. Another example of how labelling can affect everyday behaviour is described by Haynes and colleagues,[37] who screened factory workers for hypertension. In those (asymptomatic) patients who were told they had 'hypertension', absenteeism from work rose by 80 per cent, greatly exceeding the 9 per cent rise in absenteeism in the general employee population during the same period. Certain diagnostic labels, therefore, if they provoke anxiety and foreboding (such as 'cancer'), are likely to act as additional stressors, especially if the person is already physically ill.

The setting

Similarly, certain *settings* (such as a hospital clinic or doctor's office) can also induce so much anxiety that it causes a physiological response, which can be misdiagnosed as disease. The two best-known examples of this phenomenon are 'white coat hypertension'[38] and 'white coat hyperglycaemia'.[39] In the former, higher blood pressure readings are found when taken in a medical setting, compared with measurements taken in the patient's home. In the latter, it is the blood glucose level that is higher when measured in the clinic, compared with a similar test carried out in the home.

The 'Type–A Behaviour Pattern'

A final example of how the cultural values of a society may contribute towards stress and disease in its members is seen in the case of coronary heart disease (CHD). This condition is believed to have a multifactorial aetiology, and a number of risk factors that predispose to its development have been described. These include a high dietary intake of saturated fats, lack of exercise, cigarette smoking, raised serum cholesterol and hypertension. However, the work of Friedman and Rosenman[40] suggests that psychosocial patterns, especially behaviour patterns and personality type, also play a role in its aetiology, particularly in susceptible individuals. In 1959 they first described the characteristics of what they termed the *Type A behaviour pattern* (TABP) – in particular, an individual's chronic struggle to achieve an unlimited number of goals in as short a time as possible. Those individuals displaying the TABP show marked aggressiveness, ambition and competitive drive; they are work-orientated and 'workaholic' people, preoccupied with deadlines and chronically impatient.[40] Their personal lives are emotionally parched and incomplete, and both family and leisure are less important to them than work and ambition. Long-term follow-up studies have shown that individuals with this behaviour pattern are about twice as likely to develop CHD as other adults of similar age without these traits (known as the *Type B* behaviour pattern).[41] According to Friedman and Rosenman, modern Western industrial society encourages the development of Type A traits, and rewards them. Those who exhibit them often become successful executives, professionals, politicians, managers, technocrats and salesmen. However, these rewards often involve constant anxiety about failure, demotion or loss of control. Appels[42] saw this type of personality as one who cannot manage or handle the pressures of the industrialized, fast-moving and achievement-orientated society and who, by this very failure, shows the characteristics of this society in an excessive way. In his study of 22 societies he found that the mortality rate from CHD was positively correlated with a cultural emphasis in the societies on the need for achievement. Waldron[43] has examined the relationship of Type A behaviour and gender within the USA, where the risk of CHD is twice as great in men as in women. She suggests that while men's excess vulnerability may be partly due to hormonal factors, cultural factors also play a part. In particular, Type A behaviour can contribute to success in traditional male roles and professions, but not in the traditional female role in society. Accordingly, parents and other socializing institutions may promote Type A characteristics in boys but not in girls, and later in life this may protect a higher proportion of the women from the risk of CHD.

Not everyone who is 'Type A' gets a heart attack, and neither are all those who have CHD 'Type As'.[44] It is therefore useful to view the idea of the TABP as a Western 'culture-bound syndrome' (see Chapter 10), embodying many of the cultural values of an industrial, capitalist society, where competition, ambition, materialism and the time-urgency of rush hours and deadlines are all part of daily life. Furthermore, this model of stressful behaviour also encompasses some of the *contradictions* within the cultural values of Western society, and the Type A individual is the living embodiment of those contradictions. On one hand, for example, he conforms to the social values of his society – to what Weber[45] terms its 'philosophy of avarice' – and is rewarded for doing so, but on the other hand his hostile, competitive behaviour is also antisocial, damaging to himself, his family, his friends and those he works with. It can be argued

297

that this paradox of values – that some forms of antisocial behaviour are being constantly rewarded by society – is symbolically resolved (at least for a while) when he is 'punished' by suffering a heart attack, and emerges from the hospital as a chastened, fragile and less aggressive Type B.[44]

Chapter 15 includes a discussion of how some immigrants to the USA, such as the Japanese, seem to be partly protected by their cultural background against the risk of both Type A behaviour and CHD, provided that they retain many of their traditional cultural values.

COLLECTIVE STRESS AND SOCIAL SUFFERING

Under some conditions, an entire population may be said to be 'under stress'. One of the most important examples of this is migration, which now involves many millions of people worldwide, and which is described in more detail in Chapter 12. However, social suffering is also particularly common in conditions of war, civil unrest, natural disasters, population movements, political oppression, economic insecurity and extreme poverty – even if these populations do not migrate. In some cases, several of these factors may operate at the same time and in the same place.

In the sense of collective suffering, the twentieth century and the beginning of the twenty-first may be seen as one of the most stressful periods in human history. In addition to two world wars, there have been numerous civil wars, interethnic strife and widespread political repression. There has been genocide and ethnic cleansing, including the Armenian massacres of World War One, the Nazi holocaust of World War Two, the genocides of Cambodia and Rwanda, the mass killings in Bosnia, Kosovo, Darfur, and elsewhere, and the many terrorist atrocities, hostage-taking and suicide bombings of recent years. The decades of the Cold War were marked by constant anxiety about a nuclear Armageddon. In addition, Desjarlais and colleagues,[46] in the *World Mental Health* report,

cited the numerous low-intensity wars, such as those that have ravaged parts of Africa, Latin America and Asia for many years, as a particular cause of considerable stress and tension at the population level. In these conflicts the aim is usually control over populations rather than territory and, as a result, violence often takes take place anywhere within the country, and can affect civilians as well as soldiers. As with other conflicts this century, these low-intensity wars have left large numbers of people with the *post-traumatic stress disorder* (PTSD) – suffering long-term symptoms of anxiety, depression, psychosomatic disorders and social dysfunction, and experiencing 'flashbacks' to traumatic events – even long after the conflict is over and the 'stress' of it has receded.[46,47] Because many of these conflicts have taken place in poorer countries, at the margins of the world economy, the access of millions of victims to medical and mental health facilities is often very limited.

In circumstances where a similar level of stress is shared by many others in the population, what is the effect of this on the individual? Does it help make their own experience less stressful in some way, or more so? And how can communities who have collectively suffered social stress heal themselves in a collective way?

According to Desjarlais and colleagues,[46] a collective healing process almost always involves people talking openly about their pain and suffering. Often the authorities have imposed a 'wall of silence' that has to be breached before healing can take place. Expressing these narratives or trauma stories, either in public or to a therapist, is one way that people can give meaning to their experience, enabling them to leave the past behind them (see Chapter 5). In South Africa, for example, Swartz[47] described the situation of the many millions of non-white people who lived under the oppressive racist system of *apartheid*. Over almost 50 years, many of them were subject to constant humiliation, social and economic discrimination, the break-up of families, arbitrary arrest, forced relocation, and sometimes torture, extrajudicial killings and 'disappearances'. Although the effects of this system on the health of the population are difficult to quantify, it has left behind a considerable legacy of social, psychological and economic problems, including poverty, violence, crime and substance abuse. In order to heal itself on a collective level, postapartheid South Africa has tried to achieve a shared 'national healing' of this stressful period by setting up a Truth and Reconciliation Commission (TRC). Its main slogan was: 'Truth: The Road to Freedom'. To a large extent, this model is based on psychoanalytic approaches to individual psychotherapy – 'finding the truth as a basis for healing'. The TRC has encouraged both perpetrators and victims to describe publicly the traumatic events that actually occurred under apartheid, and their role in it, in order to get either amnesty or compensation. However, Swartz points out that national healing, although essential, may not necessarily heal individual victims. In some cases the revelations at the TRC may prove cathartic to those who take part in them, but in others they have the opposite effect – reminding people of distressing events, and making them feel even worse as a result. In either case, an individual's response both to suffering ('stress') and to national healing, even if it is part of a more collective experience, is often idiosyncratic, difficult to predict and, like other forms of stress response, marked by non-specificity.

REFUGEES AND STRESS

As will be described in more detail in Chapter 12, one of the commonest form of collective stress today is to be found among refugees. Many of them will have witnessed or personally experienced acts of extreme violence, sometimes including sexual abuse. As well as loss of home, property and possibly loved ones, they will also have experienced a major psychosocial transition. Some of them will be suffering from what Eisenbruch terms 'cultural bereavement': grieving for the loss of all the familiar cultural reference points that defined who they were and how they were to live their lives. They will also have lost their livelihood, their sense of security and continuity, and even their sense of self. Many will encounter hostility among their host populations. Others will experience outbreaks of infectious diseases and other health problems. There may also be alcohol or drug abuse, or different forms of antisocial behaviour, especially among the youth. Overall, flight from one's home under these circumstances is likely to lead to major physical, emotional and cognitive distress, and often long-term PTSD.[47] among refugee populations. To a certain extent, some protection for the refugees may arise from the social support available to them, especially if this comes from family, friends, people from their own community or voluntary workers. Religious figures and traditional healers may also play a positive role. In some cases, religious faith or ideological conviction can also help ameliorate the stress of their situation. Given the vast scale of many refugee situations today, both individual and collective healing may only be possible on a relatively small scale. For many individual refugees, true healing can only begin when they return home safely or when they become reconciled to a new life, in a new country.

LAY MODELS OF STRESS AND SUFFERING

In the past few decades the concept of 'stress' outlined above has increasingly entered popular discourse, and is now commonly used in books, magazines, radio, television programmes, as well as the Internet. Lay concepts of stress are often those of a diffuse and invisible force, somehow mediating between individuals (and their mental and physical state) and the social environment in which they live and work.

The lay concept of stress can be regarded as one of the most pervasive and multidimensional folk illnesses of contemporary Western society. More importantly, in a modern, more secular age it is also one of the most widely used metaphors for human suffering, and especially one that places responsibility for that suffering outside the individual. Like 'heart distress' and 'sinking heart' (see Chapter 5), lay notions of stress blend together into a single image, a cluster of negative feelings, emotions and physical sensations, in the presence of certain social, cultural and economic circumstances. In doing so, it has absorbed older, more traditional models of misfortune and unhappiness, especially where they originate outside the individual. It has become a secularized version of more supernatural concepts, such as witchcraft, sorcery and other forms of interpersonal malevolence, as well as of fate, divine punishment and possession by malign spirits. Modern images of stress provide a fascinating illustration of how Selye's original concept has entered popular culture and blended with older models of misfortune, becoming a point of overlap between popular, medical and religious explanations for human suffering.

In the author's study[12] carried out in Massachusetts, USA in 1984, 95 per cent of a sample of patients with psychosomatic disorders blamed their condition and personal suffering on 'stress', though they varied widely on what they meant by this term. It was variously described as:

- an invisible force in the environment, pressing down on the individual (to be 'under acute stress')
- an invisible and malevolent force, usually produced by other people, that enters your body and then causes disease ('stress can cause my bronchi to spasm', 'stress goes to the weakest organ. I let it get to me and eat me away')
- something that 'builds up' inside you unless you can get it out ('a good relationship can make you stay healthy, because you can ventilate a lot of stress').

'Stress' explanations are just as common in the UK too. In one study[48] in 1998 of 406 patients in an English general practice, 53 per cent of them blamed their illnesses on different types of 'stress', which they thought could be relieved by medical explanations of their condition and by discussion of their symptoms.

In English-speaking countries, a number of recurrent images or metaphors associated with the word 'stress' can therefore be identified. Each is a metaphor for a sense of personal suffering, and often of helplessness. Many of them overlap with lay concepts of 'nerves' (see below). Most of these metaphors, though not all, are drawn from the artefacts and technology of everyday life: heavy objects, machines, cars, batteries, electrical wires, strings, rubber bands, kettles, crockery and pottery. Some of them refer to the stress itself, others to reactions to the stress. Among the most common of these metaphors are:

1 Stress as a heavy *weight*. In this image, stress is conceived of as a heavy invisible weight, burden or force that somehow 'presses down' on the individuals from above – especially onto their chest, head or shoulders – and which they have difficulty in carrying. Examples include 'to be under a lot of stress', 'to be under pressure', 'to be under tension', to 'have things piling up on top of me' and 'to have a lot on one's mind' (or 'on one's plate').

2 Stress as a *wire or line.* In this image, the nerves are described as if they were a series of wires, lines, rubber bands or strings (similar to violin or guitar strings). For example, some people are 'highly strung', 'taut', 'tense', 'tightly wired' or 'at the end of their tether', while others have nerves that 'snap', or have become 'frayed' or 'jangled'.

3 Stress as *internal chaos*. Here the image is of some uncontrollable internal disorder, chaos, change or movement within the body. Examples include 'to be churned up', 'to be all mixed up', 'to be all shook up' or to have 'butterflies in the stomach'.

4 Stress as *fragmentation*. Here the image is of an object that fragments under stress, almost as if it were a plate or earthenware pot. Examples include 'to crack up', 'to fall apart', 'to break', 'to feel shattered' or 'to go to pieces'.

I now understand why people get dogs, who shouldn't

5 Stress as a *malfunctioning of a machine*. In this image, the body and self are seen as a machine or engine that can no longer function. Examples include to 'have a nervous breakdown', 'to be burnt out', 'to grind to a halt', 'to crash' or to 'need one's batteries recharged'.

6 Stress as *depletion of a vital liquid*. Here the image is of the depleted level of some vital fluid, such as blood or breast milk, or, in an overlap with point (5), of fuel or steam. Examples include 'to feel drained' or 'empty', to feel 'sucked dry', to 'run out of gas', to be 'running on empty', to 'run out of steam' or to be 'at a low energy level'.

7 Stress as *inner explosion*. This image, drawn largely from the Age of Steam, conveys the idea of the build up of an internal force or pressure which, in the absence of some safety valve, suddenly and dramatically explodes. Examples include 'to get it off one's chest', 'to burst a boiler', 'to blow one's top' or 'to blow a gasket'.

8 Stress as *interpersonal force*. This image is similar to (1) above, but includes the idea of one person somehow causing (consciously or unconsciously) another person to feel stressed or to get ill. Examples include 'my boss gives me a lot of stress', 'I get a lot of stress from living with her', 'she gave him a nervous breakdown' or 'he broke his mother's heart'.

The frequent use of mechanical or machine metaphors to describe ideas of stress is also linked to another common contemporary image in both stress literature and popular discourse: the dangerous, disease-producing nature of 'modernity' itself. This idea of modernity as being pathogenic is not, in itself, modern. In 1897, for example, the famous physician Sir William Osler described 'arterial degeneration' as resulting from 'the worry and strain of modern life', and from 'the high pressure at which men live, and the habit of working the machine to its maximum capacity'.[49] Much of the contemporary New Age and other metaphysical movements also see modern life, modern diets and urban living as inherently stressful.[50] As one

American woman stated to McGuire[51] stress 'has to do with some kind of thing that's very much a part of our Western culture – accomplishment-oriented, striving, being seen, having a big voice … Making it, striving, getting ahead, that kind of thing. Really makes us crazy and makes us sick'. Often, these ideas are associated with a sense of nostalgia for some more 'natural' way of living – for a preindustrial, more communal non-competitive and notionally stress-free 'Garden of Eden'.

'NERVES'

One of the commonest folk images of suffering, found in many different forms and in many different cultures, is the idea of 'nerves'. It seems to be particularly common among women, especially in Europe, North and South America and all the English-speaking countries, and usually overlaps with lay concepts of stress. Like stress, it incorporates physical, psychological and social experience into a single image. It also places the emphasis on an ostensibly physical phenomenon: the malfunctioning of a diffuse part of the body vaguely described as 'the nerves'. As illustrated earlier, these can be conceptualized in many different ways. However, unlike in the stress model there seems to be more emphasis on *internal reasons*, within the individual, for their emotional suffering or illness and their vulnerability to the stress of daily life. Thus some people are just born with 'weak nerves' or 'bad nerves', some inherit them from their parents and others acquire them in childhood or adulthood (when their nerves were 'frayed', 'shattered', 'broken', or 'shot to ribbons' by some traumatic event). In each case, 'nerves' are blamed for predisposing the individual to ill health. As one 72-year-old asthmatic woman stated, 'A nervous person gets asthma. All through my life I never thought I was a nervous person, but I must have been. Behind it all there must have been a case of nerves'.[12]

Anthropological studies of 'nerves' reveal that it is not a single image, folk category or culture-bound syndrome. Neither is there a clear and

How was stress expressed in pre-industrial society?

consistent set of symptoms associated with it. Rather, the concept of 'nerves' can only be understood in terms of the specific and local social context in which the word is used; for example, as a way of explaining an individual's personality, or their emotional, physical or social reactions to certain events. One problem is that physicians often misinterpret the significance of 'nerves' and the vague symptoms associated with it. As Finkler[52] points out, they often 'objectify and separate the disorder from the patient's experience in which the disorder is embedded', and assume that it is caused by physiological malfunction. By concentrating on the 'disease' rather than the 'illness' dimension of 'nerves', they may therefore miss its true significance and how it can be treated.

Case study: *nervios* in San José, Costa Rica

Low[53], in her 1981 study in San José, Costa Rica, found that both men and women, of all ages and from all social classes, could be afflicted by 'nerves' (*nervios*). In a culture where family links and the *tranquilidad* (tranquillity) of family life are very important, it is often a symptom of family discord or disruption of the family structure. For example, a crisis of *nervios* may be precipitated when a son marries an undesirable woman, when a child is born illegitimately, or when a sudden bereavement occurs. People also blame their own *nervios* on a poverty-stricken childhood, an alcoholic father or a mother who was unwed when she gave birth to them. It can manifest in a variety of vague physical and emotional symptoms, including headache, insomnia, vomiting, lack of appetite, fatigue, anger, fear and disorientation. All of these indicate that the individual feels out of control, or separated from body or self. It is thus a culturally sanctioned way of signalling to others that something has gone wrong with family relationships, and that they need sympathy and attention. Overall, the belief in *nervios* is a way of 'encouraging culturally

appropriate behaviour and an adherence to cultural norms', especially those that reinforce family relationships and thereby enhance family cohesion.

Case study: nevra among Greek immigrants in Montreal, Canada

Dunk[54] in 1989 described 'nerves' (*nevra*) among Greek immigrants in Montreal, a form of somatization found mainly among women. An attack of *nevra* manifests as a feeling of loss of control, of 'being grabbed by your nerves', which then 'burst' or 'break out'. At the same time there is often screaming, shouting, throwing things and hitting one's children. Often there are vague physical symptoms, such as headaches, neck pain, shoulder pain and dizziness. Sufferers from the condition commonly use the expression 'my nerves are broken!'. Its cause can be related to the specific conditions of the immigrants' lives, including: economic pressures, crowded living conditions, the effects of migration upon the family, gender-role conflicts and the women's double burden of running a home and going out to work. It is thus a culturally constituted metaphor for distress, and a cry for help; it can be viewed as a realistic way of coping when responded to positively by family members and others.

As the two case studies indicate, lay models of stress and 'nerves' are highly variable. They cannot be fully understood without taking into account the context in which these terms are used. Part of this context involves those traditional explanations for misfortune that have been absorbed into these modern models of stress or 'nerves'. In other cases, as with the *Ataques de nervios* of Latino immigrants, described in the previous chapter, the wider picture must be taken into account, especially the social, political and economic context in which these immigrants find themselves. Overall, the concept of 'stress', although based originally on a limited, mechanistic model, has become one of the most pervasive images of human suffering of the modern world.

KEY REFERENCES

4 Selye, H. (1976). Forty years of stress research: principal remaining problems and misconceptions. *Can. Med. Assoc. J.* 115, 53–7.

7 Young, A. (1980). The discourse on stress and the reproduction of conventional knowledge. *Soc. Sci. Med.* 14B, 133–46.

8 Pollock, K. (1988). On the nature of social stress: production of a modern mythology. *Soc. Sci. Med.* 26, 381–92.

9 McElroy, A. and Townsend, P.K. (1996). *Medical Anthropology in Ecological Perspective*, 3rd edn. Boulder: Westview Press, pp. 252–6.

10 Parkes, C.M. (1971). Psycho-social transitions: a field for study. *Soc. Sci. Med.* 5, 101–15.

11 World Health Organization (1971). Society, stress, and disease. *WHO Chron.* 25, 168–78.

15 Ader, R., Cohen, N. and Felten, D. (1995). Psychoneuroimmunology: interactions between the nervous system and the immune system. *Lancet*, 345, 99–103.

19 Engel, G. (1968). A life setting conductive to illness: the giving-up-given-up complex. *Ann. Intern. Med.* 69, 293–300.

25 Marmot, M. (2004) *Status Syndrome*. London: Bloomsbury, pp. 1–36.

36 Waxler, N. E. (1981). The social labelling perspective on illness and medical practice. In: *The Relevance of Social Science for Medicine* (Eisenberg, L. and Kleinman, A. eds). Dordrecht: Reidel, pp. 283–306.

46 Desjarlais, R., Eisenberg, L., Good, B. and Kleinman, A. (1995). *World Mental Health*. Oxford: Oxford University Press, pp. 47–50, 116–35.

47 Swartz, L. (1998). *Culture and Mental Health: A Southern Africa View*. Oxford: Oxford University Press, pp. 167–88.

See http://www.culturehealthandillness.com for the full list of references for this chapter.

RECOMMENDED READING

Ader, R.A., Cohen, N. and Felten, D. (1995) Psychoneuroimmunology: interactions between the nervous system and the immune system. *Lancet* 345, 99–103.

Hahn, R. A. (1997) The nocebo phenomenon: concept, evidence, and influence on public health. *Prev. Med.* 26, 607–11.

McElroy, A. and Townsend, P.K. (1989) *Medical Anthropology in Ecological Perspective*, 3rd edn, Chapter 7. Boulder; Westview Press.

Helman, C. G. (1987) Heart disease and the cultural construction of time: the Type A behaviour pattern as a Western culture-bound syndrome. *Soc. Sci. Med.* 25, 969–79.

Pollock, K. (1988) On the nature of social stress: production of a modern mythology. *Soc. Sci. Med.* 26, 381–92.

Young, A. (1980) The discourse on stress and the reproduction of conventional knowledge. *Soc. Sci. Med.* 14B, 133–46.

RECOMMENDED WEBSITES

Health and Safety Executive (UK): http://www.hse.gov.uk/stress

National Institute for Occupational Safety and Health (USA): http://www.cdc.gov/niosh/topics/stress/

12

Migration, globalization and health

This chapter deals with two inter-related subjects – *globalization* and *migration*. It discusses how each of these, particularly migration, can have major effects on the health and health care of populations all over the world.

GLOBALIZATION

What is globalization? The sociologist Anthony Giddens[1] describes it as 'those processes that are intensifying worldwide social relations and interdependence'. They result from 'complex economic and social ties that link countries and people around the world'. Globalization is created by 'the coming together of political, social, cultural and economic factors'. It makes possible the rapid movement of people, ideas, goods, services, money, and information across the globe in an increasingly short period of time.

In the modern world, individuals, groups and nations are all becoming more interdependent than ever before in human history. Many of these new connections between the *local* and the *global* are the result of major advances in worldwide telecommunications (such as satellite TV), information technology (such as the internet), and transportation (such as cheap jet air travel). The effect of these innovations is to link people more closely together, enabling them to communicate, share information, or trade with one another even though they may be many thousands of miles

apart. Cultures are increasingly interacting with one another, with the possibility of ideas and practices from one – such as beliefs about illness, or forms of treatment – being integrated into another.

As Giddens also notes,[1] globalization is facilitated by the increasing integration of the world economy, especially of what he terms the 'knowledge economy' or 'weightless economy', based on the global transmission of information. It is also advanced by the growing numbers of intergovernmental organizations (IGOs) and international non-governmental organizations (NGOs), both of which now reach far beyond national borders. At the same time, the growth of large transnational corporations (TNCs), responsible for a third of all world trade, are major influences in international financial markets.

Globalization has many positive social effects, but also many dangers. All this interconnectedness can come at a price. A virus appearing in one country, for example, can swiftly be transported to another on a jet aircraft; a financial crisis in one part of the world, can easily trigger a similar crisis in another. Globalization has also been blamed for widening the gap between rich and poor, both globally and locally, and thus being damaging to health. In many cases it may benefit only the better-off, since not everyone in a community owns a cellular telephone, has enough money for an airfare or access to the internet, or can afford to invest in global financial markets. For many people, globalization also means the relentless spread of Western cultural and economic power to the rest of the world, often at the expense of local cultures and ways of living.

In terms of health care, globalization can have the positive effect of spreading information on the latest medical research, transporting medical techniques, equipment and pharmaceuticals to where they are needed, and connecting people suffering from the same disease in a worldwide patient support-group (see Chapter 13). Because many people are now developing a global perspective, this can also increase their awareness of environmental dangers to health, such as global warming, and the threat of global pandemics, such as acquired immune deficiency syndrome (AIDS), severe acute respiratory syndrome (SARS) or avian influenza. On the other hand, it can help spread these same diseases, as well as environmental pollution.

GLOCALIZATION

One way of confronting globalization is by *glocalization*: integrating local and global concerns by 'localizing' (or 'indigenizing') global forces and influences, and thereby 'taming' them in the process. An example, described below, is the way that Ayurvedic medicine from India, imported into Germany, has been subtly changed to fit in with local German cultural expectations of medical care. The same process, whereby influences from abroad are 're-framed' to fit in with the local culture, is seen in the very different ways that biomedical institutions (such as clinics or hospitals) are designed and run in different countries, with different cultural backgrounds (see Chapter 4). This applies also to imported cuisines, fashions of dress, types of self-medication, and the various forms of 'alternative medicine'.

Globalization is thus never unidirectional or unstoppable, and there are many different ways of resisting its hegemonic influence over daily life. Neither does it ever effect all members of the population equally, for – at least in poorer countries – its influence will be most felt by the privileged elite who have access to the internet, travel and global

finance.[2] Many of the poorer parts of the population will continue to live their local lives, based on their local traditions and ways of behaving.

Another counter-force to globalization is the growing tendency of individuals, communities, or even whole countries to resist it hegemonic forces (sometimes called 'McDonaldization')[3] by returning to a focus on their own local (sometimes very traditional) worldview and ways of doing things.[1] In some cases this may involve a return to extreme religious fundamentalism, or to extreme national xenophobia.[4] On a much more benign level, in many Western countries it has involved a return to an emphasis on more 'natural' forms of treatment (such as herbalism, massage or 'health foods') which are seen as symbolizing the health, innocence and purity of a preindustrial past. Some forms of 'natural treatment', such as yoga, meditation, shiatsu or reiki have been imported for other countries for this purpose.

MIGRATION

One of the most important components of globalization is *migration* – a word I have used to describe not only the global movement of people, but also of ideas, objects, services, ideologies, and forms of healing. The main types of migration of interest to medical anthropologists are listed in Table 12.1.

MIGRATION OF PEOPLE

Overview of global migration

Huge and unprecedented numbers of people are now moving across the globe, from one region to another and sometimes back again, in search of work, refuge, pleasure, or a new life. This migration can be either *external* (across national borders), or *internal* (within national borders). In 2002 the United Nations Population Division (UNPD)[5] estimated that about 175 million people (2.3 per cent of the world's population) lived

Table 12.1 Types of migration

People
   Migrants
   Refugees
   Health professionals
   Tourists
Healing systems
Pharmaceuticals and drugs
Microorganisms and environmental risks
Body parts
Cuisines
Religions
Weapons
Information
Capital, jobs and debt

outside their country of birth, of which about 15–20 million were refugees, and that the rate of migration has been rising steadily in the past few decades: from 75 million in 1965 to 84 million in 1975, and the 175 million of today. Given the current rate of increase in world population, it is predicted that there will be about 230 million migrants in the world by the year 2050.[6] An interesting change in migration patterns is that about 48 per cent of migrants are now women, and this proportion is rising as more women migrate on their own, a phenomenon the International Organization for Migration[6] calls the 'feminization of migration'. In terms of distribution, about 60 per cent of all the world's migrants now live in the more developed countries, and 40 per cent in less developed regions.[5] Most of the migrants live in Europe (56 million), Asia (50 million) and North America (41 million).[5]

Voluntary and involuntary migration

Many of these people are *voluntary migrants*, choosing to leave their homes and countries in search of better economic prospects, higher standards of living, improved access to education and health care, and a brighter future for their children (Figure 12.1). However, there are also many millions of *involuntary migrants*, forced to flee their homes due to war, political upheaval, persecution, economic distress, or natural disasters. In the past, the African slave trade between the fifteenth and nineteenth centuries was one of the largest involuntary migrations in history, with many millions of Africans being transported as slaves to European colonies in the Americas and the Caribbean.

Figure 12.1 Throughout the world many people are on the move looking for a better or safer life in another country. (Source: World Health Organization, *World Health*, No. 6, November–December 1995. Reproduced with permission.)

Today, the United Nations High Commissioner for Refugees (UNHCR) is the international body that cares for most involuntary migrants (though many others are cared for by other organizations and UN agencies). Data from the UNHCR[7] indicates that by the beginning of 2005, the total number of these migrants 'of concern' – that is, people who required their assistance – had risen to 19.2 million (from 17 million the previous year). One-third (6.9 million) of them were located in Asia, while 4.9 million were in Africa, 4.4 million in Europe, 853 300 in North America, 2 million in Latin America, and 82 400 in Oceania. The UNHCR divided the total number of migrants that they were caring for into five different categories:

- *Refugees* – 9.2 million people who have fled persecution in their own countries to seek safety in a neighboring country (a fall of 4 per cent over the previous year). In 2004, the top refugee-hosting countries were Iran (1 046 000), Pakistan (961 000), Germany (877 000), Tanzania (602 000), and the USA (421 000)
- *Asylum seekers* – 839 200 people who fled their own country, and then applied for legal protection and material assistance in another country. In 2004, a total of 676 400 people applied for asylum worldwide, two-thirds of them in Europe
- *Internally displaced persons* (IDPs) – 5 574 000 people caught up in similar situations to refugees and who fled their homes, but who remained within the borders of their countries of origin
- *Returnees* – 1 494 500 refugees who have returned home after the conflict has subsided, and some stability has been restored, Between 2002 and 2005, 5 million refugees returned home, 3.5 million of them to Afghanistan, though many of these still required the assistance of the UNHCR
- *Stateless persons* – about 2 053 100 worldwide.

Internal migrations

As well as the IDPs mentioned above, migration now frequently takes place within the borders of a country for economic reasons. This is part of the phenomenon of *urbanization* described in Chapter 18, where people from the countryside move to the more attractive economic prospects that exist (or that they believe exist) in the big towns or cities. The most dramatic example of this is the Peoples Republic of China where, following the economic changes of the past few decades, an estimated 100–150 million people from the rural hinterlands have moved into towns and cities to find work,[8] especially in the booming coastal provinces of Guangdong, Beijing, Shanghai, Liaoning, Tianjin and Jiangsu.[9] This rural–urban population movement has been described as one of the largest flows of labour migration in human history.[9]

Another special group of internal migrants are those forcibly displaced from their homes and villages, due to large-scale economic development projects, such as building a large dam (e.g. the Aswan High Dam in Egypt, or the Kariba Dam in central Africa), or clearing an area for nuclear weapon testing.[10] People displaced by their government in this way are usually compensated, and resettled elsewhere, but still often yearn for their lost homes for years, or even decades afterwards.

Temporary versus permanent migrants

Some migrants leave their homes with the intention of making a permanent move to the new country, region or city, especially for economic reasons. However, many others who move to a different place are *temporary migrants*, who have every intention of eventually returning to their homes (if this is possible). This large group includes: involuntary migrants such as refugees, political exiles and emigrés, as well as voluntary migrants such as migrant labourers and seasonal agricultural workers; foreign business-people and students; diplomats and armed services personnel; expatriate professionals on short-term contracts; itinerant merchants or nomads (such as the Bedouin); people working for international governmental or non-governmental organizations; and the large numbers of tourists. One special group are 'ex-expatriates': people who have lived or worked abroad for a period of time, and who often find it difficult to readjust to their own country, and to their previous lifestyle.

Illegal or undocumented migrants

One large group of migrants are those who are illegal or undocumented, lacking genuine travel documents and/or work permits. Some have been smuggled across national borders by 'human traffickers', others have travelled on their own. No precise statistics exist for their number, though the United Nations Development Programme has estimated that there are about 30 million of them worldwide.[11] In most countries these illegal migrants are in a particularly vulnerable position. Their lives are often precarious and difficult, and they are exposed to official and public hostility, legal harassment, economic exploitation, physical violence, as well as poor health and inadequate medical care. Unlike 'legal' migrants, they often lack the assistance of official bodies, or of international aid agencies such as the UNHCR.

'Static migration'

In some circumstances, one can 'migrate' socially and economically, without actually changing locality – a process I would call *static migration*. For example, a person who was born poor but who then makes money (or wins a lottery or other prize) and rises rapidly in the social scale, even without actually leaving their home village, town, or neighbourhood, can be considered a type of social migrant. Often this rise in social status can be a major emotional transition, involving considerable stress: new insecurities, new anxieties and pressures, possible alienation from family and friends, the fracturing of old relationships, and so on. Dressler,[12] for example, has described the types of stress response (such as a rise in blood pressure, or psychosomatic symptoms) that are often associated with modernization, economic development, social change and upward social mobility in some communities in the Caribbean and the USA. In many cases economic development raises expectations, fuels competitiveness, increases dissatisfac-

tion and widens the gap between rich and poor. In this situation, both those who rise socially and those who fail to do so can suffer from considerable stress, although for different reasons and in very different ways.

Another example of 'static migration' can happen to long-term residents of an urban area if it becomes settled by large numbers of migrants from a different country, region or ethnic group. Gradually they find the atmosphere, sounds and smells of their neighbourhood changing out of all recognition. While some of the original inhabitants may welcome this development, others may find themselves feeling increasingly 'foreign' in their own homes. For some elderly people in particular, this may feel like a sort of 'migration' or 'culture shock', even though they have not physically changed locality.

MacLachlan and colleagues[13] use the term *temporal acculturation* to describe the psychological effects of these types of culture change, over time, on those native to a country. In their study in Ireland, they found that those who identified with, and adapted to, the realities of the 'new Ireland', and the many major social changes that have recently occurred there, had the lowest rate of mental health problems, while a higher rate was associated with those who would not accept these changes, and in fact denied that they had actually taken place.

The new population diversity

An important result of migration is the growing cultural and social *diversity* now found in almost every city in the Western world. This partly results from the desire of many of today's migrants (unlike in previous generations) to retain their own cultural or religious identity, rather than lose it by assimilating into the 'host community'. According to the UNDP, 'Globalization is quantitatively and qualitatively reshaping international movements of people, with migrants going to high-income countries and wanting to maintain their cultural identities and ties with their home countries'.[11] This process is facilitated by major technological advances such as the global communication network and cheap air travel, both of which enable them to maintain close contact with their countries of origin.[11] This desire to retain their own identity can also apply to minority populations born in the new country, even after several generations.

An example of this new diversity is found in Britain. In 2000 a study[14] found that only two-thirds of London schoolchildren spoke English as a home language, and that they spoke a total of 307 languages. From 1991 to 2001 more than 1.1 million people moved to live and work in the UK, and by 2001, 4.3 million people (7.53 per cent of the population) had been born outside the UK, including 494 850 from the Republic of Ireland, 941 384 from south Asia (India, Pakistan, Bangladesh, Sri Lanka), 262 276 from Germany, and 155 030 from the USA.[15] At the same time, tens of thousands of British people have moved to live abroad. One estimate in the *Sunday Times* newspaper, based on official figures, is that there are 14.2 million British nationals living abroad, made up of emigrants, their descendants, and others entitled to British nationality.[16] As well as several million living in Australia, Canada and South Africa, these figures included approximately 500 000 living in the USA, 500 000 in Spain and 200 000 in France.

In the USA, too, cultural and ethnic diversity are features of the twenty-first century. According to the National Multicultural Institute (NMI),[17] in 2005 almost one in three Americans identifies themselves as belonging to a racial or ethnic minority, and nearly one out of every five school aged children in the USA speak a language other than English at home. In four states (California, Texas, Hawaii and New Mexico) members of ethnic and racial minorities accounted for more than half of the total population.[18] California had the largest Hispanic and Asian populations (12.4 million and 4.8 million, respectively) in the USA, while the largest black population (3.5 million) was in New York.[18] The NMI predicted that by the year 2050, one quarter of the total U.S. population will be Hispanic, and half of the total U.S. population will be 'people of color.'[17]

In many Western countries immigrant groups and minorities are unable to join the mainstream culture, even if they wish to, owing to economic, social or religious discrimination. In some cities they find themselves confined to marginal, low-income ethnic ghettoes, often on the outskirts of town, with high rates of unemployment, crime and deprivation. Illegal or undocumented migrants are usually in the most marginal position of all.

'The Age of Diasporas'

Globally, the twentieth and twenty-first centuries might well be termed the *Age of Diasporas*, though many of these – such as the Jewish, Irish, Greek, Armenian, and Lebanese diasporas – have existed for much longer. Almost all countries now have large numbers of their citizens (often numbering many millions) living scattered abroad in other countries. As well as the British diaspora mentioned above, the Chinese diaspora has been estimated at about 30–50 million people,[11] while the Indian diaspora – made up of Non-Resident Indians (NRIs) and Persons of Indian Origin (PIOs) – has been estimated at 20 million or more.[19] The London *Times* newspaper estimated that in 2006 there were 25 million Russians living outside of Russia, in countries that were once part of the Soviet Union, such as Ukraine, Belarus, Latvia, Lithuania, and Kyrgystan.[20] Different migrant groups tend to concentrate in different countries and in different parts of the world. Within Europe, for example, 92 per cent of Algerian immigrants live in France, while 81 per cent of Greek immigrants live in Germany.[11]

Many diasporic communities have formed new identities in their own right, even though they often keep up links with their country of origin. In some cases this can lead to an intense, sometimes very extreme, political or religious involvement with their home countries, as exemplified by 'the investment of diasporas in independence movements and civil warfare in their homelands'.[10] From a medical anthropology perspective, the significance of these diasporas is that many individuals within them may choose to retain their original cultural and religious views of health and illness (Chapter 5), their traditional dress and sense of body image (Chapter 2), their dietary practices (Chapter 3), and even their own traditional healers (Chapter 4).

Refugees

Refugees are involuntary migrants, forced to flee from their homes because of war, revolution, social disorder, economic crises, 'ethnic cleansing' (as in the former Yugoslavia), or natural disasters (such as the Asian tsunami). There are different estimates of the numbers of refugees: in 2002 the UNPD estimated that there were 16 million of them worldwide, with the largest numbers in Asia (9 million), followed by Africa (4 million), and the developed world (3 million).[5] In 2000 Europe hosted 2 million political asylum seekers (many of whom are not yet classified as 'official' refugees), four times more than North America.[11] In the UK, for example, over 110 000 people entered the country in 2002 to seek asylum, a 250 per cent increase in five years.[21] In the mid-1990s the UNHCR estimated that about 80 per cent of all refugees were women and children[22] In official terms, refugees are defined by the fact that they cross national boundaries into another country in search of refuge, but in addition to these 'official' refugees, there are an estimated 20 million people who have been displaced from their homes, but who still remain *within* the borders of their own countries[22] – over 5 million of these IDPs are cared for by the UNHCR.[7]

As described in more detail below, being a refugee, whether external or internal, can have very negative effects on one's physical and mental health, as well as on one's social relationships.

Composition of migrant populations

Although many migrants move to a new country as part of a family unit, there are some situations where the migrant population consists mainly of men, or mainly of women, or even of children. Some of these special types of migration are described below.

Migration of men

A high proportion of men migrate on their own rather than as part of family units. Many go from poorer countries to work in the developed world – usually in agriculture, industry, mining or construction – in order to support their families back home. Others remain in their own countries, but move to other regions or cities in search of work. An example of a largely male migration are the tens of thousands of African men who go from southern and central Africa to work in the gold mines of Johannesburg, South Africa. Many of the jobs available to migrant men are low-paid and low-status, but also dangerous, and they may be at risk of injury or death from unsafe working conditions.

Most male migrants will return to their homes eventually, but some will try to remain in the new countries and to raise enough money to bring their families across to join them – a process known as 'chain-migration'. Others may marry or cohabit with local women. As described in Chapters 1 and 16, male-only migration sometimes carries health risks such as recourse to prostitutes, with a higher incidence of sexually transmitted diseases (STDs) such as AIDS. Males also migrate from one country to another, at least for a limited period of time, as part of armed forces. As well as the obvious risks of warfare that they encounter, service personnel also often have a higher risk of contracting STDs while away from home.

Migration of women

While most women migrate as part of family units, there are increasing numbers of women migrating independently to other countries. Most of them come from Asian countries such as the Philippines, Indonesia and Sri Lanka, but many also come from Africa and Latin America. In several countries now, the majority of migrants going abroad are female. In 2000, for example, 70 per cent of Philippino migrant workers were women, often living abroad without their families and sending money back to support them.[6] In Indonesia, according to the United Nations International

Research and Training Institute for the Advancement of Women (INSTRAW), 72 per cent of the labour migration is female, many of them working abroad in the domestic service area, while in Italy about 50 per cent of domestic workers come from countries outside the European Union.[23] Female migrant workers are major sources of foreign currency to their home countries, through remittances sent to their families. In Sri Lanka in 1999, for example, they contributed 62 per cent of the more than US $1 billion sent home that year as private remittances.[6]

Female migrants tend to move to the richer countries of Europe and North America, as well as to Asian countries such as Japan, Malaysia, Singapore, and Hong Kong (where there are an estimated 200 000 women migrant workers, many working as domestic helps,[24]) and to Saudi Arabia and other parts of the Gulf (in 2003 there were 140 000 housemaids working in Kuwait, mainly from Sri Lanka, India, the Philippines and Bangladesh).[25] Most of these migrant women work as domestic workers, hospital workers, or as carers of children or elderly people. Others find themselves working in low-paid jobs in unregulated parts of the economy – such as factories or farms – where they are subject to economic and social exploitation, and sometimes to sexual harassment. Some even find themselves forced into prostitution,[6] which may put them at risk of diseases such as AIDS.[24] Since the end of the Cold War, large numbers of young women from Eastern Europe and the former Soviet Union have been brought illegally into Western Europe by 'human traffickers', to work as prostitutes against their will. Also, unknown numbers of women from both Asia and the former Soviet Union, have been imported into western Europe as 'internet brides': to marry the men they 'met' over the internet. In recent years, another largely female migration is that of nurses and other health professionals, moving from poor to rich countries, a situation described below.

Where men go first to a new country, establish themselves, and then bring their wives and families to join them ('chain migration'), this may act to the disadvantage of the women. On arrival, they may find that their husbands have become more acculturated than they are and more fluent in the local language, and this may increase their sense of isolation, especially if they are confined to the home.[26] Their children, too, may become rapidly assimilated and increasingly speak only the new language. In some cases, the women may find that their husbands have even acquired another 'wife' in the interim. In later years, if their husbands die, and the children leave home, this may lead to further isolation, and resulting depression, especially if they are still not yet bilingual, or are unemployed.

Migration of children

Several migrations of children, unaccompanied by adults, have taken place in history. Many of these child migrations have originated in the UK, though estimates of the total number of children involved vary. The process began in 1618 when a group of destitute and orphaned children were sent from England to Richmond, Virginia, and ended in 1967 with child migrants being sent to Australia.[27] In the nineteenth and twentieth centuries, many other children were sent to various parts of the British Empire. Between 1869 and the early 1930s more than 100 000 British children, known as the 'Home Children' – most of them orphaned, or from impoverished backgrounds – were sent to Canada to solve the colony's farm labour shortage or to work as domestic servants.[28] The Australian Parliament website estimates that between 1922 and 1967 about 150 000 children with an average age of 8 years and 9 months were shipped from Britain to help populate the British Dominions of Canada, Rhodesia, New Zealand and Australia with 'good white stock'; 5000–10 000 of these children went to Australia, most of them sent to charitable or religious institutions.[29] Separated from their families and backgrounds, many of these British child migrants suffered emotionally and physically from this experience.[27]

Another child-only migration took place just before World War Two. Between 1938 and 1940 the British Government permitted 10 000 children below the age of 17, most of them Jewish children, to come to the UK as refugees from Nazi Germany, Austria, Czechoslovakia, and other European countries. In a process known as the *Kindertransport*, they were sent from the Continent to England in sealed trains, and then re-settled.[30] Most of them never saw their parents again, as they were murdered in the Holocaust

Today, most child migrants are adoptees (usu-ally brought to Western countries from Asia or Latin America), children sent to relatives to be edu-cated abroad, child soldiers conscripted into vari-ous armies (especially in Africa), and child refugees and asylum seekers.[31] Many of this last group are orphans and arrive at their destination unaccom-panied by any adult relatives, such as the large numbers of 'unaccompanied minors' that arrived in Europe and North America from South-East Asia after the Vietnam War. Various organizations, both non-governmental and governmental, have been set up to deal with these refugee children, including the US government's Office of Refugee Settlement, which runs an 'Unaccompanied Refugee Minors Program'. Refugee children, espe-cially from war zones, often have major mental health problems, including the 'cultural bereave-ment' described below.[31]

Migration of health professionals: doctors and nurses

One result of the growth of international labour markets, is the large number of doctors and nurses moving from poorer countries to work in richer ones. It is a controversial process, because while profiting the new country (the 'brain gain') it of often leaves the poorer countries denuded of their health professionals (the 'brain drain'). Furthermore, because medical and nursing training is so expensive, these countries are indirectly 'sub-sidizing' the rich ones by paying for the education of their health professionals. Both of these processes may seriously undermine their already impoverished and overstretched health-care sys-tem, and this fact indicates that education must

also be accompanied by opportunities for employ-ment, if such a migration is to be avoided.

Many health professionals have migrated from the Philippines over the years. During the mid-1970s, for example, 13 480 physicians were work-ing there, but another 10 410 Philippine-trained physicians were working in the USA. In addition, an estimated 15 000 nurses leave the Philippines to work abroad every year, and they can now be found in over 30 different countries.[32]

Medical migration can also take place between the rich countries themselves: in the decade 1990–2000, a net total of 3720 Canadian physi-cians moved to work abroad, mostly in the USA.[32] However, most of the foreign physicians working in the USA come from poorer countries. In 2004 they included 5334 from sub-Saharan Africa, including 478 trained in Ghana.[33] Reviewing the literature on medical migration, Bach[32] notes that in 1972, a total of 6 per cent of the world's physi-cians were working in another country, 86 per cent of them in five developed countries: Canada, USA, UK, Australia and Germany. Since 1972, the rate of this medical migration has increased even fur-ther, as has the migration of nurses. In 2000 it was estimated that about 100 000 American nurses were trained abroad, and that 25 per cent of American physicians were graduates of foreign medical schools.[32]

In the UK the situation is similar. In 2002–03 there were about 12 000 foreign nurses registered in the UK,[32] while in 2004, out of 212 356 regis-tered doctors in the UK, 61 551 of them had been trained abroad, including 9152 trained in sub-Saharan Africa – about a third of them from South Africa.[33]

Bach[32] points out that the decision to migrate is not only the result of individual factors: one has also to include the role of organizations, such as hospitals, government departments, or private recruitment agencies. These agencies (sometimes in opposition to official government policy) actively go out to developing countries to entice health pro-fessionals to work for them.[32] Although many migrant health professionals do well in their new countries, others report being underpaid, denied promotion, given lower status or more difficult jobs, or being actively discriminated against.

The following case study, compiled for the British medical charity MedAct, deals with one particular medical migration: from Ghana to the UK.

Case study: migration of doctors and nurses from Ghana to the UK

Mensah and colleagues[33] have reviewed the migration of health service personnel from Ghana to the UK. Since the 1970s over 50 per cent of all doctors trained in Ghana have subsequently emigrated to elsewhere. In 2004 there were 293 Ghana-trained physicians and 1021 nurses working in the UK. Those health professionals that have migrated have done so in search of higher income, better working conditions, and new qualifications. Many of the nurses have been actively recruited by UK nursing agencies to work in the private sector. While many Ghanaian medical migrants do benefit financially from the move, and are able to send remittances back home, there are often negative consequences for them. These can include high living costs, strains on family relationships, and unpleasant experiences in the workplace, such as racism, abuse, bullying, undervaluing of skills, and lower pay rates. On a national level, this medical migration can also have serious effects, undermining the entire health-care system back in Ghana. Globalization has blurred the boundaries between the UK and Ghanaian medical systems, leading them to become increasingly integrated with one another – but as migration is largely one-way, it is to the detriment of Ghana. They point out that that although 'health care professionals who have migrated to work in the UK were trained in Ghana at Ghanaian public and private expense: the benefits of that training are being experienced elsewhere'. It is the UK National Health Service that is 'using resources it has not created through investment, to the benefit of its users'. Many of these resources come from poorer countries that have supplied the UK with migrant doctors and nurses. They estimate that it currently costs about £220 000 to train a doctor in the UK and £37 500 to train a nurse, so that this migration would imply a saving to Britain in training costs of about £65 million from the employment of Ghanaian doctors, and £38 million from the employment of Ghanaian nurses. Thus the savings to the UK are enormous and, in effect, a poor country is now subsidizing a rich one (but without being compensated for this). The authors see this as an example of aid in reverse, and that 'the subsidy is perverse and unjust, because it worsens the existing inequity in access to health care at a global level'.

Migration of tourists

The mass movement of people in search of holidays, relaxation, health or adventure is a relatively new phenomenon. Tourism is a temporary form of migration, but one that now has major local and international ramifications. It is now a multimillion dollar global industry, employing many millions of people. It can also be detrimental to health.

World tourist trends are monitored by the World Tourism Organization (WTO), a special agency of the United Nations, with a membership of 138 countries as well as tourism associations, local governments, and private sector companies. The WTO describe the growth of global tourism as 'one of the most remarkable economic and social phenomena of the past century'. Measured by the number of 'international arrivals' (people arriving in a country from outside its borders) they estimate that this number has risen steeply from 25 million in 1950 to 763 million in 2004. During that period, the rates of international tourism have risen especially in Asia and the Pacific (13 per cent a year), and in the Middle East (10 per cent a year), compared to Europe (6 per cent) and the Americas (5 per cent).[34]

The economic impact of tourism is enormous, especially on poorer countries. In 2003 the WTO estimated that it represented 6 per cent of the total worldwide export of goods and services.[35] For poorer countries, tourism can be a mixed blessing. On one hand it brings in foreign exchange but on the other it can sometimes act like a 'cash crop' (see Chapter 3), taking people off the land, away from food production and making them more dependent on the cash economy. This is because the tourist industry is vulnerable to global fluctuations in demand and supply, and is highly sensitive to local events such as natural disasters, terrorist attacks, crime or civil unrest. Over-development and crowding of some tourist sites can damage the local environment, reduce social cohesion, introduce drug-taking and other types of antisocial behaviour, and put a strain on local health-care facilities.

Some tourists travel specifically to enhance their health, to spas, thermal springs, hydrotherapy centres, or 'health farms'. Many Mediterranean and Middle Eastern countries now offer this 'therapeutic tourism', claiming its benefits for a variety of ailments, such as arthritis and skin disorders (such as the beneficial effects of the Dead Sea waters on psoriasis). The London *Times* estimates that each year about 150 000 foreigners seek treatment in Indian hospitals for non-emergency health problems, such as hip- or knee-replacements, taking advantage of the lower cost of India's advanced medical services.[36]

Health risks of tourism

Tourism itself carries many risks, including death, injury and disease. It may result in jet-lag or sea-sickness, or actual physical injury in sports such as swimming, deep-sea diving or skiing. There are also potential dangers from local crime, terrorism, political unrest, air and rail crashes, the abuse of alcohol or drugs, natural disasters (such as the Asian tsunami), poor sanitation or water supply, food poisoning, insect bites, deep vein thrombosis (DVT) after long-haul flights, or being exposed to local endemic diseases such as malaria, yellow fever, dengue or tick-bite fever. On an emotional level, tourists may experience marital or inter-generational conflict, or suffer from depression, anxiety, or homesickness, especially if their vacation fails to become the enjoyable 'symbolic inversion' of everyday life that they had expected (see Chapter 10). Finally, certain types of specialized tourism, such as 'sex tourism' bring with them the dangers of the exploitation of underage boys and girls, as well as of the spread of AIDS and other STDs.

OTHER TYPES OF MIGRATION

This section deals with different types of 'migration': not primarily of people, but rather of objects, drugs, ideas, money and belief systems. They are spread by special types of migrants, such as traders, salespeople, arms dealers, publishers, journalists, religious evangelists, information technology specialists, bankers, representatives of transnational pharmaceutical firms and expatriate health professionals, as well as by immigrants, tourists, refugees and other migrants. Aided by the spread of global travel and communication networks, they are an intrinsic part of the process of globalization. They can also have major effects on global health, including on cultural concepts of health, illness and medical care.

Migration of healing systems

Globalization involves the spread of medical concepts, equipment, and techniques of diagnosis and treatment across the world. Since the beginning of colonialism, Western biomedicine has been exported to countries in Africa, Asia and Latin America. Today, it is increasingly being marketed to countries there that cannot afford all its expensive, drugs, laboratories, pharmaceuticals and technology, such as computed tomography (CT) or magnetic resonance imaging (MRI) scans. Importing advanced medical equipment into poorer countries may not be economically sustainable, if they cannot afford to use or maintain them. Without further economic aid, it may make them permanently dependent on the suppliers of this technology (often transnational private companies) for spare parts, maintenance, and repair.[4]

Globalization has also spread different types of health systems (such as fee-based, welfare state or socialized health care) from one a country to another. In some cases, as Whiteford and Nixon point out,[37] health-care systems transplanted to another country (such as importing a fee-for-service system into a poor developing country), may not be sustainable or 'fit in' with the local social and economic circumstances, and may have a negative effect on public health.

Within the industrialized world, forms of healing have long between exported between countries, including homeopathy from Germany in the nineteenth century and osteopathy from the USA in the twentieth century. Also, many forms of psychotherapy and counselling have begun in one Western country, and then found adherents in others (see Chapter 10). They include psychoanalysis (whether Freudian, Jungian or Kleinian), cognitive behaviour therapy, gestalt therapy, transactional analysis, psychosynthesis and various forms of body-oriented psychotherapy.

The global spread of biomedicine has influenced local traditional healers, many of whom 'borrow' some of its powerful healing symbols (such as stethoscopes, white coats, syringes, prescriptions, or pharmaceuticals) for their own purposes, and use them within their own systems of healing. Examples of this are the growth of 'injectionists' in many developing countries (Chapter 4), and the case of 'Dr John', the Xhosa healer in Transkei, South Africa (Chapter 9). In both cases, the spread of Western biomedicine has helped to create new syncretic forms of healing: a creative mix of old and new, scientific and magical, local and imported.

In the other direction, a variety of traditional healing forms, including ways of preserving health or achieving relaxation, have been imported into Europe and North America, especially from Asia. They include: acupuncture, moxibustion and other forms of traditional Chinese medicine (TCM); reiki and shiatsu from Japan;[38] yoga, transcendental meditation and Ayurvedic medicine from India; and traditional herbal remedies from Tibet and Korea. In addition, Native American 'neo-shamanism' is becoming increasingly popular,[39] as are various forms of 'spiritual healing' from Africa and the Caribbean. As well as the importation of large numbers of traditional and religious healers from these countries (see Chapter 4), it has led to the development of syncretic forms of medical practice among Western doctors themselves. An example of this are the 11 000 German physicians who also practice acupuncture,[40] and the growing interest in Ayurvedic medicine in that country, as described in the following case study.

Case study: Indian Ayurveda practitioners in Germany

Frank and Stollberg[40] studied the reasons for the growth and popularity of Indian Ayurvedic medicine in Germany since the 1980s. There are currently nine Ayurvedic health centres in the country, and approximately 100 medical doctors and 25 *Heilpraktikers* (non-medically qualified healers) who practice it, mostly within the Maharishi Mahesh Yogi organization. This rise partly results from Germany's long tradition of non-orthodox medicine, including naturopathy and homoeopathy (invented by a German physician, Samuel Hahnemann), and the relatively liberal attitude of the authorities. However, most patients in the study were drawn to Ayurveda mainly by their negative view of biomedicine, and its medications, especially their side-effects and limited efficacy. Most patients were recommended to a particular practitioner by close friends or relatives, but once they had consulted them they became 'converted' to Ayurveda. They generally had a positive experience of its gentle approach, pulse diagnosis (an 'utterly convincing, slightly magical experience'), special massages *(panchakarma)*, nutritional advice and 'natural' plant-based medicines. They also liked its longer consultations (30–60 minutes), and its more personalised approach that focused more on their individual needs, feelings and lifestyles than their biomedical physicians ever did. Overall, they saw Ayurveda as more 'natural' than medicine, and as 'strengthening' the body rather than just treating its diseases.

The authors suggest that Ayurvedic notions of 'purifying' or 'cleansing' the body (by dieting or massage) make sense to these patients, is because they resonate with traditional German ideas of *Entschlackung* or 'purification' – ideas that have been prominent since about 1900, and the beginnings of the natural healing movement (*Natuurheilkundebewegung*). Despite this, they still chose biomedicine for medical emergencies, acute illness and surgical conditions. 'You should have a healthy mixture of natural medicine and biomedicine', one person said.

Ayurveda in Germany, however, is different from Ayurveda in India. In adapting to German needs and outlook, it has dropped some of its more drastic treatments such as violent purging. Thus, this process of adaptation to local forms ('glocalisation') means that such foreign healing systems 'do not cross geographic boundaries without being changed', and local cultural conditions always ensure that 'transcontinental diffusion involves transformation and hybridisation.'

Migration of pharmaceuticals and drugs

The spread of Western pharmaceuticals, alcohol and tobacco, into many parts of the developing world – and the problems this has caused – have been described in Chapter 8. A counter-tendency is the export of remedies and drugs from developing countries to the Western world and elsewhere; for example, the globalization of Asian medicines and treatments. The popularity of TCM in the West has already been described (Chapter 4), but Hsu[41] describes how these Chinese medicines have also become popular in Tanzania. Known locally as *dawa ya Kichina*, many of them are produced by large pharmaceutical firms in the Peoples Republic of China, and then exported to Africa.

In addition to these legal medicinal substances, there is another movement of drugs from the developing world: the huge and lucrative trade in illegal drugs, such as heroin, cocaine and marihuana, from countries in Asia, Latin America and the Caribbean to feed the needs of the many hundreds of thousands of addicts, especially in Europe and North America.

Migration of microorganisms and environmental risks

Worldwide airline networks and other forms of transport, now make possible the rapid spread of microorganisms from one part of the globe to another, carried by infected individuals. This includes insect vectors (such as mosquitoes), infected foodstuffs (such as meat contaminated by bacteria) and infected pet animals or birds (as in rabies or avian 'flu). The rapid global spread of AIDS (Chapter 16), SARS, various strains of influenza, and even 'airport malaria' (Chapter 17), are all examples of this growing threat to global health.

In addition, threats to the environment and human health such as air pollution, acid rain, global warming or the spread of nuclear radiation (as after the Chernobyl disaster) are not confined within national borders. They can spread rapidly from one region to another: for example, the overuse of aerosols in one country, causing depletion of the ozone layer, may end up increasing the risk of skin cancer in many others.[4] Similarly, the overuse of resources (especially non-renewable energy sources) by industrialized countries can have effects on the environment way beyond their borders – and a similar process is occurring in the rapidly-developing economies of Asia.[4]

Migration of cuisines

The globalization of cuisine has already been described in Chapter 3. It is manifested by the international spread of 'ethnic' foodstuffs, restaurants, recipes, and modes of cooking. All this is a growing feature of most Western countries, as is the creation of new syncretic dishes, such as the

'Chicken Tikka Masala'[42] or 'chicken curry pizza' now available in the UK. Acting in the other direction is the 'nutrition transition' in countries undergoing socio-economic development, with a shift towards a less healthy diet of processed, 'fast', or 'convenience' foods, which are high in calories, fat, salt and additives. The globalization of food as a packaged product also has implications for the quality and freshness of that food, and can have a negative impact on local cuisines and nutritional health. There are also major health implications in the worldwide shift in infant-feeding practices, especially the decline of breast-feeding among migrant communities, or communities undergoing 'Westernization'. Both the 'global obesity epidemic' and the recent rise of eating disorders (such as anorexia nervosa) in developing countries can be linked to the globalization of foods and dietary habits, as well as of notions of ideal body image.

Migration of body parts

Chapter 2 described the growing international trade and 'commodification' of body organs used for transplantation. In many cases this trade is illegal, and results in the movement of large numbers of organs, such as kidneys, from impoverished donors in the developing world to recipients in the richer countries of the northern hemisphere. Scheper-Hughes[43] describes this as 'bio-piracy', and as just another example of global inequality and exploitation of the poor by the rich. She points out that donors in the developing world may be forced to part with a kidney or other organ because of their poverty, since it is the only 'collateral' that they possess.

Migration of information

According to Giddens[1], the new communication technologies (such as the internet, emails, telephones, video-conferencing, radio and television) all 'facilitate the 'compression' of time and space' by connecting individuals in real time, even though they may be many thousands of miles apart. Thus, as predicted by McLuhan,[44] the world has become compressed into a 'global village' – though this

process involves mainly those with access to these new technologies.

The migration of information can have major effects on people's sense of identity, resulting in either an erosion (or strengthening) of local identity. It may result in new forms of 'hybrid identity', composed of elements from different cultural sources.[1,11] Some may choose a global (often religious) form of identity, rather than a local one. In some cases this can spread messages of extremist religious or political movements among geographically scattered populations. All of this process of information flow may provoke conflict or hostility between different groups, but it can also produce cooperation. Overall, as Kirmayer and Minas[2] suggest, in an age of global information flows 'the distant may be more familiar and frequented than the physically close'. They suggest therefore that 'it be more useful to think of cultures in terms of information flows and of individual communities, even persons, as local eddies in the flux of a global system'. In terms of health, while information technology may spread information about the latest medical research, techniques and treatments (Chapter 13), this may sometimes cause unrealistic expectations of what medicine can achieve. In many cases global communications may help migrant groups keep in touch with their cultures of origin, including with their traditional views of health, illness and misfortune.

Some of the effects of the global flow of medical information is described in Chapter 13, in the case of telemedicine.

Migration of religions

Historically, religions have spread across the globe, often replacing the local faiths that they have encountered. Buddhism spread from India where it began into many other Asian countries, and both Christianity and Islam have been spread by conquest as well as by persuasion. In Latin America there are now many different syncretic religions – mostly a blend of Catholic, African and indigenous elements. They include *Umbanda* and *Candomblé* in Brazil, *Santeria* in Cuba and *Vodun* (or *Vodou*) in Haiti. In recent decades, this process of the migration of religions is increasing in speed and complexity. Not only do many migrants carry their religions with them (an estimated 15–20 million Muslims have settled in western Europe since World War Two), but religions are also spread by missionaries, books, the media and the Internet. Different forms of Buddhism have become increasingly attractive to many in the industrialized world, while in recent decades evangelical Protestant groups, especially from the USA, have been proselytizing widely in Latin America, Africa, Europe, the Pacific and elsewhere. Religious conversion may have a major impact on health and involve new ways of explaining illness and misfortune, new attitudes towards medical treatment, lifestyle, forms of dress, food taboos, and the use, or avoidance, of some 'chemical comforters'.

Migration of weapons

Some of the dimensions of the international arms trade, as well as the huge profits made from it, and its enormous cost in terms of death and injury will be described in more detail in Chapter 18. This global industry includes both the legal and illegal trade in small arms (such as assault rifles or AK-47s), light weapons (such as mortars and machine guns), larger weaponry (such as aircraft or missile systems), and landmines – now produced by firms in 48 different countries, and with large numbers already laid down in countries such as Cambodia, Afghanistan and Mozambique. Much of this trade flows from rich countries to poorer ones, where it can fuel local conflicts and destabilize already fragile economic and social systems. Since World War Two, 85 per cent of all major armed conflicts have taken place in poorer countries, and many of the casualties of these conflicts have been civilians, especially women and children.[45]

Migration of capital, jobs and debt

As noted above,[1] globalization can widen the gaps between rich and poor, both between and within countries. It can also blur national boundaries, and transfer power away from national governments (and their medical systems) to more distant international and transnational organizations and companies. On a local level it can have negative impacts on local industries and businesses, by 'exporting' (or 'out-sourcing') their jobs to countries where labour costs are much lower (and often with less protection for workers), and the profits for investors are much higher. Goods produced cheaply in this way may 'flood' the markets elsewhere, causing local unemployment, economic recession, increased poverty, and a reduction in health status (see Chapter 1). Many poorer countries are heavily in debt to the developed world, and much of their meagre incomes are spent on debt repayments, instead of social and economic development. On a global level, Whiteford and Nixon[37] argue that the strong control exerted by international bodies such as the International Monetary Fund and the World Bank, as well as international trade agreements such as GATT, APEC and NAFTA, can limit the development of strong, independent national governments and their ability to care for their own populations.

BENEFITS OF MIGRATION

Migration can cause physical and emotional problems but it can also bring considerable benefits to the migrants, their families and their communities back home. It may bring an immigrant family even closer together, and strengthen the emotional bonds between them. For refugees and other involuntary migrants from areas of conflict, benefits such as safety from persecution or physical danger are obvious, while for more voluntary migrants the move to a big city may have many other advantages summarized by that old English saying 'City air makes man free'. Not only may they improve their economic position, but they may also get access to better education, health-care facilities, sports facilities, and types of entertainment. They may encounter new ideas, new options and lifestyles, new views of the world, and have a greater sense of autonomy and of personal and social security. Women migrants may find that they have more options, than they would have had in their more traditional countries of origin, The children of migrants may take great pride in their membership of two cultures, and in being bilingual.[46] If they do well financially, migrants may be able to send money back to support their families back home, or even bring them across to join them. For poorer countries, these remittances to family and community can be a major source of foreign exchange. Overall, it has been estimated that remittances sent home to developing countries by migrants (sometimes known as 'migradollars') rose from $30 billion in 1990 to nearly $80 billion in 2002.[11]

HEALTH RISKS OF MIGRATION

Overall, each type of migration – whether voluntary or involuntary, permanent or temporary, legal or illegal – carries with it its own specific range of health problems and risks, and its own specific needs in terms of medical care. They are described in more detail later in this Chapter.

Whatever its benefits, migration can be a traumatic experience for the migrants themselves. It can involve the loss of individual identity, community structures, traditional leaders, religious authorities, and the abandonment of important local landmarks such as ancestral graves or religious shrines. For refugees, in particular, there is often a loss of autonomy, especially in reception and resettlement camps. All of this can affect the mental and physical health of migrants, as well as their relationships with other people.

For those who find themselves living in the cities of the developed world, often in deprived neighbourhoods, their health risks may resemble those of longstanding ethnic minorities in those countries. In the USA, for example, Betancourt and colleagues[47,48] describe how ethnic and racial minorities in the USA suffer disproportionately from cardiovascular disease, hypertension (see below), diabetes, asthma and cancer, as well as

other conditions. Some of the risks to migrant health also resemble those that afflict the urban poor in many less developed countries, as well as poorer countries undergoing 'Westernization'.[12] Several of these new health risks, resulting from economic and cultural globalization, are described elsewhere in this book. They include: the 'global obesity epidemic' (Chapter 3), with its resultant increase in diabetes, heart disease, cancers and eating disorders; the worldwide spread of legal and illegal pharmaceuticals and drugs, including alcohol and tobacco (Chapter 8); the increased rates, especially in urban areas, of human immunodeficiency virus (HIV)/AIDS and other STDs (Chapter 16); and exposure of the migrants to diseases such as malaria (Chapter 17), dengue fever and tuberculosis (Chapter 18). They also include a variety of mental disorders and stress symptoms, and social disruptions such as increased rates of marital breakdown, domestic violence, teenage pregnancy, sexual abuse, and the overuse of alcohol or drugs (Chapters 10, 11 and 18),

An early example of research into the effects of migration on physical health, was the following study of hypertension:

Case study: effects of migration on blood pressure

Cassell[49] in 1975 reviewed the research done on the effects of migration on blood pressure. In one study, the blood pressure of black migrants from the Southern USA to Chicago was compared with that of Chicago-born blacks. It was found that the longer the period of city life, the higher was their blood pressure. In another study, the blood pressures of inhabitants of the Cape Verde Islands (off West Africa) were compared with those of Cape Verdeans who had migrated to the eastern USA. The immigrants showed higher pressures at each age, and a sharper difference between young and old than did the islanders. Other studies showed higher rates of hypertension among Irish immigrants to the USA (32 per cent) when compared with their brothers living in Ireland (21 per cent). In Cassell's view,[49] the findings of these studies are unlikely to result from genetic differences between those who emigrate and those who stay behind, but possibly may result from genetic differences in the susceptibility to environmental influences among individual migrants. These influences include physical factors such as caloric intake, physical activity and salt intake, and the absence of certain parasites and diseases in the host country that, in the country of origin, usually cause wasting, anaemia and a fall in blood pressure. However, psychosocial factors also play a part, particularly the disappearance of a coherent value system and its replacement by different values and different situations, where the migrant's traditional way of coping with life is no longer effective.

MENTAL ILLNESS

Migration (whether internal or external) often seems to carry with it an increased risk of mental illness, though the reasons for this are complex, and not fully understood. Often this risk is not only higher than the native-born population in their new country, but also higher than that of their countries of origin. The evidence for this is based on higher rates of admission to mental hospitals, and higher indices of alcoholism, drug addiction, suicide and attempted suicide. These risks seem to affect some groups of migrants, but not others. However, as some authors[50] have pointed out, studies of the mental health of immigrants are difficult to interpret unless one controls for factors such as age, social class, occupational status and ethnic group on one hand, and culturally biased diagnostic methods on the other. Unless this is done, it cannot be demonstrated clearly that there is a significant association between migration and the rates of mental illness among migrants.

Desjarlais and colleagues[22] point out that being a migrant does not, on its own, necessarily lead to mental illness. A number of *other* factors are also relevant, including external factors such as employment status, housing conditions, and the reactions of the 'host' society. Such factors as xenophobia, discrimination, racial prejudice[51] (both individual and institutionalized) and racial harassment are all likely to contribute towards the immigrant's mental and physical ill health, as are the economic and political conditions prevailing in the host community. To this one can add personality factors, the cultural background of the migrants, and their original reasons for migrating.[26]

In the late 1960s, in his study of mental illness among immigrants to Australia, carried out in Victoria, Krupinski[52] found that depressive states were particularly common among British and Eastern European migrants, and the latter group also had the highest rate of schizophrenia. Overall, immigrants showed a much higher rate of psychological instability than exists in the Australian-born population. More recent studies also suggest that some immigrant groups are more vulnerable to certain mental disorders and other illnesses than others. For example, according to Fitzpatrick and Newton,[53] Irish immigrants in England and Wales have a health status as poor as, or worse than, some of the other ethnic groups from south Asia or the Caribbean. In particular, they have increased rates of suicide, alcohol abuse and mental health problems, as well as of ischaemic heart disease, obesity, diabetes and other physical disabilities. Furthermore, these health problems, and a higher overall mortality, have been found to persist in the Irish community into the second and third generations after migration.[54]

Where mental illnesses do occur among migrant populations, they may range from depression (often presenting as somatic symptoms, such as 'pains everywhere') to acute psychotic breakdowns, self-neglect, suicide attempts, drug or alcohol abuse, domestic violence, and antisocial behaviour, especially among the youth.[10] Some may become deeply withdrawn or emotionally 'numb'; others may 'freeze' their identity at the moment that they left their homes, never put that experience behind them, and never 'move on' psychologically. Colson[10] describes, for example, how some groups of refugees may develop such a shared sense of grievance that it can totally dominate their lives, and never let them adjust to their new reality, and get on with their lives.

Among elderly migrants to the UK and USA, a higher rate of some mental health problems have been reported, including depression and dementia.[55] In a recent study in the UK, Livingston and Sembhi[55] found that rates of dementia among elderly Afro-Caribbean immigrants were higher compared with Whites and to people from ethnic-minorities born in the UK. This may be related to higher rates of hypertension and diabetes in this group, as well as to their migrant status, socio-economic deprivation and social isolation.

Impact of migration on family structure

Migration can either strengthen, or fragment an immigrant family, and this in turn can affect the mental health of its members. In many cases migration has a positive effect, by enhancing family cohesion, cooperation and emotional closeness. In others, external forces such as discrimination, unemployment, the demands of the casual labour market, or the dispersal of family members by the housing authorities, may all lead to a break-up of a previously close extended family.[56]

Within the family, new family dynamics often appear after migration. The family may gradually become bicultural, bilingual or even tricultural and trilingual, with the cultural world-views of grandparents, parents and children becoming very different from each another. The generations may differ not only in language facility, but also in cultural expectations, and communication between them may become increasingly difficult. Children born and raised in the new country, but who are unable to communicate with their immigrant grandparents, can lose contact with their own cultural traditions. Also, marital conflicts may arise from shifts in gender roles, while intergenerational conflicts may focus on issues such as religious obser-

vances, use of alcohol or drugs, sexual behaviour or choice of marriage partner.

Migration involves, above all, a major sense of *discontinuity* in everyday family life. Traditional and habitual ways of doing things, of relating to other people and understanding the world, somehow do not seem to work any longer. The migrants often find themselves in limbo, separated from their homelands, yet feeling not quite at home in their new environment. Unfortunately, many of the people they encounter, both personally and officially, may not understand this. According to Colson,[10] migrants are 'people in transition, who are uneasy about themselves in a world that ignores their desire and need for continuity'.

'Inversions' of migrant family structure

The discontinuities of migration are especially marked if the family comes to an urban environment in the developed world from a very traditional, rural environment back home. In that case, their move might involve what I have termed *inversions* of their previous life, social roles and world-view. Each of the four may have major, often negative effects, on the health of some or all of the family members.

1 *Generational inversion* – a situation where the children born or raised in the new country, understand its language, culture and technology better than their parents. In an inversion of the usual power relations between generations, this gives them a new power over their parents, and over inherited tradition. It is the parents (or grandparents) who are now dependent on the young for knowledge of the world, not the other way round. When immigrant parents rely on their children to act as interpreters to health professionals, this may cause considerable embarrassment; for example, when a young son is asked to translate his mother's intimate gynaecological or sexual symptoms to the doctor or nurse. However, Green and colleagues[46] argue that bilingual child interpreters in the UK should not be seen only as acting

inappropriately, but more as 'active social agents', who often take pride in their bilingualism and in their ability to help their parents. Despite this, they found that translating more complex medical histories to a doctor was often problematic for them, especially if it involved using technical or anatomical terms, and problems also arose where there was conflict between the parent and the health professional, which the child was expected to mediate.

2 *Gender role inversion* – occurs in some more traditional communities, when the women of the family become more independent after immigration. They may want, for example, to have a career outside the home, to acquire an education, or, in the case of young women, to choose their own marriage partner. In the UK, a number of so-called 'honour killings' of young girls have taken place among some traditional south Asian communities, carried out by parents who have disapproved strongly of their daughter's choice of boyfriend or fiancé. In some communities, the woman of the family may become the only breadwinner – particularly if her husband cannot find employment or is disabled – and this may cause resentment and conflict at home. Colson[10] suggests that some men are more adversely affected by refugee status than women, as the dependant life of a refugee often involves a loss of their prior status as decision-makers, as well as bread-winners. She describes cases where refugee women took on roles previously in the 'male domain', and as a result the men had little to do, became listless and depressed, and sometimes violent.

3 *Time inversion* – a situation where the past (in the 'Old Country') seems to be much more important than the present, or even the future. It occurs especially when that future is uncertain, and even threatening. It is a state of continuous nostalgia, spent thinking constantly of the 'Old Country', regretting the move, and grieving for what has been lost instead of focusing on what has been gained. For the younger members of the family, especially those born in the new country, this process may be very unsettling for them, and even emotionally destructive.

4 *Space inversion* – a situation where, especially in the first years after migration, the proportion of unfamiliar space occupied by the migrant seems to be much greater than that of familiar space – the geography and landscapes of the Old Country, kept alive by memories, reminisces, old photographs and old documents. 'There' becomes much more real and important than 'here'. In this case, the migrant is still 'living', to some extent, in what Parkes[57] calls their previous 'life space', rather then in their present environment. As in inversion (3), this may be emotionally difficult for the children, trying hard to adjust to the new country, and to make their new lives there. Kirmayer and Minas[2] point out that, thanks to mass media, global telecommunications (such as satellite TV) and air travel, for many migrants 'the distant may be more familiar and frequented than the physically close'. In a globalized world, this phenomenon will probably become more common, and people's identities will be made up increasingly of both global and local elements.

The overall effect of these four 'inversions' – as well as of other changes in language, dress, diet, religion, social behaviour and standards of modesty – may well be to decrease migrants' sense of identity, as well as family cohesion, and thus the degree of social support that it offers its members. The 'inversions' act by reducing the authority of parents and grandparents, diminishing the power of tradition, increasing marital and intergenerational conflict, and altering key life-cycle rituals (see Chapters 6 and 9). Together with the negative effects of the 'host' environment (such as social rejection, racism, discrimination and unemployment) they can induce mental distress, and, in some individuals and groups, greatly increase their sense of confusion, anomie, alienation and anger.

Refugee health

Much of the research on migrant health has concentrated on *refugees* – before, during and after they have fled from their own homes. Unlike voluntary migrants, refugees frequently have had no chance to prepare psychologically (and practically) for this sudden move, or to anticipate its consequences. A hasty flight may leave them little time to take provisions, money, clothes, furniture, valuables, family heirlooms, or religious objects with them. It may also separate family members from one another, and they may be forced to abandon elderly or ill relatives as they flee. Agrarian communities have to leave behind not only their homes, but also their crops, livestock and equipment. All these factors can have serious long-term consequences for refugee mental health.

Physical and psychological disorders

Burnett and Peel[58] have reviewed the studies on refugee health. They report that refugees generally suffer from a higher incidence of physical and mental health problems than the general population. In the UK, for example, one in six refugees is reported to have a physical health problem severe enough to affect their life, and two-thirds have experienced anxiety of depression. In a study of 115 refugee schoolchildren in Oxford, UK, Fazel and Stein[21] found that almost one-quarter of them had some significant psychological disturbance, greater than other children from the same ethnic minorities, and three times greater than the national average.

Burnett and Peel[58] also cite several other studies from the USA, Australia and Europe, which illustrate the sorts of health problems that refugees may bring with them. Many of them have experienced periods of malnutrition, poor hygiene and sanitation, as well as physical or psychological trauma. As a result, they may have more physical injuries, as well as diseases such as tuberculosis, hepatitis A, meningitis, HIV/AIDS, benign tertiary malaria, *Helicobacter pylori* infections, and a variety of intestinal parasites. Higher rates of diabetes, hypertension and coronary heart disease have also

been reported among refugees from Eastern Europe.[58] In Thailand, Bodeker and colleagues[59] report that refugees from Burma (Myanmar) have been found to have higher rates of tuberculosis, malnutrition, respiratory infections, HIV and drug-resistant malaria, as well as psychosocial disturbances resulting from violence and displacement.

In psychological terms, refugees may suffer from anxiety, depression, panic attacks or agoraphobia as result of their earlier experience of forced migration, as well as of their current situations (especially if this involves discrimination or isolation). In social terms, different types of social disruption may arise in refugee families' communities, from marital breakdown and domestic violence, to substance abuse as a coping mechanism. Like other migrants, they may also suffer from *cultural bereavement* (see below).

Migration and mental health: theories of causation

Why is migration sometimes associated with a higher risk of mental illness?

As Desjarlais and colleagues[22] point out, migration alone does not necessarily lead to poor mental health. Many *other* factors – before, during or after migration – are also relevant, including the migrant's experience, personality, resources, age at migration,[55] cultural background, employment status, housing conditions and degree of social cohesion, as well as the reactions of their 'host' community.

Although migration (whether between countries or within them) does seem to carry with it an increased risk of mental illness, the exact reasons for this are complex and not fully understood.[55] As pointed out earlier,[50] studies of the mental health of immigrants are often difficult to interpret unless one controls for many other factors, including age, social class, education, occupational status and ethnic group on one hand, and diagnostic methods which may be culturally biased on the other. However, where rates of mental illness *are* higher among migrants, one needs to explain exactly why this is so and why it seems to be higher in some communities but not in others. This section deals with six different conceptual ways of approaching this problem:

- Multi-migration
- Push–pull
- Selection-stress
- Host *versus* migrant
- Psychosocial transitions
- Cultural bereavement

Multi-Migration

Migration can be psychologically (and physically) traumatic– especially for refugees – because moving from one country to another often involves *several* different types of migration simultaneously – a process I would term *multi-migration*. Thus the move might involve not only a change of countries, but also the transition from a small rural village with its traditional practices and religious world-view, to the noisy, colourful, confusing chaos of a big Western city, with all its loneliness, anomie, and temptations: a shift from a constricted, but known world to an exposure to a wide range of alternative lifestyles and sexualities, as well as to drugs and alcohol. In their new environment, migrants may encounter unfamiliar climates and habitats, different ways of earning a living, new forms of leisure activity, and very different types of family structure and social organization. They may also encounter considerable hostility from the 'host population', at both the individual and official levels. Their move might also involve a shift from a familiar world where a particular religion is a key part of their life, to one dominated by a completely different religion – or by no religion at all. Thus migrants from traditional societies often enter a new environment where almost all the building-blocks of their previous world – family, locality, religion, gender roles, occupations – no longer play such an important part, and are no longer valued. The resultant 'culture-shock' can be very traumatic, and can affect their psychological and physical health, as well as their relationships

with one another. The possible dimensions of multi-migration are listed in Table 12.2.

Table12.2 Multimigration

Village	$\rightarrow$	City
Rural	$\rightarrow$	Urban
Religion A	$\rightarrow$	Religion B
Religious	$\rightarrow$	Secular
Social class A	$\rightarrow$	Social class B
Climate A	$\rightarrow$	Climate B

Push–pull

The emphasis here is on *why* the migrants left their homes in the first place: whether their migration was voluntary ('pull') or involuntary ('push'). In reality, these two pathways to migration often overlap: one may be 'pushed' to migrate from an impoverished country by poverty, while at the same time feel 'pulled' towards new economic opportunities elsewhere. Each of these motivations can result in emotional problems for the migrants, and their families. 'Pull' migrants (often called 'economic migrants') may experience major disappointments if they fail to succeed in their new environments; they may also feel that they have let themselves down, as well as their families.[25] 'Push' migrants may experience difficulties in adjusting to their new environment due to constantly grieving over the past, and always wanting to be somewhere else. Often they carry a 'fixed' and over-romanticized picture of their homeland, which can make it difficult for them ever to readjust to the present reality – or even to the reality back home, if they were ever to return there. In both 'pull' and 'push' migration, though, the role of new *context* – and whether it is welcoming or hostile, generous or exploitative – will also have major effects on mental health.[22]

Selection-stress

Cox[60] has summarized three hypotheses that seek to explain the high rate of mental illness among migrants:

1 Certain mental disorders incite their victims to migrate (the *selection* hypothesis).
2 The process of migration creates mental stress, which may precipitate mental illness in susceptible individuals (the *stress* hypothesis).
3 There is a non-essential association between migration and certain other variables, such as age, class and culture conflict.

In the first group, restless and unstable people are believed to migrate more often, in an attempt to solve their personal problems. In another study in Australia in 1965, for example, Schaechter[61] found that 45.5 per cent of non-British female immigrants admitted to a psychiatric hospital within 3 years of migration had suffered an established mental illness before migration. If 'suspected cases' of mental illness before arrival were added, the figure rose to 68.2 per cent. Other studies, from different parts of the world, have shown that a certain percentage of immigrants *do* have a history of previous mental disorders in their countries of origin. For example, Zahid and his colleagues[25] in 2003 found that psychiatric morbidity among migrant housemaids in Kuwait was two to five times higher than the native female population. Among the significant risk factors for psychiatric breakdown they found a previous history of mental as well as physical illness, in their home countries. Other risk factors, especially among Sri Lankan housemaids, were a lower level of education, and a non-Muslim background.

The concept of 'stress' (Chapter 11) is often used to describe the pressures and difficulties that the migrants encounter in their new environment. However, as Littlewood and Lipsedge[62] point out, in their study of mental illness among immigrants to the UK, these disorders result from the complex interplay of many different factors, including both 'stress' *and* 'selection'. These include material and environmental deprivation such as overcrowding, shared dwellings, lack of amenities, high unemployment and low family incomes, as well as racial discrimination, and conflict between immigrants and their local-born children.

Language difficulties also play an important part, especially among female immigrants who arrive later in the country than their men folk and who are often confined within the home and family. For example, a study in Newcastle[26] in 1981 found that 58 per cent of Pakistani women spoke little or no English, and 15 per cent of men and 66 per cent of the women had received little or no schooling and were entirely illiterate. These socio-economic factors, coupled with the stress of culture change and the influence of selection, explain much of the increased rates of mental illness among first-generation immigrants. A further factor, mentioned earlier, is that diagnostic and admission rates in psychiatry may reflect political, racial or moral prejudices, and misinterpret the immigrants' cultural beliefs and reactions to their plight as evidence of 'madness' or 'badness'.

Host versus migrant

Here the emphasis is not on the migrant population, but on the *host* community. Do they welcome the newcomers, or do they resent them? Do they discriminate against them, or even attack them physically? Are they willing to give them jobs and homes? Will they allow them to integrate, or insist that they live apart – often in less desirable areas – with members of their own community? Is the host community racist in outlook, whether on an individual or institutional level?[51] All these factors can impact on the refugees, their health status,[63] and whether they are willing, or able to integrate. Mestheneos and Ioannidi,[64] for example, reviewed attitudes towards refugees in 15 member states of the European Union (EU). They found that although most of these states were now multi-ethnic, they had a variety of official policies, ranging from exclusion to integration, from assimilation to a *laissez-faire* acceptance of cultural pluralism. The refugees, however, felt that widespread racism and ignorance, at both the personal and institutional levels, were the most fundamental barriers to integration in the EU that they encountered, and this had a major emotional impact on them and their families. Those from well-educated or middle class families felt particularly humiliated by their loss of social status, especially when their qualifications were not recognized in their new country.

Psychosocial transitions

Migration from one region or culture is often a traumatic experience because it involves major disruptions in what Parkes[57] has termed the individual's 'life space' or 'assumptive world': that is, 'those parts of the environment with which the self interacts and in relation to which behaviour is organized; other persons, material possessions, the familiar world of home and place of work, and the individual's body and mind in so far as he can view these as separate from his self'. It is these comfortable assumptions that are so violently shattered in the case of involuntary migrants, such as refugees, especially if those changes happen quickly, involve a large proportion of the migrant's 'life space' and are irreversible.[57] Major 'psychosocial transitions' can affect voluntary migrants as well, of course, though their effects may be less severe – especially if the migrants have the option of one day returning home.

Cultural bereavement

The experience of migration, as a profound 'psychosocial transition', is analogous in some ways to bereavement or disablement. Eisenbruch[31] has coined the term *cultural bereavement* for those groups of people who have suffered a permanent traumatic loss of their familiar land and culture. This applies especially to unwilling migrants such as exiles and refugees, suddenly uprooted during war or persecution. The stressful changes that such a group may undergo in its collective grief are analogous to those suffered by individual mourners; like them, the grieving for the lost home and past may last for many years, or even a lifetime. Also, like other forms of bereavement, there may be pathological and atypical grief reactions, ranging from severe depression or withdrawal, to drug or alcohol abuse, psychosomatic disorders, domestic violence or other forms of antisocial behaviour. As described below, migrant communities often evolve many different strategies to prevent, or reduce, their feelings of 'cultural bereavement'.

Cultural bereavement not only occurs after physically moving from one country or region to another, it can also take place in the circumstances of 'static migration' described above.

VARIATIONS IN MENTAL ILLNESS RATES AMONG MIGRANTS

Within both migrant populations and ethnic minorities, certain groups seem to have different rates and forms of mental illness. According to Littlewood and Lipsedge[62], 'there appear to be no simple explanations for the different rates of mental illness applicable to all minority groups'. In the UK, some factors seem more significant in some groups than in others, and the best way to compare groups would be to add up all these negative factors – selection, stress, multiple deprivations, language difficulties, loss of status (both social and professional), clash between old and new cultural values, and so on, to find a 'score' indicating the risk factors for that community. For example, they note how West African students seemed particularly vulnerable to mental illness owing to dissatisfaction with British food and weather, to discrimination, economic and legal difficulties, experience of the 'typical British personality', sexual isolation, more mature age, middle-class aspirations and fear of withdrawal of their grants if they fail their examinations. Those with the lowest rates of mental illness, the Chinese, Italians and Indians, had in common a great determination to migrate, migration for economic reasons, an intention to return home, little attempt at assimilation, and a high degree of entrepreneurial activity. Immigrants who were forced to leave their countries as refugees and who cannot return were, in contrast, likely to have a higher rate of mental illness.

In his 1967 study, Krupinski[52] examined some of these variables among immigrant groups in Australia; he related their high rates of mental illness to the fact that many were single young men migrating from the UK and western Europe, among whom there was a proportion of already unstable persons (including some chronic alcoholics arriving from the UK). The stresses of migration seemed to affect migrants from southern and eastern Europe especially, particularly those in the latter group who had suffered traumatic experiences in World War Two, or loss of occupational status in Australia. Seventy per cent of East European migrants with university degrees now belonged to a lower socio-economic class, compared with only 20 per cent of British graduates. Krupinski also found that schizophrenia occurred most frequently among male immigrants 1–2 years after arrival, while in females the peak was found after 7–15 years. The late onset among females was ascribed to the onset of menopause, and the ending of the maternal role with the departure of grown-up children. In addition, a high proportion of female non-British immigrants could not speak English even after many years in the country, especially those from southern Europe. As with the Pakistani women in Newcastle,[26] their social and linguistic isolation was believed to contribute to their high rate of mental breakdown.

Pathogenic and protective factors

Within the migrant community, some cultural attributes may actually be dangerous to their health and social functioning. These may include a rigid division among the sexes, the social isolation of women, multiple religious taboos and prescriptions, hostility to the 'host' society, residential patterns which encourage several generations of a family to live in the same house, intergenerational conflicts, and extreme pressures on children to succeed financially, academically or socially (an example of the 'culturogenic stress' described in Chapter 11).

Conversely, some factors do seem to protect migrants against some, if not all, of these mental health risks. These can include:

1 If they migrate as a family unit, rather than as individuals.

2 If after migration the family remains as a coherent, constant unit of support for all its members.

3 If they have entrepreneurial ambitions and skills.

4 If they have financial resources to pay for education, decent housing, and medical care.

5 If they have fluency in the new language, as well as numeracy.

6 If they have education, and portable professional, intellectual or physical skills.

7 If they have local family or other contacts in the new country.

8 If they have a coherent religious or cultural world view, especially if this reinforces family cohesion.

Some of the self-help strategies that migrant communities evolve to protect themselves psychologically, are described in more detail below.

Personality factors also play a part. Some migrants are more positive and proactive in their approach, others less so. Many successful migrants are good 'social strategists', have personalities that enable them to reach out to others, and have the ability to build up supportive social networks. Others are more introverted, shy and vulnerable, and less able to adapt to new situations and to new challenges. However as Mestheneos and Ioannidi[64] point out, positive personality factors, even when they are present, may not be sufficient for success, as the refugees also need the support of social and other institutions in their new country. If these are absent, hostile or difficult to access, 'the process of integration becomes very hard, condemning many to social marginality or even social exclusion.'

Mental health problems among migrants to the UK

Some of the mental health problems reported among immigrants to the UK, especially in the first generation, have been examined in the following studies.

Case study: mental illness among immigrants in Manchester, UK

Carpenter and Brockington[65] in 1980 examined the incidence of mental illness among Asian, West Indian and African immigrants living in Manchester. It was found that the migrant populations had about twice the first admission rate to mental hospitals that British-born subjects had, especially those migrants aged 35–44 years, and also Asian women. Schizophrenia was particularly common among the immigrants, especially with delusions of persecution, a phenomenon noted in many other studies of migrants. The authors hypothesized that 'social and lingual isolation... insecurity and the attitudes of the milieu are the explanations for the development of persecutory delusions'.

Case study: psychiatric admissions to hospitals of foreign-born people in Bradford, UK

Hitch and Rack[66] in 1980 studied the rates of first admission to psychiatric hospitals in Bradford, and found that foreign-born people had substantially rates of higher mental illness than British-born people. The rates of psychiatric breakdown of a sample of Polish and Russian refugees in Bradford were measured 25 years after they had settled in the UK. While both had higher rates of mental illness (especially schizophrenia and paranoia) than the UK-born population, the Poles had a higher rate than the Russians. The most vulnerable group was the Polish females. The authors suggest that the difference between the immigrant groups was due partly to minimal cohesion among the Poles, and also to a strong sense of national, ethnic identity among the Russians (many of whom were Ukrainians). This ethnic social support not only afforded protection against environmental stress, it also bestowed identity, though the Russians appeared to have maintained this identity more

than the Poles. Many years after migration, though, both immigrant groups were especially vulnerable to first-time mental illness. The authors suggested that 'the combination of wartime experiences and culture shock may have been met with adequate coping mechanisms, but nevertheless rendered the personality vulnerable to later stress'. In middle age, when children have moved away from home and spouses or relatives have died, an immigrant who still speaks broken English and has no English friends will become particularly vulnerable to environmental stressors, with the consequent danger of mental or physical illness.

Case study: attempted suicide among immigrants in Birmingham, UK

Burke, in three studies published in 1976, examined the rate of attempted suicide among Irish,[67] Asian[68] and West Indian[51] immigrants in Birmingham. His findings indicate that immigrants have a higher rate of attempted suicide than the populations in their countries of origin, and this applies particularly to female immigrants. In Birmingham, those born in Northern Ireland or the Irish Republic had about a 30 per cent higher rate than the native population (as measured in Edinburgh), and higher rates than both Belfast and Dublin. Other indices of stress, such as the rates of alcoholism, drug addiction or mental illness, were also raised in this immigrant group. Asian immigrants (from India, Pakistan and Bangladesh) had a lower rate of attempted suicide than the native-born population, but their rate was higher than that of their countries of origin, especially among females. Burke points out that language difficulties for women may play a major part in this, since Asian men have usually migrated several years earlier, and have had a greater opportunity to learn the language and familiarize themselves with English culture. Female immigrants are often expected to remain at home, and there is also some culture conflict for younger Asian women and girls between the values of home and those of school or workplace. Among West Indians, too, attempted suicide was less common than in the native-born population, but West Indian women had a higher rate than women in the Caribbean; that is, the 'stresses that follow immigration and contribute to attempted suicide are more likely to affect women than men'. Part of the stress on young West Indians arises from the insecurity of low paid jobs, fear of not being able to cope financially and emotionally, housing difficulties, and the absence of the extended family in an urban setting. All of these 'may effectively reduce the tolerance of immigrants in withstanding these stresses'.

Case study: suicide levels among immigrants in England and Wales

Raleigh and Balarajan[69] in 1992 analysed national suicide rates among 17 immigrant groups in England and Wales for the years 1979–83. Using mortality data on male and female immigrants aged 20–69 years, they found that many immigrant groups, especially Poles, Russians, French, Germans, South Africans, Scots and Irish, had much higher rates of suicide than the native population of England and Wales. The rates among Scottish and Irish immigrants aged between 20 years and 29 years were particularly high. Other groups, such as migrants from the Caribbean, the Indian subcontinent, Italy, Spain and Portugal, had much lower rates than the national average. However, when the suicide rates of these various communities were compared with those of their countries of origin, they were found to be very similar. This was particularly true of male immigrants, but less true of females, especially from Ireland and Poland. The authors thus concluded that, as suicide levels in the immigrant groups differed less from levels in their home countries than from levels in England and Wales, 'the findings do not suggest that migration increases the risk of suicide'. Although they agreed that 'the economic and

social changes associated with migration can often be stressful', they suggested that 'reaction to such stress is conditioned by the social and cultural attitudes inculcated in the country of origin'.

Limitations of these studies

It should be emphasized that these four studies in the UK, carried out from 1970s to the 1990s, dealt predominantly with the first generation of immigrants, people who were born outside the country. They do not necessarily apply to those born and raised in the UK, whose experiences and degree of acculturation are likely to be different from those of their parents – even though, as mentioned above, higher morbidity rates can still continue in some communities for two or three generations after migration.[53] In addition, while all the studies seem to indicate higher levels of certain physical, emotional and social problems among first-generation immigrants, there are some inconsistencies among them. Burke's studies,[51,67,68] for example, indicate higher levels of attempted suicides among immigrants to the UK, while Raleigh and Balarajan[69] found actual suicide levels no higher among the immigrant population – although they did note that from 1970 to 1983 in England and Wales, suicide rates did significantly increase among some immigrant groups, especially those born in Russia, Ireland and South Africa. Furthermore, there are apparently wide variations in how different groups respond to the experience of migration. While these studies are useful in illustrating the high level of stress among immigrants, they do not provide enough data on how the cultural practices and world-view of immigrants – and of the host community itself – actually interact in the migrant situation. For example, which cultural traits in immigrant communities protect them from stress or predispose towards it? Do some cultural groups migrate less 'stressfully' than others? Is the status of temporary migrants (such as *gastarbeiters*) less or more stressful than that of permanent migrants, exiles or refugees? What are the effects of racial discrimination and racial prejudice, both individual and institutional, on immigrants' mental and physical health? Are some host cultures more 'stressful' to immigrants than others?

Another factor, described in Chapters 10 and 15, is that the medical and other authorities in the host community determine whether deviant behaviour among immigrants is regarded as 'mad' or as 'bad', because classifying people in these ways can significantly influence morbidity statistics among immigrant populations.

MANAGEMENT OF MIGRANT MENTAL HEALTH PROBLEMS

PSYCHOTHERAPY

In the industrialized world, many migrants who experience mental distress may find themselves referred to psychotherapists, counsellors, or psychiatrists as these particular health professionals are often in the frontline of caring for migrant communities. However, each of these approaches may, for different reasons, be unsuccessful in relieving the migrants' distress. For example, one problem with psychotherapy is that this form of Western 'talking therapy' or 'symbolic healing' (see Chapter 10) may be quite inappropriate for some clients from traditional societies.[58] First, its focus only on the individual, and not on the family or community, may be quite unfamiliar to clients from a more group-based society. Second, the 'hydraulic model' of some psychotherapy ('Let it all come out, don't bottle it up'), as well as the notion of revealing traumatic experiences or intimate secrets to a stranger may all be seen as incomprehensible, embarrassing, humiliating, or even dangerous. Clients may believe that talking about a traumatic event can even cause it to happen again, by attracting witchcraft, the 'Evil Eye' or the attention of malevolent spirits (see Chapter 5). It may also cause one to 'lose face' to a stranger, to be shamed by having to 'wash one's dirty linen in public', and reveal intimate family secrets, especially about early upbringing, or the behaviour of one's parents. For some men, being a refugee with little control over their own lives, may already seem an emasculating experience: talking about it to another man may make them feel even worse.

Psychotherapy for migrants, therefore, always has to be sensitive to these cultural concerns, especially to the unique and traumatic experiences of being a refugee. Therapy may require the services of a trained interpreter or advocate,[58] the use of community support groups, or even the use of religious figures or traditional healers. Sveaass and Reichelt,[70] for example, described the problems of doing family therapy for refugee families in Norway, and how they may be overcome. As well as the usual personal and family issues, they point out that these refugee families are often 'emotionally overburdened', not only by their past traumatic experiences, but also by now living in a context where they feel powerless, lack 'cultural competence', are financially dependent and have little social support. Dealing with them requires sensitivity, empathy, a willingness to advise on practical issues, and the creation of a 'safe space' where therapeutic work can take place.

Some migrant clients may be unfamiliar with the basic concepts of Western psychotherapy, ranging from assumptions about the causes of present-day emotional suffering lying in early childhood, to the very existence of the 'subconscious'. They also may not understand, or misinterpret, some of the spatial metaphors for the psyche commonly used in modern psychology, such as 'boundaries', 'containment', 'projection', 'introjection', 'suppressed emotions', 'inner world' or 'safe space'.

Psychotherapists also need to respect different cultural ways of dealing with psychological suffering, even if they differ from their own. As Burnett and Peel[58] point out, 'every culture has its own frameworks for mental health and for seeking help in a crisis'; for example, 'Mozambican refugees describe forgetting as their usual cultural means of coping with difficulties'. Ethiopians call this 'active forgetting'. This, of course, is very different from the 'active remembering' so characteristic of Western psychotherapy.

PSYCHIATRY

The practice of psychiatry is increasingly influenced by globalization and migration. Kirmayer and Minas[2] see this as happening in three ways. (1) It affects both individual and collective identity, in ways that can lead to a sense of anomie, and to 'the 'creolization' of identity and of cultural idioms through which emotional distress is communicated'. That is, not only do people have a new, mixed identity, but their ways of expressing distress (especially to health professionals) may also involve a mixed, confusing 'language of distress', borrowed from several different backgrounds. To deal with this, they predict 'the emergence of a *mestizo* psychiatry open to hybridization of identity and the corresponding elaboration of theories of psychopathology and treatment'. (2) Through the impact of economic inequalities which often accompany globalization, and which produce the social conditions (such as poverty, unemployment, poor housing, or discrimination) where psychiatric conditions can increase; and, most subtly, (3) by 'the shaping and dissemination of psychiatric knowledge itself'. That is, policy makers may ignore the role of social factors such as poverty, economic inequality, and underdevelopment in causing psychiatric problems, and the spread of Western psychiatric concepts may support this approach: 'psychiatric science may inadvertently collude with social forces that seek to reframe political and economic issues as problems of individuals'. This is the process of 'medicalization', already discussed in Chapters 4, 5 and 8.

Psychiatric treatment of migrants, especially the elderly, may also be difficult owing to difficulties in access, as well as cultural factors that can influence the presentation, help-seeking behaviour, and acceptability of psychiatric treatment.[55]

TRADITIONAL HEALING

For refugee populations, especially those still in reception or resettlement camps, Western ways of diagnosing and treating psychosocial problems may be inadequate. Instead, refugees may prefer their own traditional healers and remedies (often in combination with Western medicine), when dealing with their mental health needs. Such folk healers can provide a greater sense of continuity, as well as a more holistic and spiritual view of human suffering. Bodeker and colleagues,[59] for example, found extensive networks of traditional practitioners (especially herbalists) among Burmese refugees in Thailand, especially in the camps along the Thai–Burma border. They point out the advantages of this for the refugees, and that 'cooperation between Western clinical services and traditional health practitioners is intimately linked with refugee health and well-being, including cultural continuity and refuge identity'. They suggest that in these situations, an integration of Western and traditional practices would be useful. Furthermore, the use of traditional health-care resources might also increase the refugees' sense of the autonomy, reduce their dependence on foreign aid and 'counter the tendency for humanitarian-assistance to establish stereotypical donor and refugee roles'.

SELF–TREATMENT AND PREVENTIVE STRATEGIES

In a more globalized and mobile world, migrant groups can now adopt a wide range of strategies to maintain their sense of identity and to reduce their feelings of 'cultural bereavement'. These overlapping strategies may include:

1 *Recreation of micro-cultural worlds* – either within their home (in terms of language, dress, furnishing, cuisine, social roles), or else in ethnic clubs or associations, women's groups, restaurants, temples, or shops. In some cases they may form ethnic enclaves within cities, such as 'Chinatown' and 'Little Italy' in New York or London's Bangladeshi 'Banglatown',

where they can celebrate their own ethnic and religious festivals, and where some aspects of the 'Old Country' (such as atmosphere, shops, music, dress, cuisine, dance, smells, tastes) have all been recreated.

2 *Exaggeration of original culture* – whereby a new syncretic subculture is created, which in some cases is an exaggeration of the culture 'back home', such as the many expatriate English communities in the former British Empire who were 'more English than the English', or some Irish-Americans becoming 'more Irish than the Irish'.

3 *Keeping up physical contact with the Old Country* by frequent trips 'home', buying property there (or a gravesite) and 'creating a name' there by constant visits to attend family weddings, funerals, or religious festivals, as well as acts of generosity to family, friends and community.

4 *Keeping up links without returning or visiting* – by sending money home as remittances, as well as photographs and videos of the family, and sending children back regularly to meet their family of origin, acquire an education, study in a religious school, or find a marriage partner.

5 *Using the media to keep in contact* – in an age of global communications, this has become much easier, and migrants can now use emails, web-cams and mobile telephones, as well as ethnic newspapers, magazines, radio programmes and satellite TV stations, to keep in contact with people and events back home.

6 *Self-help or mutual support groups* – such as the *dertlesmek* support groups of Turkish migrant women in Belgium, or the Ethiopian Health Support Network or the Cypriot Advisory Service in the UK (see Chapter 4). These can provide social, psychological and financial support, as well as information on the new country, its laws and customs.

7 *Maintaining a 'Myth of Return' but never actually returning* – a pattern which may protect the migrant in the short term, but may have nega-

tive psychological effects years later, when they finally realize that owing to age, infirmity, political changes or other factors they will never return 'home' to their own community and country.

8 *Returning to live in the Old Country* – a pattern that is becoming more common with the advent of cheap air flights and the ability to remit pensions and other income back to the 'Old Country'. This *circular migration* is becoming more common, though in some cases migrants may choose to leave for a third country, rather than return to their country of origin.

9 *Creating a 'new life' by rejection of the Old Country and culture of origin* – a process where the migrant makes a conscious effort at compete cultural and social assimilation, and strives to develop a new sense of self by a process of 'cultural amnesia': that is, by refusing to speak in their native language, changing their name, converting to another religion, or inter-marrying with the local population. This option is more likely in the newer 'melting pot' countries, rather than in traditional European society.

For each individual migrant, these various strategies may or may not be successful. As mentioned earlier, their success also depends on a variety of other forces far beyond the control of the individual, including personality variables, unemployment, available housing, shifts in official policy, and the overall attitude of the 'host' environment towards the migrants in their midst. Because of the sharp rise in global population movements, all these factors are likely to become much more important in the future.

KEY REFERENCES

2 Kirmayer, L.J. and Minas, H. (2000) The future of cultural psychiatry: an international perspective. *Can. J. Psychiatry* 45, 438–46.

5 United Nations Population Division (2002) *International Migration 2002*. New York: United Nations.

7 United Nations High Commission for Refugees (2005) *Basic Facts: Refugees by Numbers (2005 edition):*. http://www.unhcr.ch/cgi-bin/texis/vtx/basics/opendoc.htm?tbl=BASICSandid=3b028097c (Accessed on 26 July 2005)

11 United Nations Development Programme (2004) *Human Development Report 2004*. New York: UNDP, pp. 83–105.

17 National Multicultural Institute (2005) *The Case for Diversity: Why Diversity? Why Now?* Washington, DC: NMCI. http://www.nmci.org/otc/default.htm (Accessed on 29 August 2005)

24 Bandyopadhyay, M. and Thomas, J. (2002) Women migrant workers' vulnerability to HIV infection in Hong Kong. *AIDS Care* 14(4), 509–21

31 Eisenbruch, M. (1988) The mental health of refugee children and their cultural development. *Int. Migr. Rev.* 22, 282–300.

32 Bach, S. (2003) *International Migration of Health Workers: Labour and Social Issues*. (Working Paper WP.209). Geneva: International Labour Office.

45 Southall, D.P., O'Hare, B.A.M. (2002) Empty arms: the effect of the arms trade on mothers and children. *Br. Med. J.* 325, 1457–61

55 Livingston, G. and Sembhi, S. (2003) Mental health of the ageing immigrant population. *Adv. Psychiatric Treat.* 9, 31–37.

58 Burnett, A. and Peel, M. (2001) Health needs of asylum seekers and refugees. *Br. Med. J.* 322, 544–7.

64 Mestheneos, E. and Ioannidi, E. (2002) Obstacles to refugee integration in the European Union member states. *J. Refugee Stud.* 15(3), 304–20.

See http://www.culturehealthandillness for the full list of references for this chapter.

RECOMMENDED READING

Colson, E. (2003) Forced migration and the anthropological response. *J Refugee Studies* 16(1), 1–18.

Desjarlais, R., Eisenberg, L., Good, B. & Kleinman, A. (eds) (1995) *World Mental Health*. Oxford: Oxford University Press, pp. 136–54.

Frenk, J., Sepúlveda, J., Gómez-Dantés, O., McGuiness, M.J. and Knaul, F. (1997) The new world order and international health. *Br. Med. J.* 314, 1404–07.

Giddens, A. (2001) *Sociology*, 4th edn. Cambridge: Polity, pp. 50–77.

Scheper-Hughes, N. (2000) The global traffic in human organs. *Curr. Anthropol.* 41(2), 191–224.

RECOMMENDED WEBSITES

United Nations High Commissioner for Refugees (UNHCR): http://www.unhcr.ch

International Organization for Migration: http://www.iom.int

Population Reference Bureau: http://www.prb.org

Refugees International: http://www.refugeesinternational.org

World Tourism Organization: http://www.world-tourism.org

13 _____ Telemedicine and the Internet

One of the most important developments in health care over the past few decades, has resulted from the development of the Internet and the World Wide Web. These have had a major impact on medical care, especially on the flow of medical information across the globe, and on the relationships between health care professionals and their patients.

THE WORLD WIDE WEB AND THE INTERNET

The *World Wide Web* (WWW) can be described as a global collection of accessible information, which can be accessed by computers linked to an enormous electronic network: the *Internet*. The WWW can be thought of as an 'information space', a 'universe of information' that is now available to hundreds of millions of people worldwide – provided, of course, that they have access to a computer and the Internet. Since the 1990s, this process has increased enormously, with an estimated 940 million people having access to the WWW in 2004,[1] and over 1000 million in 2006, of which 35.7 per cent were in Asia, 28.5 per cent in Europe, and 22.2 per cent in North America.[2] Despite this, many people in the developed world – especially the poor, and the less well-educated – still fall on the wrong side of the 'digital divide',[3] with little or no access to the Internet, or even knowledge of it.

Many people use the Internet to find information about health and medical issues. Access to health information is now one of the commonest reasons for going online. By 2003, for example, an estimated 70 million Americans had searched the WWW for health-related information,[4] while in Japan by 2001, an estimated 50 per cent of physicians and 22 per cent of patients were using the Internet to obtain health information.[5]

Many Internet users are looking for information on specific health problems, including mental health issues, that affect them or their families. Others use it to communicate with other people suffering from the same condition, as part of an online patient support group, or with their own doctors or other health professional. Many of these developments, which are having a profound impact on the culture of medical care, are part of the growing phenomenon of *telemedicine*.

TELEMEDICINE

WHAT IS TELEMEDICINE?

Telemedicine refers to the transfer of information about health between sites, and between people. Over the past 20–30 years it has become increasingly common in many different countries.[6] Unlike the traditional face-to-face consultation (sometimes called a 'F2F' or 'FTF' consultation) between a health professional and a client, telemedicine is health care at a distance. For Coiera,[7] its essence is 'the exchange of information at a distance, whether that information is voice, an image, elements of a medical record or commands to a surgical robot.' It is thus 'the remote communication of information to facilitate clinical care.' More broadly, according to Craig and Patterson,[6] the concept of telemedicine 'encompasses the whole range of medical activities including diagnosis, treatment and prevention of disease, education of health-care providers and consumers, and research and evaluation'. The simplest, and probably earliest form of telemedicine is the telephone consultation between patient and doctor. However, with the development of much more advanced technologies – in computers, satellite telecommunications, radios, videophones, web-cams, videoconferencing, and mobile telephone networks – a whole range of new forms of communication are now possible between people who may be living many thousands of miles apart. In each case, telemedicine should ideally not be seen as is not a form of health care in its own right, but rather as *supplementary* to the health care given by one person (the health professional) to another (the patient).

Craig and Patterson[6] see the main indications for telemedicine as a means of improving access to health care, and the quality of that care as: (1) where there is no alternative (such as emergencies in remote locations), and (2) where it is better than existing services (such as the use of teleradiology by remote rural hospitals). In technical terms, they divide telemedicine first into whether the information transmitted is *prerecorded* and then sent after a pause (like an email), or *synchronous* (like a telephone conversation or videoconference), where immediate interaction between the parties is possible; and second, by the *medium* of communication used (whether it is text, audio, still images, or video pictures).

Telemedicine programmes have been increasing steadily over the past decade, especially in the more industrialized world. By 1999, more than 40 states in the USA were developing telemedicine programmes, and there were more than 70 electronic medical networks in use nationwide.[8] Overall, between 1996 and 2001 the number of telemedicine programmes in the USA increased from 90 to 205.[9] Outside the USA, in 2005 there were 52 major telemedicine programmes, including ten in Canada, nine in Australia, and nine in the UK.[6] Telemedicine is especially useful in very large countries such as Australia and Canada, with relatively dispersed and remote populations who sometimes have limited access to health-care facilities, or to sources of information such as medical libraries. In recent years, it is increasingly being used in poorer, developing countries, especially in more remote, rural areas.

Two related concepts to telemedicine, especially in nursing, are *telecare* (sometimes called *telenursing*), which is 'the provision, at a distance, of nursing and community support to a patient',[6] and *telehealth*, which is 'public health services delivered at a distance, to people who are not necessarily unwell, but who wish to remain well and independent'.[6]

TYPES OF COMMUNICATION PATTERNS

Within telemedicine there are many potential types of communication between these parties, and among them. Each one is mediated in a rather different way by a machine, whether that machine is a telephone, radio, computer, video camera, fax machine, or any other. In each case, the machine plays a different role depending on the type on interaction, who is involved in it, and the direction of flow of the information. The six main types of communication in telemedicine are illustrated in Table 13.1

Professional ↔ Machine ↔ Professional

Here telemedicine is used to connect health care professionals with one another, in order to consult, share information or research findings, or get advice about specific clinical problems. It is used particularly at the interface between primary care

Table 13.1 Types of communication in telemedicine

(1) Professional ↔ Machine ↔ Professional
(2) Professional ↔ Machine ↔ Patient
(3) Patient ↔ Machine ↔ Professional
(4) Patient ↔ Machine ↔ Patient
(5) Professional ↔ Machine ↔ Database
(6) Patient ↔ Machine ↔ Database

doctors or nurses, especially those in remote locations, and hospital-based specialists, often a great distance away.[7,10]. Example of this process of *teleconsultation* is the videoconferencing link between local general practitioners and ophthalmologists in Finland to discuss specific clinical cases (*teleophthalmology*),[11] and a *teledermatology* programme in Turkey, in which images of skin lesions are sent to dermatologists elsewhere for their diagnosis.[12]

This type of telemedicine can use a variety of communication media, including sending emails and digitalized images, but videoconferencing is increasingly popular to conduct case-conferences, or to share research findings with medical colleagues in different localities. It includes the various forms of *telediagnosis*, especially *teleradiology* and *telepathology*. Here, images of X-rays, computed tomography (CT) scans, electro-cardiograms, blood test printouts, or other pathology test results, are transmitted to specialists in another location who will then interpret them, and advise on what further action is to be taken. Today, teleradiology is probably one of the forms of telediagnosis that is most integrated into modern clinical practice.[6]

Professional ↔ Machine ↔ Patient

Here the machine is used by health professionals to communicate with their patients, or even to treat them. The oldest form of this is the telephone consultation between professional and patient. In their review of the subject, Car and Sheikh[13] point out its many advantages, including giving medical advice, doing triage (deciding whether or not the patient needs urgent treatment or referral), following-up on the progress of an illness or on missed appointments, and giving information about preventive health strategies (such as the date that immunizations are due). However, they point out that clinicians need to acquire specific skills of communication, in order to make telephone consultations most effective.

More recently, there has been the development of a number of clinical practices, run entirely on the Internet by 'cyber doctors', which provide 'virtual house calls' and give online medical advice and information.[4]

The main forms of this type of telemedicine outlined below are *tele-education*, *telecare*, and *telesurgery*, while *telepsychiatry* and *cybertherapy* are discussed in another section.

Tele-education

An important use of telemedicine is in health education (*tele-education*). For example, Yip and colleagues[14] describe how in Hong Kong a group of patients with type 2 diabetes received health education on their diabetes, transmitted to them from the diabetic centre of a district hospital, and there was high patient satisfaction with this *telediabetes* education. According to Yip,[15] linking the diabetic patient by telemedicine (telephones or videophones) to the multidisciplinary team of diabetic specialists in a clinic or hospital, can mean frequent and direct interaction between them, and more opportunity to give the patient support, and to monitor their progress. Overall, it means shifting care from hospital or diabetic clinic to wherever the patient is located, and for the patient this can result in an increased sense of autonomy ('*tele-empowerment*'),[16] control, and confidence in managing of their own disease. Interactive videoconferencing has also been used for community health education. Reznik and colleagues,[17] for example, describe it use in delivering health education messages about the causes, prevention, and management of asthma to a group of mainly Latino immigrants in an inner-city area of the Bronx, New York.

Telecare and telemonitoring

With patients who are elderly, disabled, or housebound with chronic diseases – home *telecare* or *telemonitoring* is increasingly being used, as it allows doctors or nurses to monitor their patient's health status, answer queries, or give them advice, without actually being in the patient's home. Ruggiero[18] notes how home health care is one of the fastest growing forms of health care, as a result of the trend towards community care rather than hospitalization, though it should always supplement, not replace, a human carer. For example, Baer and colleagues[19] examined how the home-care of chronic leg wounds or ulcers could be improved if the home-care nurse photographed the wound with a digital camera, then transmitted the images to a senior specialist wound-care nurse for advice and a treatment plan. Monitoring can also be done by machines, such as those that monitor the patient's blood pressure,[20] pulse rate, blood glucose, or respiratory function, and then transmit their findings directly to a specialist for assessment. In a study in Rome, Italy by Maiolo and colleagues,[21] patients with severe respiratory disease and on oxygen therapy, were monitored at home for their arterial oxygen saturation, and heart rate. The patients did the measurements twice weekly, and the results were transmitted automatically to the hospital's processing centre, via a normal telephone line, and then checked by a respiratory physician. After 12-months of this telemonitoring, it was found that the number of hospital admissions and acute home exacerbations decreased by 50 per cent and 55 per cent respectively, with large savings in the cost of hospitalization.

Telemonitoring can also be used for patients that are already in hospital, such as those in an intensive care unit, and whose vital signs and general appearance can be monitored by nurses in another location, using monitors attached to the patient's body, or by closed-circuit television cameras (CCTV).

Not all nurses, however, are happy with the non-tactile aspects of telecare, with its absence of 'body work', once so characteristic of most nursing practice.[22]

Telesurgery

Here surgeons in one location operate on a patient in another: the actual surgery being carried out by the use of robots, controlled by the surgeons via electronic and telecommunications links – a process known as *telerobotic surgery*.[23] Theoretically, this might allow types of surgery, such as hip replacements, to be carried out on patients in areas where surgeons are few, provided, of course, that the right equipment and local medical staff and facilities are available on site. On 7 September 2001, the first transatlantic surgery (a laparoscopic cholecystectomy) was performed, when surgeons in New York successfully removed the gall bladder of a patient in Strasbourg, France – 7000 km away – by remote control, using the Zeus Robotic System.[23] Despite this, many technical drawbacks still remain in telerobotic surgery, including a lack of tactile feedback for the surgeon, and the problems of maintaining a secure, continuous electronic connection between surgeon and robot.

Patient ↔ Machine ↔ Professional

Here the technology is primarily used by patients to communicate with health professionals. It includes using the telephone, Internet or radio to consult with a doctor or nurse, report on the progress of an illness or treatment, book hospital or clinic appointments. It can also include *telepharmacy*, where drugs are ordered directly from a pharmacy over the Internet.[4] In some cases the Internet has also been used by infertile couples to order sperm or ova, to arrange surrogate pregnancies, or to make enquiries about adopting children from other countries. In Britain, the official 'NHS Direct' telephone service, run by the National Health Service (NHS) provides a 24-hour telephone system, run by specially trained nurses, to provide health advice, information and reassurance to the public (see Chapter 18).[24] For many of those who use it, it is a useful adjunct to the NHS, and if necessary the nurses who run it can refer callers to a hospital, or to their doctor, for further treatment

Patient ↔ Machine ↔ Patient

Here people suffering from particular physical or mental diseases, or who have personal problems or lifestyle issues, can communicate with others with similar experiences. This can take the form of a world-wide patient support group, in the form of an online 'chat room' or 'notice board', or else posting personal diaries ('*web-logs*' or '*blogs*') on the Internet for others to respond to. Some of these blogs may take the form of a narrative of personal suffering (a *pathography*), detailing the history and development of their own particular disease process.

Communication between members of the group may be synchronous and in 'real time', depending on the technology available, and whether the members are all living in the same time zone. Online support groups often form a virtual 'community of suffering' (see Chapter 4), with a shifting transnational membership, which exists only in cyberspace, though sometimes its members may have the opportunity to actually meet face to face. They can bring many benefits to their members – especially those with chronic diseases – including emotional support, the sharing of experiences, specific advice, the exchange of medical information, social contacts, and a lessening of the sense of social isolation.

An example of an online patient community, described by Lasker and colleagues,[25] is the PBCers Organization – an organization of people, mainly women, who suffer from primary biliary cirrhosis (PBC), a relatively rare autoimmune liver disease. It provides and electronic mailing list, support and information, for those with the disease and their families, and is also involved in fund-raising, advocacy, and educational programmes.

Problems of online support groups and chat rooms

Chat rooms for those with similar lifestyles, sexual preferences or health problems can obviously bring many benefits to those who use them, but they may also bring dangers. In a study in The Netherlands, for example, Hospers and colleagues[26] found that many of those using online gay chat rooms subsequently had sex with the men they had met there ('chat dates'), and that almost 30 per cent of those who engaged in sex with these men reported 'inconsistent safe sex behaviour', which put them at risk of sexually-transmitted diseases, such as HIV/AIDS. Furthermore, the level of unprotected sex increased as the number of sex partners met through chat rooms increased. They suggested, therefore, that gay chat rooms could be used as a way of spreading health messages about the dangers of spreading HIV/AIDS and the need to practice safe sex.

The anonymity of online chat rooms can also enable some users to create their own fantasy identity or fictional 'self', a fact which may be used by paedophiles and other criminals to 'cyber-stalk' vulnerable young people they meet in these chat rooms. Chat rooms and some websites may also promote unhealthy lifestyles, or attitudes to health. In 2005, for example, *TIME* magazine reported the existence of about 500 'pro-anorexia' websites, which promoted the idea that anorexia nervosa is less of a disease, and more of a 'life-style choice'.[27]

Professional ↔ Machine ↔ Database

Here health professionals consult online medical libraries, journals or textbooks, via a variety of Internet search engines, to enquire about specific diseases and their diagnosis and treatment, or to find out the latest research findings or clinical guidelines. The databases may be held within a particular medical institution, or in another part of the country, or even another country. Consulting these databases may be recognized as a part of a physician's continuing medical education (CME). In the future medical information, and even textbooks, may be downloaded from the Internet or programmed into either desktop computers or handheld personal computers (PDAs or personal digital assistants). Overall, the use of online information by clinicians is increasing, as illustrated in the following case study.

Patient ↔ Machine ↔ Database

Here patients access a database for information about a particular disease or medical treatment. This access can be either *active*, where the user interacts with the programme, following a number of cued steps to get the specific, personalized information they need (such as the diagnosis or treatment of their own condition), or *passive*, where the user cannot interact with the web-site (usually an online library), and can only use it to obtain information. An example of the former, described by Diefanbach and Butz[29] is the Prostate Interactive Education System (PIES), an interactive multimedia software programme which helps patients and their families get detailed information about all aspects of early-stage prostate cancer, and thus helps them make informed decisions about treatment. Other examples are a Swiss website providing an individualized smoking-cessation programme, including fact sheets, booklets, personalized counselling letters and monthly email reminders,[30] and the MoodGYM programme of cognitive behaviour therapy described below.[31]

More passive forms of access to websites are useful for health education (tele-education), and for giving people information about specific diseases and their treatments, and about the side-effects of medications and treatments. They can also provide information on local resources available (such as a list of self-help groups, or the addresses of nearby doctors, clinics or hospitals). Websites dealing with various types of cancer are among the most widely used.[32] It was estimated in 2003 that, in the developed world, an estimated 39 per cent of cancer patients were using the Internet directly, for information and advice, while another 15–20 per cent of cancer patients were accessing it's information indirectly, via family or friends.[33]

In the UK, the government-funded NHS Direct Online (Chapter 4) provides both an information service and also a personal query service. Websites that give information on specific medical conditions are also particularly useful in times of public health crises, such as the anthrax and bioterrorism scares in the USA in 2001, for providing information to the public, though the information provided on health-related websites may not always be reliable.[34]

Both forms of access to online databases, because they are impersonal, anonymous and confidential, might appeal to people with stigmatized or unconventional lifestyles, or those concerned about personal issues such as sexual health or orientation, contraception, pregnancy, or emotional or relationship problems.

The role of the mass media

Any discussion of telemedicine should be placed against the background of a cultural shift in how many people now acquire knowledge about health matters. In recent years the role of the mass media – radio, television, newspapers, magazines – in transmitting health-related information to the public, has been steadily increasing.[35] While on the one hand, the media can rapidly spread 'health scares' and 'food scares' (see Chapter 3) throughout the population, they can also have more positive effects. Radio serials, television 'soap operas' and films can all increase public knowledge of specific health issues, and even destigmatize certain conditions (such as autism, in the 1988 film *Rainman*). In both cases, it could be argued that because the mass media, especially radio and television, are increasingly seen as important and authoritative sources of health knowledge by the public, this will make people more receptive to using telemedicine, and to acquiring medical knowledge online. In telemedicine, on the other hand, Hjelm[36] suggests that because our perceptions of the computer monitor are influenced by our experience of watching TV, a teleconsultation between doctor and patient might well be experienced as not quite 'real' by either party. It may, in fact, be seen as being more 'fiction' than reality.

Overall, though, the growing importance of the mass media represents a major cultural shift away from the more traditional, personal ways that people used to acquire knowledge about health matters – from their parents, relatives, friends, neighbours, as well as from religious figures, community elders, traditional healers, and health professionals. Instead, they are beginning to rely more and more on *impersonal* sources of health knowledge, such as the mass media, the Internet, books and magazines.

TELEPSYCHIATRY, TELEPSYCHOLOGY AND CYBERTHERAPY

Telepsychiatry has become an important, though controversial, application of telemedicine. It is rarely used on its own, but almost always combined with a personal consultation with one or more health professionals. It is mostly used in remote rural areas where psychiatric facilities are limited,[37,38] but also in institutions such as prisons,[38] where psychiatrists are few, and patients cannot easily be transported to a clinic. It has been used for case-conferences, staff education and liaison, as well as in actual clinical care – diagnosing psychiatric conditions at a distance,[38] carrying out psychotherapy and assessing progress after treatment. The concept of telepsychiatry should also include online support and discussion groups for people with mental health problems,[39] and telephone counselling helplines for emotional crises, such as those in the UK run by the Samaritans or ChildLine (a free helpline for children and young people).

Telepsychiatry is particularly useful for very large countries with scattered population centres and limited psychiatric resources. For example, in South Australia – an area covering about 948 000 km², with a population of only 1.4 million – the South Australia Rural and Remote Mental Health Service use of telepsychiatry is well-integrated into its clinical practice, and is widely accepted by both patients and health professionals: especially for emergency consultations, inpatient liaison, follow-up and support after discharge from hospital, and for professional education and conferences.[38] In Canada, Urness and colleagues' review[9] of 14 telepsychiatry services also found that they were well established, though they varied in scope and complexity with some just operating within a hospital or mental health clinic and others dealing with a much wider geographical area. They were used for a variety of clinical and educational purposes, and dealt with a wide range of psychiatric problems, from severe psychoses to eating disorders, from psychological testing to the management of autism.

Research is still ongoing into the long-term clinical efficacy of telepsychiatry. Zaylor's review of the subject[8] has suggested that it *is* both effective and cost-efficient for certain groups of patients, and that clinical outcomes from interactive television (IATV) consultations were not significantly different from those with personal consultations, and he concluded that 'one could treat moderately to severely ill patients using IATV without any in-person interaction from the clinician'. The long-term efficacy of this approach, though, still needs to be assessed, as does the possibly negative effect of the technology itself on patients suffering from certain mental conditions such as paranoid psychosis.

Cybertherapy: online psychotherapy

Can psychotherapy or counselling be carried out online? Can the various forms of 'talk therapy' or other types of 'symbolic healing' (see Chapter 10) take place at a distance by telephone, email, videophone, or other method? Some authors argue that despite its limitations, *cybertherapy* – also known as *e-therapy* or *remote psychotherapy* – can be a useful adjunct to conventional face-to-face psychotherapy, especially in extending psychotherapy and counselling services to those with little access to them.[39,40]

Suler[40] lists the full range of technical possibilities now available to psychotherapists and counsellors, in the developed world. These include: video-conferencing; telephone consultations; one-to-one emails or 'text chats'; text messaging (via mobile telephones); online group therapy using emails, 'message boards', or 'chat rooms'; online patient support groups; online self-help programmes; online psychological assessment instruments; online experiential programmes (such as computerized counselling or relaxation techniques); informational websites on mental health issues; audio-recordings and film; and personal websites or online journals. Faced with this wide range, he suggests that psychotherapists may well adopt a 'multimedia cybertherapy' approach utilizing several of these techniques, usually in combination with face-to-face psychotherapy. He has also examined some of the pros and cons of 'psychotherapy in cyberspace', since each form of cybertherapy has both advantages and disadvantages. For example, when client and therapist communicate by typing text (emails) to one another, it becomes possible to schedule appointments, even

where people live in different cities or countries. Written records of the conversation are more accurate and some clients people actually become more honest and expressive when they cannot be seen, while other clients may prefer a written style of communicating about personal issues to actually speaking openly about them to another person.

On the negative side, communicating by texts implies a degree of literacy and typing skills in both parties. It excludes important face-to-face cues such as voice tone, body language and physical appearance. For some clients, the lack of a physical presence may reduce the sense of intimacy, trust and commitment in the therapeutic relationship. In addition, sending messages to and from client and therapist in 'real time' provides less 'time for reflection' for both of them. Despite these several disadvantages, Suler[40] suggests that while – in traditional psychotherapy – it is the therapist–client relationship that heals, online psychotherapy can offer *other* types of therapeutic relationship that have a similar effect.

Online psychotherapy seems to be especially useful for certain categories of people, where there is no alternative. Dunaway[39] suggests that, as well as being low cost, it is useful for the elderly, disabled or house-bound, those who have time-constraints, such as busy professionals, and those who are 'uncomfortable with the stress or stigma of traditional face-to-face counselling'. However, she notes that this type of psychotherapy may create many new problems, such as issues of patient confidentiality, quality control, licensing of practitioners, malpractice insurance and reimbursement by health insurance companies.

Videoconferencing in cybertherapy

In psychotherapy, videoconferencing has been particularly useful for interactive communication between people who, for whatever reason, cannot be present in the same room,[41] and is increasingly used within some hospitals and mental health clinics.[9] It has been found to be particularly useful in family therapy,[41] where a videoconference can be used in addition to traditional methods of therapy, especially in situations where family members are living far apart. In northern Finland it has been used as a way of connecting up all those involved in the therapy, including family members, psychologists, social workers, teachers, and local authorities all of whom may be living or working in different locations, very far from one another.[41] In child and adolescent telepsychiatry, Pesämaa and colleagues[42] also found that it was useful for education and training, conducting case-conferences, consulting with a specialist in another location, as well as for consultations with the patient and/or their family members.

Cognitive behaviour therapy in cybertherapy

One particular type of psychotherapy – *cognitive behaviour therapy* (CBT) – seems to be well adapted to being used both online and in self-help books ('bibliotherapy'), as well as in face-to-face interactions.[31] Using it online is also cost-effective. In South Carolina, USA, Cluver and colleagues[37] used CBT for therapy ('teletherapy') with terminally ill cancer patients, using a videophone which allowed visual and speech interaction between therapist and client, even though they were in different locations. Their study found that patients were satisfied with the teletherapy, as well as with face-to-face encounters. Although there were some concerns about confidentiality, they concluded that overall 'psychotherapy delivered via videophones can be used in place of traditional face-to-face therapy, without any loss of patient satisfaction.'

Cognitive behaviour therapy has also been used in interactive computer counselling programmes, which may be accessed directly on a computer or via the Internet. In the UK, Manchandra and McLaren[43] report a positive outcome from using CBT via an interactive video, with a lessening of anxiety and better social functioning. This was despite the absence of non-verbal cues, such as eye contact, facial expression, and touch. In Australia, Christensen and colleagues[31] analysed the usage, and visitor satisfaction of MoodGYM, a free Internet-based CBT site, designed to treat and prevent depression in young people. The site included behavioural training modules, a personal workbook, interactive games, and feedback forms. Over 6-month session, the site recorded 817 284 'hits' and 17 646 interactive sessions. They found that there was a significant reduction of depression and anxiety scores among those who progressed through all the modules in order, and had longer exposure to the site. However, they concluded that, owing to the limitations of the research design 'we cannot conclude that the mental health program was responsible for the changes in mental health symptoms'.

Limitations of cybertherapy

The long-term effects of cybertherapy, both individually and culturally, still need to be assessed. Will the integration of machines into psychotherapy prove to be useful in the long-term, or will it lead to even greater alienation between clinician and patient? Will many people see it as too impersonal and detached a form of communication? Will this type of psychotherapy be equally useful for all cultural groups worldwide, or is it mainly suited to those living in the industrialized world? On this point, it should be noted that cybertherapy may not be appropriate for many people whose cultural (or familial) background is more tactile, interactive and less individualistic. As described elsewhere in this book, in healing encounters many social and cultural groups expect various forms of non-verbal communication, such as touching, embracing, dancing, or kneeling to take place For them, any proper healing ritual should involve a whole range of sensory modalities in addition to sight and sound, which may include touch, taste, texture, smell, body heat, body odour, dance, synchronized movements, music, incense, chanting and special forms of clothing. Healing should take place in a specific spatial and social context, and should usually involve the participation of other people.

Ironically, the growing view in many industrialized countries of the computer as an anthropomorphic 'second self',[44] and as a powerful ritual symbol in doctor–patient consultations, may make it easier for some people to accept it a 'healer' or 'adviser' in its own right, and thus facilitate their acceptance of cybertherapy. For these people the computer itself seems to have become more than just a technological tool or inert lifeless object. It has also acquired a more mysterious and 'mystical' function as a secularized icon, idol, or oracle which one consults in moments of suffering or uncertainty – a semi-alive source of wisdom, knowledge, or even healing.

CRITIQUES OF TELEMEDICINE

Despite its growing popularity, many questions have been raised about telemedicine: Is it effective? Is it, safe, practical and worthwhile?[45] Is it cost-effective? What are its weaknesses, as well as its strengths? According to Coiera[7], the actual scientific evidence for the effectiveness of telemedicine still remains quite weak. From a medical perspective, one reason for this is the lack of reliable scientific studies on the subject. According to Hailey and colleagues,[46] in telemedicine 'good-quality studies are still scarce and the generalizability of most assessment findings is rather limited'.

Hjelm,[36] too, concludes that as yet 'there are limited data on the clinical effectiveness and cost-effectiveness of most telemedicine applications'. However, he does list the many potential advantages of telemedicine in the future, such as improving access to information and health services, enhancing professional education, and reducing health-care costs. He sees benefits in situations such as home telemonitoring of people who are elderly, chronically ill, and housebound, especially those with diabetes, hypertension, or on dialysis; telemedicine would enable them to be treated at home, rather than in hospital. Telemedicine could also be used in the form of video-links between professionals within a hospital, to discuss cases or pathological findings, while video-links could be used to allow patients, primary-care professionals, and health specialists to meet together in a 'virtual clinic'. However, Hjelm[36] also points out

the various disadvantages of telemedicine, including the depersonalization of health care, with a resultant breakdown in the relationship between patient and health professional. Relationships between health professionals themselves may also break down, as staff at the remote site might see their autonomy as being threatened, and their role being delegated to being mere technicians or camera-operators. There are also issues concerning confidentiality, the quality and reliability of online health information,[47] as well as organizational and bureaucratic difficulties.

In 2002, Hailey and colleagues[46] did a systematic review of 66 scientific studies on telemedicine, carried out between 1966 and 2000. Fifty six per cent (37) of them suggested that it had advantages over alternative approaches, 36 per cent (24) saw some disadvantages, or were not convinced of its efficacy, and 8 per cent (5) found that other approaches were preferable to telemedicine. Overall, they found that the most evidence for its effectiveness was in teleradiology (especially in neurosurgery), teledermatology, home telecare and telemonitoring, 'telemental health', transmission of echocardiographic images, and some medical consultations. In Miller's analysis of 38 studies from several different countries in 2001, 80 per cent were favourable towards telemedicine as a means of doctor–patient communication, except for its absence of non-verbal cues including touch.[48] Overall, despite the shortage of reliable research on the subject, Taylor[45] concluded, in 2005, that there was now sufficient evidence that telemedicine was a safe alternative to conventional care 'in a variety of situations and for a number of clinical conditions'. However, he noted that 'reliable evidence that it is a practical and cost-effective alternative is, at the time of writing, harder to find'.

TECHNICAL PROBLEMS

Telemedicine raises a number technical problems, many of them still unresolved.

One is that the equipment needed is often very expensive,[45] as is the cost of powering, maintaining and repairing it, and of the personnel required to secure it against theft and damage. Major commercial interests are involved in promoting telemedicine, and Taylor[45] points out that much of the current information on telemedicine is actually coming from the manufacturers of that same equipment.

Other technical problems are those of quality control, such as the accuracy and reliability of digital images transmitted online in teleradiology,[49] and the possibility of patients' confidential information being illegally accessed by 'hackers' or other 'cyber-criminals'. In poorer countries with a less developed infrastructure, there are also the problems of maintaining the equipment, getting an adequate supply of spare parts and having a reliable and continuous source of power, whether from a national electricity grid, generators or batteries. In some places there may be the danger of damage or theft of electricity cables or radio masts, or there may be atmospheric conditions that interfere with satellite or radio communications.

Another issue is that the actual information supplied on specific websites or databases may be of low quality, or not completely reliable. Much of this information is uncontrolled and unregulated.[47] In some cases, it may even have been posted there by commercial organizations such as the pharmaceutical industry or the manufacturers of telemedical equipment, both of whom have the ulterior motives of selling their products and services, as well as improving patient care. The huge volume of health information now available online, and the multiplicity of web sites, can also produce the problem of data-overload. As much of this is in the form of raw or even conflicting data, it may be difficult for untrained or inexperienced people to sift them according to reliability, and to understand the relevance of all this data to their own unique, individual situations. Pure 'information' or 'data' – without the personal experience, wisdom or understanding to interpret and make use of it – can sometimes do more harm than good, as in the case of *cyberchondria* described below.

EFFECTS ON THE PROFESSIONAL–PATIENT RELATIONSHIP

To Anderson and colleagues,[4] the Internet has basically a positive effect on public health, and 'the potential to transform the organizational structure and delivery of a variety of health services'. They suggest that the growth of 'consumer culture' in most Western countries, with its trend towards a more informed and critical consumer, is impacting positively on the doctor–patient relationship. Together with the growth of the Internet as a source of medical information, it has reduced the power of doctors *vis-à-vis* their patients, and allowed those patients to become more active, informed, and self-reliant participants in their own treatment.[4] Also, because of its anonymity, they see the Internet as being particularly useful for those who have highly personal or embarrassing queries about their health. In some cases, however, the Internet has also led people not to consult their doctors at all, even when seriously ill, or to self-diagnose in an inappropriate way.

ANTHROPOLOGICAL PERSPECTIVES: THE ROLE OF CONTEXT

From an anthropological viewpoint, telemedicine can be criticized from several different points of view. In particular, it usually does not provide data on the wider context of the patient's ill-health and suffering, including their personal experience, living conditions, and socio-economic level, as well as their family, community, religious and cultural backgrounds. Furthermore, it excludes a variety of sensory modalities such as touch, smell, and body heat, as well as a wider view of body language, posture, gesture, movement and facial expression, which are often intrinsic to close communication between people. Telemedicine can thus provide clinicians with only a limited, and reductionist view of human suffering – an abstracted image of the ill person very similar to the 'disease' perspective described in Chapter 5.

Furthermore, in telemedical consultations the actual technology used – whether video-cameras, computers, microphones, monitoring machines, or web-cams, cannot be regarded merely as neutral objects. Like the physician's desktop computer (see below), they themselves are a part of the ritual context of the healing event, and over time often become healing symbols in their own right.

Telemedicine is an example of what Hall[50] terms 'low-context communication', where most of the information transmitted between the parties is in the explicit medium itself (the computer or video screen, the X-ray photograph, or image of a CT scan or body part). This contrasts with the 'high-context communication', which is characteristic of most types of healing and healing rituals worldwide (see Chapter 9), where much of the 'information' passing between healer and client is not explicit. Instead, it is 'encoded' or hidden, either within the physical setting of the encounter itself (the 'external context'), including in a variety of 'ritual symbols', and specialized settings (such as a shrine, or clinic), or internalized in the prior experiences, expectations, cultural assumptions, beliefs and prejudices of both parties (the 'internal context'). Telemedicine excludes, therefore, much of the information that makes a deeper level of inter-personal communication possible, including the wide variety of cultural, social, and individual factors mentioned above.

When information is transmitted online, it is never 'culture-free'. For one thing, even the physical technology used is always part of a social, cultural and economic context. This usually includes the people who design, sell, install, explain, maintain and repair the equipment – as well as their attitudes, belief systems and behaviours. At the same time, for individual users of the equipment, especially if they come from very different social and cultural environments, the same visual information is not necessarily always 'seen' and 'understood' by them in exactly the same way. As in the various psychological projection tests, such as the Rorschach, different people sometimes 'see' and interpret visual stimuli differently, even when presented with the identical image, because they bring to the experience their own individual perceptions, assumptions, expectations, prejudices, anxieties, and fears, many of them derived from their cultural background. The same possibility of differing perceptions and interpretations of visual information, applies both to the computer monitor and to the video screen (see Chapter 10).

From the patient's perspective, part of the social context of telemedicine is their own level of education, since making use of online health information implies some degree of literacy, as well as an understanding of the inner logic of computer programmes. It may also require numeracy skills, and the ability to understand complex statistical notions such as those of 'risk' or 'probability' (see Chapter 15).

Another issue relates to users' attitudes towards texts, whether these are on paper, parchment or a computer screen. Does their specific cultural or religious background see texts as especially authoritative objects, and as the main source of reliable information? Does it see texts as largely irrelevant, since most of the important wisdom about everyday life, including about health, is expected to originate from other people – parents, family, friends, religious leaders, traditional healers – as well as from personal experience?

The cultural context of Internet use

Making use of the Internet, and of telemedicine, are not 'context-free' or 'culture-free' activities. Like all other human activities they are always embedded in a particular cultural *context* of time, place, social relationships, and world-view. For example, behaviours and forms of inter-personal communication such as 'texting', 'blogging', and 'web-surfing' have all become common aspects of modern industrial culture, and in turn are helping to create new forms of social organization.[51] Furthermore, the actual content and approach of websites – including those dealing with health matters – can always be regarded as cultural products. The language that they are written in, the jargon they use, their visual design and arrangement, and the internal logic and organization of the website itself all draw on certain personal and cultural assumptions of their programmers and web-designers. In that way, websites often express some of the underlying themes, assumptions, and prejudices of that cultural background, as illustrated in this case study.

Case study: cultural assumptions on UK web sites for breast and prostate cancer

Seale[52] has analysed the gender stereotypes that underlie popular UK websites for breast cancer and prostate cancer. On breast cancer sites, women were portrayed as having to make decisions about matters *other* than their immediate treatment, such as their future fertility, their childcare problems, the difficulties of telling their children about the diagnosis and their physical appearance. They were also expected to sometimes change their minds, to have the right to opt out of the decision-making process, and to consult fully with families in friends. In contrast, men with prostate cancer were portrayed as more isolated, less connected to family and friends, and more obliged to take an active and decisive role in making decisions about treatment (even to see themselves, rather than their doctors, as being the chief decision-makers), and to make those decisions without consulting with their families and friends. There was no discussion of the many stresses this decision-making might cause the men, and few personal stories of their cancer experience were given. Thus, Seale suggests that clinicians should be aware of the role of the underlying gender expectations 'that men and women feel obliged to consider when making decisions about their cancer treatments'. These underlying stereotypes may help explain to clinicians why some men with cancer do not fully consider the views of their family, do not take non-medical factors into account, and find it difficult to let doctors influence their decision-making; while for women with cancer, they may explain why they may seem indecisive, may want to opt out of decision-making, or to make treatment decisions based on other criteria.

SOCIAL EFFECTS OF TELEMEDICINE

Although telemedicine makes possible communication between people separated by great distances, it also 'individualizes' and isolates the experiences of illness and medical care. Use of a computer terminal usually (though not always) involves one person at a time, and thus telemedicine is very different from a face-to-face encounter with a real doctor or nurse, and from the public, more communal forms of healing practiced by traditional healers (see Chapter 4).

In terms of sensory input, telemedicine's limitation is that it only includes the modalities of sight and hearing, which both 'extend' the central nervous system by the use of video and audio technology.[53] At present, telemedicine does not include any other sensory modalities such as body warmth, smell, movement, or facial expression. With the exception of 'telesurgery', it also does not include touch (though 'haptic' technology, responsive to tactile cues, is currently being developed). Most importantly, as described above, it excludes the role of a healing *context*, and of the specific spatial, temporal, theatrical and sensory dimensions so characteristic of healing rituals found worldwide (see Chapter 9).

The social effects the WWW are likely to be significant, especially in the health field. In particular, it likely to have some effect on the balance of power and knowledge between health professionals and their patients.[4] This may result not only in the empowering of patients, but also in the 'deprofessionalization' of medicine itself. Like Coiera,[47] Gerber and Eiser,[54] suggest that Internet access has led to a more informed and educated patient population, with increasing numbers of people accessing health-related websites: by 2001 about 52 million people in the USA had searched the WWW for health and medical information (and this number rose to 70 million by 2003).[4] They point out that this process can undermine the physician's previous monopoly of medical knowledge, and their authoritative status, even though most patients still expect their physicians to take responsibility for making medical decisions. This increase in lay knowledge may impact on the doctor–patient relationship and on medical decision-making. For example, before consulting their doctor, patients may already have formed opinions about which treatments they prefer and those they do not, and arrive at the consultation as an 'informed decision-maker'. They suggest that this should lead not to conflict, but to a shared or 'participatory' decision-making model in the consultation. Furthermore, as many websites include inaccurate information, the physician's role should be to recommend to patients particular websites (an 'Internet Prescription') that are more reliable, or they may even create their own practice website. However, they admit that 'it is yet uncertain whether efficiency improves or declines when patient-acquired Internet information is brought into the decision-making process'.

Telemedicine may also have some negative social effects on particular groups of people. For example, Sinha[55] argues that while the aim of telemedicine is ostensibly to reach out into rural areas, it has often done so at the cost of further concentrating more health specialists and resources into urban areas. At the same time, its ability to reach into closed communities (such as prisons, and military installations), without removing patients from there to a clinic or hospital elsewhere, can further isolate members of those communities from mainstream life. Finally, Sinha points out that while telemedicine has many benefits for patients (such as reducing costs and making health care more accessible to remote populations) in the USA many vested interests, including government, the technology industry and some parts of the medical profession, have all been making considerable profits from the practice of telemedicine, and from the equipment used within it.

NEW 'SYNDROMES' OF THE COMPUTER AGE

The increased use of the Internet is not without its negative effects on psychological and physical health, and several new 'disorders' have been described in recent years. Psychological disorders include such new 'syndromes' as 'cyberchondria', which is a type of hypochondria in which people become anxious from health information that they have gathered from the Internet, often misdiagnosing their own minor complaints as major illnesses. In 'Internet addiction', individuals become psychologically dependent on accessing and interacting with certain web sites, especially for gambling, games, auctions, pornography, or 'cybersex', and may suffer some psychological withdrawal symptoms if they are unable to do so. It also includes those who compulsively chat online, or do compulsive web-surfing or database searches Both these conditions might be considered emerging 'culture-bound disorders' of the computer age (see Chapter 10).

Physical disorders associated with frequent computer use include conditions such as pains of the hand, wrist, neck or back, postural problems, repetitive-strain injury (RSI); carpal tunnel syndrome (CTS), eye-strain, and headaches.[56]

TELEMEDICINE IN THE DEVELOPING WORLD

At present, telemedicine is largely the preserve of the richer parts of the world. Many poorer countries simply cannot yet afford the expensive equipment, which has then to be transported to remote areas. They also lack trained staff to operate it, a reliable electricity supply and telephone or satellite links, and ways of securing the equipment against theft or damage. Despite this, telemedicine does have many applications in poorer countries with limited health facilities, provided that the technology used is simple and low-cost. In order to improve health status in these countries, especially in sub-Saharan Africa, Odutola[57] suggests that investing more in information technology would narrow the 'digital divide', lead to sustainable 'low-cost, area-wide, and effective dissemination and retrieval' of health information and improve both the health status and sense of empowerment of these poorer communities. In some countries this process is already underway. For example, since 1998 telemedicine has been developing in Uzbekistan, a country with significant health and environmental problems, with the support of the Ministry of Health, NATO (North Atlantic Treaty Organization), and a UK charitable trust.[58] It involves telecommunication links between the National Centre of Emergency Medicine (NCEM) in Tashkent and clinical departments in 13 regions, 17 ambulance teams and approximately 700 doctors throughout the country.

Three other examples of the use of telemedicine in poorer areas of the world, with less developed healthcare infrastructures are given below.

Case study 1: telemedicine in Dhaka, Bangladesh

Vassallo[59] and colleagues in 2001 described a successful telemedicine link between the Centre for Rehabilitation of the Paralysed (CRP) in Dhaka, and a variety of medical specialists in neurology, orthopaedics, rheumatology, nephrology and paediatrics working in the UK and Nepal. Using digital cameras and an email link, images of patients, X-rays, electrocardiograms, or other tests, were sent to the specialists for advice and a second opinion. In 70 per cent of referrals, initial email replies were received by the CRP within 1 day of referral, and 100 per cent were received within 3 days. Referral was judged to be successful in 89 per cent of cases, in terms of clarifying the diagnosis, changing the treatment, or reassuring the patient.

Case study 2: telemedicine in Arkhangelsk region, Russia

Sørensen and colleagues[60] in 1999 described the use of telemedicine in Arkhangelsk region, north-western Russia, which is an area about the size of France but with a population of only 1.5 million. Beginning in 1994, telemedicine links were established between medical specialists at the regional hospital in Arkhangelsk, and hospitals in remote areas, such as Kotlas (700 km) and Velsk (500 km), and later with local hospitals in Koryazhma, Nyandoma and Severodvinsk. From these remote centres, still pictures taken with a digital camera of patients' notes, X-rays, electrocardiograms, and laboratory tests and sent either as email attachments, or directly from computers (via the VIDA still-image system) to the specialists, for an opinion. Given the enormous distances in north-western Russia, and the high cost of transporting patients to Arkhangelsk, this was a more cost-effective way of getting a specialist opinion on these patients, and thus enabling them to be treated at their local hospital. The same system, but incorporating telephones with a loudspeaker, has been used for distance learning and the exchange of information between the doctors in Athkangelsk and medical colleagues in Tromsø, Norway.

Case study 3: telemedicine in Alto Amazonas, Peru

Martinez and colleagues[61] in 2004 studied the development of a rural telemedicine system in the Peruvian province of Alto Amazonas, an area twice the size of Belgium. It is an undeveloped region with few roads (95 per cent of health-care facilities are accessible only by river), and only 2 per cent of the province's health-care facilities have telephone lines. Health care is provided by a network of local rural 'health posts' linked to regional 'health centres'. Since 2000–01, equipment for radio communications (VHF, HF and WiFi) has been installed in 39 localities: a provincial hospital, seven health centres, and 31 health posts. Staff in the local health posts can now transmit voice messages (especially for emergency cases), as well as email message to the health centres, which in turn can then communicate via the Internet with medical authorities in the capital city, Lima. The study illustrated the usefulness of this link-up for a variety of purposes: consultations with specialist physicians; giving epidemiological surveillance reports; ordering medical equipment; distance learning for staff; and relaying information to the authorities on outbreaks of disease, natural disasters, or medical emergencies. It also reduced the time needed to evacuate emergency cases to hospital, and in 28 per cent of these cases the use of the system was life-saving for the patient. Overall, telemedicine helped to improve the diagnostic and therapeutic capacity of the health posts.

THE PHYSICIAN'S DESKTOP COMPUTER

For an increasing number of people today, the computer has become a taken-for-granted part of daily life, one of the most widespread symbols of the modern, industrialised world. For some it has become even more than that: a source of ultimate knowledge, an adviser, teacher, oracle, healer, guide, ritual object or even a sort of secular deity.

As described in Chapter 4, modern medicine is characterized by the growing power – symbolic, as well as technical – of the machine. One machine in particular, the desktop computer, has now become one of the most pervasive tools of the modern doctor, often intrinsic to the processes of diagnosis, treatment and communication. Its use is particularly widespread in office and outpatient practice. By 1995, for example, 80 per cent of UK general practitioners (GPs), 70 per cent of Danish GPs, 60 per cent of Swedish GPs, and 40 per cent of Dutch GPs were using desktop computers in their offices for storing medical records.[62]

Computers are now not only used for storing patient data, organizing appointments or sending out bills, connected to the Internet, they are also used by doctors to access up-to-date information on the latest medical treatments, research findings, and new types of drugs, including drug interactions and side-effects.

EFFECTS OF THE DESKTOP COMPUTER ON DOCTOR–PATIENT CONSULTATIONS

Despite these many advantages, it is important to consider the psychological and social impact of the desktop computer on the doctor–patient relationship. Does its presence have a positive or a negative effect?

While some studies, such as that by Hsu and colleagues[63] have reported mainly positive effects, others have given more ambiguous results. Rethans and colleagues,[64] for example, in their study of 263 patients in The Netherlands, found that 96 per cent felt that relationships with their family doctor were as easy and as personal after the computer was introduced, as they had been before. However, 66 per cent of them expressed some anxiety that their privacy was less secure now that their medical files were on a computer. Greatbach and colleagues,[65] in a study of GP consultations in Liverpool, UK, found that the computer did have subtle, adverse effects on doctor–patient interactions. These included the doctor's tendency to become preoccupied with the machine and to pause or delay conversations with the patient while consulting it, thus reducing eye-contact time with them as a result. The patients, too, changed their behaviour by stopping speaking at various points, to avoid interrupting the doctor while he was typing into the computer. On a more positive level, though, the computer did allow the possibility of 'collaborative readings', where both parties could look at the screen together, and then discuss the material presented on it.

In a Danish study, Als[62] found that computer use reduced the amount of time during which the doctor interacted with the patient. Furthermore, the doctors often used the computer for other, less medical purposes: for example, as a way of getting 'time-out' by breaking off the conversation to consult it, especially when they needed to rest, or to solve a problem. Others used it to change the form or rhythm of the conversation, such as interrupting the patient in mid-sentence, by beginning typing on the keyboard. Only in a minority of consultations did the doctors actually explain to the patient why they were using the computer at that particular moment. Interestingly, in about one-quarter of the consultations, the doctor also used it as what Als terms a 'magic box', by pointing or nodding to it, when presenting medical facts, plans or conclusions to the patient, even though these 'facts' were not shown on the computer screen. In Als's view, the machine has thus become a symbolic source of authority in its own right.

THE DESKTOP COMPUTER AS A RITUAL SYMBOL

As a physical object, the computer, with its sleek rectangular shape, and shiny surfaces of metal, glass or plastic – is both a product and expression, of a mass-production society, and of an advanced level of science and technology. Its use implies a degree of technical and economic development, and a certain level of infrastructure, such as a supply of electricity or batteries, as well as of modems, telephone lines, fibre-optic cables and access to global telecommunication systems. Furthermore, as much of the information it provides is text-based (though it often includes graphics or videos), it also requires some degree of literacy (and numeracy) from the user, as well as an understanding of the function and design of its software programmes.

As described above, the desktop computer can also be regarded not only as a useful, technical object – and one of the key icons of modernity – but also as a *ritual symbol* (see Chapter 9). In many developed societies, it has become as intrinsic to the rituals of modern healing as the physician's white coat, the diplomas on the wall, the glass cabinets of medical instruments, and the rows of impressive-looking medical textbooks on the bookshelf (see Figure 9.1). To many patients, it has become a symbol of the healing power of their doctor, connecting him or her to all the hidden powers, and extensive knowledge of modern medicine itself. This symbolic power can remain invested in the computer, as it rests on the physician's desk, irrespective of whether or not it is part of a particular doctor–patient interaction, or even whether or not it is actually switched on.

Some of the possible associations of the physician's desktop computer as a ritual symbol are listed in Table 13.2.

THE 'CYBER-BODY' AND THE 'CYBER-SELF'

In the past 50 years the growth of television, radio, and the Internet, have all had subtle effects on modern notions of the 'body' and the 'self'. Some

Table 13.2 Some associations of the physician's computer as a ritual symbol

A sign of modernity
A sign that the doctor is high-tech and 'up-to-date'
An authoritative source of knowledge and advice
A link to the greater, hidden powers of Medical Science
A link to a worldwide network of medical authorities in other parts of the country, or the world
An external 'brain' with enormous powers of memory, logic and calculation
A repository of all current medical knowledge and research: the 'collective mind' of the medical profession
A reservoir of knowledge about the patient, and their personal medical history
An objective, unemotional adviser, diagnostician, and prognostician
A reliable 'second opinion' or 'second physician' with more knowledge and experience than any individual doctor
A powerful 'healer' or 'healing object' in its own right

of these effects may also be seen in telemedicine, and may even be the result of it.

THE 'CYBER–BODY'

McLuhan[53] argued in the 1960s that television and radio had become 'extensions' of the human body, and of its central nervous system, and with their aid people could now 'see' and 'hear' events that are taking place at that moment many thousands of miles away, thus turning the world into a sensory 'global village' In the same way, a computer linked to the Internet can also function as a new type of 'sensory organ', with the ability to collect data and images, and exchange messages with people all over the world. All these new technologies have created, for many people, a new sense of their own body, and of its boundaries.

Marshall[66] has identified 'boundary anxiety' – whether of the self, family, ethnic group or country – as a major concern of the modern Western world. In particular, 'boundaries between groups and methods of maintaining boundaries seem insecure and focuses of anxiety'. This applies as much to boundaries against out-groups (such as immigrants and refugees) as to boundaries between work and home, and internal psychological boundaries. In his study of the members of an online 'chat room', he found that the 'bodyless communication' between them had led to even more 'boundary vagueness', and to an altered sense of the body. Members spoke of an 'immersion experience' while they were online, in which they lost awareness of their own physical body, and their online 'body' seemed to be 'ghostlike' and 'immaterial' – a light and ethereal being that was not bounded by ordinary space or time, and could travel instantly all over the world, and at any time. It was a body 'free from restriction or the "resistance of the Real", and hence from "materiality"' because online one could never act physically on the bodies of other people. The 'online life' of the group itself was also characterized by 'imprecise, crossed or broken boundaries' since members could leave or enter it at any moment, without the others knowing whether or not they were still 'present' and 'listening in'. It was also difficult to exclude anyone from the chat room. Marshall suggests that this process may increase 'boundary anxiety', and that one method of dealing with these new boundary problems was to rigidly enforce the boundaries, or polarities, between the individual's 'net persona' and their real-life identity, and thus re-establish a new Cartesian sense of a split self. In a secular age, such a 'virtual' online body may well take the place for some people of the concepts of 'soul', 'spirit' or even 'mind'.

The body as information

In many other ways, the human body is increasingly being seen as existing also in a 'virtual' form. An example of a virtual body is the Visible Human Project (VHP), described in Chapter 2, which was begun in 1989 by the United States National Library of Medicine. This consists of an online library of digital images of normal adult male and female anatomy, based on numerous MRI and CT scans, and anatomical images. Both the VHP and the Human Genome Project (HGP), described in Chapter 2, are reconceptualizations of the body as *information*, which is potentially available to any user of the Internet. As Sandelowski[22] put it: 'The body in these projects is data come to life on our computer screens'; 'the VHP and the HGP allow repeated excursions into virtual bodies without actually penetrating any body at all'. Both are examples of what she terms the new 'posthuman body' or 'a disembodied informational structure with no clearly defined self,' and both result in 'the disappearance of the humanist body, of the flesh-and-blood encasing of a unique and stable self'.[22]

Both the Internet and telemedicine may also increase the sense of a body that can be reduced merely to information (although this information is rarely personal, cultural or spiritual) which can be stored, and then transmitted by the Internet, radio, or telephone from one machine to another. This phenomenon is paralleled by some of the developments in genetics, where the body has been increasingly reconceptualized as a collection of hidden 'genetic codes' of information about that person's genetic inheritance, and their future risks of disease: information that can only be 'decoded' by medical science and technology.

Seeing the body primarily as information makes possible the blending of two different discourses of contagion: that of biological viruses and that of computer viruses. Parikka[67] points out that both are now spoken of as if they were 'information diseases' – one carrying a particular genetic code, the other a particular software programme – and both are typical of a society and economy which focuses increasingly on producing information, rather than goods. In Thacker's view[68] our culture increasingly thinks of computer 'viruses' in biological terms, as if they were 'material' objects that could somehow 'infect' machines, just as biological viruses can infect a living organism. At the same time, epidemiologists are trying to understand and predict how epidemics spread, by utilizing mathematical studies of computer networks (Figure 13.1), including mapping the way that computer viruses spread through an online network, from computer to computer.

A final development of the increasingly close relationship between people, computers, and the Internet, is the growing idea of the modern body as a *cyborg*: the fusion of human being and machine, already described in Chapter 2. In telemedicine, too, the possibility exists that both health professional and patient will increasingly come to see each other, and themselves, as essentially part-machine, a process that has been called 'cyborgization'.[66]

THE 'CYBER–SELF'

In the long term, increasing familiarity with computers and the Internet may well lead to a redefinition what constitutes a human being. As Turkle[44] notes, for many people today the computer has become a 'second self', an anthropomorphic 'thinking machine' outside of the body. At the same time, our culture of computation has begun to influence our own ideas of the human mind, and of the human 'self'. Thus she poses the two questions: 'What happens when people consider the computer as a model of human mind?' and 'What happens when people begin to think they are machines?' Increasingly, it seems, many people now see the mind as merely a 'software programme', located within the 'hardware' of the skull: an entity that is capable of being 're-programmed' under certain conditions. To Turkle, another implication of this view of 'mind as

Figure 13.1 Communication technology is increasingly being used to monitor the spread of diseases across the globe. (Source: World Health Organization, *World Health*, No 2 March–April 1998. Reproduced with permission.)

microprocessor' is that it leaves one with a 'decentralized' self, a sense that there is actually no 'I', no 'me', no unitary 'conscious actor' at the core of one's being, just a collection of actions and processes.[44] This sense of the hollow self is also accompanied by the feeling of being 'run' from the outside, just as machines are controlled and powered by something beyond themselves. She sees the recent development of 'home pages' on the web, which contain a collection of disparate images and facts about the owner, together with 'links' to other web sites, as an attempt to create 'new notions of identity as multiple yet coherent'.[69]

van Dijck[51] has discussed the social significance of the emergence since 1966 of online diaries or journals known as *web-logs* ('blogs'), with an estimated 10 million 'bloggers' or users of weblogs in the USA by 2004. This digital diary is sometimes extended into a more extensive *life-blog*, sometimes linked (as a *link-blog*) to many similar life-blogs to form a vast, virtual 'blog-community'. Many use life-blogs for creative expression, others to exchange information, or to disclose personal issues and concerns. In the interactive and participatory format of the Internet, blogs are both the sharing of personal disclosures and ideas 'with both known and anonymous audiences', in a reciprocal way. Overall, van Dijck suggests that these interlinked blogs, and the sharing and reciprocity that they involve, can be the means by which 'a blogger simultaneously fashions her identity and creates a sense of community'. In the modern world, with its constant flux, and the decline of many stable communities, blogging is helping to 'create a new type of cultural knowledge and social interaction', and the reciprocity that it involves will produce 'a profound reorganisation in social consciousness'.

Thus not only is the Internet process producing new definitions of 'community', it may also be producing a new sense of 'self'. For some individuals, the development of a 'virtual' self online, by creating personal web-pages and autobiographical 'life-blogs' – in the 'safe space' of cyberspace – may well be very therapeutic.

KEY REFERENCES

2 Internet World Stats (2006) *World Internet Usage and Population Statistics*: http://www.internetworldstats.com/stats.htm (Accessed on 21 February 2006)

4 Anderson, J.G., Rainey, M.R. and Eysenbach, G. (2003) The impact of cyberhealthcare on the physician-patient relationship. *J. Med. Systems* 27(1), 67–84.

6 Craig, J. and Patterson, V. (2005) Introduction to the practice of telemedicine. *J. Telemed. Telecare* 11, 3–9.

8 Zaylor, C. (1999) Clinical outcomes in telepsychiatry. *J. Telemed. Telecare* 5(Suppl. 1), S1, 59–60.

18 Ruggiero, C., Sacile, R. and Giacomini, M. (1999) Home telecare. *J. Telemed. Telecare* 5, 11–17.

23 Tang, J.C. (2003) Telesurgery – the way of the future? *McMaster Meducator* Issue 2, 15–18; http://www.meducator.org/archive/20030319/telesurgery.html (Accessed on 27 June 2005)

26 Hospers, H.J., Harterinck, P., van den Hoek, K. and Veenstra, J. (2002) Chatters on the Internet: a special target group for HIV prevention. *AIDS Care* 14(4), 539–44.

36 Hjelm, N.M. (2005) Benefits and drawbacks of telemedicine. *J. Telemed. Telecare* 11, 60–70.

46 Hailey, D., Roine, R. and Ohinmaa, A. (2002) Systematic review of evidence for the benefits of telemedicine. *J. Telemed. Telecare* 8 (Suppl. 1), S1, 1–7

52 Seale, C. (2205) Portrayals of treatment decision-making on popular breast and prostate cancer web sites. *Eur. J. Cancer Care* 14, 171–4.

54 Gerber, B.S., Eiser, A.R. (2001) The Patient-Physician Relationship in the Internet Age: Future Prospects and the Research Agenda. *J. Med. Internet Res.* 3(2), e15.

66 Marshall, J. (2004) The online body breaks out? Asence, ghosts, cyborgs, gender, polarity and politics. *Fibreculture* Issue 3; http://journal.fibreculture.org/issue3/issue3_marshall.html (Accessed on 5 July 2005).

See http://www.culturehealthandillness.com for the full list of references for this chapter.

RECOMMENDED READING

Coiera, E. (2003) *Guide to Health Informatics*, 2nd edn. London: Arnold, pp. 261–318.

Powell, J. and Clarke, A. (2002) The WWW of the World Wide Web: Who, What, and Why? *J. Med. Internet Res.* 4(1), e4.

Sinha, A. (2000) An overview of telemedicine: the virtual gaze of health care in the next century. *Med. Anthropol. Q.* 14(3), 291–309.

Taylor, P. (2005) Evaluating telemedicine systems and services. *J. Telemed. Telecare* 11, 167–77.

Turkle, S. (1997) *Life on the Screen: Identity in the Age of the Internet*. London: Simon and Schuster.

RECOMMENDED WEBSITES

Fibreculture Journal: http://journal.fibreculture.org

International Society for Mental Health Online: http://www.ismho.org

Journal of Medical Internet Research: http://www.jmir.org

14 New bodies, new selves: genetics and biotechnology

This chapter deals with the cultural impact of recent developments in medical science – particularly in *genetics* – on attitudes to health, illness, and human behaviour. In many countries, especially in the industrialized world, these developments are having an important influence on how people understand concepts such as 'body' and 'self', as well as 'risk', 'ageing' and 'disease'.

As public awareness of genetics has gradually increased, the 'double helix' model of DNA (deoxyribonucleic acid) structure, first described in 1953 by Watson and Crick, has become one of the most iconic images of the modern age (see Figure 14.1).

For some people, many of the research findings of genetics raise fundamental questions about the human condition, and about the nature of 'personhood': What is a 'person? When does a 'person' begin? When does a 'person' end? Some of these issues will be examined in this chapter.

GENETICS

THE GENETICS REVOLUTION: A NEW PARADIGM

The decades between 1940 and 1970 saw the establishment of an influential new paradigm within biology: *molecular biology*. Its development was aided by a number of new scientific technologies such as X-ray crystallography, electron microscopy, and radioactive tracing.

A major initiative within molecular biology has been the Human Genome Project (HGP),[1] an international project to 'map' the entire genome of the human organism. The *genome* of an organism is its

Figure 14.1 The double-helix structure of DNA. One of the most iconic images of the modern age.

entire genetic material or DNA. In technical terms, it consists of 'all the DNA contained in an organism or a cell, which includes both the chromosomes within the nucleus and the DNA in mitochondria'.[1] The HGP was completed in 2003 after 13 years work, and at a cost of about US $3 billion.[2] Its aim was to identify all of the approximately 20 000–25 000 genes in human DNA, and to determine the sequences of the 3 billion chemical base pairs that make up human DNA.[3] This type of study – of genes, their functions, and their relation to health and illness – is known as *genomics*. It is 'the science of genomes – more specifically, their sequencing, mapping, analysis, study and manipulation'.[4]

Rheinberger[5] sees this growth of molecular biology, especially genomics, as a major revolution in scientific thinking, with effects as significant for medicine as the rise of Germ Theory in the late nineteenth century, and the development of antimicrobial drugs in the 1940s. He points to the possibility of a 'molecular takeover of medicine', and the many implications of this development. He suggests that genetic research carries with it certain assumptions about the human condition, particularly about human behaviour, relationships, and the origins of disease. In its approach to the relative influences of 'nature' and 'nurture', and 'biology' and culture', genetics represents a major 'paradigm shift' towards biological explanations, both within medicine, and within the social and behavioural sciences.[5]

'NATURE' VERSUS 'NURTURE'

Mauron[6] has identified an underlying '*genomic metaphysics*' within molecular biology: a set of assumptions about human life that characterize much of genetic research. In particular, 'the belief that the genome is the ontological hard core of an organism, defining its distinctive traits, its individuality, as well as underpinning its membership in a particular species'. For each individual human being in a more secular age, therefore, the genome has become the 'secular equivalent of the soul'.[6,7] He points out that in traditional humanism, the 'biological nature of humans' ('*Nature*') was seen as a given – 'the most stable element, the most strictly determined and the most inflexible' – whereas the human spirit (and behaviour) was seen as changeable and perfectible, especially by education ('*Culture*'). However, the HGP and associated developments in 'genetic engineering' means that the human species can no longer be defined by 'an immutable biological nature embodied in the genome'.[6] For the first time 'Nature', too, is mutable, and alterable by human ideas, actions, technologies and science; that is, by our 'Culture'. In a sense, biology is no longer separate from culture; the ability to change biology means that Nature becomes part of culture, and the notion of an 'autonomous and sovereign 'self'[6] (or 'person') somehow separate from Nature, becomes less important, and less easy to define.

Rheinberger,[5] too, notes that the traditional dichotomy between 'Nature' (internal, fixed, immutable) and 'Nurture' (external, changeable, environmental), that is, 'between 'biology' and 'culture', is breaking down. Nature (including human nature) is now seen as almost as 'alterable' as environment always was. To Cetina,[8] this could represent the end of the humanistic project of the eighteenth century Enlightenment, with its ideals of the progress of human reason, and the improvement of human society. She sees the collapse of belief in salvation by society, as well as by reason, as having resulted in an increasing focus on the individual and on the individual's body (and genome). In the modern, secular, post-Enlightenment age, only *things* can be transformed, not people or society. This new 'culture of life' focuses on transforming nature, rather than society or culture. Instead of a growth in reason, or an improvement in social conditions, it offers a new view of the 'human individual as enriched by genetic, biological and biotechnological supplements and upgrades'.[8] By these various 'performance enhancements' – changing the body by bioengineering, nanotechnology, information sciences, and cognitive research – they are also helping to break down the distinctions between humans and machines.[8]

GENETIC DETERMINISM

Another major aspect of the new paradigm is the shift towards *genetic determinism*, and the associated view of the body as primarily an *informational system*. From this perspective, the human organism is primarily 'a medium of communication and control', whose function is determined by 'genetically enshrined instruction'.[5] An individual's genes produce information (its 'genetic code'), which then help build the body and make it function. To Rheinberger, the 'central dogma' of this new view of the body can thus be summarized as: 'DNA makes RNA, RNA makes protein'.[5]

The shift towards viewing the body primarily as *information* (in this case, genetic information) is similar to the *posthuman* body described by Sandalowski[9] (see Chapters 2 and 13), which is also understood as 'a disembodied informational structure with no clearly defined self'. In the wider society, this way of thinking is contributed to by increasing exposure to computer technology, and computer imagery. Thus an individual's genetic inheritance is sometimes described as if it were a 'software programme' that can be modified, under certain circumstances, by scientists, doctors, and 'genetic engineers'. Similarly, the body, as portrayed in the HGP, can also be seen as another example of a 'posthuman' body': an informational system but without any reference to information on that individual's psychological, social or cultural context.

For some genetic determinists, there is also a belief in a hierarchical, linear structure of human nature, with much of it being determined by genes. For Mauron this represents a shift in our modern conceptualization of what constitutes 'a person' since it is now the genes that are in control, not the mind.[6] This rather mechanistic approach[2] can be criticized for downplaying the role of psychological, cultural and environmental factors in shaping

human identity. It also raises questions about the role of the HGP itself,[10] and its medico-legal implications.[11]

Rheinberger[5] sees this new 'genetic determinism' as part of a much wider project, the 'global, irreversible transformation of living beings, animals and plants, towards deliberately engineered beings'. Events such as the cloning of 'Dolly' the sheep in 1996, and the increasing development of genetically modified (GM) crops in agriculture, are part of this process.

At its most extreme, genetic determinism overemphasizes the influence of genetic factors on human behaviour, intelligence, gender, ethnicity, sexuality, and unconventional lifestyles, as well as on physical and mental health. For most modern geneticists, though, it is the interplay of biological and environmental factors that is ultimately important in the development of the human body, in both health and disease.[12]

'GENETICIZATION'

Advances in molecular biology, especially the HGP, raise the possibility of what has been called the '*geneticization*'[7,13] of many aspects of human life, including medicine and psychiatry. Geneticization entails a shift in the ways that 'human nature' and behaviour are understood: away from cultural, educational, environmental, and socio-economic influences ('nurture') towards inner, biological mechanisms ('nature'). This trend overlaps with the wider phenomenon of 'medicalization' described elsewhere in the book.

Geneticization is likely to play an increasingly important role in both psychiatry and medicine, with more research into the links between genetic inheritance, susceptibility to disease. In psychiatry, Kirmayer and Minas[14] have warned of the limitations of the 'biologization' of the subject, and the view that brain dysfunction lies at the base of all psychiatric and behavioural disorders, and that culture and other social factors are mere 'window dressing'. Despite this, neuroscientists are currently carrying out research on the possible links between genetics and different types of mental illness (including schizophrenia). At this point, however, the exact relationship between these two phenomena is still unclear, but is likely to be exceedingly complex.[15]

More broadly, concern has also been expressed about the possible 'geneticization' of ethnicity,[7] disability,[16] sexual non-conformity, criminal behaviour and even of human culture and social organization.

GENETICIZATION AND IDENTITY

In recent decades, social scientists have become concerned that widespread public knowledge of genetics may be subtly changing people's notion of individual and group *identity*, as well as cultural ideas of 'personhood'.

'Personhood'

Mauron[6] has pointed out that the very idea of 'personal identity' 'entails an element of constancy amid the drift of time and change'. But what exactly is this constant element? For some it is their biological (or genetic) identity, and for many who take this view, especially from a religious perspective, 'personhood' begins at the moment of fertilization. This view of the 'zygote-as-person',[6] whereby a new person with the full range of human rights comes into existence at fertilization, is now an issue of major religious and political controversy, and has strongly influenced the pro- and anti-abortion debate.

An alternative view, common in the social and behavioural sciences, is that personhood is 'made' or developed over time. It is a social process, rather than a specific point in time, that can sometimes take many years, and usually involves the family, community or society into which one is born. Kaufman and Morgan[17] note that, in many cultures, newborns are considered to be 'unripe, unformed, ungendered, and not fully human', and that 'producing persons is an inherently social project.' As described in Chapter 9, most individu-als therefore go through a series of ritualized 'social births' that gradually confer full membership of the society on them.

Other aspects of personal identity are also not entirely genetic. Gender identity, for example, is not entirely due to the influence of the X and Y sex chromosomes. As described in Chapter 6, it also includes psychological, social, and cultural dimensions.

In their view of 'gender', 'race' and personal identity, anthropologists generally do not believe that 'biology is destiny', but rather that human nature results from a complex interaction of biological, psychological, social and environmental influences.

'Folk genetics'

All human groups have ways of defining their own identity, and differentiating themselves from others. These define who is kin, and who is not; who is 'one of us', and who is not. They also have ways of explaining the variety of human abilities, talents, characters and moral behaviours, both within groups and between them. Often this is based on the supposed inheritance of those qualities from parents or ancestors.

These types of folk explanation – for both group identity, and personal characteristics – could be termed *folk genetics*. On the individual level they often include statements such as: 'He got his musical talent from his grandfather', 'He's very creative; he takes after his father', 'His bad temper comes from his mother's side of the family'. In the case of negative traits, they may speak of them as being 'in the blood', or 'it runs in the family'. For some people, this type of folk genetics is an important way of explaining not only individual talents, intelligence and character traits, but also mental illness, criminality, and immoral behaviour. On a national or ethnic level, folk genetics invokes notions of a shared biological heritage (such as owing allegiance to the same 'motherland') as well as shared strengths, abilities and destiny.

Davison[18] describes how in the UK, folk notions of inheritance see individuals as the result of equal contributions from both 'sides' of their family. This applies to both biological and social characteristics, and includes physical attributes (such as hair colour, eye colour, body build or specific ailments), 'constitution' (whether 'strong' or 'weak'; whether there is a tendency to longevity (or to get ill), and 'personality' (disposition, emotional outlook, behavioural style). An implication of this is that when genetic screening reveals the likelihood of a disease developing later in life, especially if that person's parent had a similar condition, the family may link this news to other supposed traits inherited from that parent (such as depression, or over-anxiety), and which they also expect to reveal themselves at the same time. This in turn may predetermine how they deal with that individual, sometimes to their detriment. Richards,[19] too, has pointed out that English folk beliefs about 'genes' are often very different to those of medical science. These usually refer more to 'the general concept of the biological transmission of characteristics between generations,' rather than to specific knowledge of genes and chromosomes, and the mechanisms and probabilities of dominant or recessive disorders.

Folk beliefs about inheritance, therefore, need to be taken into account in understanding how people respond to genetic screening, as well as to news of inherited disorders.

'Liminal beings'

One result of the advances in medical technology and molecular biology is the emergence of a new group of 'liminal beings'. They are what Kaufman and Morgan[17] describe as 'new forms at the margins of life': beings 'who hover in an ambiguous zone between life and death'. Included here are people who are severely demented or deeply comatose for a long period, and who have thus undergone a type of 'social death'. In biology it also includes other beings that are 'not-dead-but-not-fully-alive', such as human stem cells, DNA samples, frozen embryos, ova and sperm. Should these tiny entities be regarded as 'persons', or as parts of persons, or merely as clumps of cells or mole-

cules?[6] And what is the precise status of, say, frozen sperm if its donors is no longer alive? Can it be used for posthumous fertilization of a living ovum without the consent of the donor? Would this be unethical? Can the cells of aborted foetuses be used for research, or even for gene therapy?

Increasingly, clinicians are turning to bioethicists, as well as to anthropologists, to shed light on these problems.

The disappearance of 'normality'

Clayton[20] sees one aim of the HGP as 'categorically determining the increasingly elusive essence of humanity'. However, this project has had the rather paradoxical consequence of revealing that there is no such thing as two 'genetically identical' human beings, as each individual gene sequence varies, and individual genomes can differ from one another by millions of bases.[20] Furthermore, no one is now completely 'normal' or 'healthy', since *all* human beings carry within their genomes some susceptible and 'abnormal' genes, as well as 'normal' ones. The boundary is thus increasingly blurred between 'normal' and 'abnormal' bodies, and between those classified as 'healthy' and those as 'ill'.

'Boundary anxiety'

'Boundary anxiety' has been described as one of the major concerns of the modern Western world,[21] where many of the traditional methods of maintaining boundaries around the 'self' and the group now seem less effective. At times of rapid social change such boundaries have become the focus of increased anxiety.

On the individual level, this could be seen as part of a wider phenomenon, whereby the modern human body is seen as subject to penetration by invisible rays, pollutants or 'germs' – a sense of personal vulnerability I have termed 'germism'.[22] It has some similarities to the 'porous self' of more traditional societies described in Chapter 10.

It is possible that the genetics revolution may actually increase this sense of fragile, porous boundaries by dissolving the 'symbolic skins' around individuals, families and groups, and between them and their environments. Already there is increasing blurring of group boundaries owing to globalization, large-scale immigration and growing cultural diversity, especially in societies where homogeneity was previously the norm.[7] Genomics research may add to this anxiety by dissolving some of the certainties of 'ethnicity' and 'race' (pointing out the close genetic similarities between different ethnic groups, rather than their differences), and by blurring the boundaries between human beings and other species (more than 98 per cent of the human genome, for example, is shared with chimpanzees).[6] Genetic screening also blurs the distinctions between 'normality' and 'abnormality', 'health' and 'illness', as described above. 'Genetic engineering', too, may imply that the body – and even human nature – is not fixed, but is malleable by science and technology, while 'genetic determinism' may result in a sense of fatalism, and a weakening of the idea of autonomy and free-will.

All of these developments may serve to undermine the notion of the bounded, autonomous *individual*, secure within their own fixed, unchanging identity.

Genetics and social relationships

Genetics is increasingly being used to establish relationships between people. Examples of this are using DNA testing to confirm (or disconfirm) paternity, or a biological relationship between siblings adopted by different families. In forensic science, it is used to trace the identity of human remains by linking their DNA structure to those of surviving relatives or descendants. In the criminal justice system, DNA samples are increasingly being used to prove guilt or innocence in criminal trials. In civil cases it is sometimes used as proof of descent from a particular individual, in order to support a claim for inheritance or property.

Those who share the same inherited disorder may form a support group, such as the many groups worldwide for those affected by Huntington's disease, or their relatives. In many cases these groups provide emotional and social support, as well as information to their members, and in the future may well come to be seen as a new type of 'kinship' or family group. Rabinow[23] predicts the likely formation of many such new groups and individual identities, based on shared genetic disorders – a phenomenon he calls *biosociality*. In the USA these new 'communities' already include the neurofibromatosis groups, whose members meet 'to share their experience, lobby for their disease, educate their children, (and) redo their home environments'.

It is possible that all these developments may reinforce in the public mind, not only the link between genetics and human relationships, but also that between human beings and their moral behaviour. In that sense they may overlap with the ideas of ethno-genetics described above. Above all, the new genetics may be instrumental in bringing about new forms of 'community', whose members are united only by similarities in their genomes.

Genetics and time

The increasing presence of geneticization is likely to cause some changes in cultural perceptions of *time*. To some extent, an individual's genome can be said to encapsulate their present, past and future, since all three are embodied within the same individual. Genetic screening carried out in the present can tell an individual something about their past, such as 'abnormal' genes inherited from their parents or ancestors, or not being biologically related to one or both parents. At the same time it carries information about their future in terms of the risks of developing certain diseases, or of transmitting them to one's offspring. This in turn may affect that individual's future marriageability, or choice of marriage partner, particularly in the case of mental illness or severe disability. In that sense, genetic screening can condense data about past and future into one message, and in the process dissolving the difference between diagnosis and prognosis (see below).

Genetics and social context

As Rabinow[10] points out, science – including molecular biology and genetics – is never 'culture-free', neither is it free of the influence of social context. On the contrary, the theories and practices of science and technology are to a great extent both 'cultural' and social enterprises. They are ways of understanding and interacting with the world that arise from, and make use of a particular social organization and cultural world-view, as well as specific financial interests, political pressures and religious traditions.[2] Thus the same technology can be used, and understood, very differently by people in different social and cultural contexts. In clinical genetics, for example, diagnoses are not made only on the basis of 'pure' scientific data about an individual's genome – often other, more subjective elements are also included. For example, Shaw[12] has described how, in a hospital genetics clinic in England, clinical diagnoses are also a social process, the outcome of negotiations between medical specialists, laboratory scientists, and clinical managers. Diagnoses of genetic disorders are made on the basis of a number of different factors, as well as data from laboratory tests, and include the professional experience and intuition of the specialists. In discussions with colleagues, and based on previous cases they have seen, they may decide from a patient's appearance that they 'look chromosomal' (a process known as 'diagnostic dysmorphology'), even if the laboratory tests are not yet conclusive. Thus in diagnosing inherited abnormalities they integrate both subjective *and* objective information about the patient's phenotype' as well as their 'genotype'.

More broadly, the Center for Society and Genomics at the University of California, Los Angeles (UCLA)[25] has pointed out that 'the human genome is inherently social; it has co-evolved with language, tools, and the domestication of plants and animals.' The effects of this co-evolution can be seen, for example, in the rising incidence of diabetes in some developing countries as they shift to Western diets and more sedentary lifestyles. This is believed to be because their metabolism had been specially adapted, over many millennia, to cope with frequent famines and unpredictable food supplies, and cannot cope with the new context in which they live. Thus, a modern approach to problems such as the increased incidence of diabetes, would be to take into account *all* possible factors – including social, cultural, and economic contexts – as well as role of genetic inheritance.

The case study that follows illustrates how, in a particular social context (in this case a commercial biobank), genetic information is converted from private data into a marketable commodity.

Case study: a commercial biobank in Umeå, Sweden

Høyer[26] described the activities of a large, commercial *biobank* - a collection of stored human tissue - in Umeå, Sweden. It currently holds 11 000 blood samples from about 85 000 people, making it one of the largest research biobanks in the world. Donors of blood samples to the biobank also have to answer a detailed questionnaire on their lifestyle and previous medical history. He described two different views of 'personhood' among the donors: some think of it as residing primarily in the information about their lifestyle (the 'narrative'), while others see it as residing in their blood (or genes). For some in this latter group, selling information on their genetic code to other parties thus 'amounts to selling the very person'.

The biobank functions to convert blood from a substance - a part of a person - into a tradable commodity: *information*. The biobank redefines genetic codes derived from the blood sample as information and then sells this information on to medical researchers, pharmaceutical companies and other enterprises. In this way, the medical biobank 'becomes an important intermediary between human life on the one side, and economics on the other, as even the term "biobank" seems to denote.'

APPLIED GENETICS

BIOTECHNOLOGY

Biotechnology is an important development in applied molecular biology. It consists of technologies that use living cells, or parts of those cells, to make products useful for agriculture, livestock farming, industry or medicine. Biotechnology uses the 'soft technology' of the cell, its structures and internal environment, to achieve its aims because it is 'on the level of *instruction* that metabolic processes are becoming susceptible to manipulation'.[5] It has been used to alter ('genetically engineer') various animal or plant species, including GM crops, and to produce a variety of medicines, pesticides, fertilizers, industrial lubricants and other useful chemicals. It has also used microorganisms to treat wastewater, and to clean up pollution caused by oil or chemical spills. The commercial applications of biotechnology are increasingly being exploited by large transnational corporations, as well as by universities and national governments.

GENE THERAPY

In medicine, *gene therapy* offers the possibility of correcting some genetic abnormalities before they can result in a clinical disease, by the insertion of 'normal' genes into individuals with undesirable mutations.[11] Rheinberger[5] quotes the prediction of Sir Walter Bodmer, former President of the Human Genome Organization (HUGO), that within the next few decades 'molecular medicine' could provide 'corrective measures' for up to 5000 clinical diseases with a genetic component, including heart disease, some cancers, genetically determined allergies, or even educational problems such as dyslexia.

HUMAN EMBRYONIC STEM CELLS

An important, though controversial, development in applied genetics is research into the possible uses of *human embryonic stem cells* (ESCs). First isolated in 1998, these cells are taken from the *blastocyst* of a human embryo, 4–5 days after fertilization. They are cells that have the potential to develop into many other types of cell, such as those in the muscles, nerves, or heart muscles, and in the future might be used to replace damaged cells, or those that have degenerated with age. These ESCs have attracted considerable controversy in recent years as to their exact status, and whether they are fully 'human' or not.

HUMAN CLONING

Cloning is the process of artificially producing two or more genetically identical cells or organisms, from a single cell. An example was 'Dolly' the sheep, produced by cloning in 1996. Of all the possibilities offered by biotechnology, human cloning is the most controversial. There are profound objections to it on religious, ethical, practical and political grounds.[27] There are also legal strictures against it, and in 1997, for example, it was outlawed by the Council of Europe's *Convention on Human Rights and Biomedicine*.[28]

BIOGERONTOLOGY

Biogerontology is the study of the biological basis of ageing,[29] as well as of methods of delaying or reversing the effects of ageing, and of extending life-expectancy: that is, of life enhancement and life extension. As described in Chapter 1, considerable research is being done in the area of 'regenerative medicine', especially using human embryonic stem cells, to try 'overcome age-related deteriorations of the body',[30] and to use cell-replacement therapies or tissue repair for many disorders which generally occur at a later age, such as diabetes, stroke, heart disease, and Parkinson's disease.[30] That is, to 'slow ageing from within'.[29]

To some extent, this 'regenerative medicine' is an aspect of what Kaufman and her colleagues[31] term the 'biomedicalization' of ageing, whereby ageing itself is seen as a sort of 'disease' which can either be treated or alleviated, or somehow 'cured'. To treat it 'the body seems open to unlimited manipulations at any age, and the emphasis of the health professions is on the management and maximization of life itself'. It offers the lure of 'growing older without aging.' However, as Bruce[27] notes, this raises a number of ethical, social and economic questions, especially about the considerable resources needed to support so many 'super-old people' in the population. There is also the likelihood of growing inequality between those who can afford the new 'life extension' technologies to increase their life expectancy (the 'time rich'), and those who cannot (the 'time poor').[32]

GENETIC DISORDERS

GENETIC DISORDERS AND CONSANGUINITY

Many genetic disorders arise as a result of *consanguinity*; that is, from relationships between individuals closely related to one another. Consanguinity increases the rate of genetic and congenital disorders among offspring, especially of the inherited diseases known as *autosomal recessive disorders*, such as cystic fibrosis, Tay–Sachs disease, thalassaemia and sickle cell disease (Figure 14.2). It also increases the rate of congenital malformations, mental retardation, blindness, and hearing impairment.[33,34] Marriage between first-cousins, in particular, increases the risk of severe abnormality and mortality in offspring by 3–5 per cent, compared with that in the general population, while in second-cousin marriages the increase is around one per cent.[33]

For these reasons, anthropological studies of marriage and kinship patterns are particularly useful. They reveal how, in some communities, people are encouraged to choose marriage partners from the same family, region, ethnic or religious group. Over several generations, this pattern of *endogamy* can lead to higher rates of many inherited genetic disorders.

Cousin marriages

Hamamy and Alwan[34] in 1997 reported a relatively high rate of genetic and congenital disorders in the Eastern Mediterranean and Middle Eastern regions. The reasons for this are complex, but they include inadequate public health measures for genetic screening, advanced maternal age at giving birth (especially in the case of very large families), and a high rate of 'traditional consanguineous marriages'. They report that the rate of first-cousin marriages (as a percentage of all marriages in that country) is 32 per cent in Jordan, 31.4 per cent in Saudi Arabia, 30.3 per cent in Kuwait, 30 per cent in the United Arab Emirates, 29.9 per cent in Iraq,

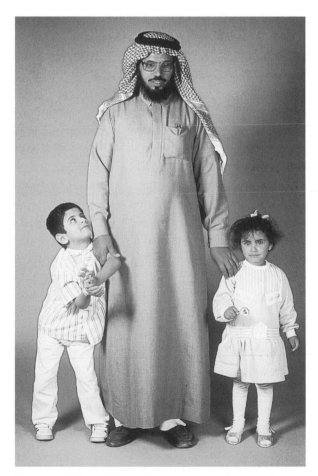

Figure 14.2 Two children with hyperphenylalaninaemia, an autosomal recessive disorder often associated with consanguinity. (Source: Nyhan, W.L., Barshop, B.A. and Ozand, P.T., *Atlas of Metabolic Diseases*, London: Hodder Education, 2005. Reproduced with permission.)

11.4 per cent in Egypt, 17.3 per cent among Muslim Lebanese, and 7.9 per cent among Christian Lebanese.[34] Some of the ways that people deal with the genetic disorders that result from this tendency towards consanguineous marriages are described below, in the case of Saudi Arabia.

High rates of cousin marriages, with resultant genetic disorders, have also been reported among Pakistani immigrants to the UK. In a 1988 study by Darr and Modell[35] of 100 British Pakistani mothers, 55 were married to their first cousins, while only 33 of their mothers had been. This suggested an increased rate of consanguinity in this immigrant community, which put them at greater risk of having children with inherited conditions such as thalassaemia.[35] According to Modell,[36] *patrilineal endogamy* is common in Pakistan, whereby women are obtained from within the extended family or tribe, and consanguineous marriages are more frequent. In Pakistan, the patrilineal family is surrounded by a larger group of relatives, the *biradheri* (brotherhood); most wives are found within this group, and marriage to a first-cousin is preferred. Modell notes that, as this custom reduces the transfer of members between families, it reinforces 'the identity of the kinship group and its distinctiveness from society in general'. In this setting, genetic diseases are also associated with less stigma, at least for the mother, since most family members are blood relatives, and the disease is often considered to already be 'in the family'. Furthermore, Qureshi[37] points out that consanguinity can also have its advantages and play a 'socially stabilizing' role for this community. It can help the family act as a cohesive unit, and the mother of an affected child can turn for help to her mother-in-law – who is also her aunt.

Case study: genetic counselling for inherited disorders in Riyadh, Saudi Arabia

Panter-Brick[38,39] in 1988 studied the parents of children with inherited disorders who had been brought to a specialist hospital in Riyadh, Saudi Arabia. Eighty-one percent of these couples were first or second-cousin marriages, and while one-third of them had experienced one to four infant deaths as a result of inherited disorders, two-thirds had had one or two affected births but no previous infant deaths. In explaining the origins of the disorder, they invoked a mixture of scientific ('genetics'), religious ('God's will') and folk explanations ('Evil Eye' or *ayn*). All attributed their child's condition to 'God's will', and Panter-Brick suggests that religion helped them to overcome feelings of helplessness, to care for their child with serenity, and even to pray for its eventual recovery. It also made possible the denial of responsibility for the disorder and, unlike in the West, only a minority of the parents acknowledged guilt for having given birth to a child that would suffer. Although two-thirds of the parents did acknowledge a possible genetic basis (*wiratha*) for the disease, only one-third were sure of this. Only a very small number could accurately remember the risks of recurrence mentioned by their doctors, or understood the precise link between inherited tendencies and actual diseases. For example, several could not understand why an inherited condition did not affect all births in the family, or affect children immediately at birth. Some knew of other cousin-marriages among their relatives that had not had affected children, and this also undermined the link between inheritance and disease. Unlike in the West, their coping strategies did not include therapeutic abortions, but did include both divorce and polygamy (in both cases, taking a new wife who might bear them healthy children). Despite the presence of inherited disorders, 36 per cent stated that they would still prefer traditional cousin marriages for themselves or for their children, though 39 per cent rejected this option. Such differences of opinion therefore 'reflects the position of Saudi families in a society undergoing rapid change'. Overall, Panter-Brick concludes that genetic counselling 'may have very little effect if consanguinity is not widely discouraged'. However, this practice is still deeply rooted in Saudi culture.

PROTECTIVE ASPECTS OF GENETIC DISORDERS

In some cases, the presence of an inherited gene may cause a particular disease, but can also protect against other diseases. The most well-known example of this is the recessive *sickle cell gene*, which, only if it is inherited from *both* parents, can cause a blood disorder: *sickle cell anaemia* (SCA) or *sickle cell disease*, which is the commonest hereditary disease in the world.[40] This can often be fatal, especially in infancy and childhood. However, if an individual is only a carrier of the recessive gene (the sickle cell *trait*), they will be healthy and asymptomatic, and also have a survival advantage in certain geographical regions. In much of equatorial Africa, for example – a region where malaria is endemic, and a deadly threat to health – the presence of this gene in the body actually protects that individual against contracting the disease, especially of the *Plasmodium falciparum* variety. Over many centuries, natural selection in sub-Saharan Africa has led to a much larger pool of people carrying this gene than elsewhere in the world. In Nigeria, for example, an estimated 25 per cent of adults are carriers of the gene, while in all of Africa there are an estimated 240 000 births of infants with SCA every year, of which about 90 000 are in Nigeria.[40] If malaria were to be controlled in those areas (see Chapter 17), then the main beneficiaries would be those with SCA, as well as the general population who do not carry the gene. If malaria is not controlled, the danger of 'gene therapy' to eradicate sickle cell trait is that more people will become susceptible to malaria.

SCREENING FOR GENETIC DISORDERS

Diagnosis of inherited genetic disorders is by *genetic screening*, carried out in specialized clinics or hospitals. Many of the people screened are healthy carriers of certain inherited diseases. In some cases, screening can be carried out prenatally on the foetus *in utero*, and show not only its gender, but also the presence of genetic abnormalities.

Genetic screening thus has far-reaching predictive powers, and can often indicate an individual's risk probabilities for late-onset disorders many years, or even decades, before the appearance of clinical signs and symptoms.[11] But what does it mean to *feel* healthy, but to be told one has a 'genetic tendency' to develop a disease? What does this do to one's sense of self, and of continuity? How does it change one's perceptions of past and future?

Genetics and 'risk'

As will be described in Chapter 15, medical and lay notions of 'risk' are often very different from one another. Epidemiological models of risk probability are based primarily on large population samples, while lay models often derive from personal or familial experience. Increasingly, however, medical science sees 'risk factors' as being embodied within the individual, especially in their genetic inheritance. According to Kavanagh and Broom,[41] these '*embodied* or *corporeal* risks', located within the bodies of individuals, are very different from both 'environmental' risks (such as pollution, nuclear waste) and 'lifestyle' risks (smoking diet, exercise). They are also different from the risks to health from poverty, inequality, and other forms of social deprivation described elsewhere in this book. Overall, genetic screening can mean locating responsibility for disease *within* individuals (or their families or ancestors), rather than in society at large.

The 'pre-patient'

What happens when a serious genetic disorder can be diagnosed, but not yet treated? Or when a completely healthy person is identified as carrying an 'abnormal' gene for a disease that will only develop in future years?

Genetic screening of healthy people has now created a new category of person: what Konrad[42] has termed the *pre-symptomatic person* or the *pre-patient*. This is an example of 'disease without illness' (Chapter 5), and of how 'paraclinical' disorders can now be revealed in healthy people by diagnostic technology, at the molecular, cellular or hormonal levels, long before they become clinical diseases (Chapter 4). Genetic screening has thus resulted in new dilemmas for both patients and practitioners. Advances in genetic diagnosis now often means a significant 'distance between the power of scientists to predict diseases and the limited ability of practitioners to cure or treat them'.[42] As technology for genetic screening is still far ahead of effective treatments, more people are being identified as being 'at risk' of a growing number of diseases, even if nothing can be done to prevent, or treat them.[41]

Huntington's disease (HD)

An example of this is Huntington's disease (HD), a serious, progressive neuropsychiatric condition that, at present, can neither be prevented nor treated. It is an inherited disease (an autosomal dominant disorder) that usually manifests itself only in mid-life (between 35 years and 45 years) with involuntary rapid movements (*chorea*), dementia, severe depression and other psychiatric symptoms, and is eventually fatal. It is transmitted by both men and women, and all the offspring of an affected individual have a 50 per cent chance of developing the disease.[43]

Because of its progressive and incurable nature, it may also take individuals many years, or even decades, to decide to have the screening test, and some people at risk refuse to take the test in the first place. In her study in British Columbia, Canada, Cox[44] described how a diagnosis of HD usually has profound implications for the individuals concerned, and for their spouses, children and relatives. Even if they know of a family history of HD, individuals at risk tend to follow many different pathways – emotional and social – towards eventually deciding to have the test. This decision is seldom completely rational, conscious or only out of self-interest. They may, for example, go for testing out of a heightened sense of responsibility to children or for its possible effect on other family members. Furthermore, as Cox and McKellin[43] point out, in genetic clinics notions of the degree of 'risk' cannot be conveyed to people only by

showing them genealogical charts of their family tree. More subjective criteria, such as emotional closeness to an affected relative, whatever their biological relationship on a family tree, might determine whether the disease ('this thing in the family') is experienced as 'getting a little closer', and therefore the individual should go for genetic screening.

The implications of diagnosis mean that the processes of diagnosis and prognosis are often fused: a diagnosis of HD is a clear prognosis, and tells the carrier what is likely to happen to them, and roughly when it is likely to happen. Konrad,[42] in her study in London, UK, found that the test converted asymptomatic people who did not know the diagnosis, and who felt completely healthy, into presymptomatic people who now knew the diagnosis and its eventual outcome. The period between becoming a 'presymptomatic' person, and actually developing the first symptoms of the disease (and thus becoming the 'embodied prognosis') is one of limbo since it might last for years or even decades.

RESPONSES TO GENETICS RESEARCH AND APPLICATIONS

Both genetic research and its many applications have been subject to strong reservations and criticism, especially about the ethical, social and economic implications. These reservations come from a number of different, though overlapping perspectives.

RELIGIOUS ISSUES

For some orthodox religious groups and individuals, many – if not all – of the applications of genetics (especially genetic engineering, gene therapy, and cloning) are seen as anathema, as 'tampering with God's will', with the scientists trying to 'play God'. For others, their objections have been based on ethical, practical, and safety issues, as well as on religious premises.

Bruce[27] has reviewed some of the ethical and religious objections to developments in genetics such as the use of stem cells, embryos and cloning – especially since the cloning of 'Dolly' the sheep in 1996, the isolation of human embryonic stems cells (ESC's) in 1998, and the publication of the first drafts of the human genome in 2000. In cloning human beings, for example, he points out that objections to it are based on three grounds: that it is wrong in principal, that it would be unacceptable because of risks to health, and that it would likely cause psychological and relational harm. He points out that reproductive human cloning is widely regarded as professionally, medically and ethically unacceptable, and was outlawed in 1997 by the Council of Europe's Convention on Human Rights and Biomedicine. Other ethical–religious issues concern the exact status of the embryo, whether or not it is fully human and whether it is right that embryos should be created *in vitro* in order to produce stem cells.[27]

CONFIDENTIALITY ISSUES

Several large *genetic databases* have been developed in recent years, in different countries and for different purposes. Some databases are used by police and other law enforcement agencies to track down criminals, or to prove guilt or innocence in a legal process. An example of this type of database is the National DNA Database (NDNAD) in the UK, created in 1996; it holds over 2.5 million samples.[45] In molecular biology, research laboratories known as *biobanks*, such as the one described by Høyer in Umeå, Sweden,[26] also hold large collections of tissue samples for genetic analysis, or for the production of pharmaceuticals or other purposes. Both types of database raise legitimate concerns about confidentiality. If the data gets into the wrong hands, then it can be misused for commercial or political purposes, or even for blackmail. For those whose genetic information is held by a database, revealing this information to others may provide details of their medical or ethnic background, of contested parenthood, or of how partic-

ular individuals are carriers of a 'defective' gene. In the last case, this may increase the stigma or discrimination that they experience,[11] and may also affect whether or not they are able to be insured, get employment, or even find a marriage partner.

CULTURAL ISSUES

Genetic research is often carried out by studying tissue samples, such as hair, blood, saliva, or other body fluids, from people who are to be screened.[11] However, Sleemboom[2] notes that in many cultures, people object to *any* part of their bodies, including body fluids, being removed for testing, especially by a stranger. Not only may these body parts be considered sacred, inviolable objects, but there may also be an anxiety that malevolent people such as witches may use them to put a curse on that individual. She notes also that in many Asian societies whose religions have a more holistic view of human life, the essence of a person cannot be reduced only to their genome. Furthermore, genetic information may be regarded as the collective heritage, and property of the *group* (family, community, tribe, or even nation) rather than of the individual. It is they who must give 'informed consent' for genetic research to take place, rather than just individuals themselves. For this more 'relational', holistic notion of self, interventions such as 'genetic engineering' interfere with 'the interrelatedness and interdependence of living beings'. In some religious groups, it may also be seen as interfering with 'fate' or with 'God's will'.

Other cultural groups may reject sperm or ovum donation as part of IVF (*in vitro* fertilization) treatment for infertility, if they come from the 'wrong' social class, caste, religion, or ethnic group, and might also reject blood transfusions or transplants for the same reason. Others might also reject all forms of *xenotransplantation* – the use of animal organs for human transplantation – as 'unnatural', and threatening to their human status (see Chapter 2).

Genetic research and applications thus always needs to be viewed within a specific cultural context, including ideas about 'nature', 'culture' and 'personhood'.

MEDICO–LEGAL AND ETHICAL ISSUES

Coleman and colleagues[11] have reviewed many of the medico-legal and ethical dilemmas, raised by genetic research and its applications. They quote from a report by the US Department of Health and Human Services that 'genetic studies that generate information about subject's personal health risks can provoke anxiety and confusion, damage familial relationships, and compromise the subject's insurability and employment opportunities'.

An example of this, noted above, is the issue of confidentiality, especially as genetics can theoretically provide a 'unique identifier' of every single individual. This information could potentially be used to stigmatize or victimize them, as well as to treat their diseases. Could employers, for example, refuse to hire individuals who carry certain genes, especially those that predispose to certain diseases,[2] or refuse to provide them with health care or life insurance? Another issue, in terms of providing 'informed consent', is whether this consent applies also to genetic material extracted (say, from a blood sample) without the knowledge or consent of the person involved.[11] Would this act constitute a form of theft?

Another problem is the possible effect – both emotional and social – on individuals who are given genetic bad news: for example, that they are a carrier of the gene for HD (see above).[43] Would this put some of these people at risk of severe depression, substance abuse, or even suicide? Coleman and colleagues[11] quote the example of the genetic mutations BRCA1 and BRCA2 genes, more common in the Ashkenazi Jewish population (1.0 and 1.4 per cent, respectively),[46] and which are associated with a statistically increased risk of breast cancer in women, with a life-time breast cancer risk of 36–56 per cent.[11] They pose the question: 'If you were one of these women, what would you do with that information?' Should the woman consider prophylactic mastectomy or prophylactic hormonal therapy, both of which carry risks of their own? Would some women prefer not to know of their increased risks, given the lack of clear preventive methods?

Finally, in some parts of Asia, prenatal diagnosis using amniocentesis and karyotyping, as well as ultrasound scans, has lead to 'prenatal gender discrimination' and even to 'sex-selective abortion', with millions of female foetuses being aborted every year (see Chapter 18). It remains to be seen whether increasing testing, before and during pregnancy, will lead to a same result, resulting in a modern form of *eugenics*.

ECONOMIC AND POLITICAL ISSUES

Here the concern is mainly about the *commodification* of the human genome. That is, the process by which people are reduced to microscopic 'units' of genetic information, which are then turned into profit by large pharmaceutical companies or other commercial concerns, often without any direct benefit to those whose genetic data is being exploited. This may include the patenting of gene sequences taken from human beings, animals and plants in a particular region. In the developing world, there is growing concern about Western biotechnology companies plundering the genomes of indigenous people, as well as those of their local flora and fauna. In particular, patenting the gene sequences of plants and herbs used as traditional remedies, and then using them for their own commercial advantage.[2] This process has been called *biopiracy* (see Chapter 18), or even *biocolonialism*.[2]

Similarly, Simpson[7] reports how in Iceland, where the DeCode or Icelandic Genome Project has been gathering genetic data on the relatively homogeneous local population, some critics of the project have claimed that 'the collective property of the nation is in effect being privatized for the commercial gain of the few'.

Another issue is that at present only the richer, more developed countries can afford the technology, equipment and trained personnel needed to run genetic screening clinics. Poorer countries cannot afford the various forms of 'gene therapy' or 'life extension' now being offered by molecular biology, especially by biogerontology.

Molecular biology, as a part of human endeavour, thus needs to be regulated by the relevant authorities. According to Sleeboom,[2] 'science cannot operate in an ethical void as it is a product of society and because the applicability of its product is relative to a socio-cultural and economic context'. In the case of genomics, increasing national and international efforts are underway to regulate genetic research and its application, and to prevent its misuse. In 1997 the United Nations Educational, Scientific, and Cultural Organization (UNESCO) unanimously approved the 'Universal Declaration on the Human Genome and Human Rights'. This declared that no research or application of the genome 'in the fields of biology, genetics and medicine, should prevail over respect for the human rights, fundamental freedoms and human dignity of individuals or, where applicable, of groups of people'.[47]

Despite this, there is still some concern and unease about where genetic research is heading, and what its long-term social effects will be. The controversy over pharmacogenetics is an example of this.

PHARMACOGENETICS

Pharmacogenetics is the study of how people's genetic make-up affects their responses to a particular drug. Its aim is to improve the clinical effectiveness and safety of that drug. In practice, this means that drugs are 'individualized', and their composition and dose are tailored to a particular individual's needs, based on their specific genetic make-up.[48,49] In some cases, drugs can also be adapted to the needs of a whole *group* of people, as well as to individuals. For example, in 2005 the heart drug BiDil (isosorbide dinitrate/hydralazine hydrochloride) was approved by the US Food and Drug Administration (FDA)

to treat heart failure specifically in African-American patients.[50]

Current research in pharmacogenetics is being carried out on drugs for a variety of conditions, including heart diseases, cancer, infectious and neurodegenerative diseases, as well as anti-depressant and drugs for pain relief.[49]

Despite these developments, pharmacogenetics has raised a number of ethical and political concerns, among both clinicians and social scientists.

ETHICAL ISSUES

As Pieri and Wilson[48] note, one ethical issue is whether this type of research favours only those with more common conditions, and excludes those whose conditions 'may not be sufficiently numerous to justify the costs associated with developing appropriate treatments'. Schubert[49] reviewed some of the other concerns about pharmacogenetics that have been expressed. They range from the overall pattern of 'geneticization', 'genetic reductionism and determinism', with the consequent danger of a 'geneticized society'. This in turn might lead to the stigmatization of certain ethnic groups, or the carriers of certain hereditary conditions. Stigmatization might also arise from newly formed groups, defined by their pharamacogenetic characteristics, such as those with severe, untreatable genetic tendencies. There is also the danger of the abuse of genetic data by governments, who might use it as a 'tool to discipline and punish citizens', or by pharmaceutical companies and other commercial interests. To prevent this, there is thus an urgent need for legislation to enforce stricter data protection.

Pharmacogenetics and 'race'

Anthropologists and others have expressed concern about whether tailoring specific drugs for specific ethnic groups may reinforce the discredited 'race' concept of the nineteenth and twentieth centuries, whereby identity, behaviour, character, morality and even culture were regarded as being predetermined by biological inheritance. For some, the concern has been that resurrecting the 'race' concept could, even indirectly, help bring back some of the abuses that followed from that approach, especially those in Nazi Germany in the 1930s and 1940s.

For many people today, 'race' remains an important folk category, a widespread though very limited way of understanding human diversity.[51] The concept of 'race' may be biologically false, but it is sometimes socially real. Simpson[7] noted how even ideas of nationhood or ethnicity often use familial terms and biological metaphors ('motherland', 'fatherland', 'mother tongue') to underlie their shared identity. However anthropologists, while they have found genetics useful for studying human origins, evolution and migrations,[52] have also pointed out the enormous genetic variations *within* different 'race' groups, as well as the close similarities among members of different ones.[51] Furthermore, the relationship of *genotype* (genetic characteristics) to *phenotype* visible physical characteristics) is not necessarily one-to-one. Many observable human characteristics – such as facial features, or body build - arise from the *interaction* of genetics *and* environment.[11] For these reasons, anthropologists have regarded 'race' as not a scientifically valid or useful concept,[53] and have focused instead on the role of social, cultural and environmental influences on human behaviour. Like other contemporary anthropologists, Cartmill and Brown[54] regard 'the race concept as biologically unrealistic, largely valueless in practice, and historically productive of suffering and injustice'.

Looked at in perspective, Simpson[7] has suggested that 'the rise to prominence of DNA as the definitive marker of human similarity and difference opens up new possibilities for "racialization"... and the essentialization of ethnicity.' It also raises 'the possibility of reworking ethnic identities as imagined genetic communities... in which the language, concepts and techniques of modern genetic medicine play their part in shaping identity, its boundaries and what is believed to lie beyond.'[7] In these 'imagined genetic communities', group identity may come to be based on shared DNA rather than on shared culture and history. This is probably more likely in communities faced with the erosion of local identities from globalization and immigration, and where genetics may be a way of conceptualizing their shared past, and 'fixing' their identity for the future.

Thus the possible danger of pharmacogenetics is that it may, quite inadvertently, reinforce the link between biology and culture,[7,48] since using ethnic or other social groups as research or treatment categories 'supports notions of their biological definition'.[48] This 'geneticization of ethnicity'[49] largely excludes the role of the social environment in creating ethnic identity, and may possibly have negative social, and political consequences.[7]

SUMMARY

This chapter has reviewed some of the emerging developments in genetics research and applications, and their ethical implications. In decades to come, these developments are likely to have a major impact on both society and culture.

KEY REFERENCES

3 Human Genome Program (2006) *History of the Human Genome Project*: http://www.ornl.gov/sci/techresources/Human_Genome/project/hgp.shtml (Accessed on 29 March 2006)

5 Rheinberger, J.J. (2000) Beyond nature and culture: modes of reasoning in the age of molecular biology and medicine. In: *Living and Working With the New Medical Technologies* (Lock, M., Young, A. and Cambrosio, A., eds). Cambridge: Cambridge University Press, pp. 19–30.

7 Simpson, B. (2000) Imagined genetic communities. *Anthropol. Today* 16(3), 3–6.

11 Coleman, C.H., Menikoff, J.A., Goldner, J.A. and Dubler, N.N. (2005) *The Ethics and Regulation of Research with Human Subjects*. Newark: LexisNexis, pp. 707–55.

13 Cox, S.M. and Starzomski, R.C. (2004) Genes and geneticization? The social construction of autosomal

dominant polycystic kidney disease. *New Genet. Soc.* 23(2), 137–646.

20 Clayton, B. (2002) Rethinking postmodern maladies. *Curr. Sociol.* 50(6), 839–51.

26 Høyer, K. (2002) Conflicting notions of personhood in genetic research. *Anthropol. Today* 18(5), 9–13.

27 Bruce, D.M. (2002) Stem cells, embryos and cloning – unraveling the ethics of a knotty debate. *J. Mol. Biol.* 319, 917–25.

28 Council of Europe (1997) *Additional Protocol to the Convention on Human Rights and Biomedicine on Prohibition of Cloning Human Beings.* European Treaty Series 168. Strasbourg: Council of Europe.

31 Kaufman, S.R., Shim, J.K. and Russ, A.J. (2004) Revisiting the biomedicalization of aging: clinical trends and ethical challenges. *Gerontologist* 6, 731–8.

34 Hamamy, H. and Alwan, A. (1997) Genetic disorders and congenital abnormalities: strategies for reducing the burden in the Region. *East. Mediterr. Health J.* 3(1), 123–32.

47 UNESCO (1998) Universal Declaration on the Human Genome and Human Rights. *Eubios J. Asian Int. Bioethics* 8(1), 4–6.

See http://www.culturehealthandillness.com for the full list of references for this chapter.

RECOMMENDED READING

Brodwin, P.E, ed. (2000) *Biotechology and Culture.* Indiana University Press.

Clark, A. and Parsons, E. (eds.) (1997) *Culture, Kinship and Genes: Towards Cross-Cultural Genetics.* Palgrave.

Kaufman, S.R. and Morgan, L.M. (2005) The anthropology of the beginnings and ends of life. *Annual Reviews of Anthropology* 34, 317–14.

Mauron, A. (2002) Genomic metaphysics. *J. Mol. Biol.* 319, 957–62.

Rabinow, P. (1996) *Essays on the Anthropology of Reason.* Princeton: Princeton University Press, pp. 91–111.

RECOMMENDED WEBSITES

Centre for Economic and Social Aspects of Genomics (UK): http://www.cesagen.lancs.ac.uk

Centre for Society and Genomics (The Netherlands): http://www.society-genomics.nl

National Human Genome Research Institute (USA): http://www.genome.gov

UCLA Center for Society and Genetics: http://www.societyandgenetics.ucla.edu/vision.htm

15 Cultural factors in epidemiology

Epidemiology is the study of the distribution and determinants of the various forms of disease in human populations. Its focus is not on the individual case of ill health, but rather on *groups* of people, both healthy and diseased. When investigating a particular disease (such as lung cancer), epidemiologists try to relate its occurrence and distribution to a variety of factors associated with most victims of that condition (such as smoking behaviour) in order to discover its probable aetiology. The factors most commonly examined are the age, sex, marital status, occupation, socio-economic position, diet, environment (both natural and man-made) and behaviour of the victims. Their aim is to uncover a causal link between one or more of these factors and the development of the disease.

Hahn[1] has compared the ways that epidemiology and anthropology approach the study of health phenomena, and how each discipline can contribute towards the other. Despite obvious differences – 'anthropologists deploy universals to arrive at particulars, epidemiologists tolerate particulars in their quest for universals' – he sees much in common between the two. Both deal with the study of *populations* rather than individuals. Both seek to understand the role of social (and other) variables in the lives of individuals and how they impact upon them. Each can offer a unique, if complementary, perspective on human health and the reasons for human disease. Although medical anthropology is more concerned with cultural variables (such as health-related beliefs and behaviours), many epidemiological concepts (such as those of probability, or 'risk factors') are increasingly of relevance to it.

Most epidemiological surveys use one of two approaches and sometimes a combination of the two. The *case–control* method examines a sample of the population suffering from a particular disease. If it is possible to demonstrate a statistically significant correlation between certain factors and the occurrence of the disease, such as a long history of cigarette smoking in those suffering from lung cancer, then a causal link can be postulated. In the *cohort study* approach, a healthy population (some of whom are associated with hypothetical risk factors such as smoking) is followed up over time, waiting for a particular disease to occur. If those associated with a particular risk factor are found to be more likely to develop the disease subsequently, then a causal link between the risk factor and the disease can be postulated. In many of these epidemiological studies, though, the precise nature of this link cannot be explained and must remain presumptive until further evidence is accumulated. In other cases, such as lung cancer and smoking, or congenital birth defects and thalidomide use during pregnancy, the aetiological link is much clearer, and can also be explained in physiological terms.

On an *individual* level, however, the notion of 'risk factors' has only a limited predictive value: for example, not all heavy smokers will develop lung cancer, not all immigrants will suffer a suicidal depression and not all 'Type A personalities' will develop coronary heart disease. In understanding why a particular individual gets a particular disease, at a particular time, a much wider range of factors – genetic, physical, psychological and socio-cultural – must all be taken into account, as well as the inter-relationships between them. This multifactorial explanation of ill health is often more useful than postulating a simple cause–effect relationship between one risk factor and one type of disease. As Kendell[2] has pointed out: 'In medicine, as in physics, specific causes have given way to complex chains of event sequences in constant interplay with one another. The very idea of "cause" has become meaningless, other than as a convenient designation for the point in these chain of event sequences at which intervention is most practicable'.

Both anthropologists and sociologists have made important contributions to the understanding of how these complex factors are related to disease, especially the role of social and cultural context. They have pointed out how variables such as social class, economic position, gender, life events and cultural beliefs and practices can be correlated with the incidence and distribution of certain diseases. Sociologists Murphy and Brown[3], for example, in their 1980 study of 111 women in London, demonstrated how both psychological and physical ill health was preceded by one or more severe life events in the previous 6 months (see Chapter 11). On a more 'macro' level, the Black Report[4] in 1982 showed how in the UK there is a relationship between social class and health, and how members of the lower socio-economic classes have poorer health and a higher mortality than their fellow citizens in the more affluent classes. In the developing world, too, there is a clear relationship between health and income. In many of these countries much of the population, already weakened by poor nutrition, will suffer from infectious and other communicable diseases. These diseases are often transmitted with the help of polluted water and food supplies, poor sanitation and inadequate housing, all of which can be improved by an adequate

income.[5] In most cases economic inequality, both within and between countries, is likely to make this situation much worse. Therefore, at a macro level, these types of economic and social factors – as well as the political organization of the particular society – must always be taken into account before considering the exact role of cultural factors in health and illness.

In the developing world, anthropological insights have been especially useful in unravelling the causes of more exotic diseases. A famous example of this was *kuru* (a progressive degenerative disease of the brain), which epidemiological studies in the 1950s found to be confined to women and children in a small area of the Eastern Highlands of New Guinea. The disease was virtually unknown among men. Various theories were advanced to explain this, but it was eventually found to be caused by a 'slow virus' infection in the brain, which was transmitted by the ritual cannibalism of dead relatives practised only by some women and children in that area.[6] For this discovery, Carlton Gadjusek was given the Nobel Prize in 1976. Other anthropological research has shed light on why people smoke, drink, take narcotic drugs, mutilate their bodies, avoid nutritious diets, reject contraceptive advice, have dangerous pastimes and follow stressful occupations or lifestyles. Marmot[7] points out how cultural factors (as well as social and psychological ones) may influence much of this risk-related behaviour. He notes how in most medical epidemiological studies the risks associated with factors such as smoking, intake of certain foods or obesity are examined, but often scant attention is paid to cultural influences shaping dietary patterns, obesity or smoking. Those studies that have looked at these cultural dimensions point out that cultural beliefs and practices are only part of the multifactorial aetiology of disease. In the case of *kuru*, for example, the virus, the social division between the sexes, and the practice of cannibalism all share in its aetiology and explain its distribution.

In many parts of the world, anthropological insights are of particular relevance in community-oriented primary care (COPC),[8] which focuses on the primary health care of individuals and families, but also looks at the health needs and health problems of their local community. Part of the continuing surveillance of the community's health involves an awareness of the role of *cultural* beliefs and behaviours in either improving health or causing disease.

These cultural factors, where they can be identified, are often difficult to quantify and are therefore less attractive to medical epidemiologists and statisticians. Neither is there a neat, measurable 'dose–response' relationship between a particular cultural factor and a particular disease, as there might be between a pathogenic organism (or chemical) and the disease that it causes. Nevertheless, despite this difficulty in quantifying cultural factors, there is sufficient evidence available to confirm their role in the development of disease, even if this role is contributory rather than directly causative. It should also be noted that, in some cases, cultural factors may protect against ill health. In the studies by Marmot and colleagues[9,10] quoted below, the rates of coronary heart disease (CHD) were compared between samples of Japanese men living in Japan, Hawaii and California. The degree of their adherence to traditional Japanese culture and world-view correlated with their incidence of CHD; it was found that the rate of CHD among the Japanese-Americans was the highest of the three groups and this matched their increasing distance from their traditional culture.

This type of study also has the value of pointing out the relative importance of genetic and environmental factors (of 'nature' and 'nurture') in the causation of disease. If three groups of Japanese with similar backgrounds have different rates of CHD, then environmental influences must somehow be implicated.

In the case of immigrant, refugee or ethnic minority communities (see Chapter 12), it is important not to overemphasize the role played by their cultural beliefs or practices in causing their poor health. This 'victim blaming' can sometimes obscure the role of the culture (and social organization) of the *host community* – the majority population among whom they live – in damaging the health of their minority communities. As McKenzie[11] points out, research indicates how racial discrimination, in particular, can adversely affect both the physical and mental health of migrant and minority communities. In the USA, UK and other European countries, studies of these groups have shown how such racial discrimination is associated with an increased incidence of hypertension, low birth weight, respiratory illness, days off work and a range of mental illnesses. These effects may be modified by individual coping styles, community structure and other factors, but the health effects of racism and inequality are a major public health issue and should therefore be of key interest to epidemiologists.

CULTURE AND THE IDENTIFICATION OF DISEASE

The cultural and social background of the epidemiologist and of the populations studied may affect the validity of the epidemiological data gathered. In that sense, epidemiology as a discipline always reflects a particular cultural view of reality, and how it should be studied. From an anthropological perspective, according to Trostle,[12] 'epidemiology is one particular system of knowledge production; it is, in short, a culture'. He notes, for example, how epidemiologists often work solely within their own familiar cultures, lack a cross-cultural perspective, and base their findings on biomedical theories of disease causation. Furthermore, some of the data they rely on, such as death certificates or definitions of race or social class, may themselves reflect cultural biases, or particular ways of classifying reality characteristic of that society, but not of others.[13] One could argue further that the use of statistical models, and overdependence on measurement – on quantitative rather than qualitative data – can also add to the 'culture-bound' aspect of epidemiological research.

One example of this are the differences in diagnostic criteria still used by epidemiologists in different countries to define particular diseases. These variations in labelling policy may give an inaccurate picture of the incidence of certain diseases in different countries. For example, Fletcher and colleagues[14] examined the apparent predominance of 'chronic bronchitis' in the UK and of 'emphysema' in North America. It was found that this was largely due to the fact that the same constellation of symptoms was diagnosed as chronic bronchitis in the UK but as 'emphysema' in the USA. Other studies among British and American psychiatrists (see Chapter 10) have shown differences in diagnostic criteria between the two groups, with American psychiatrists diagnosing schizophrenia more readily than their British counterparts. A similar study[15] showed apparent sharp differences in the incidence of schizophrenia in France and the UK. First admission rates to psychiatric hospitals for this condition, for patients below the age of 45 years, were much higher in France; however, they were much lower after that age. The study suggests that the different incidence of the disorder in the two countries is more apparent than real, and caused largely by diagnostic bias. French psychiatrists are reluctant to diagnose schizophrenia after 45 years of age, while more likely to diagnose it under 45 years, when 'the French concept of schizophrenia... seems to encompass a variety of chronic states that would be excluded in the United Kingdom for lack of symptoms'.

Another study[16] also showed marked differences in the rates of diagnosis of various diseases by doctors in five European countries. These differences, it was suggested, may either be the result of actual variations in disease morbidity in the five countries, or they may be caused by differences in the ways doctors in those countries actually interpret and diagnose certain symptoms and signs.

Zola[17] points out how the perceived incidence of a disease in a particular community depends on its actual incidence, but also on the degree of its recognition (by patients or doctors) as being something 'abnormal'. In the latter case this depends on the social context in which the disease occurs, and whether there is a 'fit' between the symptoms and signs and the society's definition of what constitutes 'abnormality'. He quotes studies illustrating how Arapesh women report no pain during menstruation, though quite the contrary is reported in the USA. Other studies, quoted by Fox,[18] have shown how congenital dislocation of the hip is considered 'normal' (though not necessarily good) among the Navaho Indians of the south-western USA, and how in 'Regionville' backache was considered 'abnormal' by the higher socio-economic groups, but not by the lower socio-economic class. Lay definitions of abnormality or disease determine, to some extent, whether these conditions find their way to doctors, and thus into the morbidity statistics. In Zola's words, 'a selective process might well be operating in what symptoms are brought to the doctor... it might be this selective process and not an aetiological one which accounts for the many unexplained or overexplained epidemiological differences observed between and within societies'.[17]

Epidemiology is directed more towards the study of 'disease' rather than that of 'illness'. Its scientific approach leads to an emphasis on 'hard' or objectively verifiable data, such as abnormal blood pressure readings, graphs, blood tests or other measurable changes in the body's structure or function. However, this excludes the many forms of illness, particularly the culture-bound folk illnesses described in Chapters 5 and 10, where physiological data are often absent. Anthropologists such as Rubel[19] have suggested that epidemiological techniques used to study such diseases as tuberculosis or syphilis can also be applied to folk illnesses such as *susto* in Latin America. These folk illnesses are perceived as 'real' by members of these societies, just as medical epidemiologists see tuberculosis as 'real'. They can also have marked effects on people's behaviour, and on their mental and physical health. In Rubel's view, the unique constellation of cultural beliefs, symptoms and behavioural changes that characterize *susto* recur with remarkable constancy among many Hispanic-American groups, Indian and non-Indian alike. By studying ethnographic case histories of those suffering from the condition, Rubel was able to isolate certain variables usually associated with each occurrence of the illness. He suggests that *susto* and other folk illnesses can be thought of as having multifactorial aetiology; that is, they result from the complex interplay of the victim's previous state of health, personality (including self-perception of success or failure in the performance of social expectations) and the social system in which he or she lives (particularly its role expectations). *Susto* occurs in social situations that the individual finds stressful, such as an inability to meet the expectations of family, friends or employers, and is 'the vehicle by means of which people of Hispanic-American peasant and urban societies manifest their reactions to some forms of self-perceived stressful situations'. While its identification rests mainly on folk perceptions and the observations of anthropologists, the techniques of epidemiology should be valuable in relating its occurrence to social, cultural or psychological variables.

CULTURAL EPIDEMIOLOGY

As Weiss[20] points out, most health-care bureaucracies and aid agencies are less concerned with cultural issues than with 'hard' epidemiological data that contribute to the calculation of *disability-adjusted life years* (DALYs). In international health policy, these have become the key indicator of the burden of disease within a country, and are the basis of the World Health Organization's annual *World Health Report*.[20] However, as the examples quoted above suggest, there can be significant difficulties in cross-cultural epidemiology, especially in psychiatry. To deal with these problem of comparing disorders across cultures, the multidisciplinary approach of *cultural epidemiology* has recently emerged.[20] An important part of this, developed by Weiss,[21] is the *Explanatory Model Interview Catalogue* (EMIC), which focuses more on studying local concepts of 'illness', and the con-

text in which they occur, rather than on medical concepts of 'disease'. The EMIC questionnaire, which has both qualitative and quantitative elements, focuses on patterns of distress (including symptoms and the social context in which they occur) within a community, as well as their perceptions of the causes of the illness, the meanings they give to it, and their help-seeking behaviour. The detailed data that it generates make it possible to both analyse and compare syndromes across cultures, and therefore to formulate more appropriate health-care interventions. For example, it is useful in identifying the stigma attached to some health problems (such as leprosy or mental disorders) – and which often make the situation much worse – and then formulating health policies to minimize that situation.[20]

Epidemiology of depression

In psychiatry, the problem of cross-cultural comparisons is particularly important (especially the dangers of the 'category fallacy', described in Chapter 10). As Patel[22] notes, there is clearly a problem when studying, and comparing depression in different cultures. Because Western psychiatry focuses primarily on *mood change* as the identifying feature of depression, it may miss other manifestations of the condition, such as multiple *somatic* symptoms, including feelings of weakness, tiredness, aches and pains, dizziness, palpitations, and disturbances in sleep pattern, and this may lead to inaccurate measurement of its prevalence within a community. Also, the Western construct of 'depression' as a condition closely linked to mood changes frequently has no clear equivalent in some non-European languages; neither may any conceptual distinction be made between 'depression' and 'anxiety'. Patel suggests, therefore, that in trying to diagnose depression across cultures, psychiatrists should strive to identify local concepts (such as *susto*) which are similar (though not necessarily identical) to the psychiatric construct of depression, rather than imposing that construct upon them. To achieve this, a number of locally developed questionnaires are being used, which are not only written in the local languages, but also take these cultural issues into account, and provide more sensitive ways of identifying depression in the community and its clinical presentations. Examples of these questionnaires include the Chinese Health Questionnaire and the Indian Psychiatric Survey Schedule.[22]

An example of the use of this more holistic approach to understanding depression, and its different manifestations, is described in the following case study from India.

Case study: cultural dimensions of depression in Bangalore, India

Raguram and his colleagues[23] in 2001 interviewed 80 patients using the Explanatory Model Interview Catalogue (EMIC) questionnaire, who were attending a psychiatric out-patients clinic at the National Institute of Mental Health and Neuro Sciences (NIMHANS) in Bangalore. All of them had been diagnosed as having depression, according to the criteria of the WHO International Classification of Diseases (ICD-9). The study found that 85 per cent of the patients presented initially with somatic symptoms (such as fatigue, aches and pains, appetite loss or sleep disturbances), rather than complaining of sadness or depression. On further probing, though, 90 per cent admitted that they did have some emotional symptoms, but only one-quarter of the sample identified sadness as their most troubling symptom. They explained their condition as resulting from many aspects of their personal and social lives, including family worries, interpersonal conflicts, financial problems, sexual issues, 'stress', 'nerves' (nara) and 'excess heat in the body'. Those who had consulted private medical doctors for this, had been dissatisfied with their treatment ('The doctor did not speak much. Just prescribed some tablets'), and with the doctor's neglect of these personal and social issues. Thus because depression is imbedded in people's experience of daily life and relationships (and is not a separate, universal, diagnostic 'disease'), the

authors suggest that 'psychological distress is not merely a state of mind, but an experiential network of social and cultural discourses that operate within any community'. To treat it effectively, one therefore needs to understand people's experiences of suffering, their belief systems and the realities of their daily lives. In poorer countries, in particular, prescribing expensive antidepressants or anxiolytics is not sufficient: 'professional frameworks for research and clinical care must be sensitive not only to professional concepts, but also to cultural contexts and the configuration of local cultural worlds. If not they are handicapped and unlikely to help.'

CULTURAL FACTORS IN THE EPIDEMIOLOGY OF DISEASE

As mentioned above, cultural factors such as specific beliefs and behaviours, can be causal, contributory or protective in their relation to ill health. In this section a number of these cultural factors are listed, many of which have already been described in more detail in previous chapters. The list is not meant to be exhaustive, but rather a selection of those factors most commonly examined by anthropologists and epidemiologists. Their relevance is illustrated later in the chapter by a number of case histories. As mentioned in Chapter 1, however, these cultural factors should not be considered in isolation or reified into independent 'things'. In every case they to be placed in a specific *context*, whether this is social, cultural, economic, or physical. This may include poverty, deprivation, social inequality, gender relations, and population density – as well as the actual physical habitat in which people live. These contexts may influence cultural beliefs and behaviours, and determine whether or not these cultural factors have a negative effect on health or not.

Economic situation

This includes:

- whether wealth is evenly distributed throughout the society
- whether the sample group is poor or wealthy relative to other members of the society
- whether income is sufficient for adequate housing, nutrition and clothing
- the cultural values associated with wealth, poverty, employment and unemployment
- whether the basic economic unit (of earning, accumulating and sharing wealth) is the individual, the family or a larger collectivity.

Family structure

This includes:

- whether nuclear, extended, joint or one-parent families are the rule
- the degree of interaction, cohesion and mutual support among family members
- whether the emphasis is on familial rather than on individual achievements
- whether responsibility for child-rearing, the provision of food, and care of the elderly, sick or dying is shared among family members.

Gender roles

This includes:

- the division of labour between the sexes, especially who works, who remains at home, who prepares the food, and who cares for the children
- the social rights, obligations and expectations associated with the two gender roles
- cultural beliefs about the behaviour appropriate to each gender (such as alcohol consumption, smoking and competitive behaviour being regarded as 'natural' for men but not for women)
- the threshold for consultation with a doctor for each of the genders
- the degree of 'medicalization' of the female life-cycle.

Marriage patterns

This includes:

- whether monogamy, polygyny or polyandry are encouraged
- whether the *levirate* or *sororate* are practised (see Chapter 16)
- whether marriage is *endogamous* (where individuals must marry within their family, kin-group, clan or tribe) or *exogamous* (where they must choose a partner from outside these groups).

In the case of endogamy there is a greater likelihood of the 'pooling' of recessive genes, with a higher incidence of such inherited diseases as haemophilia, thalassaemia major, cystic fibrosis and Tay–Sachs disease.

Sexual behaviour

This includes:

- the age of first sexual relationships
- whether promiscuity, premarital or extramarital sexual relations are encouraged or forbidden
- whether these sexual norms apply to men, to women or to both
- whether special sexual norms (such as celibacy or promiscuity) are applied to restricted groups within the society (such as nuns or prostitutes)
- whether recourse to prostitutes is socially acceptable or not
- whether homosexuality, both male and female, is tolerated or forbidden
- whether certain sexual practices (such as anal intercourse) are regarded as acceptable or not
- whether there are taboos on sexual intercourse during pregnancy, menstruation, lactation or puerperium.

Contraceptive patterns

This includes cultural attitudes towards contraception and abortion. A taboo on both of these enlarges family size, and in some cases may have a negative effect on maternal health. Certain forms of contraception or abortion may also be dangerous to maternal health, including indigenous forms of both. Attitudes to the use of condoms and other forms of barrier contraception may influence the spread of sexually transmitted diseases such as chlamydia, gonorrhoea, syphilis, hepatitis B and acquired immune deficiency syndrome (AIDS).

Population policy

This includes cultural beliefs about the optimal size of the family (such as the 'one child' policy in China) and the gender of its children – the incidence of infanticide and illegal or self-induced abortion may be related to these beliefs. Wagley[24] described a Brazilian Indian tribe, the Tenetehara, who believe a woman should have no more than three children and that these should not be all of the same sex. If a woman with two daughters gives birth to a third, the third daughter is killed. Over time, such beliefs can affect the size and composition of local communities. It also includes whether having many children is seen as a sign of full adulthood, masculinity or femininity.

Pregnancy and childbirth practices

This includes:

- changes in diet, dress or behaviour during pregnancy
- the techniques used in childbirth and the nature of the birth attendants
- the position of the mother during labour
- care of the umbilical cord (in some cultures, neonatal tetanus can result from the practice of applying dung as a dressing to the newly cut umbilical cord)[25]
- customs relating to the puerperium, such as social isolation or the observance of special taboos
- whether breast or artificial infant foods (such as powdered milk) are preferred.

Child-rearing practices

This includes:

- the emotional climate of child-rearing – whether permissive or authoritarian
- the degree of competitiveness encouraged among children (which may be related to

mental illness, suicide attempts and development of the 'Type A' coronary-prone behaviour pattern in later life)
- the degree of physical or emotional abuse regarded as 'normal' by the society[26]
- initiation rituals carried out after birth and at puberty (such as circumcision and scarification).

Body image alterations

This includes:

- culturally sanctioned bodily mutilations or alterations, such as male or female circumcision, scarification, tattooing, ear and lip piercing, foot binding and forms of cosmetic surgery (such as augmentation mammoplasty operations)
- cultural values supporting or discouraging certain body shapes, such as slimness, tallness or obesity, especially among women.

Diet

This includes:

- how food is prepared, stored and preserved
- whether there is any gender bias in how portions of food are allocated
- the utensils used in cooking and storing food
- whether food routinely contains contaminants (such as aflatoxins)
- whether food is symbolically classified into 'food' and 'non-food', 'sacred' or 'profane', or 'hot' and 'cold', irrespective of nutritional value
- whether vegetarianism or meat-eating is the rule
- whether special diets are followed during pregnancy, lactation, menstruation and ill health
- whether dietary fads and fashions are common
- the use of Western foodstuffs (with high salt, fat and refined carbohydrate levels) in non-Western communities as a sign of 'modernization'.

Dress

This includes:

- cultural prescriptions about forms of dress appropriate for men and women, and for special occasions
- fashions of dress, such as tight dresses or corsets, high-heeled or platform-heeled shoes – which may relate to the incidence of certain diseases or injuries
- body adornments, such as cosmetics, jewellery, perfume and hair dyes, which may cause skin diseases.

Long dresses that cover much of the body may predispose to certain conditions; for example, the Underwoods[27] related the long dress and veil worn by women in Yemen, as well as their confinement to 'harems', to their increased rate of osteomalacia, tuberculosis and anaemia. In the UK, lack of sunlight combined with a vegetarian diet, confinement to home and long dresses are believed to contribute to high rates of osteomalacia in Asian females.[28]

Personal hygiene

This includes:

- whether personal hygiene is neglected or encouraged
- whether, and how often, hair is washed or cut
- how often clothing is changed
- whether rituals of washing and purification are carried out on a regular basis
- whether bathing arrangements are private or communal.

Housing arrangements

This includes:

- the construction, siting and internal division of living space
- whether this space is occupied by members of the same family, clan or tribe
- the number of occupants per room, house or hut (which may influence the spread of infectious diseases)
- how indoor space is allocated by age, gender or marital status

- how the living space is heated or cooled in different seasons of the year
- whether anti-mosquito screens are integrated into the construction of windows and doors, or used to divide up internal living space.

Sanitation arrangements

This especially concerns:

- the modes of disposal of human wastes
- who carries out the disposal
- whether wastes are routinely buried or not
- whether wastes are disposed of near residences, food supplies, bathing areas or water sources.

Occupations

This includes:

- whether men and women follow similar or different occupations
- whether certain occupations are reserved for particular individuals, families or groups within the society, as in the traditional caste system in India, or the former apartheid system in South Africa
- whether certain occupations have a higher prestige and obtain greater rewards in some societies (such as the Type A executive in Western society)
- the use of certain techniques, such as traditional methods of hunting, fishing, agriculture or mining, which are associated with a high incidence of accidental death, trauma or infectious diseases
- some modern industrial occupations that are also associated with certain diseases (such as pneumoconiosis in coal miners, bladder cancer in dye workers, silicosis in metal grinders or mesotheliomas in asbestos workers).

Religion

This includes:

- whether a religion is characterized by a coherent, reassuring world-view

- whether it requires such religious practices as fasts, food taboos, ritual immersions, communal feasts, circumcision, self-mutilations or flagellation, fire-walking, or mass pilgrimages, all of which may be associated with the incidence of certain diseases.

Mass pilgrimages, for example, may be linked to the outbreak of infectious diseases such as meningitis or viral hepatitis.

Funerary customs

This concerns especially:

- how and when the dead are disposed of, and by whom
- whether the corpse is buried or cremated immediately or displayed in public for some time (which may aid the spread of infectious diseases)
- the sites of burial, cremation or display of the corpse and whether these are near residences, food or water supplies.

Culturogenic stress

This includes:

- whether culturogenic stress (and the nocebo effect) is induced, or aggravated, or sustained by the culture's values, goals, hierarchies of prestige, norms, taboos or expectations
- whether the culture fosters 'workaholism', or more relaxed attitudes to daily life
- whether there is conflict between the social expectations of one generation and those of the next.

Migrant status

This includes:

- whether the immigration was voluntary ('pull'), as with economic migrants, or involuntary ('push'), as with refugees
- whether migrants have adapted to their new culture in terms of behaviour, diet, language and dress

- whether they are subject to discrimination, racism or persecution by the host community
- whether their familial structure and religious world-view remain intact after migration
- whether they have access to their familiar religious figures or traditional healers
- the culture of the host community, especially its attitude to immigrant populations.

Seasonal travel

This includes regular, seasonal patterns of mass migration, whether of tourists, pilgrims, nomads or migrant workers. While nomads usually migrate as a community, tourists and migrant workers often migrate as individuals or in small social units. In both cases, absence from community, family and home may sometimes predispose to high rates of alcoholism and/or sexually transmitted diseases (such as AIDS and hepatitis B). It may also expose them to other diseases if, for example, they migrate from a colder climate to one where malaria is endemic.

Use of 'chemical comforters'

This especially includes:

- cultural values associated with smoking, alcohol, tea, coffee, snuff, prescribed and non-prescribed drugs, and the use of hallucinogens as sacramental drugs
- the use of intravenous 'hard' drugs by an addict subculture and the prevalence of needle-sharing among those groups (relevant to the spread of both hepatitis B and AIDS)
- the use of more contemporary 'designer' drugs, such as 'Ecstasy'.

Leisure pursuits

This includes:

- the various forms of sport, recreation and tourism
- whether these involve physical exercise or not
- whether they are competitive or not
- whether they are associated with the risks of injury or disease

- whether they involve prolonged exposure to sunlight (and ultraviolet radiation).

Domestic animals and birds

This includes:

- the nature and number of pets and domestic livestock
- whether they are kept within the home or outside it
- the degree of direct physical contact between individuals and these animals.

Various viral illnesses have been linked to domestic pets, such as benign lymphoreticulosis ('cat-scratch fever') and psittacosis ('parrot fever'), and protozoal diseases such as toxoplasmosis, transmitted by cat faeces.

Self-treatment strategies and lay therapies

This includes all the treatments used within the popular and folk sectors described in Chapter 4, such as the use of herbal remedies by traditional healers, patent medicines, special diets, bodily manipulations, injections and cupping. Lay healing that takes place in a public ritual, rather than a private consultation, may predispose to the spread of infectious diseases. Certain alternative therapies, such as acupuncture, may be implicated in the spread of hepatitis B and other infections. It also includes cultural attitudes to medical treatments and preventive strategies, such as antibiotics, oral rehydration therapy and immunizations.

SUMMARY

This section summarizes some of the cultural factors that may be of relevance to epidemiologists. Many of them have already been discussed in more detail earlier in this book. It should be noted, however, that in many cases of disease, several cultural factors actually coincide – such as occupation, use of 'chemical comforters' and dietary preferences, some of which may be pathogenic to individuals, while others may be protective. For example, a case–control study of laryngeal cancer in Shanghai,

China,[29] found that cigarette smoking was a major risk factor in both sexes (86 per cent of the male cases and 54 per cent of the females), as was the intake of salt-preserved meat and fish, while for men, occupational exposure to asbestos and coal dust was a definite risk factor. In contrast, a high intake of garlic, fruits (particularly oranges and tangerines) and certain dark green/yellow vegetables protected all groups against getting laryngeal cancer.

The importance of some of these cultural factors to the study of the origin and distribution of disease is illustrated in the following case studies.

Case study: cervical cancer in Latin America

Cervical cancer is a well-documented example of the role of cultural factors – in this case, sexual norms and practices – in the distribution of a disease. Various studies have shown it to be rare in nuns and common in prostitutes. It is extremely uncommon among Jewish, Mormon and Seventh Day Adventist women. Women with cervical cancer are more likely to have experienced early commencement of coitus, early marriage, multiple sexual partners and multiple marriages. Although the exact cause of cervical cancer is still unknown, it is believed to be multifactorial in origin, and there is a strong suspicion that a viral infection – human papilloma virus (HPV) – might be implicated.[30]

It was originally thought that a woman's sexual behaviour alone could determine her risk of cervical cancer. However in 1982, Skegg and colleagues[31] pointed out that its incidence was very high in Latin America, where women were expected to have only one sexual partner in their lives, and strong cultural sanctions existed against their having premarital or extramarital sexual relationships. They suggested that, if the hypothesis of the infective origin of cervical cancer was correct, then in some communities a woman's risk of getting the disease would depend less on her sexual behaviour than on that of her husband or male partner. One should therefore look at the patterns of sexual behaviour in a society as a whole, especially the sexual habits of the *men*. On this basis, they postulated three types of society:

1 'Type A', where both men and women are strongly discouraged from pre- or extramarital relations (for example, Mormons or Seventh Day Adventists)
2 'Type B', where only women are strongly discouraged from extramarital sexual relations but men are expected to have many (especially with prostitutes), as in many Latin American societies and in Europe last century
3 'Type C', where both men and women have several sexual partners during their lives (as in modern Western 'permissive society').

The incidence of cervical cancer is lowest in Type A and highest in Type B societies. In Type A groups, such as Jews, Seventh Day Adventists and Mormons, the low incidence could result from endogamous marriage and monogamous patterns of sexual behaviour, as well as from low recourse to prostitutes. Conversely, in Latin America recourse to prostitutes is common. In one study quoted by Skegg and colleagues, 91 per cent of male Colombian students reported premarital intercourse, and 92 per cent of these men had experienced intercourse with prostitutes. The authors suggest that this might account for the high incidence of cervical cancer in Latin America, as the prostitutes could act as a reservoir of infection. Similarly, the decline in mortality from the disease in the UK and USA (Type C societies) may be result from changing patterns of sexual behaviour among men, with less recourse to prostitutes in a more 'permissive' society.

Case study: cultural practices and hepatitis B

Brabin and Brabin[32] in 1985 reviewed the role of cultural factors in the transmission of the hepatitis B virus. The level of infection by the virus varies widely between countries, ethnic groups, tribes and even neighbouring villages. Part of the reason for this is a number of cultural factors, including sexual behaviour patterns, family and marriage patterns, and cultural changes affecting women and their childbearing age. For example, the risk of infection with the virus varies with the level of promiscuity, and the spouses of promiscuous partners are therefore at greater risk from infection, which is particularly important in the case of pregnant women. They point out that marriage patterns that permit extramarital relations, polygamy, frequent divorces or the exchange of partners may all contribute to spread of the virus, as may widespread recourse to prostitution, especially in tropical countries. Family patterns involving frequent adoption of children and their movement between households, and the movement of women in marriage between villages, may also provide channels for the spread of infection. In contrast, marital patterns that forbid marriage between different communities or segments of a community may confine the infection to certain geographical or ethnic pockets; for example, Chinese immigrants in the UK and USA and Fijian Indians all have low levels of HBsAG, characteristic of their homelands. Finally, social changes such as war, migrations and social upheaval may break down barriers that contained the virus in a local environment and spread it further afield. Since the prevalence of hepatitis B antigen (which correlates with the rate of vertical transmission of the virus) declines with age, most vertical transmission occurs when women bear children at a younger age. Cultural changes that produce a later age of marriage and childbearing will therefore reduce this transmission, and the spread of infection. The authors conclude that, especially in the case of hepatitis, 'interpretation of epidemiologic data in non-Western societies demands a cultural perspective if modes of transmission are to be correctly defined and intervention planned'.

Case study: coronary heart disease among Japanese in Japan, Hawaii and California

In a number of studies in the 1970s, Marmot and colleagues[9,10] examined the epidemiology of coronary heart disease, hypertension and stroke among 11 900 men of Japanese ancestry living in California, Hawaii and Japan itself. The aim was to identify the influence of non-genetic factors on these three groups, by comparing disease rates of the two migrant groups and those of Japanese who had not emigrated. They found that there is a gradient in the occurrence of coronary heart disease (CHD) between the three groups, with the lowest rate in Japan, intermediate rate in Hawaii and the highest rate in California. The influence of other risk factors commonly associated with high CHD rates, such as hypertension, diet, smoking, weight, blood sugar and serum cholesterol levels, was examined. It was found that the gradient in the incidence of CHD could not be explained only by the presence of these risk factors (for example, those who smoked similar amounts in the three groups still showed a gradient in the incidence of CHD). However, the incidence of CHD *was* found to be related to the degree of adherence to the traditional Japanese culture they were all brought up in. The closer their adherence to these traditional values, the lower was their incidence of CHD. Within California, those Japanese-Americans who had become most westernized in outlook had higher rates than those immigrants who followed their more traditional lifestyle. Marmot and Syme[10] point out that 'these results support the hypothesis that the culture in which an individual is raised affects his likelihood of manifesting coronary heart disease in adult life', and that this relationship of culture of upbringing to CHD 'appears to be independent of the established coronary risk factors'. In the case of the Japanese, the cultural emphasis is on group cohesion, group achievement and social stability. In this cultural group, as in other traditional societies, it is suggested that 'a stable society whose members enjoy the support of their fellows in closely knit groups may protect against the forms of social stress that may lead to CHD'.

Case study: cultural practices and parasitic diseases

Alland[33] examined the relationships between certain cultural practices and the incidence, distribution and spread of parasitic diseases. Although published in 1969, most of his findings still apply today and are also relevant to infectious diseases. He notes how the arrangement of living space, the type and arrangement of houses and the numbers of people per room or house may all influence the spread or containment of disease. The social isolation of certain subgroups, such as within a rigid caste system, may affect the spread of epidemics into certain communities. Population movements, such as a nomadic lifestyle, also help to spread parasitic and other infections, sometimes through the wider distribution of their human wastes. Certain cultural practices that separate man from the extra-human environment of some parasitic organisms also help reduce infections. For example, the practice of digging deep latrines (as opposed to discharging waste products into rivers or streams) offers protection against those parasitic infections that are spread by urine or faeces. Contamination of water supplies is also prevented by its location far from domestic animals or human habitations, and by the separation of drinking sources from water used for bathing or laundering. Other cultural practices, such as frequent spitting, may increase the spread of viral and other infections through the community. Patterns of visiting the sick, or attending large public rites or festivals, may also be related to the spread of epidemics. Certain agricultural techniques, such as the cultivation of rice paddies, may increase the danger of schistosomiasis and other parasitic infestations. Certain forms of dress, such as tailored clothing, apparently provide a better environment for lice or fleas to live in than do loose togas, while the sharing of clothing within a family may also spread these infections. These and other cultural practices may influence the distribution of a wide range of parasitic, bacterial, viral and fungal infections.

Case study: AIDS and sexual practices in urban Brazil

Parker[34] in 1987 studied sexual attitudes and practices in urban areas of Brazil, in relation to the growing incidence of acquired immune deficiency syndrome (AIDS) in that country. Based on his fieldwork, he criticized the assumption that 'sexual practices are constant cross-culturally – that sexual behaviour is largely unaffected by its specific social and cultural context'. He pointed out that models of AIDS transmission (and therefore of prevention) developed in the USA and Western Europe may be inappropriate to the Brazilian cultural context. The assumption that there are just three types of sexual behaviour – heterosexuality, homosexuality and bisexuality – with clear boundaries between these groups does not reflect Brazil's complex cultural reality. For example, not all homosexuals are regarded as being really 'homosexual'. Brazilian culture differentiates between the active, penetrating partner (the *homem* or 'man'), and the passive 'woman' (known as the *viado* or *bicha*). Social stigma attaches mainly to the latter, while the *homem* can have sexual relations with either women or men, 'without sacrificing his masculine identity'. The same distinction applies also to the more active male prostitutes (the *miche*), as opposed to the more passive transvestites or *travesti*. In popular thought, therefore, 'the category of *homossexuais* or "homosexuals" has generally been reserved for "passive" partners, while the classification of "active" partners in same-sex interactions has remained rather unclear and ambiguous'. This ambiguity can in turn undermine preventive strategies and health education that are directed only against the more obvious *viados*.

Another significant feature in Brazil is the widespread practice of anal intercourse, both between men and men, and between men and women. It is also common between male clients and female prostitutes. In adolescence, too, anal intercourse is common, mainly in order to avoid both unwanted pregnancy and rupture of the hymen – still an important sign of a young woman's sexual purity. The apparently frequent incidence of anal intercourse among different groups in Brazil thus 'makes the epidemiological picture of AIDS there quite distinct from the picture in Europe and the United States'; these patterns 'significantly change the definition of "high-risk" groups in Brazil and may well further the spread of AIDS to the population at large'. Thus, Parker concluded that epidemiological research on AIDS should recognize the disease as 'simultaneously a socio-cultural and biological phenomenon', and that preventive strategies should always take this into account.

MIGRATION AND HEALTH

In addition to the conditions just described, one other set of cultural factors is becoming increasingly important in the contemporary world; the effects on health of migration. There is now a considerable body of research that links migration and refugee status to an increased incidence of certain illnesses, both mental and physical, though the exact link between migration and illness is not clear. These studies (some of which were quoted in Chapters 11 and 12) indicate, for example, a higher incidence of mental illness, attempted suicide and hypertension among some immigrants, compared with the incidence of these conditions in the host countries and in their countries of origin. As with coronary heart disease among Japanese-Americans, it appears that the cultural lifestyles of both immigrant and host communities as well as the fit (or lack of fit) between the two, coupled with the economic situation of the country and its attitudes towards newcomers, may all contribute towards the increased incidence of these stress-related conditions.

VARIATIONS IN MEDICAL TREATMENT AND DIAGNOSIS

Epidemiological techniques can also be used in the study of differences in the diagnostic and treatment behaviour of doctors from various countries. Some of the differences between British and American and between British and French psychiatrists in the frequency with which they diagnose schizophrenia and affective disorders have already been described in Chapter 10. In the case of medical treatments, the rate of a particular treatment (such as tonsillectomy) in two countries can be compared with the actual prevalence (in both countries) of the condition (in this case recurrent tonsillitis) for which the treatment is usually prescribed. If the rate of tonsillectomies is much higher in one country, in the absence of a proportionately higher rate of tonsillitis, then it can be inferred that cultural influences on both doctor and patient are responsible for this. Obviously, both economic and technological factors, as well as the supply of both medical manpower and hospital facilities, play a part in this phenomenon, and such a study is more valid if carried out between countries with similar levels of social and industrial development.

Case study: comparison of surgical rates in the USA, Canada and England and Wales

Vayda and colleagues[35] compared overall surgical rates in Canada, England and Wales, and the USA in the period 1966–76. In particular, they examined the relationship between:

1 Operative rates per 100 000 population in each of the three countries.
2 Selected resources (surgical manpower and hospital beds).
3 National priorities, as measured by percentage of gross national product (GNP) spent on health care.
4 Disease prevalence, as measured by mortalities for selected diseases for which surgery is one form of treatment.

The rates of 10 common operations were computed in the three countries and compared. These operations were: lens extraction; tonsil surgery; prostatectomy; excision of knee cartilage; inguinal herniorraphy; cholecystectomy; colectomy; gastrectomy; hysterectomy; and Caesarean section. During the 10 years studied, overall surgical rates in England and Wales were found to have remained constant, while Canadian rates were also relatively constant, but rates in the USA increased by about 25 per cent. Canadian rates, though, continued to be 60 per cent higher than the British rates, and the USA rates, which were 80 per cent greater than those in England and Wales in 1966, were 125 per cent greater than those in England and Wales in 1976. Caesarean sections increased in all three countries from 53 per cent to 126 per cent. In 1976 about 12 per cent of all Canadian and American births were delivered in this way, but the rate in England and Wales was only 7 per cent. Hysterectomy rates were twice as high in Canada and the USA compared with the British sample. In comparing the availability of hospital beds, the British sample had the lowest number (and the lowest number of operations) of the three in 1976, and while Canada had 30 per cent more hospital beds than the USA, overall operative rates in the USA were 40 per cent higher than in Canada. In the decade under study, England and Wales spent about 5 per cent of their GNP on health care, Canada spent about 7 per cent and the USA about 9 per cent. The study could find no clear correlation between operative rates in the three countries and the availability of either hospital beds or medical manpower; neither were they related to differing mortality rates (as a measure of prevalence) of the selected diseases between the countries. Instead, the differences were caused by 'differing treatment styles and philosophies of patient management', the different value systems of these countries, the priority they assign to health care (as reflected in the percentage of GNP allocated to health care), and changes in technology (especially the increase in cardiac, vascular and thoracic surgery in the USA and Canada). The authors note that 'differing operative rates are more a reflection of consumer and provider preferences; consequently, outcomes must be measured in terms of quality of life and postoperative morbidity rather than by mortality'. This is because most operations done are elective or discretionary, and not done for any potentially fatal condition; this explains why the differences in operative rates were not related to differing mortalities from the selected conditions. The study demonstrated, therefore, that 'at least three industrialized Western countries have tolerated substantial differences in their frequencies of surgery without consistent unfavourable outcomes'. To some extent, therefore, the cultural values of the surgeon, the patient and the society in which they live play a part in determining the frequency with which surgery is used as a treatment for certain conditions.

LAY EPIDEMIOLOGY AND CONCEPTS OF 'RISK'

Because epidemiology is the study of groups, and of risk factors at the population level, it is sometimes difficult to apply its findings to any particular individual case. Similarly, it is difficult for some individuals to relate these findings to their own lives when their own personal experience tells them otherwise. For example, they may have read repeatedly that smoking causes lung cancer and

heart disease, yet know of several heavy smokers in their own families who have lived to a ripe old age.

The way that people assess their own *future risk* of illness has been called *lay epidemiology*. In a study in Wales, Davison and colleagues[36] showed the similarities and differences between lay and medical models of heart disease, especially of the risk of being a 'coronary candidate' or 'coronary prone' individual. They showed how an individual's understanding of the causes of heart disease drew on information derived from several different sources: the media, books, magazines, newspapers, contact with health professionals and the opinions of those around them, as well as from their own personal experiences (see Chapter 4). Based on this, their list of people most 'at risk' included: heavy smokers or drinkers; 'worriers by nature'; people 'under strain'; fat or unfit people; people with a red face or grey pallor; people with 'heart trouble in the family'; or those who eat excess rich or fatty food. These explanations, a combination of personal characteristics and lifestyle, were usually invoked retrospectively to explain why someone they knew had suffered a heart attack. The list was so wide, though, that 'almost any type of person could be a candidate'. To explain why some 'low-risk' people get ill, while some 'high-risk people remained healthy, they drew on alternative folk concepts of 'luck', 'chance', 'fate' or 'destiny'. Heart disease was seen as unpredictable – a 'random killer' and a condition 'famed for its caprice'. This rather fatalistic approach ('It never seems to happen to the people you expect it to happen to') raises problems for public health authorities who advocate mass population screening for 'risk factors', or major health-education campaigns, especially when they give specific advice such as 'don't eat saturated fats and you will avoid a heart attack'. Like lay models, epidemiological concepts of risk are limited 'because most fatal heart attacks happen to people outside the high-risk group', and because they cannot predict whether or not a particular individual will, or will not have a heart attack. These difficulties of applying population models to individual cases are becoming well known to the public, and are an important influence on lay epidemiology.

Individual notions of risk are also influenced by the wider cultural and social context. One aspect of this, first described by Crawford,[37] is the growth of 'healthism', especially among middle-class people in industrialized countries. This movement places the origin of health problems not in the environment or wider society, but in individuals themselves. Each person is seen as responsible for maintaining their own health (with a 'healthy lifestyle'), and disease is therefore largely their own fault. According to Crawford, 'by elevating health to a super value, a metaphor for all that is good in life, healthism reinforces the privatization of the struggle for generalized well-being'. For some people, 'healthism' can be seen as a secularized religion, a new moral discourse, where an 'unhealthy lifestyle' has now replaced a 'sinful life' (see Chapter 5). It is also a consumerist movement,[38] closely linked to the growing 'lifestyle', 'health food', 'fitness' and vitamin industries. Despite the advantages of a 'healthy lifestyle', the problem is that 'healthism' may ignore larger social causes of ill-health such as poverty, inequality, over-crowding, or pollution, by placing the 'risk' of ill-health firmly within individual behaviour.

Developments within medicine also influence individual concepts of risk. One aspect of this is the increasing medical emphasis on individual 'risk factors' as leading to disease. Mass screening campaigns, such as those for cervical smears, aim to relate population concepts of 'risk factors' (in this case, for cervical cancer) to individuals within those populations. However, Kavanagh and Broom[39] point out that this may sometimes have negative results. In cases where only a few abnormal cells are found, considerable anxiety may be caused to women who are told they now have 'precancer'. This now becomes an 'embodied risk', one that originates within her own body and not from without. Dealing with this sense of something alien or 'other' within the body 'involves a complex translation of a fact about the population into terms that are personally meaningful'. This type of situation is an inevitable result of the increasing sophistication of medical technology (Chapter 4) but is also an example of 'disease without illness' (Chapter 5).

Despite this, the concept of 'risk factors' has become a key feature of modern biomedicine. For example, Skolbekken[40] has analysed the number of times that the terms 'risk' or 'risks' was mentioned in the titles or abstracts of British, American or Scandinavian medical journals, over the period 1967–91. He found a significant and rapid increase in the numbers of 'risk-articles' over that period; these were 'rising in numbers much faster than the general increase in the total number of published articles'. The highest rise in this 'risk epidemic' was in epidemiological journals, where about 50 per cent of articles published between 1986 and 1991 were 'risk-articles'. Skolbekken points out that 'risk' is no longer associated only with major illnesses, such as heart disease, cancer and human immunodeficiency virus (HIV)/AIDS, but is now applied to a much wider range of circumstances. One of the dangers of this is that 'if we are to are to believe the epidemiological risk constructions, there seem to be few, if any, things in life that are purely healthy or unhealthy'.

I have used the word 'germism'[41] to describe this pervasive modern sense of vulnerability, of invisible external dangers that can attack or invade the body's boundaries at any time, whether these are microbes, pollution, radiation, climatic conditions, or even social change itself. To deal with this growing sense of risk – and the anxiety over areas of life over which one has no control – people increasingly focus not only on a 'healthy lifestyle' but also on exerting control over small areas of their life over which they *do* have control: the care of their bodies, their diet, clothing, car, house and garden, as well as their personal relationships.[42]

Trostle[43] uses the terms 'popular epidemiology' or 'community epidemiology' to describe a situation where communities themselves take the initiative in identifying and monitoring health risks in their own environment (such as pollution, radiation or a disease outbreak), and then bring this information to the attention of public health officials, epidemiologists, academics, politicians or the media. They may compile maps, for example, showing the prevalence of a particular disease in a particular neighbourhood, such as clusters of cancer cases near to a certain factory, or toxic waste dump. In many cases these community findings are eventually examined in more detail by professional epidemiologists whose research into the matter may, or may not, confirm them.

Concepts of personal risk management

An individual's concept of 'risk' depends to some extent on the significant social groups that surround them. Douglas,[44,45] in her 'Cultural Theory', has identified four different world-views, and ways of behaving, which depend on the types of social groupings of which individuals are part, and the role of those groups in their daily lives. This classification is based on two axes (or continua): *group* – the degree of closeness and interconnectedness of the group (these are essentially face-to-face groups not large groupings such as the Catholic Church), including the intensity of experiences that members share within it; and *grid* – the degree to which the behaviour of members is constrained by the rules and customs of the group. Each of the four types is associated with different values, attitudes and world-view, including how they respond to severe ill health. Although these are ideal types, in practice people may share the characteristics of more than one type. The anthropologist Gerald Mars[46] has made a useful adaptation of Cultural Theory to explain the range of attitudes towards health 'risks', and personal risk management. His model describes four different ways of explaining ill-health when it occurs, and of preventing it in the future. They are:

1 *High group – High grid* – people who have a hierarchical view of the world, with a high respect for authority (including of doctors), and whose behaviour is tightly constrained by the rules of the group (whether work, family or leisure). They are generally conservative and traditional in outlook, and reluctant to change behaviour. To them, disease strikes when you break the rules, especially those derived from higher sources (such as doctors or religious leaders). Illness is commonly explained as having 'done something wrong', such as 'not following the doctor's advice'. In traditional societies, severe events such as death in childbirth might be explained as: 'she got ill, because she must have committed adultery'. Risk avoidance, therefore, means following the rules.

2 *High group – Low grid* – people who are generally part of smaller groups, with an egalitarian view of the world. They tend to reject all hierarchies and distrust authority. Within the group there are few barriers between people, but this is combined with a deep suspicion of the world outside the group. All bad things and contagions are believed to come from beyond the group's borders. Thus, these people often see health risks as originating from 'outside', blaming it on outside forces, whether witchcraft, pollution, microbes, nuclear wastes, invisible rays, globalization, or 'Big Business'. They also tend to distrust health messages from authorities such as the government or the medical profession. Risk avoidance is based on forms of behaviour loosely shared by the group, such as vegetarianism, certain diets, meditation, or other 'alternative' strategies.

3 *Low group – High grid* – people who are generally isolated, powerless and anomic. They are often poor or working in jobs where they have little autonomy or choice. There are very few social connections between them and other people in their situation, but their lives are strongly constrained by many outside forces: the government, local authorities, police, employers, landlords and politicians, as well as by levels of unemployment or economic recessions. Because they have little sense of control over their personal lives, they tend to have a fatalistic attitude towards health risks ('You can't do anything to prevent a heart attack,

when your time has come, it just happens'). They tend to ignore health advice from the authorities and those 'above them'. Risk management is very partial and inconsistent, because they believe that life is a gamble, and that ill-health results largely from 'fate', 'bad luck' or 'the luck of the draw'.

4 *Low group – Low grid* – people who lead highly individualized, independent lives, often as entrepreneurs in business or the creative professions. They tend to be very competitive and connected to other people only in loose networks, which they use for social benefits or advancement, and do not feel strongly constrained by outside social pressures. They tend to be open to the latest health fad or fashion, such as the very latest treatments, diets or 'miracle cures'. Their view of risk is more personalized, and they tend to blame ill-health on themselves and their own behaviour ('It's your own fault, if things go wrong'). Like type 2, they have little respect for hierarchy and authority, and their risk-management strategies mean that they are always willing to 'shop around' for a better treatment, or for a 'second opinion'.

Obviously these four groupings are ideal and abstract types, and there is much overlap between them. Like epidemiological models, they cannot be easily applied to any individual case. Nevertheless they do help us understand why some health promotion campaigns, however well-designed, may fail to reach all members of the population, or to be understood by them in a similar way.

KEY REFERENCES

4 Townsend, P. and Davidson, N. (eds) (1982). *Inequalities of Health: the Black Report*. London: Penguin.

6 Gadjusek, D.C. (1963). Kuru. *Trans. R. Soc. Trop. Med. Hyg.* 57, 151–69.

7 Marmot, M. (1981). Culture and illness: epidemiological evidence. In: *Foundations of Psychosomatics* (Christie M.J. and Mellett, P. G. eds). Chichester: Wiley, pp. 323–40.

15 van Os, J., Galdos, P., Lewis, G. *et al.* (1993). Schizophrenia sans frontieres: concepts of schizophrenia among French and British psychiatrists. *Br. Med. J.* 307, 489–92.

17 Zola, I.K. (1966). Culture and symptoms: an analysis of patients' presenting complaints. *Am. Soc. Rev.* 31, 615–30.

19 Rubel, A.J. (1977). The epidemiology of a folk illness: *Susto* in Hispanic America. In: *Culture, Disease and Healing: Studies in Medical Anthropology* (Landy, D. ed.). London: Macmillan, pp. 119–28.

21 Weiss, M.G. (1997) Explanatory Model Interview Catalogue (EMIC): framework for comparative study of illness. *Transcult. Psychiatry* 34, 235–63.

22 Patel, V. (2001) Cultural factors and international epidemiology. *Br. Med. Bull.* 57, 33–45.

34 Parker, R. (1987). Acquired immunodeficiency syndrome in urban Brazil. *Med. Anthropol. Q. (New Ser.)* 1, 155–75.

36 Davison, C., Smith, G.D. and Frankel, S. (1991) Lay epidemiology and the prevention paradox: the implications of coronary candidacy for health education. *Sociol. Health Illness* 13(1), 1–19.

39 Kavanagh, A.M. and Broom, D.H. (1998) Embodied risk: my body, myself. *Soc. Sci. Med.* 46(3), 437–444.

40 Skolbekken, J.A. (1995) The risk epidemic in medical journals. *Soc. Sci. Med.* 40(3), 291–305.

45 Douglas, M. (1986) *Risk Acceptability According to the Social Sciences*. London: Routledge and Kegan Paul.

See http://www.culturehealthandillness.com for the full list of references for this chapter.

RECOMMENDED READING

Hahn, R. A. (1995). *Sickness and Healing: an Anthropological Perspective*. New Haven: Yale University Press, pp. 99–128.

Janes, C., Stall, R. and Gifford, S. (eds) (1986) *Anthropology and Epidemiology*. Dordrech: Reidel.

Trostle, J. (2005) *Epidemiology and Culture*. Cambridge: Cambridge University Press.

Weiss, M.G. (2001) Cultural epidemiology: an introduction and overview. *Anthropology and Medicine* 8(1), 5–29.

RECOMMENDED WEBSITES

Centers for Disease Control and Prevention (USA): http://www.cdc.gov

World Health Organization: http://www.who.int

16 The AIDS pandemic

Acquired immune deficiency syndrome (AIDS) is one of the deadliest diseases of the modern age, and a major threat to global health. Anthropology can play a major role in understanding the social, cultural and economic contexts in which it occurs, and help design strategies to both prevent and manage the pandemic.

OVERVIEW OF THE PANDEMIC

According to Mann and colleagues,[1] by 1992 164 countries had reported cases of AIDS to the World Health Organization WHO). In 2004 the Joint United Nations Programme on human immunodeficiency virus (HIV)/AIDS (UNAIDS) in its annual

AIDS Epidemic Update estimated that there were 39.4 million people living with HIV (37.2 million adults and 2.2 million children under 15 years), that 4.9 million people (4.3 million adults, 640 000 children) had become newly infected with the virus that year, and 3.1 million people (2.6 million adults, 510 000 children) had died that year from the disease (see Table 16.1).[2] The greatest regional prevalence of HIV was in sub-Saharan Africa; although it has just 10 per cent of the world's population, it was home to 60 per cent (25.4 million) of those living with HIV (Figure 16.1). While some countries such as Uganda had shown a decline in rates, there has been a marked increase in southern Africa. South Africa now has the highest number of people living with HIV in the world, with an

Table 16.1 Global human immunodeficiency virus (HIV) prevalence and mortality figures for acquired immune deficiency syndrome (AIDS) by region, 2004

Region	Adults and children living with HIV	Adult and child deaths caused by AIDS
Sub-Saharan Africa	25.4 million	2.3 million
Asia	8.2 million	540 000
Latin America	1.7 million	95 000
North America, West and Central Europe	1.6 million	23 000
Eastern Europe and Central Asia	1.4 million	60 000
Middle East and North Africa	540 000	28 000
Caribbean	440 000	36 000
Oceania	35 000	700

The Joint United Nations Programme on HIV/AIDS (UNAIDS)/World health Organization (WHO) (2004).[2]

estimated 5.3 million by the end of 2003.[2] Largely owing to AIDS, life expectancy at birth has dropped below 40 years in nine African countries: Botswana, Central African Republic, Lesotho, Malawi, Mozambique, Rwanda, Swaziland, Zambia and Zimbabwe.[2] Throughout sub-Saharan Africa, women are disproportionately affected by HIV; on average there are 13 women living with HIV for every 10 infected men, and the gap between the genders is increasing.

In the richer countries of North America, Western and Central Europe, the picture is also alarming. In 2004 there were a total of 1.6 million people living with AIDS in these regions, with 64 000 newly infected with HIV, and 23 000 deaths caused by AIDS (3101 of them in Western Europe).[2] Among young aged 15–24 years it affected 0.1 per cent of females and 0.2 per cent of males. Despite widespread health education programmes in these countries, UNAIDS conclude that 'prevention efforts are not keeping pace with the changing epidemics in several countries', as new sections of the population are becoming infected: as well as men who have sex with men, and injection drug use, an increasing proportion of people, especially women, are being infected through unprotected heterosexual intercourse.[2] For many women, a major risk factor is that their partners may not disclose to them that they are HIV positive. In addition, different sections of the general population, especially those in areas of socio-economic deprivation, are now suffering a much higher rate of infection. In the USA, for example, an estimated 40 000 people are newly infected each year, but the epidemic is now disproportionately lodged among African-Americans (who accounted for about 25 per cent of all AIDS cases in 2003), and especially African-American women (about 72 per cent of new HIV diagnoses among US women).[2]

Not only is AIDS dangerous in its own right, having a compromised immune system also puts people with AIDS at risk of other diseases. These

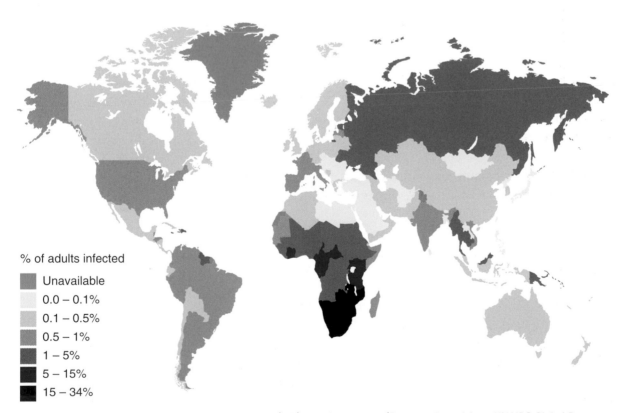

Figure 16.1 Worldwide human immunodeficiency virus (HIV) prevalence rates. (Source: adapted from UNAIDS Global Report 2006, 'A global view of HIV infection' (2005).)

% of adults infected
- Unavailable
- 0.0 – 0.1%
- 0.1 – 0.5%
- 0.5 – 1%
- 1 – 5%
- 5 – 15%
- 15 – 34%

co-morbidities are especially evident in poorer countries where treatment may not be available or affordable. They include diarrhoeal diseases, pneumonia, herpes zoster, tuberculosis and malaria, which contributes synergistically with AIDS to a higher morbidity and mortality, in areas where both diseases are prevalent, especially in sub-Saharan Africa.

In the developed world, the majority of people who need antiretroviral treatment do have access to it; many now receive treatments such as highly active antiretroviral therapy (HAART). As a result, there is now a significant extension of life expectancy and quality of life among people living with AIDS, and deaths from the disease have stayed relatively low. However, UNAIDS warn of two potentially dangerous trends. First, that in many countries many people with HIV infections remain undiagnosed: for example, they estimate that in the UK about one-third of people with HIV do not know their own serostatus and are likely to discover it only once they actually get an AIDS-related illness. Second, 'there is worrying evidence of antiretroviral drug resistance among some newly HIV-infected individuals in Western Europe'. They suggest, therefore, that 'the main challenges are to provide early and effective treatment and care to all HIV-infected people, to rejuvenate prevention efforts and adapt them to the changing patterns of the epidemic, and to reduce the psychosocial, economic and physical repercussions of HIV infection'.[2]

Acquired immune deficiency syndrome is not only unique from a biological point of view. Because its spread is so clearly linked to certain patterns of human *behaviour*, especially sexual behaviour, it is truly both a biological and a socio-cultural phenomenon. As such, any attempt to control its spread cannot focus only on the search for a vaccine or a pharmacological cure. It must also take into account the complex social, cultural and economic environments in which the disease is embedded, and which may either help or hinder its spread.

The following section outlines some of the many ways that research in medical anthropology (and other social sciences) can, and already has, contributed towards an understanding of these various socio-cultural factors.

METAPHORS OF AIDS IN THE WESTERN WORLD

Acquired immune deficiency syndrome is not just a disease. Like the plague, cancer and tuberculosis before it, AIDS in the popular perception has become a *metaphor* – or rather a cluster of metaphors – and a vehicle for expressing many of the fears and anxieties of modern life. Their use in the media, and in both medical and popular discourses, may play a political role, stigmatizing and alienating even further those groups (such as homosexuals, drug addicts or immigrants) said to be most at risk of the disease.[3] Thus Frankenberg[4], in his analysis of the portrayal of AIDS in modern literature, points out that 'the paradox that AIDS is popularly seen both as a disease of the few and other, and as the ultimate threat to the many and same'. These ways of talking about AIDS, and the prejudices and the fears associated with them, can undermine attempts to identify, treat and control the disease, and to offer its victims the care and compassion they deserve. Thus the moral and ideological attitudes of a society towards AIDS are just as relevant to its control as is the search for an effective vaccine. As Clatts and Mutchler[5] note, it is therefore important to examine 'what society does to people with words and the images the words evoke'. They note that a culture's metaphors play a prominent role in defining the identity of ourselves, and of others, and how we relate to one another. In the USA, the discourse on AIDS has often defined the victim as the ultimate 'other' – 'alien, antisocial, unnatural, dangerous and threatening'. They describe how, gradually, the images of illness and evil have merged, until to say someone 'has AIDS' is also to say that they are 'dangerous and untouchable', and their disease a manifestation of their inner 'moral evil and/or mental illness'. Stigmatized groups such as homosexuals and drug addicts are often associated with images of a personality type that is 'compulsive, out of control, and maladjusted'. Clatts and Mutchler point out that this identification of AIDS only with the deviant 'other', as well as overconfidence in the powers of medicine to cure the disease, may be dangerous, since it 'has lulled the American public into believing that they are "safe" so long as they adhere to the virtuous venting of desire'.

Powerful and negative metaphors of AIDS were particularly common during the early years of the epidemic. They are less prevalent today in most developed countries, even though HIV/AIDS still carries a significant stigma in many other parts of the world. In North America and Western Europe of the 1980s and early 1990s, a number of recurrent images or metaphors of AIDS could be identified, particularly in the lurid headlines of the popular press, and which included the following:

1 AIDS as a *plague* (sometimes even called 'the gay plague').[6] This image echoed those of medieval pestilence or plague mentioned above; that is, of an invisible, spreading destructive force that brings with it chaos, disorder and the breakdown of ordered society, family life and interpersonal relationships.

2 AIDS as an invisible *contagion*. In this image, apparently based on older folk models of infectious diseases, AIDS was viewed as an unseen influence transmitted by virtually any contact with an infected person, whether this contact is with the body surface, body wastes or even with the air that they breathe. This invisible influence could occur at work, school, home or even at church. Like medieval theories of disease, it was as if the sufferer were surrounded by an infected miasma, or cloud of poisonous 'bad air', which caused disease in others nearby. Implicit in this image was the idea that the sexual lifestyles of sufferers from the disease might also be contagious to those around them.

3 AIDS as *moral punishment*. In this image, victims of the disease were usually divided into two groups: those who were 'innocent' (the accidental recipients of blood transfusions,

such as haemophiliacs and children, and the spouses of those who were bisexual or who engaged in extramarital sex); and those who were 'guilty' (such as homosexual men, bisexuals, promiscuous people, prostitutes and intravenous drug users).[7] This particular image of AIDS is still prominent in some popular press coverage of the disease.

4 AIDS as *invader*. This is an image that usually included themes of xenophobia and foreign invasion, since it often involved prejudices against foreigners, immigrants and tourists, especially Africans, Haitians and others.

5 AIDS as *war*. This image may be linked with the previous one, where AIDS was seen as a war waged on conventional society by immoral lifestyles, promiscuity, foreign influences and stigmatized minorities (such as gays, prostitutes, immigrants or drug abusers); here, heterosexual victims of the disease were sometimes depicted as if they were 'collateral damage' – innocent civilian casualties caught up in the crossfire of a war.[8]

6 AIDS as a *primitive* or pre-social force or entity. This was a similar image to that of cancer described above, but characterized more by images of childlike hedonism and unrestrained and unconventional sexuality.

Although these metaphors are much less commonly used today (at least in the Western media), they still remain potent in many communities worldwide. When attached in popular discourse to the very word 'AIDS', they have often been used for political purposes, especially to stigmatize even further certain groups in society, such as homosexuals, immigrants and drug abusers. However, from a medical anthropology perspective, these metaphors are dangerous for many reasons, and especially because they may impede any rational assessment of the risks of the disease and how it is to be recognized, controlled, prevented and treated. Watney[9] has noted how the 'moral panic' and prejudice in most media commentary on AIDS makes any rational evaluation of the disease very difficult, since these prejudices 'heavily overdetermine all discussion of the virus'. Cominos and colleagues[10] also pointed out that the only way to prevent person-to-person transmission is by education, 'which is only effective if predicated upon in-depth understanding of prevailing knowledge, attitudes and practices related to HIV infection in diverse societies and subgroups'. However, such research on the transmission of AIDS will not be possible if the stigmas and metaphors attached to it make many people unwilling to come forward for diagnosis and treatment.

Another danger of AIDS metaphors is that the imagery of moral punishment and the overemphasis on stigmatized subcultures such as gay men or intravenous drug users may prevent AIDS patients from getting the compassionate care and medical treatment that they deserve. For example, Cassens[6] has described the serious social and psychological consequences that gay men diagnosed as having AIDS often have to suffer, including rejection by family or others. At a time of major psychological stress they may also have to undergo what may be termed a 'social death' of isolation, and the withdrawal of social support (see Chapters 9 and 11).

Therefore, as the examples of AIDS and cancer illustrate, under some circumstances certain serious medical *diseases* can also become forms of *folk illness*, and this can seriously impair the recognition, diagnosis, management and control of these conditions.

CULTURAL REPRESENTATIONS OF AIDS

Acquired immune deficiency syndrome is a global disease, but different human groups differ widely in their understanding of its origins, significance and modes of spread, as well as in the meanings they ascribe to it. This is a further example of the split between 'disease' and 'illness' described in Chapter 5. In many ways, AIDS has become the pre-eminent folk illness of the modern age, absorbing, in each local context, a variety of indigenous images, metaphors and cultural themes. As in all forms of human misfortune, these provide answers to questions that people ask themselves, such as 'why *me*?' and 'why *now*?'

In many countries now, widespread publicity about AIDS has led some anxious or depressed individuals to develop what may be termed *folk AIDS*. This is a type of illness without disease that has also been termed 'pseudo-AIDS'[11] or 'AIDS neurosis',[12] and in which people become convinced that they have the disease, even though there is no medical evidence for this. One reason for this, as Miller and colleagues[11] point out, may be that the early symptoms of AIDS, such as lethargy, loss of appetite and weight and excessive sweating, are similar to those of anxiety and depression, and some individuals may thus misinterpret them. In Japan, Miller[12] has reported the widespread incidence of 'AIDS neurosis' – the first case being reported in 1985 – with many officials convinced that it is 'a distinctly Japanese illness'. She quotes one AIDS counsellor as saying: 'Japanese are at much greater risk for developing AIDS neurosis, than they are of getting AIDS'. The syndrome is usually characterized by somatic complaints, depression, sleep disturbances, suicidal ideas and the delusion, despite evidence to the contrary, that they are HIV seropositive.

In other contexts, cultural representations of AIDS may be a blend of medical and indigenous beliefs – a physical disease but also a punishment for sinful behaviour. For example, Ingstad[13] described how, in Botswana, traditional healers knew of AIDS, but saw it as just a new form of *meila*, a folk illness caused by the breaking of certain sexual taboos (see below). In the USA, Flaskerud and Rush[14] found similar beliefs among some African-Americans, with AIDS being seen as 'punishment for sin', a result of breaking religious and moral laws, especially those against homosexuality or extramarital sex. These cultural representations are not static, however. Anthropologists have shown how they can change over time as new information (often from health education programmes) is received and then blended with older, more traditional beliefs, as illustrated in the following case history.

Case study: changing concepts of AIDS in Do Kay, Haiti

Farmer[15] described how concepts of acquired immune deficiency syndrome (AIDS) (*syndrome d'immunodéfiecence acquise*, or *sida*) gradually changed during the period 1983–89, in the rural village of Do Kay, Haiti. In 1983–84, the village had heard only vague rumours of a 'city disease' (*maladi lavil*); very few knew how it was transmitted, or how serious it was. By 1985–86, and drawing on folk models of illness causation, the idea had become common that *sida* was a 'sickness of the blood', something that 'spoils your blood, and makes you have so little blood that you become pale and dry'. Partly owing to public health programmes, these beliefs gradually became linked to vague understandings of *sida* as caused by an irreversible pollution resulting from blood transfusions or same-sex relations, as well as by weakness from overwork in the city, or by travel to the USA. In 1987, a consensus about the symptoms of *sida* had begun to develop, especially its association with diarrhoea and tuberculosis. That same year, the first resident of Do Kay fell ill with the disease; this was widely blamed on a 'sent sickness', or sorcery, due to envy. The victim's family consulted a voodoo priest, who confirmed this, and identified certain individuals responsible for it. When another villager fell ill with the disease, though, most did not believe that she actually had *sida*, as she was considered 'too innocent' to be the victim of envy. By 1988–89, after both villagers had died and a third had fallen ill, a consensus about the disease had developed in Do Kay. *Sida* was seen as two entities, both caused by a microbe: a 'natural' illness, caused by sexual contact with someone who 'carries the germ', and an 'unnatural' illness sent by sorcery from a malicious person. Condoms were helpful against the former, but useless against the latter. The 'unnatural' *sida* could only be prevented by using charms that could 'protect you against any kind of sickness that a person would send you'.

Thus, as Farmer pointed out, over the 6-year period 'the term *sida* and the syndrome with which it is associated came to be embedded in a series of distinctly Haitian ideas about illness'. These in turn link the sudden appearance of the disease to wider social and political issues, which he described as 'the endless suffering of the Haitian people, divine punishment, the corruption of the ruling class, and the ills of North American imperialism'.

PUBLIC AND PROFESSIONAL KNOWLEDGE OF AIDS

In many parts of the world, increasing numbers of education programmes have tried to disseminate knowledge about AIDS to the public. However, for a variety of reasons, large numbers of people are still unaware of how it is transmitted, how it can be prevented, and the types of symptoms to look out for. Even if they have been told, they may not understand the underlying concepts; in some communities, for example, not everyone is familiar with the germ theory of disease, and therefore they may not be sure what exactly is meant by 'a virus'. Neither do they understand how this tiny, invisible, intangible entity can cause them to be ill.

Misconceptions about AIDS are still common, though they were more so in the 1980s and 1990s, than they are today. In a study in Walsall, UK, in 1988 for example, Smithson[16] found good general knowledge of AIDS (90 per cent had got their information from television and 80 per cent from newspaper articles), but also some significant misconceptions about how it could be spread. Twenty-six per cent, for example, thought they could get it from giving a blood donation, 16.1 per cent from sharing crockery or cutlery and 15.6 per cent by using a toilet previously used by an AIDS patient. As part of the same study, health personnel (such as nurses and laboratory technicians) were asked the same questions: 17.8 per cent of them also believed AIDS could be caught by donating blood and over half were fearful that they could catch AIDS from patients. In another study of 399 individuals in San Francisco, New York and London, Temoshok and colleagues[17] found that a general fear of AIDS, as well as antigay prejudice, was associated with a low knowledge of AIDS; there was a lower level of knowledge and higher level of general fear of the disease in London, compared with San Francisco, with New York intermediate between the two. From this study, however, it was 'not clear whether fear and… prejudice promote ignorance, or whether ignorance increases fear and prejudice'. In either case, knowledge of the disease is not enough; the role of irrational fears and prejudices is also important in determining whether people change their behaviour or not.

Snow[18] in 1993 described how, in some poor urban neighbourhoods, African-American folk beliefs also ascribed AIDS to 'toilets', 'filth', 'touching', 'kissing' and 'mosquitoes'. Some see it as evidence of 'bad blood' ('So many things can go wrong with your blood; like AIDS, a lot of things will give you impure blood'), others as the result of 'lowered resistance' to impurities, poor health habits, exposure to cold, improper nutrition, or 'a body weakened by menstruation'. The belief that mosquitoes can transmit the disease has also been found in Namibia, as has the notion that asymptomatic carriers are not infectious.[19]

Knowledge about how to prevent AIDS is particularly important among the young, though it may not necessarily be translated into action. In Brazil, for example, the largest and most populous nation in South America, 26 per cent of its population is under the age of 20 years, and AIDS is an increasing health problem.[20] In a large study of a student population (aged 13–22 years) in Porto Alegre, southern Brazil in 1993, De Souza and colleagues[20] found that while 95 per cent had high levels of knowledge about the physiology of reproduction, this did not always translate into safer sex precautions. While 42 per cent of the sample had already had a sexual relationship, and 35 per cent had sex at least once weekly, 52 per cent of them did not take any systematic or regular contraceptive precautions. Whatever the reasons for this, the authors conclude that this situation places many Brazilian teenagers at a high risk for unwanted pregnancies, as well as for sexually transmitted diseases such as AIDS.

Although such studies of beliefs about AIDS and its prevention may be useful in providing a baseline for future health education, anthropologists have often warned that beliefs and behaviours are not necessarily identical; people may not actually do what they say they do (see Chapter 19). Research indicates that knowledge of risk does not, in itself, always result in a change of behaviour, as shown by the many people who continue to smoke, drink and drive under the influence of alcohol, despite knowledge of the many risks involved.[16] The psychological reasons for this 'split' are complex, and often ill understood. On a social level, as illustrated below, factors such as gender inequality and poverty play a major role. On an individual level, the reasons may include a belief that one is 'lucky' or 'blessed' (and thus immune to danger), a subconscious desire to be damaged or killed or even a craving for the excitement of risk-taking. As one study of the sexual behaviour of young men in a Thai village put it, 'HIV provides another opportunity to test their invulnerability; to display a badge of courage to their friends'.[21] Thus, studies of beliefs and behaviours often require further anthropological investigation in order to understand why people behave (or do not behave) in a particular way, despite the health education messages that they have been exposed to.

SOCIAL DIMENSIONS OF AIDS

People diagnosed as having AIDS (or as being HIV positive) often become the victims of discrimination and prejudice, or even of violence. In extreme cases, this social rejection may lead to the 'social death' described in Chapter 9. Anthropological studies can provide baseline data on the attitudes, prejudices and stereotypes about AIDS held by the rest of the population, and the degree of stigma attached to it. Katz and colleagues,[22] for example, interviewed a group of 433 adults – mainly nurses, medical students and chiropractic students – in New York City in 1987 about how they perceived sufferers from serious diseases, including AIDS. The study revealed that AIDS is a 'severely stigmatizing condition', and for all groups in the sample the status of AIDS sufferers was as 'social deviants who are seen as themselves responsible for having this disease'. In Owambo, Namibia, Webb[19] also found that AIDS was a highly stigmatized disease, and that many believed that 'those who are infected will knowingly infect others, either deliberately through some malicious motive, or as a result of their inability to remain abstinent'. As Temoshok and colleagues[17] note, there are 'cultural differences in the degree of interaction with and prejudice against the higher risk groups based on fear of the disease'. Data on these differences, therefore, can be used to design public education programmes that aim at decreasing ignorance of the disease, and irrational fear of it. However, stigma does not attach only to the so-called high-risk groups and individuals in society. Stanley[23], in her study of white middle-class women with HIV, has shown how in the USA (as elsewhere) stigma extends also to all parts of the population who are HIV positive, irrespective of their sexual orientation, gender, economic status or ethnicity.

One growing area of research is into the *social networks* of those with HIV. Not only is this useful in tracking the spread of the virus, but it enables understanding of the social context of at-risk behaviours, such as syringe-sharing or unprotected sex. Thus Parker and her colleagues[24] have investigated the sexual networks of HIV-positive men in London, in order to identify how at-risk behaviours help spread the virus. Certain situations, such as sex between older and younger men, or between male prostitutes and their clients, were identified as particularly likely to spread the infection throughout a much wider network of people. In New York City, Neaigus and colleagues[25] have shown how the 'risk networks' of intravenous drug users often overlap with their social networks; that is, people shared syringes mainly with those with

whom they were already closely involved. Thus 70 per cent injected or shared syringes with a spouse or sex partner, a close friend or someone that they knew fairly well. This implies that changing risk networks can be very difficult, since these networks are an important part of addicts' daily lives (see Chapter 8). However, these same social ties with other drug-users can be a useful route – in the form of peer pressure and emotional support – through which to spread messages about the ways to reduce high-risk behaviours. For example, these ties can be used to develop a collective self-organization of drug injectors, 'in order to make HIV risk reduction a permanent feature of drug injectors' subculture'.

Anthropologists can therefore often help identify the social networks, self-help groups and other community resources that can be mobilized to help those with AIDS, and which can then be integrated into their long-term treatment. This is particularly important in cities since, in Western countries especially, AIDS is predominantly an *urban* disease. By the end of 1991, for example, nearly 20 per cent (37 436) of all AIDS cases identified in the USA were reported in New York City, which was second only to San Francisco in the cumulative numbers of cases per 10 000 population.[26] Despite their anomie, urban environments offer some advantages over rural ones for people with AIDS: greater concentration of medical resources; more developed support networks and self-help groups; and a greater tolerance of diverse lifestyles. They also facilitate the development of gay subcultures, with their own practices and view of the world. In some cases, this subculture may be detrimental to health. In the USA in 2001, the Urban Men's Health Study[27] identified a high prevalence of recreational drug use (52 per cent) and alcohol use (85 per cent) among urban gay men, and this could have major consequences for their health. While their rate of alcohol use was comparable to other urban men, their rate of drug use was higher than that of the general male population.

Health education programmes therefore need to take into account both the social and cultural diversity of urban populations, and the many different kinds of community support available for those with the disease.

SEXUAL PRACTICES AND BEHAVIOUR

The spread of AIDS is closely linked to sexual behaviours, but this intimate area of human relationships has always been notoriously difficult to study. In recent years, however, a number of anthropological studies have begun to remedy this situation, and have provided useful data for public health programmes. These studies reveal that patterns of 'normal' and 'abnormal' sexual behaviour (heterosexual and homosexual) differ widely between, and within, different societies. For example, anal intercourse has been reported as being relatively common among both heterosexuals and homosexuals in Brazil,[28] compared with some other countries. Another example is the significant variation found world-wide in the incidence of extramarital sex, and the fact that in most societies it is commoner among men than among women (see Chapter 6); this is a crucial fact, because in many parts of the world AIDS is increasingly becoming a heterosexual disease.[21] Furthermore, where such double standards of sexual morality exist, with women (but not men) expected to be chaste, faithful and virginal at marriage, women may be put at risk from their husband's behaviour, especially their recourse to prostitutes.[29]

In Mexico, Carrier[30] describes the significance for AIDS prevention of the cultural values of urban (and mainly *mestizo*) males. These include the importance of family, manliness (*machismo*), strict gender roles, the dichotomization of women as being either 'good' or 'bad', and the shame attached to homosexuality. As in Brazil,[28] the sharp division of gender roles means that there are two distinct groups of homosexual men: those that play the active, insertive 'masculine' (*activo*) role, and those that are passive (*pasivo*) and penetrable. Only the second group is considered to be truly homosexual, as well as 'feminine'. The *activo* group is not stigmatized as homosexual – 'the mas-

culine self-image of Mexican males is thus not threatened by their homosexual behaviour as long as the appropriate role is played and they also have sexual relations with women'. That is, 'although involved in bisexual behaviour, they consider themselves to be heterosexual'. The emphasis on *machismo* encourages males to have 'multiple, uncommitted sexual contacts which start in adolescence' as a sign of manliness. In contrast, the dichotomization of women into 'good' (virginal, faithful, respectable) and 'bad' (those who have already acquired a 'spoiled identity') is accompanied by constraints on female sexual behaviour that can last 10–12 years, from adolescence to young adulthood. During this period it is the 'bad' women who are sought after; they may play the role of prostitute (*puta*), lover (*amante*) or common-law wife. In some cases, homosexual partners may offer 'a free or certainly a lower-cost alternative to whatever female partners are available'. Carrier also points out that after marriage, 'male extramarital relationships may be only with females, but they may also include or be only with males'. Overall, he concludes that 'more sexually active single males in Mexico have had sexual intercourse with both genders than have Anglo-American males'. In terms of preventive strategies, he suggests that, as most bisexual and homosexual men live with their families, a national health education campaign should focus on the family rather than individuals, educating the family about the importance of safer sex practices by their members. Another useful strategy, given widespread poverty in some areas, would be increased availability of free or low-cost condoms, as well as of spermicidal lubricants (for those playing the *pasivo* role).

ATTITUDES TO CONDOM USE

Despite decades of advice about the need for 'safe sex', and the value of condoms in preventing HIV infection, many people in high-risk groups still continue to reject them. In some cases this is because of the condoms being unavailable or unaffordable (Figures 16.2 and 16.3). In others it may be due to certain cultural attitudes towards them. As Whitehead[31] notes, condoms often have a 'symbolic power' or socio-cultural meaning in different communities, which can affect people's response to them. Schoepf[32] described some of the widespread folk beliefs about condom use, and their supposed dangers for women, in parts of Central and East Africa. These include infections, permanent sterility and even death, should a condom break and remain inside the vagina. In Uganda, Obbo[33] described how these fears have had a major effect, since some women see condoms as threatening to their reproductive health. In a society where there is social pressure on them (as on men) to prove their fertility, where barren women are pitied and

mothers are respected, and where women gain access to social status and resources by marriage and child-bearing, the risks of condom use seemed high. Added to this was the opposition of some Ugandan churches, and the authorities' belief that easy availability of condoms promotes promiscuity. Elsewhere, Preston-Whyte[34] has described other folk beliefs, in South Africa, about how the condom itself may cause AIDS, or that because it holds bodily fluids these may be mis-used by sorcerers.

Men in many countries reject condom use for a number of reasons, often related to beliefs about its effect on reducing sexual sensation ('taking a shower in a raincoat'). In other cases, these beliefs may be related to other aspects of masculine identity. In a study of urban, low-income African-

Figure 16.2 Street poster in Cambodia promoting safe sex and the use of condoms to prevent acquired immune deficiency syndrome (AIDS). (Source: © Sean Sprague/Panos Pictures. Reproduced with permission.)

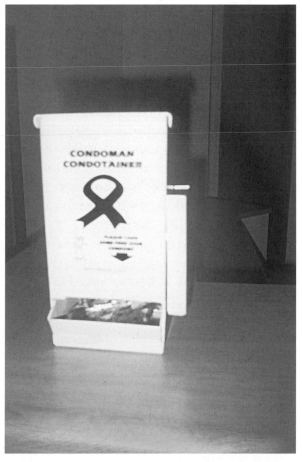

Figure 16.3 A condom dispenser in a primary care clinic in Transkei, South Africa.

American men in Baltimore, Whitehead[31] found that barriers to condom use may be linked to:

- ideas about the importance of fathering children, as part of male identity
- sexual prowess, and conquests, as evidence of masculine attractiveness
- economic capability, as an attribute of masculine status and power.

In this community, as in many others world-wide, men's core identity and sense of self-esteem (especially that of younger men) may lead them to take many risks in their daily lives. Not using a condom is just another form of risk-taking behaviour, among many others.

Women are often reluctant to initiate condom use, in case they are seen as being too sexually experienced and too 'forward' in their behaviour.[35] Others may feel that to suggest a condom may threaten the survival of their relationship, damaging intimacy by suggesting that they don't trust their sexual partner. But another major issue here is the differential in *power* – physical, social and economic – between women and men in many societies. Often younger or poorer women feel unable to resist the pressure from men not to use a condom.[21] This is particularly the case with prostitutes, who in any case may use condoms with clients, but prefer not to use them with in their more intimate relationships with boyfriends (see below).

The easy availability of condoms, combined with a greater knowledge about AIDS, does not necessarily result in a decrease in sexually risky behaviour. For example, Kapiga and Lugalla[36] examined the sexual behavior and use of condoms of a sample of 10 000 people in Tanzania, between 1991/2 and 1996. During that period both the government and non-governmental organizations (NGOs) had actively promoted the use of condoms, as an important part of AIDS prevention. However, there was only a modest increase in condom use (from 9.3 per cent to 15.2 per cent) during those years, and little change in sexual behaviour. In fact, there was some evidence that

increased condom use, especially among younger people, was correlated with a greater level of high-risk sexual behaviour, such as having other sexual partners outside of marriage, or outside a steady relationship. This pattern was less marked, though, among more educated women. The study points out that 'it is important to realize that simply targeting groups of people who are likely to practice high-risk behaviours without changing the social environment within which such people live is unlikely to be effective.' In Tanzania this includes poverty, increasing unemployment, and gender inequality.

PATTERNS OF FEMALE AND MALE PROSTITUTION

In many parts of the world, prostitution, both male and female, is an important source of HIV infection,[37] as it is of other sexually transmitted diseases. Like other forms of human behaviour, prostitution can only be fully understood in terms of the specific cultural and social *context* in which it appears. For example, the Western model of 'career' (or full-time) prostitution, tacitly tolerated by the authorities within a red light district, may not be applicable elsewhere. In many poorer countries, prostitution is a more complex phenomenon. It may involve, for example, what may be termed 'episodic prostitution', where, for economic reasons, women (and less commonly men) sell sex before or during marriage, or after being widowed or divorced. Their prostitution career may last only a few months or years, interspersed with marriage and/or childbearing. Thus, prostitutes are not a homogeneous group, and within the same city or region several different types of prostitution may be found. Carrier[30] notes how a study in Mexico identified nine different types of prostitutes selling their services to male clientele from all social classes: 'street walkers; itinerant travellers; dance hostesses and barmaids; taxi girls; professionals living in brothels; semi-professionals; lovers (*amantes*); call girls; and companions for parties or vacations'. Each of these types of commercial sexual activity offers different types of risk of AIDS transmission, and may well require a different form of intervention.

In most settings, *poverty* and the economic dependence of women are major causes of female prostitution, especially in its 'episodic' form. They may be widowed, divorced or abandoned by husbands, and forced into it to feed their families, or their husband may be too sick or elderly to work. In some parts of Africa they may have to repay the 'bridewealth' paid for them by their husband, after getting divorced, or if they do not wish to be 'inherited' by their dead husband's brother (see below). In their personal lives they may thus be wives, mothers or grandmothers, and have other sexual relationships that are not in any way commercial. In other cases, as described by Webb[19] in northern Namibia, 'transactional sex' may be a much more informal arrangement between adolescent boys and girls, or between a girl and an older man. In this case the girls do not, in any way, consider themselves to be prostitutes. Prostitution, however, is not the only economic strategy available to women in poorer regions; as Pickering and Wilkins[38] found in the Gambia, West Africa, there are other ways that divorced or widowed women can make a living, which do not involve selling sex, such as working as a laundress, hairdresser or cook, or selling groundnuts, fruit or alcohol.

Lyttleton[21] described how in Thailand urban dwellers earn nine times the income of rural people, and many 'commercial sex workers' from these poor villages will spend several years in Bangkok building up capital before returning to their villages to raise a family. In the rural areas themselves, commercial sex, though less common, also exists, and a more permissive attitude to sex has spread from city to countryside. In some cities, too, young female students occasionally sell sex at discos or in their dormitories.

Even if prostitutes are willing to adopt 'safe sex' practices, their clients (who have the ultimate economic control in the situation) may object. For example, Leonard's study[37] of 50 male clients of female prostitutes in Camden, New Jersey, showed that 29 had refused to use a condom. Despite being aware of the dangers involved, they tried to 'minimize' this risk by various strategies, including choosing a woman who looked 'clean', 'well-groomed', relatively inexperienced, or free of drugs. Others preferred oral to vaginal sex, believing it to be safer. Thus, because 'condom use is one of the most important points of negotiation for disease prevention between sex partners', AIDS prevention programmes should target not only prostitutes but their clients as well. However, as Waddell's study[35] in Perth, Australia suggests, even if prostitutes are willing to use condoms with clients, they may still refuse to use them in their more intimate relationships with boyfriends or husbands.

As well as female prostitution, male and bisexual commercial sex are a feature of several societies. These include different forms of male prostitution, such as the 'masculine' (*miche*) and more 'feminine' transvestites (*travesti*) in Brazil[28] and the *activo* and *pasivo* in Mexico.[30] In societies with a sexual double-standard (as in many parts of Latin America and elsewhere), where adolescent and young adult males are encouraged to have sex but their female counterparts are not, the risk of prostitute use may be increased. Similarly, in several parts of Africa[39] a late marriage age for men, often combined with the need to accumulate a large 'bridewealth' to pay a prospective wife's father, may also increase this risk.

Thus, interventions to reduce HIV transmission in prostitution need to take into account the economic, social and cultural context in which this type of behaviour takes place. They also need to consider the intimate emotional relationships in which prostitutes are involved, and their possible role in the transmission of the disease.

INTRAVENOUS DRUG USE AND NEEDLE-SHARING

In the USA, intravenous drug users (IVDUs) are the second largest at risk group for AIDS.[40] Of the

41 960 new cases of AIDS reported in 2000, 28 per cent were associated with the intravenous use of drugs.[41] In many other industrialized countries, the situation is similar; in Edinburgh, UK, for example, an estimated 60 per cent of the injecting drug users in the city are now HIV positive. In Spain, the spread of intravenous drug use in the population since 1978 has also lead to a wider diffusion of the AIDS virus throughout the country.[42] Increasingly, IVDUs have become an important source of HIV exposure for the heterosexual population.

Detailed ethnographic studies indicate that IVDUs, and the addict subcultures that they form, are *not* homogeneous; they vary in motivations, attitudes, sexual behaviours, social networks, the actual drugs they use and the techniques of injection that they employ. In most cases, however, the sharing of needles is a major source of HIV infection, though it sometimes overlaps with other at risk behaviours. Page and colleagues[40] studied 230 injecting drug users, most of them African-American, living in poor neighbourhoods in Miami, Florida. Of the sample, 104 were found to be HIV positive, and this was clearly correlated with their practice of needle sharing. In preparing for injection, not only were needles often shared among them, but many also cleaned their syringes in the same jar of water or drew their drugs from the same receptacle. In addition, 136 of the sample had, at one time or another in their lives, traded sex for money; of these people, 45 (33 women and 12 men) had worked as prostitutes for periods ranging from a few months to several years before the study began.

In 1989 in another study of 438 IVDUs in San Francisco, USA, Newmeyer and colleagues[43] found that more than 90 per cent of them admitted to recent sharing of needles and syringes (though only 9 per cent of the sample were HIV positive). While 86 per cent said they cleaned their needles between sharing episodes, this was not done consistently, and much of this cleaning consisted of only a simple water rinse. Part of the reason for needle sharing was that at that stage (1985–86) there was a chronic shortage of needles, as public policy made

it illegal to possess them (unless for certain 'medically arranged circumstances'). Newmeyer and colleagues suggest, therefore, that IVDUs could prevent the spread of AIDS in four ways: by stopping drug use completely; failing that, by not injecting the drugs; if injecting, by not sharing needles and other equipment; and by disinfecting the injecting equipment that is being shared. Their research indicated that only the last option would be acceptable to most IVDUs, and that it could be done effectively by cleaning the equipment with household bleach. They also concluded, however, that because 'changing sexual practices of IVDUs will be more difficult than changing their needle-using behaviour', the focus of interventions should be mainly on the latter.

Sibthorpe,[44] in a study in Oregon, USA, in 1992, examined the reasons why so many IVDUs refused to use condoms and practise 'safe sex'. Of the 161 drug users interviewed, the vast majority did not use condoms regularly (but 58 per cent of the sample saw their risk of contracting HIV as zero or slight). The use of condoms correlated with the types of sexual relationships they were involved in; the greater the social (and emotional) distance between partners (such as that between prostitute and client), the more likely they were to use them. In more intimate relationships, though, there was resistance to them; not using a condom was equated with love and trust – the very basis and proof of intimacy. Thus some prostitutes would use condoms with clients, but not with their husbands or boyfriends ('that's my man, that's the difference'). In this situation, the condom can thus be seen as a form of 'symbolic skin' (see Chapter 2) and a barrier to intimacy between these two people. Sibthorpe points out that in the USA, AIDS prevention has focused on the 'personal responsibility model' of risky behaviours, rather than on the relationships in which they occur. Because sex within an intimate relationship is 'one of the bases of human social relations', condom use in these close relationships can be deeply threatening to both partners, signifying either guilt or suspicion and calling into question 'the commitment, attachment, and exclusivity' of the relationship. She therefore concludes that the 'greatest gains in safer sex practices can be expected in those relationships that only minimally affirm social bonds', while in more intimate relationships, changing to condom use may be much more difficult.

Thus, as Page and colleagues[40] warn, 'inter-community variations in self-injection practices are potentially infinite, and each variant may be accompanied by different kinds of risks of HIV infection'. For this reason, strategies developed for one country, region, city or community may not be completely appropriate for another, and specific local conditions must always be taken into account.

A further issue is that some other forms of drug-use, where drugs are not actually injected, may increase the risk of HIV. For example, Sanchez and colleagues[45] report the case of heroin-sniffers in South Florida, USA, whose risk of contracting HIV is increased by other forms of behaviour related to their heroin use, such as having sex with multiple partners (including with IVDUs), insufficient use of condoms and prostitution in order to pay for their drug habit.

TRADITIONAL AND ALTERNATIVE HEALERS AND AIDS

Studies of health care pluralism (see Chapter 4) in both richer and poorer parts of the world are also relevant to AIDS research. As in other serious diseases, such as cancer, chronic pain or disability,[46] for which medicine can offer no 'quick fix', many AIDS patients may choose to use different types of self-treatment or to consult with traditional or alternative practitioners. Self-treatment is especially common in the industrialized world (see below). In a study in gay men with AIDS in West Hollywood, California, USA,[47] for example, while 92 per cent were currently using biomedical treatments, 69.2 per cent were also using one or more alternative therapies at the same time, and a further 19.3 per cent had used them in the past. Thus, only 11.5 per cent had never made use of any form of alternative therapy.

In some cases, communities may consult traditional or religious healers in an attempt to prevent the disease striking in the first place, and these healers may become useful allies in controlling the spread of the disease. In Botswana, Ingstad[13] describes how the various traditional Tswana healers – such as the *ngaka ya diatola* ('doctor of the bones'), *ngaka ya dishotswa* ('doctor of herbs') and *profiti* (a 'prophet' of the Independent African Churches) – often have different attitudes to the origins and treatment of AIDS. Some see it as a 'modern disease', which traditional medicine is unable to help. Others see it as a 'Tswana disease', a version of *meila* (an indigenous folk illness) that they could treat by traditional methods. In this condition, disease and misfortune are ascribed to the breaking of sexual taboos, which forbid intercourse within certain periods of time, such as during menstruation or shortly after childbirth. This makes men vulnerable to 'pollution' originating within the female body (in her blood), which the man can then transmit to any other women with whom he has intercourse. As with AIDS, blood and semen are seen as the vehicles for transmission of the 'pollution'. Ingstad suggests that in the future Tswana traditional healers may have an important role to play in AIDS prevention by, for example, encouraging the use of condoms: 'Advocating condoms as a way to prevent *meila* probably carries more incentive than advocating them to prevent pregnancy or other sexually transmitted diseases'.

Green[48] points out that elsewhere in Africa there is also an urgent need for a closer collaborative relationship between traditional healers and the health authorities, especially where doctors and nurses are in short supply. He notes that the healer' new role will require some education and training, and that they would be especially useful in: (1) referring cases of sexually transmitted diseases (STDs) to the health system; (2) identifying and locating the sexual partners of clients infected with STDs; (3) advocating the use of 'barrier' methods of birth control, such as condoms, as well as of spermicides; (4) influencing sexual behaviour towards more faithful, single-partner relationships; (5) influencing people to adopt less risky sexual practices (such as 'thigh sex') as an alternative to penetrative sex; and (6) providing counselling and emotional support to clients with HIV and AIDS, and their families.

In terms of the treatments for AIDS offered by non-medical healers in different cultures, further studies are urgently needed on their efficacy (or lack of efficacy). It should be noted, however, that in some cases folk definitions of efficacy might be different from those of biomedicine. For example, both religious and secular forms of symbolic healing (see Chapter 10) may be very helpful to sufferers and their families, since they may be able to 'heal' the individual, even if they cannot 'cure' the disease. Conversely, other forms of folk and alternative healing may have a more negative effect on health. Injectionists, acupuncturists and those who practise ritual scarifications, bleeding or 'cupping' may all inadvertently help the spread of the disease. In either case, anthropology can contribute towards an understanding of the social, psychological and physical effects (on the immune system, for example) not only of secular folk remedies such as herbs, massage, moxibustion, but also of the different forms of symbolic healing practised world-wide.

Finally, it is possible that some IVDUs regard themselves, however perversely, as 'healer's, in their own right, seeing the drugs that they ritually inject into themselves and others as a form of medicine for the physical and psychological symptoms of withdrawal. In that sense, they are acting as what may be termed 'auto-injectionists'.

Case study: alternative approaches to treating HIV/AIDS in the USA

O'Connor[49] has described the many forms of self-treatment and alternative strategies being used in the USA in the mid-1990s, especially by gay men in the PWA (people with AIDS) community. Since the mid-1980s there had been a well-organized grass-roots response to the epidemic, with the proliferation of self-help organizations and networks of information. They aim not only to help those with the disease, but also to promote further research and different forms of treatment, especially as conventional medicine seems to offer little but palliation. She describes dozens of alternative or complementary forms of self-treatment, including:

- nutritional approaches, such as macrobiotic and yeast-free diets, the 'Immune Power Diet', food supplements, antioxidants, and megadoses of vitamins or minerals
- herbal treatments, such as echinacea, ginseng, garlic, St John's wort, aloe vera, astragalus or Bach flower essences
- homoeopathic treatments, such as nux vomica for severe nausea, or arnica for muscular pains)
- traditional Chinese medicine, both herbal preparations and acupuncture
- New Age holistic approaches, such as guided imagery, visualization, therapeutic touch, *reiki*, *Qi Dong* or crystal healing
- psychological and metaphysical approaches, such as religious healing services, prayer, and positive thinking to increase 'psycho-immunity'
- conventional pharmaceuticals used in 'unofficial' ways, or before being given official approval (such as 'underground drugs' obtained from 'guerrilla clinics', treatment study groups or from abroad).

O'Connor points out that most of these treatments are intended to *supplement* rather than supplant conventional medical treatment. For the PWAs, they are ways of taking personal responsibility for their health, and asserting their rights and expertise in their own condition and its treatment.

BODILY MUTILATIONS AND ALTERATIONS

As described in Chapter 2, many of the forms of bodily mutilations practised world-wide can involve risks to health. Among those that may help spread the HIV virus are tattooing, scarification, circumcisions,[50] ear and lip piercing, and the sharing of blood in ceremonies marking membership of a cult or 'blood brotherhood'. Rituals where blood is regularly spilt – by self-flagellation or piercing of the skin – may also sometimes be implicated. All forms of bodily mutilation should therefore be taken into account when planning an AIDS prevention programme. Where a particular cultural group is unwilling to abandon these practices, aid workers may be able to convince them to use sterile needles and instruments and disinfectants (for circumcision or scarification, for example), and to supply these free of charge where necessary. Not all bodily mutilations may be dangerous though: recent research suggests that, in some circumstances, male circumcision can offer some protection against HIV infection.[51]

PATTERNS OF MIGRATION AND THE SPREAD OF AIDS

Studies of regular patterns of population movement, such as those of migrant labourers, seasonal farm workers, truck drivers, travelling businessmen or tourists, are relevant to an understanding of how AIDS spreads within and between different countries. Where people (usually men) migrate as individuals rather than as part of an established family unit, there is a greater risk of acquiring sexually transmitted diseases, including AIDS. For example, Webb's study[19] of the Owambo region of Namibia indicated a number of transmission routes of HIV infection linked to population movements. These included:

- migrant labourers working in mines and urban areas in the south of the country, who had sexual relations there during their absence from home
- traders and truck drivers who travelled regularly along the main trunk road from the south (HIV infection tended to cluster in areas closest

to the roadside, where traffic densities were greatest)
- military personnel stationed at various bases in the area (many of whom had previously lived in Zambia and Angola, during the war for independence).

In Thailand, too, Lyttleton[21] described how large numbers of seasonally migrating workers (including prostitutes) as well as about 200 000 truck drivers 'many of whom ply the length and breadth of the country, stopping at the many truck-stop brothels', may also aid the spread of the disease. As well as these more regular population movements, the creation of refugees, especially the mass uprooting of people by war or civil unrest, may also be related to an increased incidence of certain diseases, including AIDS (see Chapter 12).

Female migrant workers, in particular, are vulnerable to sexual exploitation and abuse, which in turn can increase the dangers of their contracting AIDS – a danger highlighted in Bandyopadhyay and Thomas's study[52] of the 200 000 female migrant workers, many from the Philippines, who are working in Hong Kong as domestic helps. In Western Europe, large numbers of women from Eastern Europe and the former Soviet Union have migrated to work as commercial sex workers in the cities of Western Europe, many of them taken there against their will by 'people traffickers', and they are particularly at risk of contracting the disease, and returning with it to their homelands. Another related issue, especially in developing countries, is the growing level of 'sex tourism', which often involves the sexual exploitation of underage girls and boys by tourists from the richer countries, some of whom may demand sex without the use of condoms.

Finally, the process of migration into cities is also important since, in some cases, social constraints on behaviour may be less powerful than they would be in small rural communities. Overcrowding, contact with people from different backgrounds and exposure to advertising and the media may all weaken these social constraints in an urban environment, and increase the incidence of alcoholism, drug abuse, teenage pregnancies and STDs, especially AIDS. In other cases, population movements to the city may follow a more circular pattern, with newly urbanized people maintaining close links with their rural roots and traditional values, and returning there regularly to visit their families, and *vice versa*.

MARRIAGE AND KINSHIP PATTERNS

In different cultures, certain patterns of kinship and marriage may sometimes increase the risk of the HIV virus spreading within a community. These include *polygyny* (one man, several wives) and *polyandry* (one women, several husbands), 'ghost marriage' and 'women marriage' (see Chapter 6). Polygyny is particularly important, since Ember and Ember[53] estimate that it is still practised in some form in about 70 per cent of human societies. In this situation, a husband who has contracted the HIV virus may thus pass it on to several women, and then on to their children. In addition, some societies which practice the *levirate* (or 'widow inheritance'), where a man is obliged to marry his brother's widow, or the *sororate*, where a woman is obliged to marry her deceased sister's husband,[53] may also be more at risk of the spread of AIDS. In the industrialized world, where the rates of separation, divorce and remarriage are greatly increasing, the effect may sometimes be similar.

AIDS AND SOCIAL INEQUALITY

Acquired immune deficiency syndrome (and other STDs) can only be understood within their particular socio-economic context, especially if it is one of economic and social inequality. That is because one of the most important influences on the disease is *poverty*, which can be both a risk factor for acquiring AIDS and a result of it. Poverty may mean that women or girls have to enter prostitution, in order to support themselves or their chil-

dren, or to pay off a family debt. In that situation it may also mean that neither they nor their clients may be able to afford condoms. Poverty can help concentrate the disease in certain areas, or in certain parts of the population. In South Africa, for example, Fassin[54] relates the extremely high incidence of AIDS in the African population to the legacy of apartheid, with its many decades of economic and social inequality. The resulting poverty and deprivation have resulted in low educational levels, unsafe and overcrowded living conditions, a greater danger of rape and of young women being forced into prostitution, and an economic pressure on men to migrate on their own to the big cities, in order to work in industry or on the mines. All of these factors add up to an increased risk of HIV infection.

In dealing with this situation many poorer countries, especially in Africa, lack basic health facilities, and often have a chronic shortage of drugs to treat the infection, and of medical personnel to administer them. They may also lack the ability to deal with the more serious co-morbidities of HIV/AIDS, such as tuberculosis, malaria, certain pneumonias, and skin lesions.

Acquired immune deficiency syndrome in turn can impoverish individuals, families, communities and even entire countries. The costs of clinics, transport, diagnostic equipment, as well as the salaries of medical and other personnel, can be enormous. AIDS can decimate the labour force of a country, and damage its educational system. In 2003 the BBC[55] reported that in Zambia 1967 teachers had been lost to the disease in 2001, and over 2000 the following year, while in parts of Malawi over 30 per cent of teachers were HIV positive. Even when available, AIDS medications are not cheap. Approaches to therapy such as HAART can involve taking 20 tablets a day or more,[56] though several countries are now trying to develop cheaper versions of these antiretroviral drugs.

Another form of social inequality relevant to the spread of AIDS is *gender* inequality: the differentials in power between men and women. As Lyttelton's study in Thailand[21] illustrated, young women may not have the power to resist the demands of their male partners to have sex without using a condom. This situation is particularly true in the commercial sex industry already described.

All these factors mean that, as part of any AIDS-prevention programme these structural inequalities, both economic and social, need to be addressed – in addition to treating medically those who have already contracted the disease.

EVALUATION OF PREVENTIVE STRATEGIES

Anthropology is useful in the follow-up or *evaluation* of preventive strategies. Because of the diversity of at-risk groups, local interventions are usually also necessary in addition to national (or international) public health campaigns.[19,21] In many communities, outreach programmes have been successful in bringing information about AIDS prevention (as well as condoms and other items) to different communities, and to particular groups of people within them. Daly and Horton[57] point out that 'the best workers are often recruited from the target group itself', whatever that is. Thus some outreach programmes have recruited prostitutes as, in effect, 'community health workers', encouraging them to distribute condoms, spread information about AIDS and refuse to have unprotected sex with their clients.

In San Francisco, community health outreach workers (CHOWs) were used to convince IVDUs of the value of sterilizing their injecting equipment with household bleach and, together with educational literature, they handed out thousands of 1-oz bottles of bleach to them. In London and other European cities, 'needle exchanges' have been set up to supply sterile needles and syringes to addicts, free of charge and with no questions asked.

In Thailand, Lyttleton[21] has described how the comprehensive National AIDS Program, begun in 1989, provides considerable information about AIDS prevention to the population, especially via the media and in schools, clinics and hospitals. At the level of the rural village, however, local custom and belief may make this information less effective in altering behaviour. In one north-eastern village, for example, the people saw some of the at-risk behaviours, including visiting prostitutes, as 'something belonging to city lifestyles' rather than their own. The overemphasis on prostitution as a source of AIDS meant that for some men, sleeping with several different village women is not 'promiscuous', unlike a single visit to a CSW (commercial sex worker). Others avoided cheaper prostitutes, whom they perceived as more likely carriers, but instead used 'good girls', such as students. So many men disliked using condoms that some prostitutes did not insist on their use on every occasion, especially if the clients were 'local government officials who pull rank', young men claiming to be virgins who wanted their first experience to be 'natural' and men regarded as 'respectable' or who were regular clients. Thus Lyttleton emphasizes that, in addition to national campaigns about avoiding at-risk behaviours, 'to understand the spread of HIV, both real and potential, the local meaning attached to these acts is essential knowledge'.[21]

Similarly, Heald[58] has criticized the official AIDS prevention programme in Botswana for not taking into account local social realities and cultural attitudes towards the disease, and for not taking into account the viewpoints of influential local traditional healers and local churches. She points out that many of the anti-AIDS billboards are in English, yet most people speak Setswana. Furthermore, the government's 'ABC' model of prevention (A = Abstain, B = Be faithful, C = Condomise) is largely designed abroad, and the language used in health education 'is the language of western science and policy' (see figure 16.4). It is also the language of individualism, and assumes a particular Western model of individual rational choice, provided only that one is given the 'facts', and told what the choices are. In real life, however, people's choices are contextual: they are often linked closely to social and economic relationships, and many people (especially women) do not have as much autonomy, or control over their lives, as the model implies. Furthermore, the very public nature of the campaign, with its open discussion of sexuality and condoms, has met resistance from the churches, as well as from many parents, who see it as encouraging promiscuity in the population.

Some AIDS prevention programmes may also fail because they assume, quite erroneously, a high level of literacy in their target population, or even access to radio or television. Others may neglect to take into account *economic* influences on behaviour, such as poor, widowed, divorced or abandoned women being forced to work as prostitutes in order to feed their families – a situation that has been called 'survival sex'[59] – or poor village girls in Thailand having to work for several years in the city in order to accumulate money for their future.[21] Other economic constraints include the inability to afford basic medical treatment, including drugs, tests, hospitalization and rehabilitation, and a lack of money to buy condoms or bleach (in the case of IVDUs) or to travel to a clinic to get them. For example, prostitutes who have many clients in a single night may be unable to afford to

supply each with a condom, even if these are available. In poorer countries the economic impact of AIDS is substantial, especially in terms of health-care costs and reduction in the labour force, and any programme must take these facts into account.

A further aspect of programme evaluation is an assessment of the role of national and international bureaucracies in education, research and the provision of medical care (see below). As well as their institutional subcultures (which may either help, or reduce their effectiveness), the economic, political[60] and religious influences on AIDS prevention programmes also need to be assessed, as do the human rights of those who have the disease.[61] The attitudes of health professionals may also have a negative effect on AIDS surveillance and treatment. Some studies have shown how many AIDS victims still distrust the medical system to provide them with effective and non-judgmental health care. For example, a study in 1994 of 632 homosexual men in England[62] found that 44 per cent of them had never informed their general practitioners of their sexual orientation, and that of the 77 who were HIV positive, 44 per cent had not told them of this fact.

On the medical side, the increasing use of treatments such as HAART (especially in the

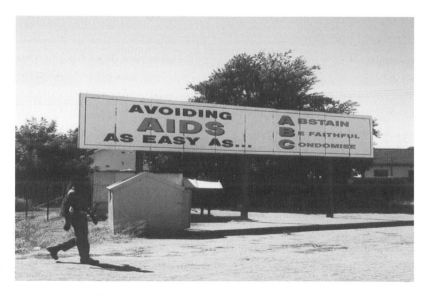

Figure 16.4 Billboard near Gaberone, Botswana promoting the 'A,B,C message to prevent AIDS' (acquired immune deficiency syndrome). (Source: © Suzette Heald. Reproduced with permission.)

developed world) is encouraging, but anthropologists need to caution the medical system about its tendency towards 'cure' rather than 'care', i.e. its over-emphasis on the physical, rather than the psychological, social and cultural aspects of ill health (see Chapter 5). This means that input from anthropologists and other social scientists is urgently needed in both the planning and evaluation of AIDS prevention programmes. Furthermore, the success of these programme should always be monitored not only from the perspective of the medical authorities, but also from that of the at-risk community themselves, and where possible they should assist in helping to design more effective interventions in the future.

KEY REFERENCES

3 Sontag, S. (2001). *Illness as Metaphor and AIDS and its Metaphors*. London: Picador.

12 Miller, E. (1998). The uses of culture in the making of AIDS neurosis in Japan. *Psychosom. Med.* 60, 402–9.

15 Farmer, P. (1990). Sending sickness: sorcery, politics, and changing concepts of AIDS in rural Haiti. *Med. Anthropol. Q. (New Ser.)* 4, 27.

21 Lyttleton, C. (1994). Knowledge and meaning: the AIDS education campaign in rural northeast Thailand. *Soc. Sci. Med.* 38, 135–46.

24 Parker, M., Ward, H. and Day, S. (1998). Sexual networks and the transmission of HIV in London. *J. Biosoc. Sci.* 30, 63–83.

30 Carrier, J. M. (1989). Sexual behavior and the spread of AIDS in Mexico. In: *The AIDS Pandemic: A Global Emergency* (Bolton, R. ed.). Reading: Gordon and Breach, pp. 37–50.

37 Leonard, T. L. (1990). Male clients of female street prostitutes: unseen partners in sexual disease transmission. *Med. Anthropol. Q. (New Ser.)* 4, 41–55.

40 Page, B., Chitwood, D. D., Prince, P. C. *et al.* (1990). Intravenous drug use and HIV infection in Miami. *Med. Anthropol. Q. (New Ser.)* 4, 56–71.

44 Sibthorpe, B. (1992). The social construction of sexual relationships as a determinant of HIV risk perception and condom use among injection drug users. *Med. Anthropol. Q. (New Ser.)* 4, 255–70.

52 Bandyopadhyay, M. and Thomas, J. (2002) Women migrant workers' vulnerability to HIV infection in Hong Kong. *AIDS Care* 14(4), 509–21.

54 Fassin, D. (2003) The embodiment of inequality. *EMBO Rep.* 4 (*Spec. Iss.*), S4–9.

58 Heald, S. (2002) It's never as easy as ABC: Understandings of AIDS in Botswana. *Afr. J. AIDS Res.* 1, 1–10.

See http://www.culturehealthandillness.com for the full list of references for this chapter.

RECOMMENDED READING

Aggleton, P. and Homan, H. (eds). (1988) *Social Aspects of AIDS*. Philadelphia: Falmer Press.

ten Brummelhuis, H. and Herdt, G. (eds). (1995). *Culture and Sexual Risk: Anthropological Perspectives on AIDS*. Reading: Gordon and Breach.

Farmer, P. (1992) *AIDS and Accusation: Haiti and the geography of blame*. Berkeley: University of California Press

Green, E.C. (1994) *AIDS and STDs in Africa: Bridging the gap between traditional healing and modern medicine*. Boulder: Westview Press/University of Natal Press.

UNAIDS (2004) *AIDS Epidemic Update*. Geneva: Joint United Nations Programme on HIV/AIDS (UNAIDS)/World Health Organization.

RECOMMENDED WEBSITES

AIDS and Anthropology Research Group: http://puffin.creighton.edu/aarg

UNAIDS: Joint United Nations Programme on HIV/AIDS: http://www.unaids.org/en/default.asp

UNICEF: Programmes to prevent HIV/AIDS: http://www.unicef.org/aids/index.php

Tropical diseases: malaria and leprosy

This chapter deals with two of the commonest tropical diseases found worldwide: malaria and leprosy. Together these two diseases account for millions of deaths each year, especially in poorer countries, and impose an enormous burden on them in both human and economic terms.

MALARIA

THE SCALE OF THE PROBLEM

Malaria is one of the world's most dangerous and widespread parasitic diseases. Its name comes from the ancient concept of the *mal aria* or 'bad air,' which was believed to cause disease in damp, low-lying areas. It is caused by parasites transmitted by the bite of an *Anopheles* mosquito. More than half the population of the world is estimated to live in areas where malaria transmission occurs to some degree.[1] The majority of cases occur in tropical Africa, but they also occur in parts of Asia and Latin America. It is especially common in poor, deprived and undeveloped regions, where it has an enormous effect on public health. According to the World Health Organization in 2005, 107 countries and territories – with a combined population of 3.2 billion people – have areas at risk of malaria transmission within them. World-wide, between 350 and 500 million people suffer from the disease each year, often severely.[2] Malaria kills between 1.5 and 2.7 million people annually, and over a

million of these deaths are in children below the age of 5 years although they also include many older children, pregnant women and non-immune travelers.[1] Although there are four types of human malaria (*Plasmodium vivax*, *Plasmodium malariae*, *Plasmodium ovale* and *Plasmodium falciparum*), most cases of malaria are caused by the *P. falciparum* and *P. vivax* parasites, and *falciparum* malaria alone causes about 1 million deaths annually.[2] Overall, malaria is responsible for 10–30 per cent of all hospital admissions world-wide.[3] Furthermore, it is often associated with several other conditions, such as malnutrition, respiratory infections, acquired immune deficiency syndrome (AIDS) or tuberculosis.

Malaria is particularly severe in sub-Saharan Africa. In 2005 the World health Organization (WHO) estimated that 60 per cent of the cases of malaria worldwide (and about 75 per cent of *falciparum* cases) occurred in this area.[2] The disease is especially dangerous to children; it is a major cause of anemia in children (and pregnant women), low birth weight, premature birth, and infant mortality. In endemic African areas, malaria accounts for 25–30 per cent of all hospital outpatient visits, 20–45 per cent of all hospital admissions, and 15–35 per cent of hospital deaths (Figure 17.1).[2]

Like other global diseases, high rates of malaria are a feature of poverty and inadequate health services. Urbanization, the growth of shanty towns, overcrowding, poor nutrition, economic inequality, civil disorder, patterns of migration and

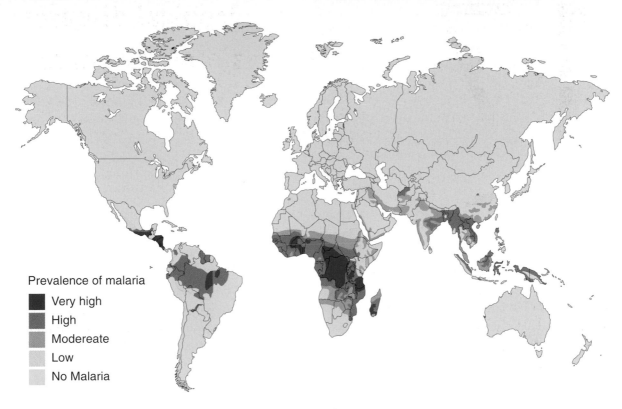

Figure 17.1 Global distribution of malaria transmission risk, 2003. (Source: World Health Organization, http://rbm.who.int/wmr2005/html/map1.htm as accessed on 1 September 2006. Reproduced with permission.)

Prevalence of malaria
- Very high
- High
- Modereate
- Low
- No Malaria

the movement of refugees, as well as the high cost of antimalarial drugs, all make the situation much more difficult to control. However, like AIDS, malaria can also help to *cause* poverty, and can be a major brake on economic development.[3] The economic loss caused by the disease in Africa alone, has been estimated at $2 billion annually.[4] Improving the living standards of ordinary people in poorer countries through economic advancement can be almost impossible without a sound malaria control policy and the allocation of appropriate funds. As well as the growing costs of treatment and prevention, adults with the disease are often too exhausted to work, and children feel too tired or unwell to study in school.[5]

To deal with this situation, the World Health Organization, together with other United Nations agencies, launched the Global Malaria Control Strategy (GMCS) in 1995. Its aim was to ensure that 90 per cent of the world's malaria-endemic

countries would implement national malaria control programmes as soon as possible. By mid-1997 this target had been met, with 47 of the 49 malaria-endemic countries in Africa completing their national plans of action, while outside Africa 57 other countries had also reoriented their malaria control programmes in accordance with the Global Malaria Control Strategy (GMCS).[1] However, these national policies are not enough. For their success, they also need economic development – in order to afford better housing, improved sewerage, more swamp drainage and more effective drug therapies – as well as community participation in all prevention and treatment strategies.

Despite all these initiatives, malaria remains one of the worst of global health problems. This is due partly to widespread economic underdevelopment and to the emergence of species of mosquito resistant both to pesticides and to the drugs that prevent and treat the disease.[6] New strategies are being developed to prevent and treat the disease. These include a reevaluation of some indigenous anti-malarial treatments. Artimisinin, for example, has been found to be effective against some drug-resistant strains of the disease. It is extracted from the Chinese medicinal herb *Artemisis annua* – known as *qinghaosu* – and the Chinese have used it as a treatment for fevers for over 1000 years.[7]

Despite these many advances in the prevention and treatment of malaria, in certain communities a variety of *cultural* beliefs and practices are also still part of the problem.

FOLK BELIEFS ABOUT MALARIA

Several anthropological studies have shown how folk beliefs can influence whether a community cooperates with a malaria control programme, whether it recognizes the early symptoms of the disease, and whether or not it accepts medical treatment for it. These beliefs also influence how people explain the origin and nature of the disease itself. Two key issues, in all of these anthropological studies, are:

- whether people connect mosquito bites with the origin of the disease
- how people interpret the significance of fever, and whether or not they relate it to malaria.

In south-eastern Tanzania, for example, Muela and colleagues[8] in 1998 found that while 98 per cent of people interviewed believed that mosquito bites did cause malaria, many also believed in *other* modes of transmission, such as drinking or wading through dirty water, or being exposed to 'intensive sun'. At the same time, the symptom of malaria most frequently reported was *homa*, or fever. However, *homa* had a broader meaning, since it could also express a general malaise or diffuse body pains. In the rainy season, when the wetness and heat favour mosquito breeding, people tended to identify *homa* with malaria. However, in the dry season, they were more likely to attribute the same fevers to hard work, exposure to the cold, or to 'intensive sun'. Furthermore, people often differen-

tiated between two types of *homa*: one caused by malaria, a 'natural' disease that was easily treated, and another 'unnatural' form caused by spirits or witchcraft (*uchawi*), which was more difficult to treat. In the latter form, witchcraft was said to cause an illness that exactly mimics malaria, but is *not* the same disease. Seventy-three per cent of mothers in the study believed that this 'fake malaria' could be produced by witchcraft, and 62 per cent that witches could make the parasites invisible. That is the reason, they believed, why hospital tests sometimes could not detect the disease, and why medical treatments sometimes failed to cure it. Where the 'hospital people' could not help, a traditional healer (*mganga*) was often called in. Even when people felt that they had the 'real' malaria, and had accepted medical treatment, they might blame witchcraft if the treatment failed or if the condition recurred or suddenly worsened. Furthermore, people with 'real malaria' often asked the question *why* – 'Why did the mosquito sting my child and not someone else's?' 'Why did it happen to *me*?', 'why *now*?' – questions that can only be answered by a traditional healer. In the case of children, virtually all their mothers in the study who suspected malaria would go first to a hospital, but if there was no relief for their children, 60.6 per cent would then turn to a traditional healer. During the *mganga*'s treatment of witchcraft, anti-malarials would not be taken, since they were considered ineffective or even dangerous at that time.

Another study[9] carried out in a different region of Tanzania in 1996 also found that people differentiated between several types of fever or *homa*. 'Malaria fever' (*homa ya malaria*) was only one of a group of mild conditions, regarded as not very dangerous, especially as the fever often came and went. It was recognized as occurring when mosquitoes were very numerous, in the rainy season between April and May. More severe fevers, known as 'fevers which do not respond to hospital treatment' (*homa zisizokubali tiba za hospitali*), were blamed on spirits, witchcraft, sorcery or other causes. They included serious childhood illnesses known as *degedege*, characterized by a sudden onset, high fever, trembling, delirium, stiffness of limbs, convulsions and a high mortality rate. People were not clear about their cause; sometimes they were blamed on spirits, but only occasionally were they ascribed to malaria. It was also believed that a child with *degedege* should not have a needle inserted into the skin as this might cause malevolent spirits to enter the body, and cause rapid death. In this region, therefore, many people did not give malaria control a high priority, as it was only seen as a mild fever. Often they did not associate their *homa ya malaria* with more serious complications such as cerebral malaria, severe anaemia or malaria in pregnancy.

In India, a study in 1997 by Lobo and Kazi[10] in Surat district, Gujurat state, also found different folk models of fever, and of the causes of malaria. As in the Tanzanian examples, fever was regarded as a disease in itself, as well as a symptom. In the three villages they studied, people recognized 30 *different* types of fever (or *tav*). However, the situation was complicated by the fact that there was a wide variation, even within the same village, in how people described these fevers, their possible cause and how they should be treated. In different villages, people described similar fevers but gave them different names – or they gave them the same name, but were referring to different types of fever. In general, though, to most people in the district, malaria was seen as one particular type of fever, of which two forms were recognized: *sado* or simple (mild) malaria, and *zeri* or 'poisonous' (severe) malaria. Lobo and Kazi point out that these two categories of folk malaria were not necessarily synonymous with biomedical malaria, and may not even overlap with it. There was wide variation in beliefs about other symptoms associated with these types of malaria (especially the *sado* form) in the three villages. For example, in one village *sado* malaria was associated with loss of appetite, lethargy, bitter taste in the mouth, drowsiness and sweating, while in another village it was associated mainly with cold, body aches, headache, 'loosening' of the body, pain below the knee, waist pain

and fluctuating fever. *Zeri* malaria was usually associated with symptoms such as a longer-lasting fever, acute shivering, weakness, severe pains, vomiting and, sometimes, convulsions. In terms of the aetiology of these malarial fevers, 59.5 per cent were not sure what caused malarial fevers, while only 34.1 per cent of the sample blamed them on mosquito bites.

These examples indicate, therefore, that folk beliefs about fevers in general, and malaria in particular, often vary widely within the same country, the same region, and even within the same village. Furthermore, in many communities there is no universal agreement that malaria is caused by insect bites; neither is there agreement on the types of fever characteristic of the disease, or the treatment appropriate for it. Therefore, any malaria control programme needs to take into account local beliefs about the disease, and how it may be prevented or treated.

Case study: Beliefs about malaria in a farming community in southern Ghana

Agyepong[11] in 1992 described beliefs about fevers, including malaria, in a farming community of the Ga-Adangbe tribe in southern Ghana. She describes *asra*, which is a symptom complex that can include fever, but also some or all of the following: chills, headaches, bodily pains, yellow eyes, a bitter taste in the mouth, deeply coloured urine, loss of appetite, weakness, vomiting, pallor of palms and soles, and cold sores around the mouth. A more serious, less common, version was *asraku*, where the person has high fever, confusion, and 'acts like a madman'. Only a small minority believed that mosquitoes could cause *asra*. Almost all members of the community agreed that *asra* was caused by contact with excessive external heat, especially from sunlight, but also from cooking, burning charcoal or standing too close to a fire. This heat causes *asra* by accumulating in the body, and upsetting the body balance by an effect on the blood. The prevailing view was that *asra* could not be prevented. It was an unavoidable fact of life, and of having to work outdoors in the harsh sunlight. Treatment for the condition mostly took place at home and only rarely at medical facilities. Home remedies included herbs to 'wash the blood of the illness', so that it was sweated out through the skin or else passed out in the urine. Only if these remedies failed did they resort to pharmaceuticals bought over the counter, such as analgesics or, occasionally, low doses of chloroquine.

ATTITUDES TO MALARIA TREATMENT

People diagnose malaria, in themselves and in others, by a number of methods. These include the clinical presentation, the season of the year when it occurs, and the personal circumstances that preceded the illness. Where malaria is endemic in a community, some form of *self-treatment* is usually common: either the use of traditional home remedies, or of pharmaceutical drugs bought from a retail outlet.[12] This approach partly results from the high cost of medically prescribed drugs[13], but also from folk beliefs about the origin and nature of the disease itself. Depending on these beliefs, the ill person may be first treated at home,[12] or else be taken straight to a hospital,[9] or sometimes to a traditional healer.[9] In most cases people move back and forth between biomedical and traditional systems, depending on their condition. The process usually begins with self-treatment, but later this is often carried out in parallel with medical treatment. Self-treatment strategies sometimes replace medical care, especially if the drugs fail to work and the patient deteriorates. In that case, a traditional healer may be consulted. In the study by Muela and colleagues,[8] for example, when a patient failed to recover or relapsed, a *mganga* would be consulted – first to diagnose witchcraft or evil spirits, then to neutralize them by rituals or herbal treatment. This in turn might pose serious problems for successful treatment, since 96 per cent of the sample believed that once herbal

medicines were begun, anti-malarials should not be given. Taking them at the same time as chloroquine was dangerous, as the effect on the patient might be too strong, and their blood 'start boiling'.

Mwenesi and colleagues,[12] in the Kilifi coastal district of Kenya, also found that most mothers who diagnosed malaria in their children first turned to over-the-counter drugs bought from a retail outlet. Twenty-nine per cent of mothers had given their children antimalarial drugs, and 30 per cent antipyretics or other medications (including antibiotics). Only 25 per cent had taken the child to a clinic, 9 per cent had given them no treatment at all and 7 per cent had given them a home remedy such as a herbal preparation of the *neem* tree (*Azadirachta indica*). The most popular choice was a combination of antipyretics and antimalarial drugs. Similarly, in southern Ghana, Agyepong[11] found that *asra* was first treated at home using a complex mixture of herbs or pharmaceuticals. The herbs were given to 'wash the blood of the illness', the drugs to treat the specific disease. Among the Mende people of Sierra Leone, Bledsoe and Goubaud[13] found that malaria was treated by certain foods or condiments (especially pepper), by certain herbs, by rubbing white chalk into the skin, and sometimes by Western pharmaceuticals. They found that many people chose these drugs on the basis of *colour*, choosing white medicines to relieve fever because they were seen as analogous to the traditional white chalk and its assumed 'bitterness', which is said to produce warmth and reduce fever. For that reason, people would accept medicines such as chloroquine, provided that it was white, or if its bitterness was not disguised by sugar coatings. But this also meant that other white or bitter medicines, such as aspirin, heart drugs, antidiarrhoeals and anti-hypertensives, would also be considered as acceptable treatment for malaria.

These studies indicate, therefore, some of the reasons why medically prescribed antimalarials may be accepted or rejected by a particular community (Figure 17.2). They also suggest why these drugs are often combined with other forms of treatment, either self-administered or from a traditional healer, in ways that 'make sense' to the community in terms of their local cultural beliefs.

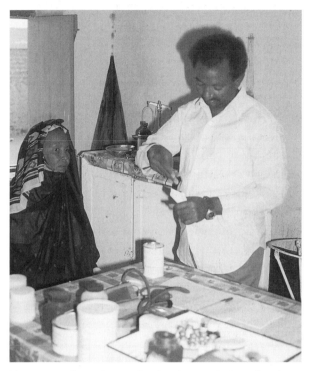

Figure 17.2 Preparing medication for a malaria patient in Sudan. (Source: World Health Organization, *World Health*, No 2, March–April 1998, page12.)

ATTITUDES TO MALARIA PREVENTION

In many communities, malaria is so common that it is sometimes regarded as a normal (if undesirable) part of everyday life, and not as something that doctors can ever prevent. Similarly, mosquitoes and their bites are such a common part of life that people may believe that nothing can be done to eradicate them.[8–11] Furthermore, preventive strategies for malaria have to take into account the fact that many people do not connect mosquito bites to the disease. If, as in Agypong's study,[11] people believe that malarial fever (*asra*) is caused by external heat, then, as one informant put it: 'There is nothing that we can do [to prevent it]. Unless you can provide us with other jobs so we do not work too hard in the sun'. Modern methods of prevention on a community level, such as better housing, screens erected across windows and doorways, drainage of stagnant water, spraying of potential reservoirs of the parasite, use of insect repellents, and bed nets impregnated with pesticide often do not make sense in terms of indigenous folk beliefs. They may also be unaffordable, especially the high cost of pesticides and anti-malarial drugs produced by the Western pharmaceutical industry.[14]

Figure 17.3 Community participation in malaria prevention. Householders in a Chinese village dip their mosquito bed nets in an insecticide (deltamethrin) to protect themselves against mosquito bites. (Source: World Health Organization/TDR/Y. Zhao, *World Health*, No. 3, May–June, 1998, page 10.)

In many communities there are well-tried traditional ways of repelling mosquitoes, to prevent their bites or the diseases that they might carry. In Gujarat, for example, Lobo and Kazi[10] have described how these methods include covering the body with sheets to protect it, or using the smoke of burning cow dung or *neem* leaves. However, they found considerable resistance to the use of mosquito bed nets. Of the 30 per cent who owned one, only 53.7 per cent used them regularly. People described them as very expensive, and as uncomfortable or suffocating, and there were often difficulties in finding a place to suspend them over the sleeping area. Also, some people (13.3 per cent) preferred sleeping out in the open, especially in very hot weather. In addition, cultural concepts of *personal space*, including who should sleep where, based on age, gender and status, made their use problematic. For example, elderly members of the family usually slept out on the verandah. This was partly because they were closer to toilet facilities, but also because of a cultural need to keep a physical distance from grown-up daughters and daughters-in-law and their children. In many households children slept in the kitchen, as it was believed that kitchen smoke repels mosquitoes. In some households, a young couple without children would sleep in the kitchen, but older couples in the sitting room. Within the houses, families slept in beds or cots, or sometimes on the floor, especially in the poorer social castes. All these variations in the location and allocation of sleeping spaces make the universal use of bed nets very difficult. As well as requiring a place to hang them from, these nets impose individual 'bubbles' of space (see Chapter 2) on communities and families who value communality and a greater sharing of personal space than is common in the industrialized world.

Thus, any attempt to get community participation in malaria prevention needs to take these cultural beliefs and concerns into account. The role of economic factors must also be considered, since many people simply cannot afford bed nets,[15] antimalarial tablets, different types of dress and more protective housing arrangements. Neither can they afford to change traditional ways of agriculture, even if this brings them into regular contact with reservoirs of mosquitoes.

MALARIA AND MIGRATION

Outbreaks of malaria are often linked to massive movements of human populations. In some parts of the world, the disease is extremely common among refugees. It is one of the main killers of people fleeing from armed conflict, especially civil wars and social unrest, in developing countries.[16] Often, these people are displaced from an area where malaria is uncommon to areas of high transmission. Having no natural immunity, they succumb quickly to the disease and its complications. This has particularly been the case in Africa, in regions where malaria is endemic and where large numbers of refugees have resulted from conflicts in Rwanda, Burundi, the Democratic Republic of the Congo, Somalia, eastern Sudan, Ethiopia, Kenya and Malawi.[16] In Asia, a similar problem has occurred among Cambodian refugees on the Thai–Cambodian border, and among refugees from Afghanistan in Pakistan and elsewhere. In these cases, medical interventions have to focus not only on bringing health care quickly to the refugee camps, but also on finding out the cultural beliefs and practices of the refugees themselves. This type of rapid research (Rapid Assessment Procedures) in emergency relief situations is listed in Chapter 19, and has been described in more detail by Slim and Mitchell.[17]

Other population movements that can contribute to the spread of the disease include tourist air travel[17] – either of sick people or of mosquitoes themselves, carried in clothing and baggage – and migrant labour. In poorer counties, particularly where there is often marked economic inequality between regions, patterns of migrant labour can expose more people to the disease. Liese,[3] for example, has described how, in Brazil, the relative poverty of the countryside leads people to seek work in towns and cities as migrant labourers. Each year, thousands of young men are being attracted to the gold rush in the Amazon basin. Many of these would-be miners or *garimpeiros* live in poor conditions, in houses without proper walls and have poor nutrition. Many suffer from malaria. Coming from the south of the country, they have never before been exposed to the disease and, having little natural immunity, it affects them severely. They transport malaria with them when they return back home to visit relatives or friends. When they have spent their savings, they trek back to the Amazon, and the process starts all over again.

In some cases, it is not people but mosquitoes that migrate between countries, and then cause malaria. This is the cause of *airport malaria*, which has been reported in countries in Western Europe, as well as in the USA, Israel and Australia.[18] It is caused by *Anopheles* mosquitoes carried on aircraft from endemic areas (in either the cabin or the baggage), which bite and infect people living or working near the airport where the aircraft has landed. According to the WHO, between 1969 and 1999 a total of 89 cases of airport malaria had been reported to them.[18]

SUMMARY

The examples outlined above illustrate, therefore, that the effective prevention and treatment of malaria requires a holistic approach. This includes economic development, alleviation of poverty, better housing and work conditions, and access to affordable antimalarial drugs, insect repellents and impregnated bed nets (Figure 17.3). It also requires an understanding of folk beliefs about the origin, nature, recognition and treatment of the disease.[19,20] This holistic approach is also important for the control of other mosquito-borne diseases such as yellow fever, dengue, and filariasis.

LEPROSY

Leprosy, or *Hansen's Disease*, is a severe, disabling tropical disease caused by the bacterium *Mycobacterium leprae*. It has been known for millennia, and was mentioned in the Old and New Testaments, as well as being recognized in ancient China and Egypt. In India, which today has the majority of the world's leprosy cases, it has a long history and was first described in 600 BC by the physician Sushruta in his treatise *Sushruta Samhita*.[21]

The disease mainly affects the skin and the nerves, but if is not treated it can cause permanent damage to the skin, eyes, nerves and limbs. The condition develops slowly, with an incubation period of 5 years, and it can take up to 20 years for symptoms to appear. It is usually treated successfully by multidrug therapy (MDT), using a combination of three drugs: dapsone, rifampicin and clofazimine.[21] The BCG (bacillus Calmette–Guérin) vaccine, used for tuberculosis prevention, also affords some protection against contracting leprosy.[22] According to the WHO,[21] more than 14 million leprosy patients have been cured in the past 20 years, and the number of people suffering from the disease has dropped from 5.2 million cases in 1985, to 286 000 cases at the end of 2004, and during that year approximately 410 000 *new* cases were detected (compared with 804 000 in 1985). Despite these improvements, leprosy is still considered to be a major health problem, and nine countries in Africa, Asia and Latin America account for 75 per cent of the total global disease burden; in particular, India, Brazil, Madagascar, Mozambique, Myanmar (Burma) and Nepal.[21] To deal with the disease, the WHO in 1999 formed the Global Alliance for the Elimination of Leprosy (GAEL) in collaboration with various governments, health agencies, and pharmaceutical companies.

LEPROSY AND STIGMA

Despite the fact that it is only mildly contagious,[21] one of the major problems of dealing with leprosy is the *stigma* attached to it. Since ancient times, those who have contracted the disease have attracted social rejection and discrimination. In India, for example, although the degree of stigma has decreased somewhat in the past 50 years,[23] Chaturvedi and colleagues[24] report that the disease still evokes 'public fear and hate', and that patients often encounter disapproval, rejection, exclusion, and discrimination. There are also still widespread cultural misconceptions about the disease, including that it is hereditary, very contagious, or the result of divine punishment.

The impact of stigma

Leprosy has a major impact on those who contract it, as well as on their families. This is due not only to the disease, but also to the stigma that comes with it. In socio-economic terms, many sufferers find themselves unable to obtain employment, and often become dependent on others for their support, or even have to resort to begging in order to survive. Overall, Thomas and Thomas[23] estimate that between 21 and 45 per cent of all people with leprosy deteriorate economically as a result of having the disease. In India, there are differences in the effects of the disease on different caste groups, with those in the lower castes experiencing more economic problems, and those in the upper castes having more social problems.[24]

Both the disease process of leprosy and its social consequences can have devastating effects on people's lives, especially on their schooling, employment, recreation, finances, and social functioning. It can affect their sex lives, their personal relationships, and reduce their chances of getting married. Often they find themselves rejected by friends, family and community, and face social ostracism, isolation, rejection and discrimination. Some in the community may seek to exclude them from workplaces, as well as from swimming pools and other public facilities, or even to confine them in 'leper colonies' (before the 1950s, pauper lepers in India were segregated by law, were barred from travelling on trains or serving in the military, were not eligible for insurance and were not allowed to inherit property).[25] Some of the patients with leprosy 'self-stigmatize', isolating themselves from social life lest their diseased skin or disabled limbs be seen by other people. Stigmatization seems to have a greater social impact on *females*, who suffer more isolation and rejection than men, find themselves ignored by their husbands or families and face an increased likelihood of divorce.[24] In one Indian study, for example, 58 per cent of women with the disease expressed suicidal ideas, while 8 per cent had actually made a suicide attempt.[26]

All this has very negative effects on the psychological state of people with leprosy, resulting in higher rates of depression, anxiety, and suicidal feelings.[24] This is correlated with their degree of physical disability, but also with the attitudes of the patient's family and community, and their levels of knowledge about the disease.

In India, Chaturvedi and colleagues[24] point out that in a dark-skinned population, anything that changes the colour, complexion, texture or appearance of the skin attracts attention, and sometimes stigma. As well as leprosy, this also applies to *other* forms of easily-visible skin diseases; these are also associated with a high psychiatric morbidity. *Psoriasis*, for example, which is characterized by scaly red patches on the skin, is also a stigmatised condition and often results in anxiety and depression among its sufferers, especially women. However, stigmatization is even more severe with *vitiligo*, a skin disease characterized by pale spots or patches of depigmentation on the skin. Chaturvedi and colleagues found that the patients with vitiligo 'have suffered the same physical and mental abuses as leprosy', with widespread discrimination against them.[24] Often they are considered unmarriageable, and women contracting it after marriage face the possibility of divorce. Sufferers are considered to have *Sweta Kushta* ('white leprosy'), and in some religious texts it is said that they had done *Guru Droh* (insulted their teacher in a previous life) and that the vitiligo was punishment for this. Because vitiligo is relatively common in India, this has major implications for public health.

In dealing with leprosy stigma in India, Chaturvedi *et al.*[24] suggest that solutions should include support and mental-health care for patients (including self-help groups and group therapy), legislation to prevent discrimination, and greater public education about the disease. However, they point out that greater knowledge about leprosy does *not* necessarily lead to positive attitudes towards leprosy sufferers, even among doctors and health educators.

In Nigeria, Awofeso[27] described a similar widespread prejudice and stigmatization that people with leprosy encounter, in a society 'that values bodily integrity, beauty, physical and economic independence'. The level of stigmatization seems to vary by region, with a greater degree in the predominately Christian south, and a relatively milder level in the predominantly Moslem north. Awofeso reported that inadequate knowledge of the disease is widespread, even among medical practitioners and nurses. As in India, stigmatization has negative effects on both physical and mental health, since the majority of leprosy-related deformities (Figure 17.4) result from patients concealing their disease until complications develop, and they are forced to seek help.

Leprosy does not necessarily attract the same degree of stigmatization in every country. For example, in 1981 Waxler[25] compared differences in attitude towards leprosy patients in India and Sri Lanka, despite very similar fears of contagion in both populations. In Sri Lanka people with leprosy also tended to withdraw to some extent from social life, but they were often able remain at home, and even continue to work. Despite some degree of stigma, she found that 'the general pattern, relative to the Indian one, is one of acceptance, or at least of tolerance.' Among the reasons for this might be a less hierarchical caste structure, and the fact that Buddhism, with its 'stress on tolerance of differences and on compassion for others', is the predominant religion of the country.

Figure 17.4 A 46-year-old widow with severe deformities from leprosy, near Kathmandu, Nepal. (Source: © M Burgess. Reproduced with permission.)

Case study: stigma of leprosy patients in Banaras (Varanasi), India

Barrett[28] studied 72 leprosy patients attending a treatment centre and street clinic in Banaras, India, from 1999 to 2001. He found that the effects of the social stigma of leprosy were 'far worse than the disease itself', and that they exacerbated both the physical and psychological effects of the disease. This stigma was also more 'contagious' than the disease itself, since it usually affected the patient's family, leading them to seclude or reject the victim, especially when the disease could no longer be concealed. Even if the disease was completely cured by treatment, the social stigma for the victim might still last a lifetime. For this reason, the leprosy patients adopted a variety of strategies to conceal their disease from others – and from themselves. These included denial, not going for treatment, covering affected areas with clothing, travelling for treatment to clinics many miles away, not adhering to the treatment prescribed or going to unofficial healers for treatment. Others tried to ignore their affected limbs, and spoke of them as if they were not really part of their body; speaking of 'the hand' (*haath*) rather than 'my hand' (*hamare haath*). As many of these diseased limbs had lost all touch and pain sensation, this often resulted in neglect, and 'dissociation' of a part of their body that required constant attention and care. Some tried to exaggerate their physical deformities even further – by surgery, self-mutilation, or wearing blood-stained bandages – in order to attract more money when begging. Overall, Barrett describes the circular relationship between stigma and physical disability, whereby stigma can cause delayed treatment, inadequate treatment or self-neglect, all of which may exacerbate even further the physical deformities caused by the disease.

FOLK BELIEFS ABOUT LEPROSY

As mentioned above, leprosy, like all other serious diseases, is associated with many different folk beliefs about what causes it, who gets it, how it should be recognized, and how it should be treated. White,[29,30] for example, studied leprosy beliefs in 1998–99 among people living in shanty-towns (*favelas*) or low-income neighbourhoods in Rio de Janeiro, Brazil (a country where about 45 000 cases of leprosy are detected each year[29] and where the incidence of the disease is second only to India). Among the folk beliefs that she found were that leprosy (*lepra*) could be contracted from other people (including from sexual relations), as well as from dogs, cats, rats, beaches, rivers, open ditches, dirt (*sujeira*), the wind (*o vento*), or from eating certain foods such as fish and pork. Several believed it could be contracted from casual contact with a leprosy patient, including from their clothes or other personal items. Some, especially from northern Brazil, believed you could get it from 'burned blood' (*sangue queimado*), which arises when the blood is 'burned' by hard liquor or strong medicines. Others believed that leprosy resulted from sorcery (*feitiço*) or 'evil eye', or was

a punishment from God, or was actually a 'life lesson' (an opportunity to learn more about suffering and compassion). There was also confusion about how to recognize the disease, and its early symptoms. The popular belief was that it was characterized by itchy patches of skin, rotting flesh, suppurating lesions and loss of limbs, but they often ignored the early warning signs, such as painless areas of depigmented skin. To add to the confusion, many of the patients had had their condition misdiagnosed by the physicians they consulted. Even when treatment was begun, some people abandoned it because of its side-effects, such as changes in skin tone, facial swelling, and weight gain.

White[30] points out, however, that ideas about leprosy causation are *not* static and often change over time, especially after prolonged contact with the medical system. One aspect of this was the renaming of leprosy (*lepra*) – with its many negative associations in folk belief – to the more neutral, less stigmatizing term *hanseníase*. In other ways, too, patients gradually assimilated some (though not necessarily all) of the biomedical concepts of leprosy – its causes, complications, treatment and prognosis – into their own belief systems. The syncretic explanatory models that emerged from this process were influenced also by government health education programmes, and by the media – especially by television.

Leprosy as a social role

Leprosy, then, is both a social *and* a biological disease, and one cannot treat one of these aspects, without also treating the other. Both stigma and disability need to be dealt with. In every society, patients *learn* how to be 'a leper', and to some extent that role is always 'socially constructed'. For example, Waxler[25] described how in Ethiopia, where the disease 'is feared and stigmatized' and believed to be incurable, many people with the disease actually stigmatized themselves, and withdrew from normal life, marriage, work, recreation, and religious activities, often ending up isolated and impoverished. She contrasts this fatalistic approach with the more active role of American leprosy patients, some of whom become 'career patients' – giving public talks, and agitating for better treatments and for a greater public tolerance of the disease. In the USA they 'learn to be the kind of lepers Americans expect', expressing values of 'activism, self-sufficiency, and change'. In each of these cultural settings, therefore, leprosy patients learn how to behave in a way consistent with the social values of that particular society.

REHABILITATION OF LEPROSY PATIENTS

Thomas and Thomas[23] describe how in the past 25 years leprosy care has shifted from the hospital to the home, from institutions to the community – an approach supported by the WHO. Modern leprosy rehabilitation has adopted a multidimensional approach, especially *community-based rehabilitation* (CBR), instead of the segregation of leprosy sufferers that occurred in the past. Because medical interventions such as reconstructive surgery are only appropriate for a small proportion of sufferers with deformities, a more comprehensive treatment for rehabilitation needs to be developed, one that requires more participation, and input, from both patients and community. In CBR patients are helped by their families and by volunteers, as well as by the health professionals (Figure 17.5). The aim of rehabilitation is not only to restore function to the patient in order to make them 'fit in' with the community, but also to change community attitudes towards the patients: to be more tolerant and accepting of people with these disabilities. This represents a shift from a purely medical approach to a more holistic approach, and one that should be more affordable, humane, and culturally appropriate. Despite major socio-economic problems in countries such as India – poverty, corruption, community apathy or rejection – this approach still offers the most viable way forward.

KEY REFERENCES

1 Trigg, P. and Kondrachine, A. (1998). The Global Malaria Control Strategy. *World Health* 3, 4–5.

8 Muela, S. H., Ribera, J. M. and Tanner, M. (1998). Fake malaria and hidden parasites – the ambiguity of malaria. *Anthropol. Med.* 5(1), 43–61.

9 Winch, P. J., Makemba, A. M., Kamazima, S. R. *et al.* (1996). Local terminology for febrile illnesses in Bagamoyo district, Tanzania, and its impact on the design of a community-based malaria control programme. *Soc. Sci. Med.* 42, 1057–67.

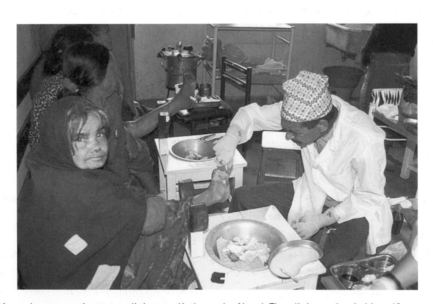

Figure 17.5 Treating a leprosy patient at a clinic near Kathmandu, Nepal. The clinic worker is himself a cured leprosy patient. (Source: © M. Burgess. Reproduced with permission.)

10 Lobo, L. and Kazi, B. (1997). *Ethnography of malaria in Surat*. Surat: Centre for Social Studies.

11 Agyepong, I.A. (1992). Malaria: ethnomedical perceptions and practice in an Adangbe farming community and implications for control. *Soc. Sci. Med.* 35, 131–7.

12 Mwenesi, H., Harpham, T. and Snow, R.W. (1995). Child malaria practices among mothers in Kenya. *Soc. Sci. Med.* 49, 1271–7.

16 Meek, S. and Rowland, M. (1998). Malaria in emergency situations. *World Health* 3, 22–3.

23 Thomas, M. and Thomas, M.J. (2003) The changing face of rehabilitation in leprosy. *Indian J. Lepr.* 75(2), 59–68.

24 Chaturvedi, S.K., Singh, G. and Gupta, N. (2005) Stigma experience in skin disorders: an Indian perpective. *Dermatol. Clin.* 23, 635–42.

25 Waxler, N. (1981) Learning to be a leper: a case study in the social construction of illness. In: *Social Contexts of Health, Illness, and Patient Care* (Mishler, E.G., Amarasingham, L.R., Osherson, S.D. *et al*, eds.) Cambridge: Cambridge University Press, pp. 169–94.

27 Awofeso, N. (1996) Stigma and socio-economic reintegration of leprosy sufferers in Nigeria. *Acta Leprol.* 10(2), 89–91.

29 White, C. (2002) Sociocultural considerations in the treatment of leprosy in Rio de Janeiro, Brazil. *Lepr. Rev.* 73, 356–65.

See http://www.culturehealthandillness.com for the full list of references for this chapter.

RECOMMENDED READING

Heggenhougen, H.K., Hackerthal, V. and Vivek, P. (eds.) (2003) *The Behavioural and Social Aspects of Malaria and its Control*. World Health Organization, Special Programme for Research and Training in Tropical Diseases (TDR).

World Health Organization (2005) *World Malaria Report 2005*. World Health Organization.

RECOMMENDED WEBSITES

Centers for Disease Control and Prevention: http://www.cdc.gov/malaria/faq.htm

International Federation of Anti-Leprosy Organizations (ILEP): http://www.ilep.org.uk/content/home.cfm

Special Program for Research and Training in Tropical Diseases (TDR) (UNICEF/UNDP/World Bank/WHO): http://www.who.int/tdr

World Health Organization, Leprosy: http://www.who.int/lep

World Health Organization, Malaria: http://www.who.int/topics/malaria/en

18 Medical anthropology and global health

Traditionally, most anthropologists have studied small-scale societies, or relatively small groups of people within a wider society. They have usually aimed at a holistic view of a particular culture or community, including how its different aspects are connected with one another – to understand, as Mars[1] puts it, 'the articulation of family and kinship organization with grass-root political power and authority, the relation of these to religious beliefs and practices, and the place taken in all these affairs by the way goods and services are produced and distributed'.

Medical anthropologists, too, have concentrated mainly on health problems at the local (and occasionally national) level. However, in recent years many of the major threats to human health – such as overpopulation, pollution, global warming, drug abuse and the acquired immune deficiency syndrome (AIDS) epidemic – can no longer be confined, or dealt with solely behind local or national boundaries. In an increasingly mobile and interdependent world, they are truly global in both their origins and their effects. Furthermore, information about these problems has also become global as telecommunications, the Internet, radio, television, jet travel and mass tourism connect more areas of the world with one another.

For these reasons, future research in medical anthropology is likely to focus not only on how certain cultural and social factors can damage individual health, but also on the health of the human species as a whole. This will involve adopting a much more global perspective – a holistic view of the complex interactions between the cultures, economic systems, political organizations and ecology of the planet itself.

Medical anthropology, as a biocultural discipline integrating both medical science and biology with the social and behavioural sciences, brings a unique perspective to the study of these global health problems. Its comparative, cross-cultural approach coupled with the collection of physical and psychological data gives it an overview of the diversity of beliefs and behaviours found worldwide, and the relation of these to health and disease.

It can also help explain the effects and causes of these global problems at the local level. To take one example, AIDS, described in more detail in Chapter 16, now poses a threat to health on a global level. Faced with this situation, detailed in-depth ethnographic studies can provide information regarding:

- how an increase in AIDS can affect the social, economic and cultural life of a particular community
- how beliefs and behaviours within that community change (or do not change) to meet this threat
- what explanations are given (in terms of local beliefs) for the origins of the disease and why some people are afflicted by it and others not
- whether sufferers from it can mobilize social support or find themselves stigmatized and rejected

- how sexual relationships, marriage patterns, family structures and religious rituals are altered by the disease
- whether changes occur in the way that different genders and generations relate to one another
- the strategies of prevention and self-care used by the community, and how these articulate with local and national medical systems
- the shifts that take place in the patterns of work, migration and residence
- the role of local and global economic factors in the origin, spread, persistence and management of the disease.

THE ROLE OF POVERTY

It should always be noted, however, that all these anthropological approaches to health problems have to take place against the background of one key issue in global health: *poverty*. Extreme poverty is the greatest killer and cause of ill health and suffering across the globe.[2] Together with economic and social inequality, it is responsible for more physical and mental ill health than any other cause.

The health risks of the poor are very different from those of the rich. Gwatkin and colleagues[2] point out that in richer countries, the proportion of older people in the population rises because of a decline in fertility rates and a decline in mortality. As a result, chronic 'non-communicable' diseases (such as heart disease, diabetes or cancer) begin to predominate as a cause of death. In 1990 chronic diseases were responsible for 56 per cent of all deaths worldwide, compared with 34 per cent from infectious ('communicable') diseases (and 10 per cent from accidents and injuries). However, rich and poor countries varied in their main causes of death. Among the poorest 20 per cent of the world's population, chronic diseases were much less important, and 59 per cent of deaths are caused by infectious diseases compared with only 8 per cent among the richest 20 per cent, where chronic diseases accounted for 85 per cent of all their deaths. Health policy should therefore focus on fighting communicable diseases as a way of decreasing the 'poor–rich gap'. Focusing resources mainly on chronic diseases will have the opposite effect, widening the gap, benefiting mainly the world's richer citizens.

THE CONCEPT OF 'GLOBAL HEALTH'

In many parts of this book, I have tried to show how definitions of 'health' vary widely across societies and cultures. A related issue, however, is the definition of 'global': What exactly do we mean by phrases such as 'Global Health', 'World Health' or 'International Health'? As Keane[3] points out, there are many *different* ways of looking at 'globality' – 'the consciousness of the world as a single place.' He identifies four different conceptual models (though they often overlap) that underlie most of the discourses of 'world health' or 'global health'. In his analysis, he uses the anthropological distinction between two types of human groups: (1) 'community' (*gemeinschaft*), a small, intimately-connected group, with a strong common feeling; and (2) 'society' (*gesellschaft*), a much larger, more impersonal group, with looser links between its members.

1 *Gemeinschaft I* – this views the world as made up of multiple, relatively closed and discrete communities, which provide the main context for their lives (a view held also by most anthropologists). In health policy, this perspective emphasizes the role of 'community resources', 'community participation', 'community leaders' and 'community health workers' (see below). Often foreign medical aid and globalization are seen as disrupting the internal balance of these communities.

2 *Gemeinschaft II* – this views the world as 'one community', irrespective of national borders, or of differences in language or culture. Each person therefore has obligations to all others in this wider global human community, in terms of our common humanity, especially if they are

ill or suffering. This approach can be said to underlie the movement for universal human rights, and international medical aid organizations such as the International Red Cross and Médecins sans Frontieres (MSF).

3   *Global Gesellschaft I* – views the world as a collection of nation-states, which are seen as the principal agents for delivering health care to the world's population. Health interventions on a global level will therefore always require the permission, and cooperation of each national government. This is the predominant approach of the WHO, which 'facilitates exchange of information and ideas between nation-states, and sets up codes of (voluntary) national health standards' for them.

4   *Global Gesellschaft II* – this is a more radical perspective, and focuses on the inequalities within the 'world system' – both within, and between societies – in economic, social, and health terms. Health is seen as contingent on upon economic well-being, and thus ill-health is tied to 'global economic dependency' and 'global patterns of exploitation'. Economic and social inequalities should therefore be the main focus of health policy. In this view, the use of traditional healers, or community health workers, is merely 'low quality health care for the poor'.

Each of these four perspectives thus implies a very different view of 'the world', and of the appropriate ways that health care should be delivered to its population. Each perspective has major ideological, policy and practical implications, for it can greatly influence not only health policy, but also the allocation of funds for local and international health care programmes.

To Keane's four groups, one could add a fifth, more contemporary view of 'world health': that the world itself has become the 'patient', and its health is now steadily deteriorating:

5   The *environmentalist* position focuses on the damage done to the planet and its biosphere as a result of human action (such as pollution,

greenhouse gases, global warming, overpopulation, destruction of the rain forests, or nuclear tests). Health policy, in the widest sense, should therefore be directed at changing the way human beings behave, in relation to each other, and to the natural environment itself.

KEY ISSUES IN GLOBAL HEALTH

To illustrate the relevance of medical anthropology to certain contemporary global health problems, a few key issues have been selected for further discussion. They are:

1   Overpopulation.
2   Urbanization.
3   Primary health care.
4   Pollution and global warming.
6   Deforestation and species extinction.

OVERPOPULATION

Overpopulation is one of the most serious global problems, and the situation is worsening every year. Despite attempts to slow it down, the world's population is still growing exponentially. In 2005 the United Nations[4] estimated that over the next 45 years the world's population would increase by 2.6 billion, from the present 6.5 billion to 9.1 billion in 2050, and that almost all this growth will take place in the poorer countries, where the current population of 5.3 billion is expected to swell to 7.8 billion by 2050. In addition to this massive population increase, energy consumption by the richer countries is increasing at an even faster rate. Overall, world energy consumption has grown from an estimated 1 terawatt in 1890 to 3.3 terawatts in 1950 and 13.7 terawatts in 1990; on average, poor people use one-tenth of the energy of rich people.[5]

Overpopulation, plus the overuse of energy sources (such as fossil fuels), is potentially a dangerous combination, with deadly results for global health. These include widespread starvation, disease, poverty and civil unrest; the depletion of valuable fossil fuel reserves; and environmental dangers such as climatic changes and global warming (due to the 'greenhouse effect'), the rise of sea-levels with flooding of coastal plains, increased heat waves and droughts, and natural disasters such as hurricanes and cyclones. Overpopulation, as well as economic development, also leads to an increased worldwide demand for *water*; in 2005 the United Nations Development Programme (UNDP) estimated that overall water use is expected to increase by 40 per cent in the next 20 years. In future decades, proper 'water resource management' will become even more important as the population increases. Currently, about 1.2 billion people lack access to safe drinking water, and 2.4 billion lack access to proper sanitation, and in both situations this can lead directly to a high incidence of water-borne infections.[6]

Family planning programmes

Various strategies have been put forward to deal with the growing problem of overpopulation, including international programmes such as those of the WHO or of the International Planned Parenthood Federation, and national ones such as the 'one child' policy in the People's Republic of China. Most of these family planning programmes have targeted women, and have aimed at increasing their awareness of the benefits of reducing family size, allowing longer gaps between pregnancies and using the various forms of artificial contraception now available. As described in Chapter 6, many women in poorer countries still prefer to use traditional forms of fertility control, such as herbs or prolonged lactation, instead of using imported artificial forms of contraception.

In 1993 it was estimated that 43 per cent of married couples world-wide are using some form of modern contraception.[7] This included 52 per cent of couples in the richer, developed world, and 27 per cent in the developing world (although in China the figure was 73 per cent).[7] In India, it was estimated in 2001[8] that 48.2 per cent of couples (in the age range 15–49 years) were practicing some

form of family planning; female sterilization accounted for 34.2 per cent, while male sterilization declined from 3.4 per cent in 1992–93 to 1.9 per cent in 1998–99. In that same period, condom use increased from 2.4 to 3.1 per cent. An estimated 30 million legal abortions were carried out world-wide in 1987, as well as 10–22 million illegal ones.[7] An emerging issue is sex-selective abortion, whereby in some Asian countries increasing access to prenatal ultrasound scans has led to selective abortion of female fetuses. In India, Jha and colleagues[9] estimate that over the past 20 years about 10 million female fetuses have been aborted, over this period, resulting in a fewer girls than boys being born in India, especially in urban areas. This is especially true in families that already have one or more daughters, but no sons.

As a form of population control and family planning, abortion can pose many dangers to health, including haemorrhage, infection and perforation of the uterus, especially in the hands of untrained personnel. It was estimated in the early 1990s that between 100 000 and 200 000 women died each year in developing countries from the complications of illegal abortions.[7]

Despite their good intentions, family planning programmes have often been unsuccessful in reducing population growth. In many parts of the world, the idea of limiting one's fertility has either been rejected outright or accepted only very reluctantly. It is thus important to recognize, as Warwick[10] points out, that the demand for family planning is *not* universal, and it is not accepted by many different cultures. There are many reasons for this.

In most cases, the meaning of family planning is closely related to the value given to children. In many cultures, having a child is the visible sign of adult status; also, for many men, the birth of a son is the ultimate proof of their virility. In those communities where starvation, poverty, insecurity and a high infant mortality rate are common, fertility is given a very high social value. Having many children is one of the few ways that people can ensure their future, especially where the state is weak, has few resources and cannot provide comprehensive care for its citizens. The traditional extended family provides its members with a small-scale society of their own. It functions as a social and economic unit, sharing in the creation and distribution of resources, providing its members with a miniature social security system and helping them with the care of children, the elderly and the infirm.

A further salient reason for the rejection of family planning is that some world religions disapprove of all artificial forms of birth control, preferring instead more 'natural' (rhythm) methods. However, at both national and local levels there are many other reasons why family planning programmes are not successful. Warwick[10] notes that 'in every country, at least one group is opposed to organized family planning for some reason', and the opposition may be based on religious, cultural, economic or political criteria. In some developing countries, for example, family planning programmes originating in the West may be seen as just another form of colonialism, imposing itself on the local culture and population and weakening them in the process. Also, in those multi-ethnic countries where there have been conflicts between different communities, such as Sri Lanka, Lebanon, Malaysia, Fiji, South Africa and India, these conflicts 'may create feelings that a large population is vital to communal survival and that family planning helps one's enemies'.[10]

Another factor influencing the acceptability of contraceptive techniques is cultural beliefs about the body, particularly the female reproductive system. These include ideas, such as those described among some low-income groups in the USA,[11] of the uterus being a hollow organ, closed throughout the month and only 'open' during menstruation. Becoming pregnant is therefore only possible just before, or just after the period when it is still 'open' (during the period itself intercourse is strictly forbidden), and therefore there is no need to take contraceptive precautions during the rest of the month.

In addition, women in many cultures see menstrual blood as 'polluting' or 'poisonous', and fear the effects of a decreased menstrual flow, when more of the 'poison' will remain within their bodies (see Chapters 2 and 6). This is one of the reasons why the contraceptive pill, which may cause lighter menses or even their cessation, has been rejected by many women world-wide. For example, Good[12] in 1977 described how in Maragheh, Iran, lighter periods resulting from use of the pill were blamed for causing women to have the folk illness 'heart distress' (see Chapter 5), and are therefore avoided. In Scott's study[13] in 1975 in Miami, Florida, many of the women interviewed saw the pill as dangerous for this same reason, fearing that the accumulated blood would cause them to have 'blood pressure', mental illness, or to be nervous or depressed. In those groups that see menstrual blood as polluting and dangerous to other people, the intermenstrual 'spotting' sometimes caused by the pill may also lead to its rejection: it might also prevent them from taking part in certain religious rituals and festivals due to their temporary state of 'pollution'.

Similarly, cultural attitudes can influence whether the intrauterine contraceptive device (IUCD) is acceptable or not. Some may welcome the IUCD, which often causes heavier periods, as a way of increasing the monthly loss of their 'poisonous' blood. Others may reject it, based on folk models of female anatomy. For example, in Jamaica, MacCormack[14] in 1985 found that some women believed the uterus and vagina to be a single tube, open at both ends, and feared that the IUCD might therefore move and get lost somewhere within the body. Snow[15], in her study of low-income African-Americans in the early 1990s, found similar beliefs about IUCDs. Because menstrual blood was seen as polluting and shameful, the idea of exposing oneself to a strange physician for the IUCD to be inserted during a period (which it usually is) was met with revulsion.

In Japan, there has been widespread public and official rejection of oral contraception. Sobo and Russell[16] ascribed this to traditional Japanese beliefs about how the human body should always be in accordance with nature, unlike the Western desire to always conquer nature. By making the fertile female body infertile, artificial contraceptives (including the pill, surgical sterilization or the IUCD) violate this relationship. The pill particularly is seen changing the body's natural ecology, depriving the body 'of the opportunity to follow its natural, self-determined rhythm'.

As well as these cultural beliefs, family planning methods can also be rejected for more practical reasons such as availability or cost, especially in areas of extreme poverty. Condoms and oral contraceptives may have to be purchased on the open market, at a price that most people simply cannot afford. Also, since all forms of artificial contraception (including sterilization) carry with them certain risks and side-effects, knowledge and experience of these within a community will obviously influence whether women are willing to accept them or not.

As mentioned above, most family planning programmes have targeted women. According to McCally,[7] 'the control of population growth appears to be in women's hands. The empowerment of women, meaning access to education, health services, employment and public health, is coming to be understood as a major determinant of fertility'. Reproductive decision-making may not, however, be only the prerogative of women. Decisions on fertility also depend on local cultural conditions, patterns of marriage and residence, and the ways that individual women are embedded in family and kinship networks. Dyson and Moore,[17] for example, point out differences in the power of women to make decisions about fertility between north and south India. According to their research, women in the north tend to marry younger than those in the south, to be more controlled by their husband's family, and to be under stronger pressure from them to produce many children, especially sons. In his study of Yemenite Jews in Israel, Weingarten[18] described how most couples only start to practice contraception after the woman's fertility has been proved by having a child. In 40 per cent of cases the method used is coitus interruptus, and because this puts all the responsibility on the man it 'saves the woman from the need to restrict her fertility, which is traditionally the source of her status'. It also, presumably, maintains the man's status as the prime decision-maker.

Family planning programmes also need to target men. At present, many of the programmes aimed at men seem mainly to emphasize the use of condoms for AIDS prevention rather than as a regular form of contraception within a relationship. Arguably, by emphasizing only the female link to fertility, some men may even be led to conclude that if fertility is solely a female issue, then so is responsibility for infertility as well (see Chapter 6). Getting the cooperation of men (as well as women) is especially important in male-dominated societies, where they make most of the fertility decisions. Among the Hausa of northern Nigeria, for example, Renne[19] describes how married women are often kept secluded within their homes. This *auren kulle* ('marriage lock') means that they have little access to contraception without their husband's permission. They have few financial resources, so cannot afford to buy contraceptives, and in any case are discouraged from visiting chemist's shops or clinics unless accompanied by their husband or an older female relative.

Because of the diversity of populations, many anthropologists have therefore concluded that there cannot be a universal model of family planning that is applicable to all parts of the world. Within many countries, different regions, religions, ethnic groups, social classes and local communities may all have very different attitudes towards family planning, and each may require a different type of programme. In some cases, especially where the population is culturally, ethnically or socially diverse, this may make a national family planning strategy difficult, if not impossible.

Thus Warwick[10] suggests that, as well as programmes at the national and international levels, local communities should also be involved in family planning programmes. This will involve regular consultations with the community, being sensitive to their cultural needs, expectations and concerns (for example, having female staff conduct interviews and examinations), and enlisting the opinions and cooperation of local religious and political leaders. It also means recognizing that 'in some regions socio-cultural conditions may not be ripe for any kind of family planning program. Life may be too precarious, the value of children too high, the politics too polarized, or the issue of fertility control too remote to make such an investment worthwhile'.

Finally, like all other forms of health aid and intervention, family planning programmes cannot take place in a vacuum. They should always be part of a more holistic approach that also involves social and economic development, such as the reduction of poverty, improved health care, better nutrition, higher levels of literacy and employment, and the reduction of maternal and infant mortality. From a global perspective, this will also involve a more equitable distribution of resources between the poorer and richer parts of the world, and a reduction of energy consumption by the latter.

The following case study from Argentina looks at how cultural beliefs about the body, sexuality and fertility may influence acceptance of modern forms of contraception.

Case study: attitudes towards contraception of two groups of women in Argentina

Molina[20] in 1997 studied attitudes towards modern forms of contraception (the pill, diaphragm and IUCD) among two groups of Argentine women: indigenous Pilagá women in the north-east, and low-income *criolla* (Creole) women who had migrated to Buenos Aires. Both groups rejected modern forms of contraception, but for different reasons. The *criollo* women were used to traditional plant-based methods of fertility control (up to 20 different plant infusions used as contraceptives or abortifacients). Furthermore, unlike the doctors, they did not see procreation as only a biological phenomenon, but as a more mystical process. They

believed that any single act of intercourse did not carry with it a risk of pregnancy because pregnancy could only result if the personal 'energy' or 'vital power' of the partners was high enough. 'Stronger' partners could conceive during a single session of intercourse, but most people had to copulate much more very frequently to achieve this result. Both parties also had to optimize their personal 'energy' levels, often with the aid of shamans or herbal medicines. The pill was rejected because it was not plant-based, and could not be classified according to taste – bitter, sour or strong, attributes on which the efficacy of a plant depends. Pills were also seen as dangerous substances that could cause unpleasant physical symptoms, such as bodily swellings, headaches, and liver complaints. Both diaphragm and IUCD were rejected because, in the *criollo* view, illness was conceived of as a foreign 'substance' located within a particular part of the body, where it causes a dysfunction. As both these internal contraceptives were placed within the woman's body, it was believed that they could therefore cause her to become 'ill', or even to develop cancer. The Pilagá women also believed that fertilization was a mystical as much as a biological event. Pregnancy was also unlikely from a single act of intercourse. Seen as inherently fertile, frequent copulation would not only cause fertilization but was also necessary for the actual development of the embryo and the placenta, for the woman herself 'is a mere vessel and contributes nothing to procreation'. Traditionally, contraceptive methods were unknown, and both abortion and infanticide were used by the Pilagá for unwanted pregnancies. In recent years, they have increasingly adopted *criollo* attitudes towards procreation, and now reject modern contraception for very similar reasons. They now use more plant-based methods, and have less resort to abortion. The Pilagá believe, moreover, that the efficacy of a birth-control method (like pregnancy itself) is not only dependent on human behaviour, but also on the deities 'who ultimately decide whether the process will be effective or not'. In both *criollo* and Pilagá populations, therefore, there is conflict between

URBANIZATION

A parallel phenomenon to overpopulation has been the massive increase in urbanization. At the beginning of the nineteenth century the world's urban population totaled less than 50 million;[21] in 2004 it was estimated by the United Nations Population Division at 3 billion, and it was anticipated that by the year 2030 this figure would reach 5 billion.[22] The proportion of the world population that lives in cities is expected to rise from 48 per cent in 2004 to 61 per cent by 2030.[22] Furthermore, this annual rate of increase would be nearly double that expected of the world population at large. Many parts of the world have now seen the development of huge 'mega-cities' (10 million population, or more) such as Cairo, Calcutta, Mexico City, São Paulo, Bombay, Jakarta and Manila, due mainly to natural increase, but also to migration of people from the countryside in search of a better life. In 2003 there were 20 of these mega-cities.[22] Tokyo, with a population of 35 million in 2003 is the world's most populous urban agglomeration, followed by New York-Newark (18.3 million), São Paulo (17.9 million), and Mumbai (17.4 million). Almost all the future growth of urban population will take place in the poorer, less developed parts of the world, with an average increase of 2.3 per cent in population during the period 2000–30, so that by 2017 the total number of urban dwellers in these countries will be roughly equal to the number of rural dwellers.[22]

Cities themselves can have a major impact on the environment. Their large areas eat up the available agricultural land, previously used for food production. They use enormous amounts of energy, and produce large amounts of pollution, sewerage, and garbage. Often they create their own 'micro-climates', especially an increased temperature over the city area (known as the *urban heat island* effect), as well as wind tunnels between high buildings, noise pollution and light pollution. They are often subject to flooding, as large areas of ground covered with concrete do not absorb heavy rainfall or the overflow from riverbanks. This in turn can lead to landslides, or the subsidence of badly built houses. Cities are also filled with cars, buses and trucks, which adds to air pollution (especially from older and poorly maintained vehicles), as well as to the incidence of traffic accidents. Large, crowded cities are also vulnerable to epidemics of infectious diseases, crime and family breakdown, incidents of social unrest and attacks by terrorist groups.

In 1985 the WHO proposed the *Healthy Cities Project*,[23] to improve urban environments throughout the world and reduce their negative effects on health. The aim was to produce clean, safe environments that would meet the needs of their populations, and create a strong sense of community by promoting a high degree of public participation in local and city government. In recent years this project has become even more urgent, given the increasing and often uncontrolled growth of cities today, especially in poorer countries.

Growth of the urban poor

The rapid growth of urbanization has also been accompanied by the rapid growth of the 'urban poor', often living in shantytowns, slums or squatter settlements 'in the shadow of the city'. Overall, in the late 1980s, the percentage of urban dwellers living in these growing slums and shanty towns varied from 79 per cent in Addis Ababa, 67 per cent in Calcutta and 60 per cent in Kinshasa to 30 per cent in Rio de Janeiro, 23 per cent in Karachi and 20 per cent in Bangkok.[24]

These communities often include large numbers of homeless people, including many 'street children', whose lives are perilous, insecure, and often very brief. Some of them spend several years living 'on the street': in a study of street children in Kathmandu, Nepal, for example, Panter-Brick[25] found that the mean duration of this homelessness was 2.7 years, but in some cases it was a much as

9 years. The urban poor face numerous health problems, often worse than those of their rural counterparts. Many of these are a combination of the problems of underdevelopment (such as malnutrition and infectious diseases) and those of development (pollution, noise, traffic accidents, etc.). Harpham and colleagues[24] described how these problems have three main sources:

1 *Direct problems of poverty*, such as unemployment, low income, limited education and literacy, inadequate diet, lack of breast-feeding and prostitution.
2 *Environmental problems*, caused by poor housing, overcrowding, inadequate sanitation and water supplies, lack of waste disposal, air pollution, traffic accidents, the siting of hazardous industries nearby and lack of land to grow food on.
3 *Psychosocial problems*, such as stress (see Chapter 11), insecurity, marital breakdown, depression, alcoholism, smoking, domestic violence and drug addiction.

These health problems are rarely confined to the slum communities themselves. In Mexico City, for example, there are so many people without proper sanitation that a 'faecal snow' often falls on the city as the wind sweeps up dried human waste.[4] As illustrated below, these overcrowded urban environments can also become breeding grounds for several infectious diseases – some spread by humans, other by vectors such as mosquitoes.

Case study: dengue and urbanization in Mérida, Mexico and El Progresso, Honduras

Kendall and colleagues'[26] study in 1991 of Mérida and El Progresso indicates how an increasing urban population, and especially the growth of slums and shanty towns, is creating new ecologies of disease. In many urban areas of Central and South America and the Caribbean, overcrowding, population mobility, pollution, poor sanitation and the accumulation of garbage are all helping the rapid spread of certain diseases. These include insect-borne diseases such as dengue, and its variant dengue haemorrhagic fever (DHF), malaria, yellow fever, elephantiasis and Japanese encephalitis. Dengue is caused by a virus and transmitted by mosquitoes, especially *Aedes aegypti* (which can also transmit yellow fever). It can cause bleeding disorders and death, and there is no specific treatment or vaccine for it at present. In urban areas, the mosquitoes breed in collections of stagnant water such as in rainwater pools, barrels, bottles, discarded tyres, flowerpots, vases and animal drinking troughs. However, many people are still unaware of the dangers posed by mosquitoes in an urban environment and of the need to take precautions against them. In Mérida, although most of the population knew about dengue from public health education programmes, some confused it with other fever-producing illnesses such as *derengue* (a disease of cattle), *deshidratación* (dehydration) and 'flu; they were also unaware that insects were its vectors, blaming instead certain 'winds' for carrying it and other febrile illnesses. In El Progresso, too, most people knew of dengue, but many confused it with 'flu, and also believed that it came from the 'winds' or from garbage rather than from mosquito bites. The authors concluded, therefore, that given the growth of urbanization and of these 'new' urban diseases, their control 'will require theoretical knowledge about the organization of urban environments and its relationship to disease, new methodologies to encourage participation and social activism in health, and increased knowledge about influencing health behaviour'.

Anthropological research in the new megacities, especially among the urban poor, can contribute to the provision of community-oriented primary care (COPC), which is a form of health care that emphasizes the importance of relating health care provision to local needs and conditions.[27] Here, its role is to assess the specific health needs and problems of a particular community, to raise awareness of the role of cultural beliefs and behaviours in their health (and health care), and to act as their advocates to the medical and other authorities where necessary. Ethnographic research can also be relevant to the planning, application and evaluation of a variety of primary health-care programmes at both national and international levels, as illustrated later in this chapter.

PRIMARY HEALTH CARE

In 1978, the WHO issued its famous declaration in Alma-Ata of 'Health for All by the Year 2000'.[28] This ambitious plan aimed to develop, throughout the world, a *comprehensive* system of primary health care (PHC). The programme was to consist, as Mull[29] describes it, of 'essential health care made universally accessible to individuals and families by means acceptable to them, with their full participation, and at a cost that they, their community and the country as a whole could afford'. As part of the comprehensive approach, health care was to be accompanied by improved health education, nutrition, sanitation, immunizations, family planning, maternal and child health, and the supply of essential drugs (see Chapter 8). Above all, it represented a move away from the curative, 'quick fix', centralized medical model towards a more preventive, decentralized and community-based strategy.[29]

This comprehensive approach was seen as crucial in tackling global health problems, especially in Third World countries. In these poorer countries, infant and child mortality rates are many times higher than those in the industrialized world. It has been estimated that 12 million children die through poverty every year,[5] many of them from preventable or treatable diseases. These deaths occur mainly from infectious diseases such as respiratory illnesses, neonatal tetanus, diarrhoeal diseases, polio, diphtheria, pertussis, measles, rubella, tuberculosis, cholera, typhoid and yellow fever.[30] Others die from parasitic diseases such as malaria,

bilharzia, leishmaniasis and, increasingly, from AIDS and hepatitis B. Most of these causes of early death are associated, directly or indirectly, with *poverty*, and can be either prevented or treated – as they have been in most industrialized countries.

Critics of the plan for world-wide comprehensive PHC pointed out its considerable cost, the shortage of available health-care personnel and the practical difficulties of community participation. Some health planners suggested instead a more *selective* form of PHC that would focus on specific health problems (such as diarrhoeal diseases), especially those of infants and children. The policy of 'child survival' became paramount, and has now been adopted in some form by most organizations involved in international health. Its strategies have been summarized by UNICEF as 'GOBI-FF,'[28–30] that is:

- Growth monitoring
- Oral rehydration
- *Breast-feeding*
- *Immunization*
- Family planning
- Food supplements.

A further '*F*' was added, for '*Female literacy*',[31] since there is evidence that higher levels of maternal literacy are associated with a decrease in both the birth rate and in infant mortality rates.[30] This is due, among other reasons, to women being able to read health-related pamphlets or information, and the instructions on containers of medicines.

Mull[29] has criticized selective PHC for its narrower approach, instead of Alma-Ata's more comprehensive strategy, and its emphasis on community participation and empowerment, it advocates 'dealing with measurable disease entities so that quantifiable results could be produced at the lowest possible cost'. He also points out that GOBI-FFF targets mainly children and younger women, while ignoring the rest of the community. Men, too, need to be involved in health-care interventions, since many may not necessarily follow their wives' or mothers' health advice. To prevent them drinking, smoking, being too competitive or adopting at-risk sexual behaviours, health interventions may have to be brought to them in the workplace or via (male) community leaders. Also, as Green[32] found in Bangladesh, although women provided the main care for children, it was the men who decided which medicine to buy if the children were ill.

Despite the conceptual split between the 'comprehensive' and 'selective' approaches to PHC, Mull[29] points out that in many international aid programmes a pragmatic fusion of the two has actually taken place; for example, a 'top-down' and selective focus on a particular health problem (such as diarrhoeal illnesses) combined with interventions that improve nutrition, sanitation, water supplies, female literacy and popular participation at the community level.

PROBLEMS OF GOBI–FFF

Some of the specific problems associated with applying each aspect of the GOBI-FFF strategy have been described in more detail earlier in this book. They include oral rehydration therapy (Chapter 1), breast-feeding and food supplements (Chapter 3), and family planning (above). In many cases, both organizational and local cultural factors may make them difficult to apply. For example, although paediatricians agree on the value of growth monitoring (mainly height and weight) as a way of identifying malnutrition or other developmental problems, it can also be seen as a Western, culture-bound way of defining 'health'. As described in Chapter 5, the numerical definitions used to define 'normality' may not match indigenous beliefs about whether a child is healthy or not. Parents may see a child as 'healthy' if he or she can smile, play, talk, respond affectionately, or perform certain domestic or ritual tasks, irrespective of their height and weight. Furthermore, some mothers may fear the envy of others if, at the clinic, their own child is found to be more 'normal' than other children, or they may fear being accused of witchcraft or 'evil eye' if the situation is reversed. The next section will concentrate mainly on immunizations and on the prevention and treatment of diarrhoeal and respiratory diseases, including tuberculosis.

Immunizations

An estimated 5 million children die each year from diseases preventable by immunizations.[29] To deal with this, the World Health Organization set up the *Expanded Programme on Immunization* (EPI) in 1974 to target six major childhood diseases: diphtheria, tetanus, pertussis (whooping cough), polio, measles, and tuberculosis. Since then rates of immunization of the world's children in their first year of life has risen from only 5 per cent in 1974 to 76 per cent by the end of 2003.[33] In 2000 the WHO launched another initiative: the Global Alliance for Vaccines and Immunization (GAVI), an international private-public partnership with the Gates Foundation and others, to raise immunization coverage in the world's 74 poorest countries, and to introduce new vaccines against diseases such as hepatitis B and *Haemophilus influenzae*, type B.[34] By 2004, with an estimated 500 million immunization contacts with children annually, it was estimated that the EPI was preventing the deaths of at least 3 million children a year, while polio was 'on the verge of eradication', and about 750 000 fewer children were disabled, blinded, or mentally retarded as a result of vaccine-preventable diseases.[33]

There are the two key problems faced in trying to immunize a large proportion of the world's population:

1 The organizational and technical problems of making vaccines available to those who need them (this includes the need for a 'cold chain', whereby vaccines remain at a constant low temperature from the place of production to the site of immunization)
2 The need to increase acceptability of vaccines, even when they are available.

The technical issues include the cost, production and efficacy of the vaccines, and how they are distributed. Organizational problems include: when and how immunization campaigns are to be put into practice; whether they should target particularly vulnerable groups or the entire population; whether they should be separate, or integrated with the rest of PHC; how communication with the community can be effectively organized; and whether local healers, such as traditional birth attendants, should be involved in the campaign. However, they point out that immunizations alone often do not reduce overall mortality rates unless *other* issues, such as malnutrition, and poor housing, are also dealt with. Overall, there is thus 'a need to be aware that immunizations do not represent a magic, or universal protection against all ill'. In terms of acceptability, they link low levels of acceptability with a number of factors, including: low socio-economic status; large families; low educational level of mothers; social isolation; and migrant status (including nomadic lifestyles). Coverage for handicapped or otherwise disadvantaged children has also been shown to be low, as has been that for girls compared with boys. In contrast, those 'predisposed to immunization' tend to believe that their susceptibility to a disease is high, that the consequences of getting it would be serious, that immunization is the most effective way of preventing it, and that there are no serious barriers to immunization.

Attitudes to immunization

Certain indigenous beliefs may either help or impede immunization campaigns; in general, in order for these to be successful they should somehow 'make sense' in terms of people's own perceptions of ill health. Nichter[36] points out that limited information combined with some local beliefs may lead to fears or false expectations of a particular immunization campaign. In his study in south India in 1992, he found that only 11 per cent of the households in North Kanara district and 28 per cent in South Kanara had a family member who had been informed as to the illness prevented by the immunization they had received. In most cases, health workers had merely told them that 'vaccinations are good for health and they prevent disease'.

Figure 18.1 An immunization session in the Philippines. Access to preventative care is a right for the individual and a necessity for society. (Source: World Health Organization, *World Health*, No 5, September–October, 1996, page 8. Reproduced with permission.)

Some pregnant women thought that vaccinations were 'tonic injections' that would cause them to have big babies, and thus difficult deliveries. Told by health workers that the vaccines were powerful 'health injections', other people thought that they were too strong for a body in a 'weakened' state, such as a child who was weak or ill, especially with fever, productive cough or diarrhoea. Others thought that vaccines, like ear piercing or ritual scarification, 'shocked' the body back to health. Other beliefs about vaccines included that they removed 'toxins' from the body, protected against all serious infectious diseases as well as mystical illnesses such as *krimi*, were 'long-lasting doses of antibiotic' that travelled all over the body to reduce illness, and reduced children's future fertility. Furthermore, many people did not trust the competence of the PHC staff administering the injections, especially if they were outsiders and not accountable to the community. Conversely, health workers in those target communities might sometimes be reluctant to give immunizations, for fear of being blamed if they failed to work or if they caused side-effects. Where side-effects to a particular vaccine do occur, mothers often reject all other forms of vaccination on the assumption that they are all 'similar', and therefore have similar bad reactions.

Nichter[36] further points out that while there are advantages in health workers' identifying a vaccine by the name of an illness with which people are familiar (such as whooping cough), this may be more difficult where the disease to be prevented has a vaguer, more diffuse clinical picture (such as a rash or fever). Also, in many cases people believe that a vaccine may protect against a specific disease or a range of diseases that they fear, even if this is not the case. For example, in their research in south Kanara, Nichter and Nichter[37] found that while 50 per cent of mothers surveyed thought that vaccinations protected their children against specific illnesses (such as polio, or tuberculosis), 28 per cent thought that they protected them against all 'big' or serious illnesses found in that community. He points out therefore that these false expectations may contribute to the perception among many people that vaccinations are not very effective.

Similar misconceptions have been reported from many other parts of the world. For example, in a study of Xhosa mothers in rural Transkei, South Africa in 2003, Helman and Yogeswaran[38] found that while their attitudes towards immunizations were generally positive, and their knowledge of polio and measles vaccines was high, there was confusion about the reasons for some other immunizations. Several of the mothers thought BCG (bacillus Calmette–Guérin) immunized against 'BCG disease', while DPT (diphtheria–pertussis–tetanus) vaccine prevented 'DPT disease' – just as the polio vaccine prevented polio (*ipolio*), and measles vaccine prevented measles (*imasisi*). They therefore did not connect BCG with tuberculosis prevention, or DPT with preventing the diphtheria, pertussis or tetanus.

Mothers may also see visits to clinics, and receiving injections, as actions that are taken only when someone is ill, not when they are healthy.[38]

Giving injections to a healthy baby may seem counter-intuitive (especially when it may make the baby temporarily unwell). One result, as in the Transkei example, was a confusion between prevention and treatment. Vaccines were said to either act by 'strengthening the child ('he will grow up strong'), preventing him getting ill ('the child becomes less vulnerable to illness'), or even by 'treating' an already sickly child ('I notice that when I gave birth to him he was not so well, but after receiving immunizations there was a difference'). Furthermore, childhood diseases, like other diseases, are usually seen as multicausal in origin (see Chapter 5) and not just caused by a particular microbe. Conditions such as polio or measles may be blamed on a variety of other factors, such as poor mothering, 'bad milk', 'dirt', witchcraft, exposure to bad weather, inadequate housing, divine punishment, or the wrath of ancestors – and these diseases cannot be prevented by immunization alone.[38]

Episodes of side-effects from a vaccine can also reduce immunization uptake. In Mozambique,[39] Cutts and colleagues found that knowledge of another child who had had a post-vaccination abscess could dissuade a mother from having her own children vaccinated. In more affluent countries, the media can play a similar role in alarming mothers about the possible dangers of immunization. For example, in the UK, in the late 1990s, there was considerably media publicity about a possible link between the measles–mumps–rubella (MMR) vaccine, and the later development of autism and Crohn's disease. Although this claim was later contested by many other scientists, the national uptake of MMR dropped significantly, especially among more affluent social classes. Casiday and her colleagues[40] found that although most parents were in favour of immunization in general, many were ambivalent about the safety of MMR, and they displayed 'a considerable level of distrust in the government's role in regulating risk.' Despite distrusting 'doctors' in general, they nevertheless trusted the advice on immunisation of their own family doctors.

437

Social and economic factors

Several studies indicate that *social* and *economic* factors in a child's family background can play a crucial role in reducing the overall level of uptake. These include: (1) low household income,[35] (2) poor levels of education,[41] (3) low level of literacy,[41] (4) large family size,[35,39,41] (5) living far from the clinic,[39,42] and (6) inability to pay for transport to the clinic.[43] The mother may also be pregnant, or unwell, or have no-one to leave her other children with, when she goes to the clinic.[38]

Other factors that can cause low uptake have nothing at all to do with the children, their parents, or families: they are the fault of the medical system itself. For example, in poor areas, clinics may be sited too far from the places where people live. There may be no easy transport to the clinic.[38,42,43] They may only be open at inconvenient times (in the Mozambique study, the clinic was only open a small number of days per week).[39] They may have rigid appointment times, which may not suit the more unpredictable, chaotic lives of poor rural people. They may frequently run out of vaccines, and then have to send the mothers and infants home empty-handed.[41] They may (illegally) charge the mothers for the immunizations and the staff in the clinics may be rude, or unhelpful, to both mother and child.[38,42]

A final issue is that the members of a community may not understand why only children, and sometimes women, are the main targets of vaccination campaigns, while men and older children are ignored. They might advance a whole range of conspiracy and political theories to explain why they, too, are not being given the powerful 'government injections' said to enhance health and protect against disease.[37]

Overall then, an understanding of both structural factors and indigenous ideas about both diseases and vaccines is crucial to the success of any immunization programme. According to Heggenhougen and Clements,[35] 'messages which contradict beliefs, habits and action which people have invested with time, effort and resources and around which people have based their lives, will require considerably more force, ingenuity, and/or repetition in order to impress than messages which agree with their way of doing things'.

An example of a closer fit between local beliefs and those of the medical system, in relation to immunizations, is this study from Burkina Faso.

Case study: acceptance of childhood vaccinations in Kéru, Burkina Faso

Samuelsen[44] in 2001 found a very high acceptance (almost 100 per cent) of childhood immunizations among mothers in the village of Kéru, Burkina Faso. This was largely due to resonances between traditional forms of 'vaccination', practiced in the village for many years, and the modern forms now being promoted by the public health system. Traditionally, mothers in Kéru would bring their babies to a local herbalist healer (known as a vaccinatrice) for the treatment, and prevention of a variety of folk illnesses. Using a razor blade to make 30–40 small incisions in a child's skin, she would then rub special herbs into them. Many of these preventable illnesses were believed to be caused by a 'weakening of the blood', so that treatments where medicines were directly mixed with the blood would reverse that process – and help strengthen the blood again. Samuelsen also points out that cicatrization with knives or razors, as well as scarification followed by 'cupping', is also practiced in many other parts of Africa, and that vaccination against smallpox was actually practiced in West Africa long before it was introduced to Europe. In Kéru there is now a two-way influence between the traditional and the public health systems' for, as Samuelsen points out, 'So-called indigenous practices are not static, but adjust and change continuously in the response to changing social and cultural conditions'. The vaccinatrice has integrated many of the approaches and self-presentation of the local public health clinic or Centre de Santé et de Promotion Sociale (SCPS), such as a once-weekly 'clinic day', waiting times, cash payment and the use of imported razor blades and needles. While the SCPS are critical of the healer's treatments and its dangers (especially infections and haemorrhage), these traditional beliefs and practices have actually increased community acceptance of modern immunizations, by reinforcing the idea that disease can be prevented by the process of immunization.

Diarrhoeal diseases

Some of the issues related to diarrhoeal diseases, and the acceptance of oral rehydration solution (ORS), have already been discussed in Chapter 1. These diseases, which kill about 5–7 million people every year, are largely linked to poverty, with the resultant poor nutrition, water supplies, housing, sanitation and garbage disposal. Before diarrhoeal illnesses can be permanently reduced, or eliminated, these socio-economic issues will have to be addressed.[45] In addition, Weiss[46] has described the many cultural explanations found world-wide about the origin, significance or treatment of diarrhoeal illnesses. For example, in many cultural groups (including in Latin America and South Asia) they are blamed on an imbalance of 'heat' and 'cold' either within the body or in the environment. In other groups, 'bad breast milk', heavy foods, dirt or pollution may be blamed. Supernatural causes (see Chapter 5) of diarrhoeal illnesses include the evil eye, witchcraft, sorcery, malign spirits, divine punishment, contact with a menstruating woman, parental sexual infidelity, or having sex during pregnancy or lactation. Indigenous treatments may involve herbal remedies, patent medicines, religious rituals, changes in diet or breast-feeding, and even 'cleansing the gastrointestinal tract with enemas, purgatives, and emetics'.

Nichter[47] stresses the importance of understanding whether communities differentiate between ordinary (usually viral) diarrhoea and the more dangerous dysentery (caused by bacteria such as *Shigella*). As well as ORS, the latter may require antibiotic treatment, and often hospitalization. He points out that in some communities the bloody diarrhoea associated with dysentery may be considered more serious than the more watery, secretory diarrhoea, but in others the situation may be reversed. In Mindoro, in the Philippines, for example, he found that the emphasis by health workers on the dangers of dehydration meant that villagers feared the (less severe) form of watery diarrhoea more than dysentery. Fever and pain, not blood in the stools *per se*, were seen as reasons for going to the clinic. In Sri Lanka, bloody diarrhoea is associated with 'heat' trapped in the body, and is treated by ingesting 'cooling substances', as well as medicines and ORS. Some people refuse antibiotics, though, which they see as 'dangerous heating agents for bloody diarrhoea'. In contrast, others refuse ORS for watery diarrhoea, 'because cultural common sense dictates drying up watery stool'.

Both community health workers and traditional healers have been used to promote the use of ORT within their communities. However, these healers are not a homogeneous group, and often vary in their knowledge of ORT and in their willingness to use it. In Montrouis, Haiti, for example, Coreil[48] found that while 74 per cent of mothers had heard of ORT, only 51 per cent of healers had. Of all the healers, 32 per cent had taught mothers about ORT, and 2 per cent had used it themselves. Midwives and 'injectionists' were more knowledgeable about ORT, and more willing to use it, than were both herbalists and shamans. Of all the traditional healers, traditional birth attendants – because of their close involvement in maternal and infant care – are probably best placed for advising mothers on the benefits of ORT.

Respiratory infections: acute and chronic

In most of the Third World, acute respiratory infections (ARIs) are one of the major causes of death in infants and young children under 5 years of age. In India, for example, an estimated 500 000–750 000 children die of these infections every year.[49] The United Nations Children's Fund (UNICEF)[50] estimated in 2000 that each year 2 million children under 5 years die from ARIs in developing countries. The ARIs most commonly implicated are pneumonia, bronchitis, bronchiolitis and tuberculosis. Like diarrhoeal diseases, they are often associated with poverty and deprivation, and sometimes complicate other childhood infections such as measles and pertussis. They are often associated with conditions such as malnutrition and malaria.

As with diarrhoeal illnesses, anthropological studies of ARIs have examined indigenous beliefs and practices, forms of traditional healing, and attitudes to medical treatments.[49] Local perceptions of these conditions are particularly important, since they may influence the point at which parents define them as potentially dangerous (and seek further help), and whether this occurs before or after the infection has had a chance to spread to the rest of the family or community. These indigenous beliefs may include, for example, notions of 'normal' and 'abnormal' ways of breathing, the significance of different types of cough, wheeze, phlegm or fever, and so on. In terms of explaining the origin and significance of ARIs, many of the lay theories of illness aetiology described in Chapter 5 also apply. Another important issue is the use of Western pharmaceuticals (such as antibiotics) bought over the counter from local pharmacies or medicine vendors (see Chapter 8), since these may lead to the development of resistant strains of bacteria responsible for ARIs. The important role of anthropological insights in developing preventive and treatment strategies for these illnesses has been recognized by WHO, with its Programme for the Control of Acute Respiratory Infections.[51]

Tuberculosis

Among the more chronic respiratory diseases, tuberculosis (TB) is the most serious. In 1991 it was estimated that about 1700 million people were or had been afflicted by the disease,[52] and that every year 8 million cases of TB were occurring worldwide, as well as about 3 million deaths from the disease, 95–99 per cent of which were occurring in developing countries.[52] A more recent survey in 2003[53] estimated that in the year 2000 there

were a total of about 8.3 million new cases of TB worldwide, and that incidence rates of the disease were highest in sub-Saharan Africa. Between 1997 and 2000, while the total number of new TB cases worldwide increased at a rate of 1.8 per cent per year, the number of new cases in the former Soviet Union increased much more quickly (6.0 per cent per year), as did those in sub-Saharan Africa (6.4 per cent per year).[53] Overall, the global burden of tuberculosis, and diseases associated with it, seems to be steadily increasing.

Tuberculosis is usually a disease of poverty, associated with poor nutrition, overcrowding and inadequate health care. Recently, however, cases of TB in the Western world have been increasing, often in poor inner-city neighbourhoods, and sometimes in association with AIDS or other diseases. In 1998 it was estimated that by the year 2000, some 1.4 million cases of tuberculosis (14 per cent of the global total) would be associated with HIV infection.[54] However, figures from the year 2000 indicated that only about 9 per cent of all new TB cases in adults (aged 15–49 years) were actually attributable to HIV infection, but the proportion was much greater in the WHO African Region, (31 per cent) and some industrialized countries, especially the USA (26 per cent). That year there were an estimated 1.8 million deaths from the disease worldwide, of which 12 per cent (226 000) were attributable to HIV infection.[53]

Attempts to treat TB and control its spread have encountered a number of social and cultural problems. According to a review by Rubel and Garro[55], the two main barriers to successful control are a delay in seeking treatment and the abandonment of treatment before it becomes effective. Cultural beliefs about the significance of early symptoms of the disease play a particularly important part. For example, a study they carried out among Mexican migrant workers in southern California found considerable delays (8.5 months, on average) between the onset of symptoms and the decision to consult a doctor. Many of them misinterpreted their early symptoms, such as cough, fatigue, loss of weight, headaches, back pains or running nose, as evidence of less serious conditions, such as *gripe* (grippe) or *bronquitis* (bronchitis), or even *susto* (see Chapter 5). Many attributed their fatigue and weight loss to hard work and lack of sleep, and initially treated themselves by smoking and drinking less, going to sleep earlier, using patent medicines and leading what they perceived to be a healthier lifestyle. A further reason for treatment delay (as well as its early abandonment) is the marked *stigma* associated with the disease in many parts of the world. The authors quote a study among Zulu people in South Africa, which found that to suggest that sufferers from TB were infectious was tantamount to identifying them as witches or sorcerers, since these were the only people in that community with the power to cause illness to other people. A study in Mexico City showed that 52 per cent of patients discharged from hospital after treatment for TB were not allowed to go home because of the hostility of their families; another showed that many patients had abandoned their treatment early because of the costs of transport to the clinic, a dread of family disintegration, and fear of rejection by their families (25 per cent of the defaulters had not told their families of their true diagnosis). Since successful completion of treatment is associated with good social support from the family, the stigma associated with the disease may be one reason why attempts to control it can fail. Other reason for failure relates to the health-care system itself, and the ways that TB clinics are organized. For example, arranging appointments at inconvenient times, repeating registration of patients at every visit, seating people in overcrowded and poorly ventilated waiting rooms, seeing them rigidly in order of registration (and ignoring any extenuating circumstances), and physicians using technical jargon when talking to patients, may all contribute to people's reluctance to come to a clinic for treatment or follow up. Thus, failure of treatment, including its cost and availability are some of reasons for the persistence of TB. In designing more effective interventions, Rubel and Garrow suggest that it is necessary to assess 'how people use

knowledge to interpret symptoms of this chronic, debilitating disease at the time that they seek help and how their help-seeking decision is influenced by financial, transport and other considerations'.[55]

Case study: folk models of tuberculosis in Dongora, southern Ethiopia

Vecchiato[56] in 1997 described folk beliefs about tuberculosis, and self-treatments, in a farming community of the Sidama people in southern Ethiopia. Despite a high prevalence of tuberculosis in that area, and despite the fact that no social stigma was attached to it, only a fraction of the cases presented themselves to the local clinic. However, most Sidama did recognize the symptoms of the disease, which they blamed either on overwork or on poor nutrition (though some accepted that it spread by contagion, or by 'inhaling dust particles'). However, 52.1 per cent believed that traditional remedies (*Sidama taghiccho*) were much more effective in treating tuberculosis than modern ones, while only 37.8 per cent preferred the latter. Traditional treatments included eating a nutritious diet (especially meat, milk and *ensete* porridge), ingesting several types of herbal remedies (mostly used as emetics, to vomit out the 'bad blood' that accumulates internally), or getting a traditional healer (*oghessa*) to apply smouldering wooden rods to 'cauterize' the diseased parts of the body, especially the chest. Vecchiato noted that one reason that antituberculosis drugs such as streptomycin were often rejected was that they have no emetic effect, and suggests that future antituberculosis programmes take into account these indigenous beliefs, and work with them where possible. As a starting point, they should acknowledge that the Sindama can accurately diagnose pulmonary tuberculosis, that they do have a sense of diseases being contagious, and that they do see the value of a highly nutritious diet when ill. He also suggests that attempts be made to discover whether traditional herbal remedies are effective in treating tuberculosis, or not.

Community resources in PHC

The emphasis in the Alma-Ata declaration on *community participation* in PHC has meant that a number of community resources have been used to facilitate PHC at the local level. These include:

1 community health workers (CHWs)
2 Community health groups
3 Traditional healers
4 Community leaders.

Community health workers

These are generally members of a particular community whose task is to improve the health of that community, often in cooperation with the health-care system or with national or international aid agencies. They may be selected by their communities, though sometimes this is done by local leaders or by outside agencies. They advise the community on preventive strategies and give advice on child care, healthy nutrition, immunizations and hygiene, as well as providing some limited curative and first-aid services; in addition, many become more general agents for change in the community, in areas outside the health field. Since Alma-Ata, many thousands have been selected and trained, in 62 many different countries, and in both rural and urban areas.[57] They include the 'barefoot doctors' in China, the 'family welfare educators' in Botswana, the 'village health development workers' in Indonesia, the 'village health volunteers' in Thailand and the 'community health agents' in Egypt. In most cases, CHWs are given a short course of training – usually a few weeks to a few months – and a small amount of equipment, such as a few basic drugs, some dressings, disinfectants, thermometer, and scales and charts for measuring the weights and heights of children. In some countries, the training of CHWs has been much more extensive, such as that of the *feldsher*,[58] or physician's assistants, in rural parts of Russia and the former USSR, who have provided some basic PHC at the village level since Peter the Great founded them in the eighteenth century, and whose training lasts up to about 2.5 years.[58]

However, the use of CHWs is still controversial. For one thing, their selection and training raises the problems of how 'community', 'health' and 'worker' are each defined. The definition of a 'community', for example, may be a bureaucratic fiction, imposed on a disparate group of people by some distant official or aid agency with little local knowledge. For one thing, these communities are not static; many are in a constant state of flux, as some people migrate in from rural areas while others leave in search of work. Neither are they homogeneous. Slums and shantytowns, especially those with a high proportion of rural migrants, often have many different communities within them – formed by people from the same village or region, or based on different religious, ethnic or social backgrounds. Each micro-community, and often each gender, may have very different attitudes to health and illness, and use a different range of traditional cures and healers (see Chapter 4).

Definitions of 'health' are also problematic since, as illustrated throughout this book, medical and lay definitions of health are often very different. Which definition, then, is the CHW meant to promote? If these workers are seen to be merely the agents of the health service, can this reduce their credibility in the eyes of their community? Finally, many of these CHWs are not 'workers' in the formal sense since most are unpaid volunteers or receive very little money for their time and effort.

Another argument against CHWs is that, with their limited period of training, they are not 'real' health practitioners, and can only provide 'second-class health care for second-class citizens'. In many cases, ill people prefer consulting a 'real' doctor, whatever the cost, effort or travel involved. A follow-up study of Tanzanian CHWs,[59] for example, found that although the community was generally in favour of them, they (and the CHWs themselves) were primarily interested in them providing curative rather than preventive services. Also, 53 per cent of the 344 CHWs interviewed had had no supervisory visit from any health agency in the previous 3 months. The combination of inadequate diagnostic and treatment skills, infrequent supervision and shortage of drugs undermined the acceptance of CHWs by their communities; despite this, they were seen as a valuable resource, and 88 per cent of those trained since 1983 were still active 5 years later.

Community health groups

Other local resources may be *community health groups*, which are organized to share information about health issues (such as the importance of family planning, breast-feeding or immunizations) and to give help to their members. Many are women's groups, especially antenatal and mother-and-baby groups, and are often facilitated by local CHWs.

Traditional healers

Traditional healers have also been promoted as an intrinsic part of PHC, and some of the arguments for and against their use have already been summarized in Chapter 4. In some cases, the roles of CHW and traditional healer may overlap, either directly or indirectly owing to familial links. In the author's study in Porto Alegre, southern Brazil, for example, the majority of the 150 community health workers (*agente de saúde*) recruited to work in the shanty towns (*favelas*) in the early 1990s

had at least one traditional healer in their family tree, though by 2006 this trend had largely disappeared. The intention of WHO has been to involve traditional healers in PHC, for example in the Essential Drugs Programme (see Chapter 8), but without causing too much disruption to local cultural patterns[60]. That is: 'the establishment of primary health care services in developing countries should not result in abrupt disruption of prevailing cultural patterns in rural communities. The work of traditional healers, for example, should be adapted and supplemented so as to ensure that innovation is successfully integrated into existing systems of care'.[60]

Community leaders

A final resource used in PHC are community leaders, or people of influence – such as local schoolteachers, religious figures or political leaders – since their cooperation might be vital for the success of any health-care initiative. In many systems of PHC, these community resources are often combined with local clinics or 'health posts' situated in villages or urban shanty towns and staffed by doctors, nurses or other health professionals, often in cooperation with CHWs. More serious cases would then be referred to regional district

Figure 18.2 A primary health care clinic in a *favela* or shanty town in Porto Alegre, southern Brazil, built and run in cooperation with the local community.

hospitals, or sometimes to more specialized hospitals elsewhere. To some extent, this shift towards a community-based PHC also means a shift away from a medical model that has become increasingly expensive, overspecialized and overdependent on technology. It also implies the development of a new kind of doctor, who sees successful PHC as not only an applied medical science, but as an applied social science as well.

The role of anthropologists in PHC

Since Alma-Ata, many anthropologists have been involved in the planning, application and evaluation of PHC programmes,[29–31] and in increasing community participation in health care. As well as their expertise in local cultures, health beliefs and practices and traditional forms of healing, Donahue[61] sees their role as 'culture brokers', mediating between the needs of local communities and those of the health-care system: 'Anthropologists can provide direct feedback to the community which they have studied. Their knowledge of the structural–cognitive systems of both the traditional and the modern medical systems allows them to find points of articulation between the two'. Mars[1] suggests that 'in an attempt to link social reality to social planning', medical aid programmes should develop a network of 'barefoot anthropologists' – and one trained anthropologist could, with the aid of locally recruited assistants, monitor up to 10 small-scale communities and facilitate a two-way communication in order to modify and influence more centralized policy decisions.

It should be stressed, however, that 'anthropologist' is not necessarily synonymous with 'Western anthropologist'. In many different contexts, especially in non-Western countries, it is those anthropologists and other social scientists that come from those countries (or even from those communities) who may be the best people to act as consultants and researchers. These people, who understand the subtleties of local custom and belief and are native speakers of the language, may be better able to avoid the 'cultural imprint of the West' inherent in many PHC programmes (see below). This type of input is crucial in community-based PHC, since these programmes have often been developed by a distant international bureaucracy in Europe or North America, or by a national urban elite with little knowledge of local conditions in rural areas or in the poorer neighbourhoods of their own cities.

Primary health care and cultural concepts of time

One important reason for the failure of health education and preventive strategies, in PHC and elsewhere, is a difference in the perception of *time* between health planners and local communities. Many of these programmes are designed by middle-class individuals and target people much poorer than themselves, and much of the health education is based on what may be termed a 'middle-class investment model'. That is, 'invest' in yourself now (by education, savings, a nutritious diet, avoiding smoking, using a condom and 'deferring gratification'), and this behaviour will result in your reaping a 'profit' (or 'interest' on your 'investment') many years in the future. In terms of health, this profit will be in the form of better physical health, a better quality of life and increased life expectancy. However, this approach ignores the daily reality of people living precarious, poverty-stricken lives. The daily, sometimes hourly, struggle for survival – for food, shelter, money and safety – of many people living in slum or shanty town communities, especially where there is no social welfare system, means that they live in a very short time-span. People living this precarious existence may not be able to plan more than a day or two ahead; to expect them, for example, to avoid smoking so that in 15 or 20 years time they will not develop lung cancer or heart disease is simply impractical, especially with adolescents and younger people, who also have a very different sense of time. As well as changing the socio-economic realities in which they are embedded, programmes in health education need to stress the short-term benefits of a change in

444

behaviour. They may also need to break down long-term health interventions into much shorter time units (such as the 'day at a time' approach of Alcoholics Anonymous) in order to reflect the way different people experience time in their daily lives.

Socio-economic considerations and PHC

As mentioned earlier, many of the health problems addressed by comprehensive PHC are the result, direct or indirect, of poverty, especially the inability to afford adequate food, housing, clothing, sanitation, garbage removal, transport and health care.[62]

For the rural poor of Third World countries, another major obstacle to health and health care is not their cultural belief systems, but the lack of any physical infrastructure, especially of roads, railways, bridges, electrical power, street lights, telephones, hospitals and clinics.[63] Poor-quality roads, infrequent or expensive public transport and long distances to travel to a clinic may all influence their ability and willingness to seek medical care. Also, within a particular country, wealthier regions may be better able to afford the infrastructure of health than poorer ones. In India, for example, the richer states of Maharashtra and Gujarat have 1.5 and 1.1 hospital beds respectively per 1000 population, while the rates for the poorer states of Bihar and Madhya Pradesh are only 0.3 and 0.4, respectively.[63] There is also a significant shortage of doctors, nurses and other health professionals in many poorer countries, and an urban bias in their distribution (see Chapter 4).

However, all attempts at improving health and preventing disease will be pointless unless larger social, economic and ecological issues are also addressed. These include the overpopulation, pollution and global warming mentioned above, but also the transnational marketing of 'chemical comforters' such as tobacco,[64] pharmaceuticals (see Chapter 8) and addictive drugs. Another issue is the enormous *inequality* in wealth and resources between different parts of the world; it has been estimated that the world's richest 20 per cent are 150 times richer than the world's poorest 20 per cent, and that the gap between the two is steadily widening[2].

The international arms trade

Finally, it is also pointless to save children from infectious diseases if they are going to be killed by crime, war or other forms of violence. According to the *Global Health Action* report of 2005–06, an estimated 191 million people died as a result of conflict in the twentieth century.[65] Furthermore, more than 85 per cent of the major armed conflicts since World War Two have taken place in poorer countries, and between 1986 and 1996 a major proportion of the people dying as a result of armed conflicts were civilians, particularly women and children.[65] The role of the international arms trade – both legal and illegal – is important here. In a *British Medical Journal* article[5] it was estimated that in 1993 developing countries were spending about $38 on arms for each person, but only $12 on health, and that the entire annual budget of the WHO amounted to just 3 hours of world expenditure on arms. As well as using up scarce resources, these arms are a major threat to human life. That same year an article in the *New York Times*[66] it was estimated that about 100 million landmines threatened civilians in more than 60 countries, and had caused tens of thousands of deaths and injuries, especially in Afghanistan and in South-East Asia (about 30 000 people in Cambodia had lost limbs, mostly from mines). At the same time, the market for these mines was worth $200 million per year, and they were being produced by some 100 companies and government agencies in 48 countries.

Huge numbers of people are killed each year by guns. Overall, the WHO estimated that in 1998, 2.3 million people worldwide died as a result of violence, and that this included several hundred thousand from gun-inflicted homicides.[67] According to the BBC,[68] the highest death toll from firearms is in Brazil, where guns kill one person every 15 minutes, and where there were 36 000 shooting deaths in 2004.

Many of the homicides caused by firearms occur in the 'gun-rich, resource poor' parts of the world such as Brazil, but this is not always the case: in 2000, for example, American males had three times the risk of dying from firearm-related injuries than did Canadian males, while for American females the risk was seven times greater.[69] Overall, the 2003 *Small Arms Survey* estimated that 639 million small arms were in circulation worldwide (one for every 10 people on the planet), that 59 per cent were held legally by civilians, and that the annual sales of global arms were $21 billion, and that the UK, France and the USA earned more from arms sales than they provided in aid to the Third World.[70] It should be noted that in many parts of the world small arms are held not only by the army and police. According to the more recent 2005 *Small Arms Survey*, for example, there were about 58–107 million small arms in the Middle East, of which the vast majority (45–90 million) were in civilian hands.[71] In 47 of 49 major conflicts between 1990 and 2000, small arms and light weapons were the main weapons used, and they caused considerable injury and loss of life.[72] As stated earlier, more than 85 per cent of the major conflicts since the Second World War have taken place in poorer countries.[72] In these countries, therefore, PHC has to take place against the background of the large stocks of arms, and of the many deaths and injuries, as well as the drain on financial resources and dangers to health personnel, that they may cause.

A related issue is that war, civil unrest and ecological disasters usually result in refugees – currently estimated as between 15 million and 50 million world-wide,[5] but mostly located in poorer countries. Some of the many physical, psychological and social effects of refugee and migrant status are described in Chapter 12.

The evidence, therefore, is that the organization of any system of PHC, whatever its ideology or origin, must always take these wider socio-economic and ecological issues into consideration. That is, in order to be truly effective, it must always have some 'comprehensive' element in it.[29]

Health–care bureaucracies and PHC

To understand any form of PHC fully, the role played in it by the culture of medicine itself must be examined (see Chapter 5), as well as that of its various institutions, such as hospitals, medical schools, government departments and the bureaucracies of international aid agencies. Each of these has its own institutional subculture, hierarchy, ideology (whether political, religious or secular) and view of health, illness and the nature of medical care. In examining PHC, therefore, medical anthropology is not just about the health beliefs and behaviours of different cultures and communities; an essential part of its perspective is an understanding of how these institutional factors can either help or hinder the successful delivery of health care.

Foster[73] points out that health professionals easily accept the premise that the principal barriers to health care lie within the target community. The assumption is that 'effective health care can be achieved only when members of traditional communities change their health behaviour. Rarely if ever is the question asked, "How can anthropologists help to change bureaucratic behaviour that inhibits the design and operation of the best possible health care systems?"'.[73] Furthermore, 'among health personnel there is a hopeful assumption that there is a right "key" which, if only anthropologists can discover it, will unlock the door to wholehearted community cooperation in primary health care activities'.[47] Similarly, Coreil[74] warns that 'studies are commissioned with the hope that social science can pinpoint a simple key element that can be manipulated in such a way to make the whole system work as desired'. The assumption is that 'if changing behaviour will result in effective primary health care, it must be community, not bureaucratic, behaviour that changes'.

Foster[75] emphasizes the enormous strides that international health agencies (such as WHO) have made in meeting the world's health needs, especially in developing countries. However, he sees many of them, although international in ideology, as bearing 'the cultural imprint of the West'. He describes three premises that underlie many international medical aid programmes:

1 That the developed world possesses both the talent and the capital for helping 'backward' countries to develop.
2 If some people have 'know-how', and others do not, those with the 'know-how' are the proper ones to plan and execute the transfer.
3 Particular institutions and modes of operation that have met the needs of the developed world are the appropriate templates for the developing world, i.e. 'the health strategies that have served the West are universal, equally suited to Boston or Bombay'.

Innovative approaches to PHC

In very large or very poor countries, some very innovative methods of delivering primary care directly to a widely scattered population have been developed. Other methods have been developed to bring health-care advice directly to the public, without requiring them to make a trip to a clinic or hospital. Examples of some of these innovative approaches are:

• *The Royal Flying Doctor Service (RFDS)*[76] of Australia was developed on national basis in 1930, and since then brings health care to remote communities, especially in the vast interior or 'Outback'. It also transports ill patients to hospital, in urban areas. In 2004 the RFDS and its 45 airplanes attended to 210,423 patients, carried out 31,231 aerial evacuations, made 58, 012 landings, and flew a total of over 19 million kilometers.[76]
• *The Phelophepa Health Care Train*[77] of South Africa, founded in 1994, travels all over the country, bringing health care to remote rural communities who have little access to primary health care. The carriages on the train contain a variety of clinics including health screening, maternal and child health, counselling, ophthalmology, dentistry and health education. Rural communities are told in advance when the train will be stopping in their local area. Each year the train operates for 36 weeks, covers 15 000 km and treats over 180 000 patients. Since 1994, 595 961 children have been screened, 6679 local volunteers have been trained in a Basic Health Education Program, and more than 7000 students (medical, nursing and others) have done voluntary work on the train.[77]
• The *NHS Direct* telephone service,[78] a part of the British National Health Service (NHS), is a 24-hour telephone helpline run by specially trained nurses, that provides free medical advice, health information, and reassurance to the public. It is part of the NHS and runs parallel with it. If necessary, the nurses can refer callers to a hospital or to their doctor for further treatment. The telephone service is supplemented by an online service NHS Direct Online, which provides health information as well as an enquiry service about specific health issues.

This section illustrates, therefore, that local realities – social, cultural, economic and demographic – and the needs and desires of local communities also need to be taken into account when designing any system of PHC. For this reason, many of the insights of medical anthropology, usually based on detailed microstudies in local communities, can be useful to those who plan, administer and evaluate primary health-care programmes. They can help design systems of PHC at the local, national and international levels, which are humane, culturally appropriate and cost-effective, and which meet the needs not only of medical bureaucracies but also of the local communities themselves and the individuals within them.

POLLUTION AND GLOBAL WARMING

In 1944, the anthropologist Malinowski differentiated between the 'basic' human needs necessary for biological survival (such as metabolism, movement, growth, health and reproduction) and 'secondary' (or derived) needs (necessary for social life).[79] These man-made 'derived needs' included systems of laws, values, religion, art, ritual, language and symbolism, but they also included material objects, artefacts and technology. With socio-economic development, 'new needs appear and new imperatives or determinants are imposed on human behaviour'. The problem is that these new culturally derived needs, such as the 'need' in Western society always to eat food with a knife and fork, to go holiday by airplane every year, or to own a motor car and a refrigerator, often become seen as if they were as 'basic' or biological as the need for food or shelter, and become difficult to do without. In looking at ecological issues, therefore, anthropological studies of these culturally derived, quasi-basic needs are important, since their constant production by advertising and industry can outstrip the planet's resources, create inequality and dissatisfaction, and be dangerous to the environment.

To take one small example, the widespread use of chlorofluorocarbons (CFCs) in both refrigerators and aerosols has been found to contribute towards the thinning of the ozone layer, as well as to global warming (the 'greenhouse effect'), both of which can seriously damage human health.[80] Although economic factors (such as the profits involved in producing, promoting and selling these products) play a major role in their popularity, so do culturally influenced beliefs and behaviours. For example, where aerosols are used as deodorants, air cleaners, hair lacquers and furniture polish, their use is clearly influenced by certain cultural values, which are constantly reinforced by advertising. In Western countries, in particular, these stress the importance of living in an odour-free environment, with an absence of both natural body odour and extraneous smells within the home. They also promote certain hairstyles and colours (particularly those suggesting a youthful appearance), and emphasize shiny, reflecting surfaces on furniture within the home as a sign of order, affluence and social respectability.

The motor car

Another more pervasive example is the motor car, an invention that has had a profound effect on human life, transforming societies, cultures, economies, landscapes and human relationships all over the world.

Although exact figures are hard to come by, one estimate is that today there are about 600 million motor vehicles worldwide, about 200 million of them in the USA.[81] However, for all its benefits, the cost of this invention has been high in human terms. Since it was invented just over a century ago, and since the very first fatal traffic accident in 1898, an estimated 20 million people have been killed in car-related accidents,[82] and many millions more have been injured – making it one of the most dangerous inventions in human history. The WHO estimate that world-wide more than 1.2 million people are killed on the roads every year, and that in 1998 over 38 million injuries were sustained worldwide by people involved in motor vehicle accidents.[83] The economic cost of these deaths and injuries is enormous; in developing countries, the WHO estimate this cost to be about US $100 billion annually.[83] Automobiles are responsible not only for direct damage to human health, but also for damage to the environment. The best-known example of this is air pollution from car exhaust fumes – mainly carbon monoxide, ozone, nitrous dioxide and hydrocarbons. In overcrowded cities with high traffic densities, air pollution can have serious and permanent effects on health, particularly on the respiratory system. In addition, the combustion of leaded fuel (banned in the USA, but still common elsewhere) can lead to the fallout of lead oxide in dust, which may then contaminate food, the soil, crops and the feed of livestock, and cause serious health problems, especially in children.[84]

The car, however, is not only a form of transport. It is also a symbolic object that has different *meanings* for different people, depending on their culture and socio-economic background, their gender and age group. It often symbolizes values of prestige, power, autonomy, individualism and mobility (both social and geographical); images often created, or sustained, by the motor industry.

As with population control, attempts to reduce air pollution from car exhausts need to take some of these socio-cultural issues into account. National traffic policies (such as enforcing lowered speed limits, subsidizing unleaded fuel, checking car exhausts, increasing car tax and banning cars from city centres) may not be the only solution. Before people can be converted from private to public and less polluting forms of transport, such as railways, not only must these be easily accessible and affordable, but it is also important to understand why so many people seek to own cars in the first place. Here, anthropological studies of the cultural roles of car ownership can be useful, as part of a national transport policy.

Case study: symbolism of the motor car in Chaguanas, Trinidad

Miller[85] in 1994 described how in the town of Chaguanas, Trinidad, the car is 'a vehicle not only for transporting people spatially but also conceptually from one set of values to another'. These new values include notions of individuality, since in contemporary Trinidad 'the car is probably the artefact which outweighs even clothing in its ability to incorporate and express the concept of the individual'. In conversation, people are sometimes identified not by name, but by the make or number plate of their cars. For young males, particularly, cars have become the means of realizing their inner fantasies of independence from family, successful seduction and sexual attraction (street wisdom insists that 'women will not look at men who don't have cars'). As a public way of expressing individuality, cars can be 'customized' by special decorations to their upholstery or exteriors, clearly marking the status and character of the owner. One result of this is 'an unwillingness to walk, once in possession of a car'; huge traffic jams are commonplace as people drive to work or school, even when it is very near to home. Thus, in Trinidad, as elsewhere, the car has become 'as well-established a vehicle for expressive identity, as it is a vehicle for transport'.

Public health measures to reduce air pollution need to take these cultural factors into account. As with advertisements for tobacco and alcohol, the constant creation of 'derived needs' – and the emphasis on meeting these only by the consumption and public display of a material object, such as a car – will have to be dealt with, before the damage to the environment becomes irreversible.

Global warming

Global warming is one of the most important features in modern life, with many serious implications, and the situation is likely to worsen in the years to come. McMichael and colleagues[86] note that during the twentieth century, the average temperature of the world increased by approximately 0.6°C, and that about two-thirds of this warming has occurred since 1975. This is due mainly to 'greenhouse gases' (GHGs), which are principally carbon dioxide (mainly from fossil fuel combustion and burning of forests), methane (from irrigated agriculture, animal husbandry and oil extraction), nitrous oxide and various man-made halocarbons (such as CFCs). Most significantly, the United Nations Intergovernmental Panel on Climate Change (IPCC) concluded in 2001 that: 'There is new and stronger evidence that most of the warming observed over the last 50 years is attributable to human activities', especially the release of greenhouse gases from fossil fuels.[86] The IPCC concluded that if no specific actions are taken to reduce greenhouse gas emissions, global temperatures are likely to rise between 1.4°C and 5.8°C from 1990 to 2100.[86]

These climate changes are likely to have major effects on human health. According to the *World Health Report* 2002,[87] these effects range from increased deaths from respiratory or heart disease caused by extreme temperatures to deaths from an increase in 'weather disasters', such as floods, droughts or severe storms. Changes in weather patterns are also likely to affect the prevalence of vector-borne diseases such as malaria and dengue fever, the seasonal incidence of various food-related and waterborne infections, the yields of agricultural crops, the range of plant and livestock pests and pathogens, the salination of coastal areas and freshwater supplies by rising sea levels, and the risk of conflict over depleted natural resources (such as water, fuels or minerals). They estimate that in 2000 climate change was responsible for about 2.4 per cent of worldwide diarrhoea, 6 per cent of malaria in some middle-income countries and 7 per cent of dengue fever in some industrialized countries. Overall, climate change was responsible for about 154 000 deaths that year.

DEFORESTATION AND SPECIES EXTINCTION

One of the major threats to global health is deforestation, especially of the rainforests. Less than 50 per cent of the area covered by prehistoric tropical rainforests still remains, but it is currently being cut down or burned at a rate of about 142 000 square kilometres per year (approximately 1.8 per cent of the total area still standing).[88] Forests – 'the Earth's lungs' – play a crucial role in stabilizing global gases, thus reducing the greenhouse effect, and in maintaining global rainfall patterns. Their destruction can result in a reduced rainfall in adjacent areas and irreversible soil erosion, causing crop failures and a fall in food production. As well as its effects on the planet's ecology, there are three other serious problems associated with deforestation:

1 *Destruction of indigenous peoples* living in forest areas, both physically and culturally, by direct violence from loggers, ranchers, miners or government officials, or by the actual destruction of their habitat and hunting grounds.
2 *Species extinction* of animals, birds, plants and microbes, including many that could be used in the development of medicines.
3 *Infectious diseases* resulting from destruction of the natural habitats and ecological niches of certain viruses or their vectors, and their release into human populations.

In many cases, anthropologists have been able to contribute a more detailed understanding of the problem. For example, they have provided considerable data on indigenous tribal groups, especially within the Third World (such as Brazilian Indians), and on how many are dying as a result of destruction of the forests in which they live and hunt or by diseases brought in from the outside world.[89] Many have acted as advocates on their behalf to government and other bureaucracies, in an attempt to stop what may amount to genocide. Frequently, they have pointed out to those living in industrialized countries that they could learn valuable lessons from these indigenous peoples; especially their respect and reverence for the natural environment and its limited resources.

Traditional medicines

The destruction of natural species, especially plant, bird, animal and microbial, poses a special threat to global health. Within the next 50 years, an estimated one-quarter of all species will become extinct, particularly those lost by the rapid tropical deforestation.[88] At the current rate, this loss of biodiversity would mean an estimated 27 000 species lost every year, or more than 74 per day. An important result of this would be the loss of many thousands of potential medicines, of use in treating many different diseases. Chivian[88] in 1993 estimated that about 80 per cent of all people living in developing countries (about two-thirds of the world's population) relied almost exclusively on traditional medicines using natural substances, mostly derived from plants; even in the USA, 25 per cent of all prescriptions dispensed from community pharmacies between 1959 and 1980 contained active ingredients extracted from plants. Many of these plants have been used by indigenous healers for centuries before the development of modern pharmaceuticals, and are still being used. In 2003 the WHO estimated that 25 per cent of all modern medicines were made from plants, first used traditionally.[90] Among the more better-known medicines that are derived from plants are quinine and quinidine (from cinchona bark),

D-tubocurarine (from the *Chondrodendron* vine), aspirin (from willow bark), digitalis (from foxglove), morphine (from the opium poppy), the anticancer drugs taxol (from the Pacific yew tree), vinblastine and vincristine (from *Vinca rosa*, the periwinkle plant),[88] and the antimalarial artimisinin (*Artemisia annua* from the Chinese herb *qinghaosu*). Over the years, anthropological studies of traditional healing and indigenous pharmacopoeias have been a useful source of information about many other plant-based medicines, their advantages and disadvantages, and how they are used by human groups in different parts of the world.[91] It has been pointed out, though, that even though traditional herbal medicines are 'natural' in origin, they can sometimes be dangerous to health, and cause a variety of allergies, toxic effects, and even cancers.[92]

There is increasing concern about the growth of *biopiracy*, which is the unauthorized, and often illegal, use of the biological resources (such as indigenous plants, crops, or animals) or of traditional remedies of methods of healing of local communities in poorer countries by large business corporations in the developed world. Often this occurs by foreign companies taking out patents on local biological resources, and then going on to develop new pharmaceutical products; the profits from this development, however, are often not shared with the indigenous communities themselves. To prevent this situation, the United Nations Convention on Biological Diversity (CBD), first presented at the Earth Summit in Rio de Janeiro in 1992, has now been ratified by 168 countries.[93] Its aims are the conservation of worldwide biological diversity, the sustainable use of this biodiversity and a 'fair an equitable sharing of benefits arising out of the utilization of genetic resources'.[93] National governments have also taken action to protect their own biological resources: in 2002, for example, India passed the Biological Diversity Bill which aimed to address 'the basic concerns of access to, and collection and utilization of biological resources and knowledge by foreigners, and sharing of benefits arising from

such access'. Before the bill, cases of biopiracy in India had included the patenting of the wound-healing properties of *haldi* (tumeric), and the hypoglycaemic effects of *karela* (bitter gourd).[94]

In 2002 the WHO launched its first comprehensive Traditional Medicine Strategy.[95] Its aim was to develop national strategies on the scientific evaluation and regulation of traditional medicines (TM) and complementary medicines (CAM). It also aimed to improve the availability and affordability of TM/CAM, including essential herbal remedies – an essential strategy, since about one-third of the population of developing countries lack access to essential medicines, and therefore 'the provision of effective TM/CAM therapies could be a critical tool to increase access to health care'. However, this had to be accompanied by further research into the safety and efficacy of these therapies.

Deforestation also carries with it the danger of the release of new infectious diseases into human populations because of the destruction of natural habitats and the disruption of delicate local ecologies. For example, the cutting down of tropical rainforests (as in the Amazon area) displaces forest rodents, who were the usual reservoir hosts of sandflies (which carry protozoa of the genus *Leishmania*). As a result, the sandflies turn temporarily to biting humans, and thereby increase the incidence of leishmaniasis, a serious disease said to affect over 12 million people world-wide.[88] Similarly, ticks, tsetse flies (carriers of African sleeping sickness) and kissing bugs (carriers of Chagas' disease, common in Central and South America, and affecting 15–20 million people) may all be released by the destruction of their usual habitats. Several viral illnesses have also recently 'emerged' from forest regions as a result of deforestation. Among them is Kyasanur forest disease (KFD), carried by *Haemophysalis spinigera* ticks, which usually feed on small forest animals in the tropical forests of southern India. With the introduction of sheep and cattle into previously forested areas, they become reservoirs of the disease, as do the humans who tend them.[88,96] As with other 'new' viral diseases, anthropologists have studied the impact of these epidemics on particular communities, as in this case from India.

Case study: community reactions to Kyasanur forest disease in South Kanara district, southern India

Nichter[96] in 1987 described Kyasanur forest disease (KFD) in South Kanara District as essentially a 'disease of development' – the result of deforestation and the rearing of cattle in the cleared scrublands between villages and forest. Many of those afflicted were poor agricultural workers, who tended these tick-bearing cattle. In the area, the local cosmology divides the universe into three realms: that of humans, that of the wild (forest) and the realm of spirits mediating between the two. Danger is inherent in any meeting between the human and spirit realms, and when the spirits are not controlled the results may be 'crop failures, epidemics, and the violent death of humans and domestic animals'. Faced with the outbreak of KFD, the villagers in the area assumed that the spirits were punishing some moral transgressions on their part, and tried to placate them by various rituals; their belief in KFD's supernatural causation was reinforced by the failure of doctors to cure it. During the epidemic, many victims refused to go to hospital, for both cultural and economic reasons, preferring instead to be treated at home by a private Ayurvedic practitioner. They feared that to die in hospital would be to have a 'bad death', and their unsatisfied spirit (*preyta*) would cause problems to their surviving kinsfolk. To appease such a spirit would then entail expensive rituals that they could not afford. Hospitalization also meant the loss of another healthy wage earner, who would be forced to help nurse the patient in hospital. In contrast, the private practitioner, although less (medically) effective, was more sensitive to popular health beliefs than the hospitals, prescribed special diets in keeping with those beliefs and was quite liberal in his administration of diazepam (Valium) to patients having a wide variety of illnesses. By treating them at home, he also helped avoid the expense of a 'bad death'. Nichter points out that, at first, government officials played down the link between KFD and deforestation, and did not sufficiently tap community self-help as a resource in dealing with the epidemic. Despite their belief in the mystical origin of the disease, the villagers' 'effort to appease this spiritual cause of KFD did not preclude an interest in controlling ticks as an instrumental cause of disease'.

In addition to loss through deforestation, many species of wildlife have been hunted almost to extinction, not as a source of food but rather for more cultural reasons. These include:

- whales hunted early in the century to provide whalebone for women's corsets
- thousands of animals shot annually on safaris in Africa to provide trophies for wealthy hunters
- sharks killed as a source of 'shark fin' soup, popular in the Far East
- foxes, mink and rabbits killed to provide fur coats for fashionable women
- rhino horns used, in a powdered form, as an aphrodisiac in parts of Africa
- elephant tusks, to provide ivory for ornaments
- tigers killed for their organs, used in traditional medicaments in India and China
- bears, hunted in parts of Asia for their gallbladders, reputed to have a medicinal value.

In each of these cases of environmental destruction, Cortese[97] points out that human belief systems are part of the problem, especially the anthropocentric view of the world that 'man is the most important of all the species and should have dominion over nature', and that the world's resources are 'free and inexhaustible'. One of the consequences of this belief, and the economic and political systems that go with it, is the present ecological crisis, and its growing threat to global health.

SUMMARY

As this section briefly illustrates, there is often a connection, direct or indirect, between the ecology of the planet, the health of its inhabitants and certain cultural beliefs and behaviours. As well as human practices that cause environmental pollution, they include deforestation, the use of nuclear power and weaponry, the extinction of many species of wildlife and the emphasis on short-term profits and political power over the long-term interests of humanity. All need to be considered by the medical anthropologist of the future, since human culture influences how those problems are produced, whether they are recognized and whether or not they are dealt with.

THE ROLES OF ANTHROPOLOGY IN A GLOBAL HEALTH STRATEGY

This chapter has outlined not only some of the global health problems that we face today, but also the inherent tension between national (and international) solutions to them on one hand, and local social and cultural conditions on the other. In other words, there is a basic *paradox* at the core of almost all global health strategies, whether they are for population control, improvement in nutrition, prevention of HIV/AIDS, encouragement of breast-feeding, or any other form of health promotion. This paradox can be expressed as:

1 Global health problems require a global health strategy.
2 No global health strategy can be universally applicable to *all* parts of the world because of the wide diversity of human population groups, especially at the local level.

Given this situation, some of the possible roles of medical anthropology in a global health policy can be summarized as follows:

1 To carry out detailed research in local communities and social groups into the social and cultural dimensions of specific health problems and diseases.
2 To provide a comprehensive database on the social and cultural composition of different communities world-wide, based on prior research by other anthropologists.
3 To study the relationship between health beliefs and behaviours in particular contexts or communities; i.e. to explore the differences between what people say they believe or do and what they actually do in practice, and explain the reasons for these discrepancies
4 To mediate between health interventions at the local level and policy makers at the national or international levels in order to adapt the programme to specific local conditions
5 To aid in these interventions at the *local* level by:
   a ensuring that the programme 'makes sense' to the community, in terms of their local social, cultural, and economic realities
   b identifying community resources (such as local leaders, religious organizations or women's groups) that can act as change agents in health education or health care, as part of a national or international programme
   c monitoring the impact of these programmes on the local community over time
   d developing a network of locally recruited 'barefoot anthropologists'[1] (research assistants) or social scientists, to assist in the planning, application and evaluation of the programme
   e providing feedback for policy makers on the progress and impact of the programme
   f adapting health education programmes to disseminate information through culturally appropriate channels within the community (such as teachers, religious leaders or traditional healers)
   g acting as advocates, or cultural interpreters, for the community to health bureaucracies and policy makers at the national or international levels
6 To organize educational programmes on the

social and cultural dimensions of health and disease for policy makers, and for other researchers.

7   To monitor the institutional cultures of national and international medical aid agencies, to improve their efficiency and help reduce ethnocentric or medicocentric bias

8   To develop and test new research instruments (such as rapid assessment procedures) to study particular health problems in specific local and national contexts (see Chapter 14).

However, all of these interventions should be based, on a realistic understanding of both the strengths and the limitations of anthropology, when applied to global health issues.

Anthropology's *strengths* include:

1   It can provide detailed knowledge of particular local human communities.
2   It can provide detailed comparative data from a wide variety of human groups world-wide.
3   Its approach to research is holistic and multi-dimensional.

Anthropology's *limitations* include:

1   Its knowledge may be too local, and too confined to specific small communities.
2   Its researchers may lack training in biology, epidemiology or psychology – all of which may be relevant to certain research problems.
3   Its tradition of lengthy ethnographic research may be inappropriate in situations where serious health crises need to be dealt with as a matter of urgency.

Despite these limitations, the aim of this chapter has been to show that anthropology can still make a very considerable and ongoing contribution to the solution of global health issues.

KEY REFERENCES

2   Gwatkin, D.R., Guillot, M. and Heuveline, P. (1999) The burden of disease among the global poor. *Lancet* 354, 586–9.

3   Keane, C. (1998) Globality and the construction of World Health. *Med. Anthrop. Q.* 12(2), 226–40.

10 Warwick, D. P. (1988). Culture and the management of family planning programs. *Stud. Fam. Plan.* 19, 1–18.

22 United Nations Population Division (2004) *UN Report Says World Urban Population of 3 Billion Today Expected to Reach 5 Billion by 2030* (Press release POP/899, 24 March 2004). New York: UNPD.

24 Harpham, T., Lusty, T. and Vaughan, P. (eds) (1988). *In the Shadow of the City: Community Health and the Urban Poor.* Oxford: Oxford University Press, pp. 40–88.

35 Heggenhougen, H. K. and Clements, C. I. (1990). An anthropological perspective on the acceptability of immunization services. *Scand. J. Infect Dis. Suppl.* 76, 20–31.

38 Helman, C.G. an Yogeswaran, P. (2004) Perceptions of childhood immunizations in rural Transkei: a qualitative study. *S. Afr. Med. J.* 94(2), 835–8.

47 Nichter, M. (1991). Use of social science research to improve epidemiologic studies of and interventions for diarrhea and dysentery. *Rev. Inf. Dis.*, 13(Suppl. 4), S265–71.

53 Corbett, E.L., Watt, C.J., Walker, N. *et al.* (2003) The growing burden of tuberculosis: Global trends and interactions with the HIV epidemic. *Arch Intern Med* 163, 1009–21.

57 Walt, G. (ed.) (1990). *Community Health Workers in National Programmes.* Maidenhead: Open University Press.

71 Graduate Institute of International Studies (2005) *Small Arms Survey 2005.* Oxford: Oxford University Press.

86 McMichael, A.J., Campbell-Lendrum, D.H., Corvalan, C.F. *et al* (2003) *Climate Change and Human Health.* Geneva: World Health Organization, pp. 6–7.

See http://www.culturehealthandillness.com for the full list of references for this chapter.

RECOMMENDED READING

Baer, H., Singer, M. and Susser, I. (2004). *Medical Anthropology and the World System*, 2nd edn. Westport: Praeger.

Chivian, E., McCally, M., Hu, H. and Haines, A. (eds). (1993). *Critical Condition: Human Health and the Environment*. Cambridge: Massachusetts Institute of Technology Press.

Coreil, J. and Mull, D.J. (eds). (1990). *Anthropology and Primary Health Care*. Westview Press.

Hahn, R.A. (ed.) (1999) *Anthropology in Public Health*. Oxford: Oxford University Press.

Inhorn, M.C. and Brown, P.J. (eds) (1997) *The Anthropology of Infectious Diseases: International Health Perspectives*. Reading: Gordon and Breach.

Nichter, M. and Nichter, M. (1996). *Anthropology and International Health: Asian Case Studies*, pp. 329–65. Reading: Gordon and Breach.

Russell, A., Sobo, E.J. and Thompson, M.S. (eds) (2000) *Contraception across Cultures*. Oxford: Berg.

World Health Organization. (2002) *The World Health Report 2002 – Reducing risks, promoting healthy life*. Genevaa: World Health Organization.

RECOMMENDED WEBSITES

Center for Traditional Medicine:
http://www.centerfortraditionalmedicine.org

Global Health Watch: http://www.ghwatch.org

United Nations Population Division:
http://www.un.org/esa/population/unpop.htm

World Health Statistics 2005 (World Health Organization): http://www3.who.int/statistics

New research methods in medical anthropology

To meet the challenges of both international and local health problems – many in need of urgent intervention – a number of new research techniques have been developed in medical anthropology, as well as in psychology and sociology. All of them aim to provide a new understanding of health and illness, especially of health-related beliefs and behaviours. Many of these take the form of *qualitative* techniques, though they are often now combined with more quantitative (or measurement-based) techniques within the same project.[1] These may include large-scale population surveys of morbidity and mortality, and of the prevalence and incidence of certain diseases. Furthermore, a problem is frequently researched using several different qualitative techniques at the same time, and as part of the same study.[2] They are drawn from a 'toolbox' of several of the data collection methods mentioned below. Often these are combined with the more traditional participant-observation technique of ethnography,[3] described in Chapter 1. Using several different techniques to examine the same research question has an important advantage. When analysing the data, a strong *agreement* between the findings from two or more of these different techniques is then usually seen as an indication (and a way of confirming) the validity of those data – a process known as *triangulation* (see below).[4]

While quantitative studies often try to discover *what* has happened in a particular situation, most research projects in medical anthropology try to

answer the question *why*?[5] Why, for example, do some people prefer traditional or alternative healers for some conditions but not for others? Why do some people change their diet during illness, pregnancy or lactation in ways harmful to their health? Why do some groups reject one form of medical treatment, but accept another? Why are some conditions regarded as diseases in one group, but not in another? Why are behaviours thought of as 'bad' in one group regarded as 'mad' in another? Why is contraception accepted by one community, but not by another? Why are levels of alcohol or drug abuse high in one cultural group, but not in another?

TYPES OF DATA

To examine any of the problems described in this book – particularly the role of health beliefs and behaviours – requires a more holistic and multidimensional approach. The researchers have to be sure that they have understood, as far as this is possible, *all* aspects of the situation being studied. To achieve this, researchers should ideally aim to examine, and then to integrate, four different types or levels of data,[6] each one collected and analysed in a very different way.

The four levels of data are:

1 What people *say* they believe, think or do.
2 What people actually *do*.

3 What people *really* think or believe.

4 The *context* of the above three points.

Examining only one form of data, such as using a questionnaire to collect statements about stated health beliefs (level 1 data), may often give a very different picture from what is actually observed in their daily lives (level 2 data). The latter data are often collected by the process of participant-observation, described in Chapter 1. Discrepancies between level 1 and level 2 data – that is, between what people *say* they do and what they actually *do* in practice – have often been reported by anthropologists. They may need to be explained by deeper, more hidden beliefs (level 3 data) – what people *really* believe at the level of their inner 'cultural grammar' (what Hall[7] terms 'primary' or 'secondary' level culture; see Chapter 1) or at the level of the personal unconscious. At this personal level, for example, doctors who advise patients of the dangers of smoking but continue to smoke heavily themselves may possibly do so because:

• they genuinely believe that smoking is harmless
• they assume that they are 'lucky', and will not get ill from smoking, even if other people do
• they actually likes the sense of danger and risk involved in smoking
• they actually want, on some level, to get ill from smoking.

Data at this level may therefore have to be inferred from levels 1 and 2, or revealed by more in-depth and more detailed studies. Although more difficult to discover, data at this level should never be ignored, since many failures of health promotion or disease prevention programmes result from these types of phenomena. Finally, data at levels 1, 2 and 3 can also be heavily influenced by the *context* in which those data were gathered, and information on this context (level 4 data) needs to be explicitly noted in any description of the research findings.[6] This may include the time, place and circumstances in which the research was actually carried out, as well as the characteristics of the researchers themselves.

INFLUENCES ON DATA COLLECTION

Unlike the traditional quantitative or 'positivist' approach to research, especially in the social sciences, *qualitative research* recognizes that certain factors inherent in the research project itself can influence the phenomena under study, and thus the types of data that can be obtained. This is particularly true in studies of human populations and their culture or social organization. In these settings, this recognition of the subjective and contextual aspects of qualitative research is a major strength of its approach, and not a weakness. This is because it provides readers of the research with much more information on which to base their evaluation of its findings and their opinion of its validity. This differs from quantitative scientific research (in the social sciences), which still commonly promotes the myth of the 'invisible researcher' (and research technique) whose presence supposedly has no influence whatsoever on the people being studied.

The major influences on data collection recognized by qualitative research are:

1 The attributes of the *researcher*.
2 The attributes of the *research technique*.
3 The *context* in which the research takes place.

The implications of this are that, in some cases, different researchers, even when using identical questionnaires, may produce very different data from the same population. Often this is due to some subtle influence of their personal attributes, such as age, gender, ethnicity, dress, body language, tone of voice, religious or political background, and so on, on the people being interviewed. In addition, each research technique also imposes its own specific influence on the people being studied, particularly on what they say and do during the study, the questions that they answer, and the ones they do not. At its simplest level, this includes research techniques such as self-administered questionnaires, which require high degrees of literacy or numeracy in the study population, or familiarity with such culture-bound approaches as the multiple-choice questionnaire. More subtly, however, it refers to the influence of, say, the visible presence of a tape-recorder or video camera in the interview, and how this may cause either self-consciousness and withdrawal in the people being interviewed, or a tendency to over-dramatize answers. Finally, the *context* in which the research is carried out – the setting, and circumstances where the data are actually gathered – may also influence the data obtained. People behave differently in different contexts, and the same questionnaire administered in a hospital ward, police cell, supermarket or in the subject's home may all give very different results.

QUALITATIVE RESEARCH METHODS

In recent years, an increasing focus has been on research methods that can collect ethnographic data in a relatively short period of time compared with the lengthy periods of traditional fieldwork or *ethnography*, though this remains a very valuable type of research. These newer techniques are becoming more popular and sophisticated. They are regarded as particularly useful in the planning, design and evaluation of health education, disease prevention, and international aid programmes. They are particularly relevant in situations where research (and policy decisions to be based on that research) need to be fairly close together in terms of time. This is the case in situations of emergency (such as refugee crises or natural disasters) or in outbreaks of infectious diseases, where rapid control can save many lives, especially among the young, elderly and vulnerable. Traditional ethnography,[3] as described in Chapter 1, which can take up to 2–3 years to complete, write-up and analyse, is simply not useful in this type of situation.

Some of these newer and more rapidly-administered research techniques are summarized in the following paragraphs.

OPEN-ENDED QUESTIONNAIRES

These can be structured, or semistructured. They may be directed at a particular research question (such as dietary taboos during pregnancy), or at a wider issue (such as beliefs about the origin, presentation and treatment of infertility). Open-ended questions are, for example, 'What causes tuberculosis?', 'Why have you become ill?', 'How do you feel about your condition?', 'What causes tuberculosis?'. Often one or more such open-ended questions are included in a more structured or even a multiple-choice questionnaire. Answers to these open questions are either written down by subjects, or recorded and then transcribed. Examples of open-ended questionnaires (clinical questionnaires) relating to the topics in this book are listed in the Appendix.

RAPID ASSESSMENT PROCEDURES

Rapid assessment procedures (RAP)[8] are increasingly popular in international medical aid and health promotion programmes. Among the best known of them are *rapid ethnographic assessment,*[9] *focused ethnographic study,*[10] *rapid epidemiological assessment*[11] and *rapid rural appraisal.*[12] In each case the research can take between several weeks and several months, and is often carried out by a team of researchers rather than a single researcher. This research is usually carried out in cooperation with the community (in fact, communal participation is necessary for *all* forms of RAPs). During the research, members of the research team each study different aspects of the community's daily life, especially their health-related beliefs and behaviours, with the aid of a booklet of standardized research questions and open-ended questionnaires. These may include their social and economic organization, gender roles, health beliefs, local folk illnesses and culture-bound syndromes, infant-feeding practices, use of traditional healers, self-treatment strategies, diet and nutrition, and housing arrangements. Other researchers will collect demographic and census data, and try to assess the health status of the community by carrying out surveys of morbidity and mortality – often in relation to specific diseases, such as malnutrition, tuberculosis or acquired immune deficiency syndrome (AIDS). Usually, the study will focus on a specific health problem or research question, such as family planning, malaria control or AIDS prevention. In the study of refugee groups, Eisenbruch[13] has also developed another type of rapid assessment procedure, the *cultural bereavement interview*. This is a way of understanding how refugees have responded to their experiences of displacement – physically, emotionally and socially (see Chapter 12).

In recent years, RAPs have been used to study aspects of infant feeding practices,[14] malnutrition,[15] acute respiratory infections,[10] women's reproductive health,[16] childhood development, human immunodeficiency virus (HIV) and AIDS,[17] immunizations, infant mortality,[18] attitudes to epilepsy[19] and community health needs.[20] For example, Pelto and Grove[10] described how a focused ethnographic study was developed for the World Health Organization (WHO) to study acute respiratory infections in children, and some of the useful findings from it. In many cases, these RAPs need to be combined with data gathered from longer-term, more intensive fieldwork, and often with more clinical or epidemiological data as well.

COLLECTION OF EXPLANATORY MODELS

Explanatory Models (EMs) of illness and misfortune (see Chapter 5) can be collected in various ways, including by the questionnaire listed in that chapter. As mentioned in Chapter 5, EMs have their limitations, but can still be a useful research tool. Other, more detailed methods of collecting health beliefs and attitudes, and the meanings that people give to their illness, include the much longer and more structured Explanatory Model Interview Catalogue (EMIC) developed by Weiss and colleagues,[21,22] and the shorter, more semi-structured Short Explanatory Model Interview (SEMI) developed by Lloyd and colleagues.[23] Bhugra[24] notes

that both types of questionnaire have been found to be particularly useful in psychiatric research across cultures: EMIC, for example, has been used by Raguram and colleagues[25] to study clinical depression in Bangalore, India, while Jadhav and colleagues have used it to study the same condition in London, UK.[26]

FOCUS GROUPS

Focus groups[27,28] are intensive interviews with a small group of people (usually 8–12), each of whom shares certain attributes. Ideally, they should not have met each other before. The focus group might be, for example, a group of pregnant teenagers, of male adolescents, drug abusers or AIDS patients. The aim is to observe and record the health-related beliefs and behaviours of this particular group of people, as revealed in the group discussion – particularly by their answers to key questions and the interactions between group members. The group is run by one or more facilitators, and proceedings are taped and then transcribed. Focus groups are often useful as part of RAPs. Some of the advantages and pitfalls of this technique are summarized by Asbury.[28]

FREE LISTING

The aim of this technique is to reveal underlying health beliefs by asking subjects to list as many items as possible on a particular subject.[29] For example, 'Tell me all the types of fevers that children suffer from', 'List all the ways that diarrhoea is treated in your community', 'Tell me all the symptoms of tuberculosis that you know' or 'List all the foods that are bad (or good) for diabetes'.

PILE SORTING

This usually follows from free listing. Subjects may be given the list of items gathered above, each of which is written on a separate card. They are then asked to sort them into piles according to certain criteria. For example, 'please put in one pile all the types of childhood fever that you think should be brought to a clinic, on another pile those you would treat yourself at home, and on another all those you think should be treated by a traditional healer'. The subjects are then asked to talk about the piles, and to describe in detail the reasons for their choices.[29]

RANK ORDERING

This is an elaboration of pile sorting, whereby subjects are asked to group the cards (compiled from free listing) into hierarchies in terms of specific criteria. For example, grouping types of childhood fever according to severity in three groups, from 'most severe' to 'moderate' to 'mild'[29].

SEMANTIC NETWORK ANALYSIS

This technique overlaps somewhat with free listing. Its aim is to reveal, often with the aid of 'free association', all the concepts, images, fears, prejudices and assumptions that are linked in people's minds to a particular word or phrase. This can include a particular symptom, disease (such as 'cancer') or diagnostic label. It is useful for the study of folk illnesses and their symbolic associations, as in Blumhagen's study[30] of 'hyper-tension' and Good's[31] description of the folk illness of 'heart distress' in Iran.

FAMILY INTERVIEWS

These are often based on the concepts and techniques of enquiry of family therapy. These concepts include that of 'family systems theory',[32] which views the family as a system of relationships that always strives for equilibrium. They aim to examine specific aspects of the family culture[33] and its relevance to health, illness and lifestyle. In this type of study, the definition of 'family' may often be quite broad, and include many non-biological members (see Chapter 10) who also play significant roles in family life.

NARRATIVE ANALYSIS

This usually includes analysis of autobiographical accounts of ill health, doctor–patient interactions, surgical operations and diagnostic tests; or of significant life events such as childbirth, bereavement or severe illness. It also includes the collection of longer life histories from some selected informants.[34] All are either written down (by the subject or the researcher), videotaped or tape-recorded. Analysis of these narratives can focus either on the structure of the story or on its meaning, or on both.[35]

COLLECTION OF MEDICAL FOLKLORE

This is the study of inherited folklore – within families, communities and wider populations – that relates to health, illness and medical care. It usually includes the collection of traditional remedies, 'old wives' tales' and methods of diagnosis. It is collected either as oral folklore (usually gathered from older members of the community) or from published texts, home-doctor books, pamphlets or advice leaflets. An example of this approach is Snow's in-depth study[36] of traditional African-American health beliefs and folk medicine.

ANALYSIS OF WRITTEN OR VISUAL MATERIAL

This material may include diaries, family photographs, historical records, census reports, maps, newspaper articles, advertisements, self-help pamphlets, shrines, wills and even novels relevant to a particular area, group of people or type of ill health.

VIDEOTAPES, AUDIO TAPES, AND PHOTOGRAPHS

These techniques are used especially in studying specific events within health care, such as doctor–patient or nurse–patient consultations, behaviour in a clinic waiting room, or the body language of health professionals or their patients. Although useful, this is a 'snapshot' technique, capturing only a moment in time. It tells little about what happened before or after the recording took place, or about the inner belief systems of the participants.

GENEALOGIES AND GENOGRAMS

These are collected from informants, and are useful for understanding the patterns of kinship and marriage within a family or community,[37] the inheritance of patterns of lifestyle (such as alcoholism, drug abuse and teenage pregnancy) or of symptom patterns within a family (the 'family symptom tree'),[38] and the origins and persistence of hereditary diseases (such as cystic fibrosis or Tay–Sachs disease).

SOCIAL NETWORK ANALYSIS

This involves compiling a chart of the network of the people associated with a particular individual.[39] It may focus on family, friends, neighbours, work associates, sexual partners, members of the same club or church, or any particular combination of these. It is especially useful in contact tracing during outbreaks of infectious diseases (including sexually transmitted diseases), in monitoring the spread of health-related information in a community, and in studies of the social support available to ill individuals. An example of this technique is Parker and colleagues' study[40] of the transmission of HIV in London by analysing the sexual networks of a sample of people who are HIV positive.

MAPPING AND MODELLING

In these techniques subjects are asked to portray – by drawings, diagrams, artwork or even sculptures – certain aspects of their daily lives or belief systems. For example, these may include drawing a map of their home, village or local community, drawing diagrams of the body's interior to show the location of organs or indicating on a standardized outline of the body (as in Boyle's study of body image among English patients)[41] the location

of bodily organs or systems. Most studies of body image have used this approach, such as MacCormack's study[42] of Jamaican women's understanding of their own reproductive systems. A combination of mapping and open-ended questionnaires – the 'drawing-interview' – was used in the COMAC Childhood and Medicines Project on childhood perceptions of illness in nine European countries, carried out in 1990–93.[43] Here each child in the study was asked to make a drawing of the last time that they were ill, and was then interviewed in depth about the content and meaning of the drawing they had made.

PROJECTIVE TECHNIQUES

These are similar to use of Rorschach and other tests in psychology. Groups or individuals are exposed to the same photograph, slide, film, model or written vignette, and are then asked to describe and comment on it. This is useful in revealing hidden assumptions about levels of understanding (level 3 data). For example, a sample of mothers may be shown a set of 10 photographs of children, some of which are visibly suffering from a particular disease, and asked to pick out and talk about which children they see as healthy or unhealthy, and how they would deal with the situation. Another projective technique – observed play with dolls (often made with explicit sexual organs) – has been used in eliciting evidence of sexual abuse from children.

STRUCTURED VIGNETTES

This technique, developed by Greenhalgh and colleagues,[44] aims to overcome what I would term *deference bias* – the tendency of some subjects from disadvantaged backgrounds to agree automatically with any question the researcher asks, especially if the researcher comes from a more affluent or educated background. The vignette is a fictional story, in the form of a tape-recording, text or even a cartoon, presented to the subject for comment. The aim is to reveal a subject's belief system (level 3 data) by noting how much he or she agrees or disagrees with the story. If a tape-recording is played, it may then be played back slowly, sentence by sentence; after each, the subject is asked, for example, 'Do you agree that this person would have acted (or thought) in this way?' Some deliberately incorrect statements may be included to check for deference bias. Presenting it as a fictional vignette reduces the element of intimidation and the desire to please the investigator.

ETHNOGRAPHY OF A MEDICAL INSTITUTION

These use traditional participant-observation techniques[45] to study the institutional culture, norms, rituals, social organization, use of language and division of labour within a medical or nursing environment. Often the researchers work within the institution for a period of time (as, say, hospital porters, nursing assistants or receptionists), in order to carry out their fieldwork. The settings could include a hospital ward, clinic, doctor's office, medical school or nursing college. Examples include Goffman's work[46] on the culture of mental hospitals, Katz's studies[47,48] of surgical rituals and the culture of surgeons in the USA, and Barrett's study[49] of how schizophrenia is defined and treated within a state psychiatric hospital in Australia.

ETHNOGRAPHY OF A FOLK, TRADITIONAL OR 'ALTERNATIVE' HEALER

This is a participant-observation study, which usually involves 'sitting in' with one or more healers and observing the ritual setting of their work, the techniques that they employ and the types of responses that their patients have to them. It often also involves trying to assess the efficacy of these techniques *vis-à-vis* those of conventional Western medicine. Examples of this type of ethnography include Kleinman's study[50] of the work of the *tângki* or folk shaman in Taiwan, Finkler's study[51] of spiritual healers in Mexico, and Simon's study[52] of a Xhosa folk healer in Transkei, South Africa.

COMPUTER ANALYSES

The chief value of these software programs lies in their capacity to analyse large bodies of text, to select out certain themes or clusters of themes and to reveal relationships between them, or between them and certain demographic or other variables.[53] Many computer programs are useful in converting qualitative data (in the form of texts or transcripts) to quantitative data (in the form of statistical analyses, models, charts, tables, graphs or diagrams). In his review of this computer-assisted analysis of qualitative data (known as CAQDAS), Seale[54] points out its advantages in terms of speed, rigour, the facilitation of team research, and the development of consistent coding schemes. There are now numerous software programs available that are commonly used to analyse data in medical anthropology. They include: NU*DIST,[54] ETHNOGRAPH,[54,55] ANTHROPAC[55,56], TEXTBASE ALPHA[55], EPISTAT, ZYINDEX[55], GOPHER[55], TALLY[55], AnSWR[57], ATLAS[54] and Nvivo,[54] which allows pictures and sound files to be associated with a project, as well as raw text.

SUMMARY

Keesing[58] remarked that anthropology is more 'concerned with meanings rather than measurement, with the texture of everyday in communities, rather than formal abstraction'. Despite this, most medical anthropology research these days usually includes collection of some *quantitative* data (such as a village census, household survey, household income studies, caloric intake, food production, crop output, infant mortality or disease prevalence) in addition to these qualitative research methods. The Peltos[59] point out that the task of the modern medical anthropologist is increasingly to develop ways of integrating qualitative with quantitative data – of articulating detailed ethnographic studies of health beliefs and behaviours with the work of epidemiologists and other more quantitative researchers.

In cross-cultural psychiatry, a series of more specialized research instruments, both qualitative and quantitative, has been developed. Mumford[60] reviewed several of these techniques, whose overall aim is to identify, analyse, measure and compare mental disorders across a variety of cultures. For example, the Bradford Somatic Inventory (BSI) was developed 'to meet the need for a multicultural inventory of common somatic symptoms reported by anxious and depressed individuals in Britain and the Indian subcontinent'.[60] Another example is the 'cultural bereavement interview' mentioned above[13].

THE QUESTION OF VALIDITY

Qualitative research techniques do have a number of limitations, in medical anthropology and elsewhere. In particular, they are labour-intensive,[61] require special training for researchers, are suitable mainly for studying small groups of people, and are unsuitable for large-scale population surveys or studies of physiological data. There is also the possibility of the sample interviewed not being typical of the population at large, and of observer bias or disagreement among researchers.[6]

In order to minimize these possible biases and maximize the validity of the research findings, the following strategies should be followed:

1 During the research, attributes of the following should be *standardized*:
   a the researcher
   b the research technique
   c the context of the research.
      This means that, as far as is possible, the same researcher (or someone of similar attributes) should carry out all the research, using the same research techniques each time, and it should be carried out in the same setting (in terms of place, time, and circumstances).
2 During the research, the *same* phenomena should be studied, using *different* research techniques (chosen from the 'toolbox'), since a high degree of agreement among these findings would be significant, and maximize the chances of validity. This process of seeking agreement or overlap among the findings from different research techniques in the same study is known as *triangulation*.[62]
3 When analysing research findings, such as a body of text produced by an open-ended questionnaire, the aim is to get the *agreement* of several researchers when coding the data and identifying underlying themes. That is, several researchers should independently read and analyse the material, then compare notes in order to identify areas of agreement among them.[61] This is also a form of triangulation.
4 When publishing or presenting the research, the time, place and precise circumstances in which it was carried out – as well as the attributes of the researcher, and of their techniques – should be fully described. This *thick description*[62] of the actual research process enables the reader to make a judgment on the validity of the findings, and to assess the degree to which they may have been influenced by the particular circumstances in which they were carried, or the particular researcher.

These new approaches to qualitative research, and the attempts to make them even more valid and reliable, are now an essential part of most social sciences.[63] They are also particularly relevant to the field of clinically applied medical anthropology as it enters the new millennium.

RESEARCH PROBLEMS IN CULTURALLY DIVERSE POPULATIONS

It should be noted however, that to some extent 'research', whether qualitative *or* quantitative, is in itself a very culture-bound concept. For many people it may also be a very unfamiliar one. The idea that knowledge and understanding of the world, and of the human condition, can best be obtained by the rigid rituals of objectivity and measurement of a research project, may seem unfamiliar, as well as quite inappropriate. For many such people, knowledge and wisdom is based on more subjective criteria, such as personal perceptions and experience, the views of family, friends or peer group, the opinions of respected religious leaders, or of religious texts or the knowledge acquired in one's own education, both informal and formal.

The 'research culture' of Western society with its underlying epistemology, its concepts of proof and validity, its emphasis on numbers, percentages and statistics, its search for objective rather than subjective truth and its ideas of experimentation and reproducibility can be seen as expressing basic, particularly Western, cultural themes. These include the emphasis on individuality, choice, social equality, cognitive skills and the ability to articulate one's thoughts and experiences to others – as well as the difference between 'objective' and 'subjective' knowledge. This culture-bound aspect is also true of many *research methods*, including some of those listed above, and which may be quite inappropriate for very culturally diverse modern societies – or for more traditional, rural societies. Some examples of the methodological and ethical problems in carrying out research in these new contexts are:

1 *Randomized controlled trials* (RCTs) may have less validity in a very heterogeneous society, with many different ethnic and cultural groups, since it may not be possible to regard the sample as 'typical' or representative of the wider population. For that reason sampling for RCTs may have to be done separately, in each of these ethnic, cultural or social groups, since they may not only vary in terms of lifestyle and outlook, but also in terms of genetic make-up.

2 *Multiple choice questionnaires* (MCQs) can impose an artificial framework on human experience. While notions of *choice* may be a key characteristic of Western, consumer society, and how our daily experience is shaped, this may not apply to all groups and individuals. For example, asked a question like 'Is the pain: (A) better, (B) worse, or (C) the same' some may reply 'All of them. You see, it's variable. Sometimes it's better, and sometimes it's worse. In other words, it's basically always the same'.

3 *Open-ended questionnaires* and open-ended interviews with individuals, especially in qualitative research, may not be appropriate for the members of some groups, for several reasons:

a The interviewees may not be literate, either in their own language or in the language of the questionnaire, or both.

b The interviewees may object to the gender, age, ethnicity, or social background of the researcher. Some women, for example, may prefer to be interviewed only by a female researcher, and even then may require the presence of a chaperone or family member.

c The interviewees may object to the setting of the research interview, and prefer a less public venue, such as their home. This can sometimes create other problems for the researcher, such as a lack of privacy or the presence of a large family.

d The interviewees may object strongly to the notion of a stranger interviewing them, especially about personal matters. They may find the whole process inappropriate, embarrassing, and even dangerous. They may fear that the information they reveal may find itself in the wrong hands, such as those of the police, immigration authorities, income tax officials, or the members of rival groups. They may also fear that answering certain questions to a stranger may cause them to 'lose face', 'be shamed' or 'lose masculinity' in the presence of this stranger. In some cases they may fear that talking about positive events may attract the 'Evil Eye' or 'witchcraft' (see Chapter 5), while talking about traumatic events may even cause them to reoccur.

e In some religious communities, it may be difficult to interview women, especially younger women, on their own without the presence in the room of a senior male family member. This in turn may inhibit the interview, especially when these males insist on answering all or most of the researcher's questions.

f In some traditional communities, especially rural ones in developing countries, a senior local leader, such as a village headman, chief, or traditional healer, may insist on being present at the interview, and this can also limit the types of data that can be collected.

g In many traditional communities, 'general knowledge' is not seen as appropriate for all members of the society. Knowledge is never general. Certain types of knowledge – for example, about health, illness, childbirth, or traditional healing[64] – are only held by certain specialized people (such as only the men, or the women), and they may not wish to share that knowledge with an outsider. The women, for example, may be the only ones who know the esoteric healing secrets of certain herbs, passed down from mother to daughter. They might therefore be unwilling to make their knowledge public, and thereby risk losing their symbolic (and often economic) power within their community.[65]

h The *deference bias* mentioned above may lead to the interviewees telling the researcher what they think they want to hear, out of respect for their higher social status.

4 *Statistical concepts* such as 'risk', 'risk factors' or 'probability', based on the Western scientific model may be inappropriate for communities whose indigenous concepts of risk are based more on personal, religious or fatalistic elements.

5 *Physiological studies* that involve, say, the removal for testing of bodily fluids, such as blood, sperm, sputum or cerebrospinal fluid may be rejected by some groups. They may perceive this removal: as being *taboo*, since these fluids are the property of the donor, and an intrinsic part of their body; as *dangerous* to the

donor, if they were to fall into the hands of malevolent people such as witches or sorcerers; and as causing a permanent *depletion* of the body's vital resources, especially where body fluids are seen as finite in volume, and non-renewable. For groups that regard their body fluids as having both a sacred power, and being non-renewable, the removal of a large amounts of blood, for example, may be regarded as 'theft' of something vital to that person, and as a process that puts them in greater danger than they were before.

6 *Informed consent*, as a concept, may be unfamiliar and even threatening to some ethnic communities. As well as issues such as illiteracy or 'deference bias', research subjects may be reluctant to sign an official-looking paper whose implications they do not fully understand. To overcome this, Dein and Bhui[66] suggest that consent be obtained not as a 'one-off' event, but 'as a continuing process of negotiation between researcher and informant', and this implies therefore 'a long-term relationship of trust' between researchers and the people that they are studying.

ETHICAL ISSUES

In any society, whether urban or rural, Western or non-Western, diverse or not, these methodological issues should always be considered together with certain key ethical questions:

1 What possible benefit will such research bring to the research subjects, their families and their communities?

2 Will the research be exploited by others, to the detriment of the subjects, and their community?

3 What might be the psychological effects be, both positive and negative, of the research project on the subjects, and on those around them?

4 Will the research findings be fed back to the community, and if so, to whom and by whom?

KEY REFERENCES

3 Keesing, R.M. (1981) *Cultural Anthropology: A Contemporary Perspective*. Austin: Holt, Rinehart and Winston, pp. 1–8.

11 Smith, G.S. (1989) Development of rapid epidemiological assessment methods to evaluate health status and delivery of health services. *Int. J. Epidemiol.* 18(2), S2–14.

13 Eisenbruch, M. (1990). The cultural bereavement interview: a new clinical research approach to refugees. *Psychiatr. Clin. North Am.* 13, 715–35.

21 Weiss, M.G., Doongaji, D.R., Wyoij, D. *et al.* (1992) The explanatory model interview catalogue (EMIC): contribution to cross-cultural research methods from a study of leprosy and mental health. *Br. J. Psychiatry* 160, 819–30.

22 Weiss, M.G. (1997) Explanatory Model Interview Catalogue (EMIC): framework for comparative study of illness. *Transcult. Psychiatry* 34, 235–63.

23 Lloyd, K.R., Jacob, K.S., Patel, V. *et al* (1998) The development of the Short Explanatory Model Interview (SEMI) and its use among primary-care attenders with common mental disorders. *Psycholog. Med.* 28, 1231–7

28 Asbury, J. E. (1995). Overview of focus group research. *Qual. Hlth. Res.* 5(4), 414–20.

35 Bleakley, A. (2005) Stories as data, data as stories: making sense of narrative enquiry in clinical education. *Med. Ed.* 39, 534–40.

45 DeWalt, K.M. and DeWalt, B.R. (2002) *Participant Observation*. Walnut Creek: AltaMira Press.

54 Seale, C. (2005) Using computers to analyse qualitative data. In: *Doing Qualitative Research* (Silverman, D. ed). London: Sage, pp. 188–207.

66 Dein, A. and Bhui, K. (2005) Issues concerning informed consent for medical research among non-westernized ethnic minority patients in the UK. *J. R. Soc. Med.* 98, 354–6.

See http://www.culturehealthandillness.com for the full list of references for this chapter.

RECOMMENDED READING

Bernard, H. R. (2002). *Research Methods in Anthropology: Qualitative and Quantitative Approaches*, 3rd edn. Walnut Creek: AltaMira Press.

Helman, C. G. (1991). Research in primary care: the qualitative approach. In: *Primary Care Research: Traditional and Innovative Approaches* (Norton, P. G. Stewart, M., Tudiver F. *et al.*, eds). London: Sage, pp. 105–1124.

Helman, C. G. (1996). The application of anthropological methods in general practice research. *Fam. Pract.* 13(Suppl. 1), S13–16.

Pelto, P.J. and Pelto, G.H. (1990). Field methods in medical anthropology. In: *Medical Anthropology* (Johnson T.M. and Sargent, C.E. eds). Westport: Praeger, pp. 269–97.

Scrimshaw, N. S. and Gleason, G. R. (eds) (1992). *Rapid Assessment Procedures*. Boston: International Nutrition Foundation for Developing Countries (INFDC).

Silverman, D. (ed) (2005) *Doing Qualitative Research: A Practical Handbook*. London: Sage.

RECOMMENDED WEBSITES

Qualitative Research for Health Programmes (compiled by Patricia Hudelson). World Health Organization: http://whqlibdoc.who.int/hq/1994/WHO_MNH_PSF_94.3.pdf

Appendix

JOURNALS AND WEBSITES

The following journal and websites, in several different countries, either publish articles on medical anthropology, or else have an interest in its concepts or research findings.

JOURNALS

Ageing and Society (UK)

AIDS Care (UK)

AM: Rivista della Società Italiana di Antropologia Medica (Italy)

Anthropology and Medicine (UK)

Bunka to Kokoro (Culture and Psyche) (Japan)

Cross-Cultural Psychology Bulletin (USA)

Culture, Medicine and Psychiatry (USA)

Culture, Health & Sexuality (UK)

Curare: Zeitschrift fur Ethnomedizin und Transkulturelle Psychiatrie (Germany)

Ethnicity and Health (UK)

Forced Migration Review (UK) (also in French, Spanish, Arabic)

Health: An Interdisciplinary Journal for the Social Study of Health, Illness and Medicine (UK)

International Migration Review (USA)

Journal of Cross-Cultural Gerontology (USA)

Journal of Cross-Cultural Psychology (USA)

Journal of Ethnopharmacology (The Netherlands)

Journal of Gender, Culture and Health (USA)

Journal of Refugee Studies (UK)

Journal of the Royal Anthropological Institute (UK)

Journal of Transcultural Nursing (USA)

Kallawaya: Órgano del Instituto Antropológico de Investigaciones en Medicina Tradicional (Argentina)

Les bulletins d'Amades (France)

Medical Anthropology (USA)

Medical Anthropology Quarterly (USA)

Medicina y Ciencias Sociales (Spain)

Mental Health, Religion and Culture (UK)

Medische Antropologie (The Netherlands and Belgium)

Transcultural Psychiatry (Canada)

Santé et Société (France)

Social Science and Medicine (UK/USA)

Sociology of Health and Illness (UK)

Viennese Ethnomedical Newsletter (Austria)

WEBSITES

Professional Organizations

AG Medical Anthropology: der Deutschen Gesellschaft für Völkerkunde (Germany)
http://www.medicalanthropology.de

AGEM: Arbeitsgemeinschaft Ethnomedizin (Germany)
http://www.agem-ethnomedizin.de

Amades: Anthropologie médicale appliqué au development et à la santé (France)
http://www.amades.net

American Anthropological Association
http://www.aaanet.org

Medical Anthropology Switzerland MAS: Commission: Interdisciplinaire d'Anthropologie Médicale (Switzerland)
http://www.seg-sse.ch/fr/commissions/ciam.shtml

Royal Anthropological Institute (UK)
http://www.therai.org.uk
Society for Applied Anthropology (USA)
http://www.sfaa.net
Society for Medical Anthropology (USA)
http://www.medanthro.net/index.html
World Health Organization
http://www.who.org

Traditional medical systems
Traditional Asian Medicine
http://www.iastam.org/home.htm
Traditional Chinese Medicine
http://www.mic.ki.se/China.html
Traditional Indian Medicine
http://www.mic.ki.se/India.html
Traditional Islamic Medicine
http://www.mic.ki.se/Arab.html

Diversity and health
American Public Health Association
http://www.apha.org/ppp/red/Background.htm
National Multicultural Institute (USA)
http://www.nmci.org/otc/default.htm
South East Sydney Ilawarra Area Health Services, NSW, Australia
http://www.sesahs.nsw.gov.au/intermulticult/links/links.htm
University of York, Department of Health Sciences
http://www.york.ac.uk/healthsciences/equality/cultural.htm
USA/UK Collaborative Initiative on Racial and Ethnic Health
http://www.omhrc.gov/us-uk/index.htm

Cultural competence in health care
Diversity Rx (USA)
http://www.diversityrx.org/HTML/DIVRX.htm
National Center for Cultural Competence, Georgetown University
http://gucchd.georgetown.edu/nccc
Office of Minority Health (USA)
http://www.omhrc.gov/clas/index.htm
http://www.omhrc.gov/cultural/
Research Centre for Transcultural Studies in Health, Middlesex University
http://www.mdx.ac.uk/www/rctsh/ccap.htm

Program for Multicultural Health, University of Michigan Health System
http://www.med.umich.edu/multicultural/ccp/tools.htm

Cross-cultural nursing
Royal College of Nursing (UK)
http://www.rcn.org.uk/resources/transcultural/index.php
Research Centre for Transcultural Studies in Health, Middlesex University
http://www.mdx.ac.uk/www/rctsh/index.htm
State University of New York Institute of Technology
http://www.sunyit.edu/library/html/culturedmed/bib/transcultural

Cross-cultural psychiatry, psychology and psycho-analysis
Association Internationale d'EthnoPsychanalyse
http://clinique-transculturelle.org
International Association for Cross-Cultural Psychology
http://www.iaccp.org
Japanese Society of Transcultural Psychiatry
http://www.jstp.net/Index_E.htm
Society for the Study of Psychiatry and Culture (USA)
http://www.psychiatryandculture.org
World Association of Cultural Psychiatry
http://www.waculturalpsychiatry.org
World Psychiatric Association
http://www.wpanet.org

Ethno-pharmacology and traditional plant remedies
European Society of Ethnopharmacology
http://ethnopharma.free.fr/index.html

Telemedicine: web-journals
Cyberspsychology and Behavior
http://www.liebertpub.com/publication.aspx?pub_id=10
Journal of Telemedicine and Telecare
http://www.rsmpress.co.uk/jtt.htm
Telemedicine and e-Health
http://www.liebertpub.com/publication.aspx?pub_id=54

Author Index

Subject Index

illness/ill-health/sickness (physical or in general) – *continued*
  folk *see* folk illness
  metaphors *see* metaphors
  narratives of *see* narratives
  patient's perspectives on 126–8
  presentation 148–9
  process of becoming ill 128
  refugees 323
  rituals of 237–8
    case studies 241–4
  smoking causing, warnings about 216–17, 217
  treatment *see* therapy
  understanding of (patient's) 153
  see also disease; health risks
imaging at distance (teleradiology) 336
imbalance *see* balance and imbalance
immigrants
  in UK
    Asian *see* Asian immigrants
    food beliefs 56, 63–6, 69
    gender role inversion 322
    health professionals 313
    infant feeding practices 72, 73, 74
    mental illness 256, 260, 321, 325, 327–30
    nutritional problems 63–6, 69
    population diversity relating to 309
  in US *see* United States
  see also migration; minorities
immune system, psychological state affecting 265, 290
immunization (vaccination) 435–9
  children 435–9
  tuberculosis *see* BCG vaccination
'immunization' properties of foods 57
  see also vaccination
impairment vs disability 35
in vitro fertilization (IVF) 41, 177, 178
incest, reproductive technologies seen as 178
India
  Ayurvedic system *see* Ayurvedic medicine
  cancer and diet 78

childbirth
  cultures 173
  pain in 192
contraception
  neem oil 182
  programmes 428
death rituals 233, 235
deforestation and Kyasanur forest disease 451–2
depression 377
diaspora 309
family structures 285
Hinduism *see* Hinduism
immunization in South Kanara 436, 437
leprosy 420–1, 421, 421–2
malaria 415, 418
pain language 188
primary health care 445
traditional medicine 91–2
Indian food cuisines in UK 76
indigenous beliefs *see* folk beliefs
indigenous forest peoples, destruction 450
individual(s)
  controlled abnormal behaviour 248–9
  epidemiological studies and 372–3
  as factor
    in health-related beliefs and behaviours 4, 127
    in illness causation 135–6
    in stress response 292
  genetics of drug responses 369–70
  stress as force between 301
individual body 23–4
industrialized countries *see* developed countries; Western countries
inequalities
  health, socioeconomic factors 5–7, 426, 434
  social, AIDS and 408–9
infant(s)/babies
  feeding practices 69–74
  mother and, conceptual separation in Western obstetrics 171
infanticide 179, 182
infections

deforestation and 451–2
  domestic animals as source of 382
  drug-resistant 105–6
  immunization *see* immunization
  lay theories of causation 136–7, 142–3
    children's perceptions 144
  parasitic *see* parasitic disease
  poverty and 434
  respiratory *see* respiratory infections
  sexually-transmitted, male circumcision and 21
  tropical 412–24
  see also germs; micro-organisms
infertility 176–9
  treatment 41–2, 177–9
informal sector of health *see* popular sector
information
  body as 351–2, 357
  online
    patient access to 339
    professional access to 338–9
informed consent 15, 465
inheritance, *see entries under* genetic
injections, folk healers' 85, 89
Institute for Complementary Medicine 112, 113
institutions *see* bureaucracies and institutions
insurance, health 126
internal migration 307
  of displaced persons 307
International Classification of Impairments, Disabilities and Handicaps (ICIDH) 35
international medical aid programmes, Western approaches 447
Internet/world wide web (and websites) 334, 467–8
  addiction to 347
  blogs 338, 353
  cultural context of use 345–6
  medical advice on 108
  medical anthropology articles 467–8
  psychotherapy 341
  self-help groups 108